# Nursing Leadership and Management:

## Concepts and Practice

*FOURTH EDITION*

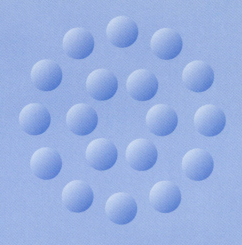

# Nursing Leadership and Management:

## Concepts and Practice

*FOURTH EDITION*

**Ruth M. Tappen**
EdD, RN, FAAN
Professor
Florida Atlantic University
College of Nursing
Boca Raton, Florida

**F. A. DAVIS COMPANY** • Philadelphia

F. A. Davis Company
1915 Arch Street
Philadelphia, PA 19103

Printed in the United States of America

Last digit indicates print number: 10 9 8 7 6 5 4 3 2 1

*Acquisitions Editor:* Joanne P. DaCunha, RN, MSN
*Developmental Editor:* Peg Waltner
*Production Editor:* Jessica Howie Martin
*Cover Designer:* Louis J. Forgione

As new scientific information becomes available through basic and clinical research, recommended treatments and drug therapies undergo changes. The author and publisher have done everything possible to make this book accurate, up to date, and in accord with accepted standards at the time of publication. The author, editors, and publisher are not responsible for errors or omissions or for consequences from application of the book, and make no warranty, expressed or implied, in regard to the contents of the book. Any practice described in this book should be applied by the reader in accordance with professional standards of care used in regard to the unique circumstances that may apply in each situation. The reader is advised always to check product information (package inserts) for changes and new information regarding dose and contraindications before administering any drug. Caution is especially urged when using new or infrequently ordered drugs.

**Library of Congress Cataloging in Publication Data**

Tappen, Ruth M.
    Nursing leadership and management : concepts and practice / Ruth M. Tappen.—4th ed.
        p. ; cm.
    Includes bibliographical references and index.
    ISBN 0-8036-0609-5
    1. Nursing services—Administration. 2. Leadership. I. Title.
    [DNLM: 1. Nursing, Supervisory—Nurses' Instruction. 2. Leadership—Nurses'
Instruction. WY 105 T175n 2001]
RT89 .T36 2001
362.1'73'068—dc21

00-059041

*To my family*
*who mean the world to me*

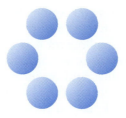

# Preface

## ● WHAT LIES AHEAD?

It is an exciting time to be in nursing. The public is beginning to understand how critical the professional registered nurse is to the quality of the health care provided to sick and well alike. Advanced practice nurses are recognized for their ability to manage a wide range of common health concerns effectively and in a manner that recognizes the uniqueness of each individual. Our profession has produced highly skilled clinicians, successful entrepreneurs, respected researchers, and savvy political leaders. The opportunities for leadership are incredible. The sky's the limit!

At the same time, however, we face many challenges. Pressures to lower costs have spurred efforts to use higher proportions of ancillary personnel. These unlicensed and non-nursing personnel require far more supervision by the shrinking number of RNs at the bedside and in management positions. Demands placed on each individual nurse have increased almost to the breaking point in some cases.

Our colleagues in related health professions are experiencing many of the same pressures. We are all being asked to better articulate what each profession and each level within that profession contributes to the health of the nation. The situation is fluid and dynamic. Shifts in thinking occur rapidly, as do shifts in how health care dollars are spent. This has direct effects on nurses' employment opportunities and career choices. In other words, they affect each individual reader, the nursing profession as a whole, and anyone who may need nursing care at some time.

As a profession, we need to be sure that we have a voice in the decisions being made, that we act as advocates for nursing and for the people who need our care. As individuals, too, each of us must clearly articulate the value of our contribution and the need for nursing care. This is leadership on a grand scale and this book will help you prepare for those challenges.

## ● THE NEW 4TH EDITION

This edition is thoroughly revised and updated. Several new contributors have been added, but others will be familiar to readers of earlier editions. A humanistic philosophy applied within an open systems framework has been the foundation for this book since the first edition and continues to be so. Some of the most basic material, which is repeated so often in the introductory sections of many nursing textbooks, has been condensed to allow for new material.

Much has been added to this new edition. This edition includes entirely new chapters on workplace ethics and on informatics. The material on workplace health and safety has been expanded to become an entire chapter; the same has been done with workplace diversity and the leadership aspects of career development. All of these changes reflect the increasing importance of these subjects in the healthcare work environment. New graphics should enhance the readability of this edition, always an important consideration in a textbook.

## ● ACKNOWLEDGMENTS

Finally, a heartfelt thank you to all who have contributed in some way to the evolution of this textbook: all the reviewers, students, educators, and colleagues who have shared their thoughts about the book and offered suggestions on how to improve it. This, too, is part of leadership: sharing your observations so others may improve their work. I wish that I could say thank you personally to each one of you. Many of you probably have no idea how valuable your input has been and the extent to which you have shaped this new edition.

Ruth M. Tappen, EdD, RN, FAAN

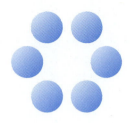

# Contributors

Cynthia Daubman, RN, MS
Poughkeepsie, New York

Phyllis George, RN, MA
Director of Public Health Nursing
Dutchess County Health Department
Poughkeepsie, New York

Patricia Z. Lund, EdD, RN
Professor
Department of Nursing
Western Connecticut State University
Danbury, Connecticut

Kimberly A. Pero, MSN, RN
Executive Director of Clinical Services
Greystone Healthcare Division

Leslie Schlienger, MSN, RN, CRRN
Administrator
Life Care Home Health Services Corporation
Delray Beach, Florida

Marian Turkel, PhD, RN
Assistant Professor
Florida Atlantic University
College of Nursing
Boca Raton, Florida

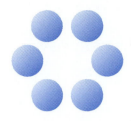

# Consultants

Paula Boley, MSN, RN
Assistant Professor
Anderson University
Anderson, Indiana

Joy Ruth Cohen, RN, PhD
Quinnipiac College
Department of Nursing
Hamden, Connecticut

Giovanna Morton, RN, EdD
Associate Dean and Professor
Marshall University
College of Nursing and Health Professions
Huntington, West Virginia

Sylvia Womack, MSN, RN
Assistant Professor
Macon State College
Department of Nursing
Macon, Georgia

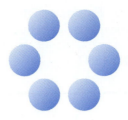

# Contents

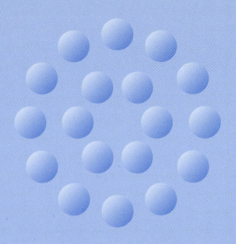

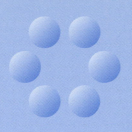

CHAPTER *1*

# Studying Leadership and Management

## LEARNING OBJECTIVES

*After completing this chapter, the reader will be able to:*

- Discuss the value of studying leadership and management for the healthcare professional.
- Define and distinguish between leadership and management.
- Use an open systems framework when analyzing leadership and management situations.

- Recognize the use of nondeliberative and deliberative mechanisms to reduce stress and avoid threatening situations in the work environment.

**H**ave you ever been thoroughly frustrated in your attempts to get other people to change? Or been puzzled by the behavior of your fellow students, nurses, or other healthcare practitioners? Or wondered how our healthcare system got to be the way it is? These questions are addressed in the study of nursing leadership and management.

## WHY STUDY LEADERSHIP AND MANAGEMENT?

The study of leadership and management is an essential part of every healthcare professional's preparation for practice. Experienced professionals often say that most of the serious problems they face in their work are not technical problems but people problems. People problems are the kind of issues that leadership and management skills can help you address.

The primary purpose for studying leadership and management is to learn how to work with people, not only as individuals but also as members of groups, teams, and organizations. Using nursing leadership and management concepts and skills allows you a greater understanding and control of events in work situations. It can impart a sense of personal power and self-direction in situations that would otherwise be confusing, frustrating, or terribly discouraging. The following are examples of what you can gain from studying nursing leadership and management. You can:

- *learn how to work well with other people.* Nurses rarely work alone. Most often, they are part of a healthcare team composed of other nursing personnel and members of other health-related disciplines.
- *advocate for one's patients and clients.* Sometimes nurses find that other members of the healthcare team are neglectful of patient needs or rights. Nurses are often in a position to see that those needs are met and people's rights respected.
- *understand nurses' position in the healthcare system.* We are working within an extraordinarily complex, ever-changing healthcare system. To function effectively, nurses need to understand the forces that affect their ability to provide the highest quality care possible.
- *bring about change.* Although stability might seem more important than change in volatile times, improvement of the way in which we deliver healthcare is an ongoing challenge. Gaining

acceptance of needed changes is vital to the improvement of health care.

- *take control of one's practice.* When coworkers or employers have a limited view of what nurses do, assertiveness and negotiation skills can help you define and expand your practice.
- *be prepared to assume leadership and management responsibilities.* Once you have become an experienced nurse, you will be expected to assume leadership and, sometimes, management responsibilities.
- *support the nursing profession.* Our profession is at a crossroads, facing unprecedented challenges as well as opportunities to expand and advance as never before. Which way will we go? The answer depends on us and our ability to assume leadership.

## Leadership and Management Defined

### Leadership

Leadership is the process of influencing others (Tannenbaum, Weschler, & Massarik, 1974). Effective leaders obtain the cooperation and resources they need to meet their goals (Chemers, 1993). These leaders inspire others through their personal trustworthiness and self-confidence and communicate a vision so compelling that it can turn self-interest into commitment to the job (Bennis & Nanus, 1985; Chemers, 1993).

Senge (1999) defines leadership as "the capacity of the human community to shape its future . . . specifically to sustain the significant processes of change required to do so" (p. 16). Leaders generate and sustain creative tension in a group, not a negative tension but a positive tension that mobilizes others' energy and enthusiasm. He emphasizes that leadership is found throughout an organization or community, noting that "diverse people in diverse positions," not just those at the top, can and must contribute to any enterprise (p. 16).

The study of leadership encompasses many facets of human behavior, including motivation, the effects of culture, leadership theories, group development, teamwork, organizational dynamics, power, and conflict. Leadership also includes skills such as effective communication, confrontation and negotiation, critical thinking, and prob-

lem solving. Other important leadership tasks are conducting effective meetings and conferences, providing meaningful evaluations, and implementing large- and small-scale changes. Leaders need to know not only why the people they work with act the way they do, but also how to influence that behavior.

> **All people have untapped leadership potential . . . leadership is there in you.**
> —Tichy, 1997

Whenever you attempt to influence people, you are exercising leadership. The attempt defines leadership—it does not always have to be successful. It is also not necessary to be designated the leader. Any member of a group can act as its leader. The following example may help to clarify this point:

> A nursing student is observing a medical team debriding a necrotic decubitus ulcer. An intern is ready to begin but the patient has not had any analgesia. The nursing student says to the intern, "The patient has not been given any pain medication or local anesthesia." The intern stops and turns to the attending physician, who immediately orders analgesia.
>
> The student exercised leadership in spite of being the most junior member of this team. If the student had thought, "Hmm, I don't think they ought to begin without analgesia," but had not said anything, the student would not have shown any leadership at all despite having had the right idea.

To be a leader you must make a decision to act; doing so requires skill, knowledge, energy, vision, and self-confidence, qualities that will be discussed in later chapters.

### Management

Management, too, is a process of influencing others, *but with the specific intention of getting them to perform effectively and contribute to meeting the organization's goals* (Drucker, 1967). Effective managers obtains and effectively utilizes the people, money, and other resources needed to get the work done (Longenecker & Pringle, 1981). Management is often described as the process of getting work done through other people.

A manager is formally and officially responsible for the work of a given group, for ensuring that the necessary amount of work is done and that it is done well. To fulfill this responsibility, the manager may be expected to hire and fire people, formally evaluate staff members, recommend raises and promotions, prepare and implement a budget, approve expenses and purchases, review the work done by staff members, assign and schedule staff members, handle conflicts, contribute technically, and plan the current and future activities of the department. As numerous as they are, these traditional management functions may not be sufficient for these turbulent times. Managers also need to be able to empower their employees, develop their creative potential, find innovative solutions to difficult problems, and be open to the demands of continuous change and reorganization (Morgan, 1997).

The study of management encompasses a broad range of knowledge and skills. It includes the principles and techniques of budgeting, project planning, staff development, and formal evaluation procedures. It also includes an understanding of management theories, of the different ways in which organizations have developed hierarchies and structured work groups, and of the internal and external factors that affect the organization and its ability to survive and grow.

Many nurses move quickly into beginning managerial or quasi-managerial positions, and they are expected to fulfill all of these responsibilities. Without adequate preparation, it is difficult to either understand or carry out the expectations of the managerial role.

## The Difference between Management and Leadership

Management and leadership are closely related, often intertwined, concepts. Management is a formal, specifically designated position within an organization. Every work group, unit, or department reports to some kind of manager. Leadership, on the other hand, is an unofficial, achieved position that may be assumed by more than one person at a time. Management is an assigned role; leadership is an attained one.

### *Leadership is action, not position.*
—*McGannon, 1997, p. 160*

Leadership and management are not mutually exclusive. Instead, they should be thought of as complementary (Napolitano & Henderson, 1998). To be a good manager, it is absolutely essential to be an effective leader. The real challenge for most managers is to combine strong leadership with strong management (Kotter, 1997). This combination is so important that some use the term **leader-manager** or **manager-leader** to emphasize the importance of the leadership aspects of management and to synthesize the concepts from both into the role of the leader-manager (Williamson, 1986; Napolitano & Henderson, 1998). The opposite is not true, however. Anyone in a group or organization can be a leader; you do not have to be in management to be a leader.

### *Most U.S. corporations today are overmanaged and underled.*
—*Kotter, 1997, p. 24*

Every healthcare professional has the responsibility to assume some leadership within his or her profession. Not every professional can or needs to be a manager, but it is still helpful to have a good understanding of the basics of management, especially when professional nurses at all levels are increasingly asked to offer input into managerial decisions. As a leader or manager, you are in a responsible position that requires that you maintain the confidence and trust of the people with whom you work. Many leadership and management strategies are quite powerful in their effect. The healthcare professional who takes advantage of the opportunities to use such strategies also assumes the responsibility to use them constructively.

## ● FOUNDATIONAL CONCEPTS FOR LEADERSHIP AND MANAGEMENT

Some concepts related to human behavior are especially relevant to the study of leadership and management. Of these, **systems theory,** which helps us find some order and make some sense of the confusing complexity of most work situations, and the categorization of **common behavior patterns** directed to reducing stress and avoiding threatening situations are presented here. Although both are probably familiar to you, the difference in this presentation is that they are applied to your actions and those of your coworkers. In the study of leadership and management, these familiar ideas are used to assist us in understanding how people interact with their environment at work.

## Open Systems: The Interaction of People with Their Environment

It has taken some time for systems theory to be accepted as fundamental to the understanding of leadership and management. Systems theory is particularly valuable in broadening our perspective and encouraging consideration of the total picture instead of just the individual details (Kerzner, 1998). A comparison of the more traditional mechanistic perspective and an open systems perspective can be found in Table 1–1.

### System Defined

A virus, a heart, a person, a group, and a community are all living open systems. Each is a whole entity having identifiable parts (components), characteristics (attributes), and a definable boundary.

*Some of the challenging concepts in systems thinking came more easily to students with backgrounds in engineering or biology—integrative disciplines, after all—and less easily to those more practiced at taking things apart, such as finance and accounting.*
—Petzinger, 1999a, p. 44

Kerzner (1998) defined a living system as "a group of elements, either human or nonhuman, that is organized and arranged in such a way that the elements can act as a whole toward achieving some common goal, objective or end" (p. 69).

To fully understand a system, it is necessary to define it in terms of three aspects: its components, its attributes as a whole, and the relationships of its components internally and externally with the environment. The **components** of a system can be almost anything: molecules, cells, organs, people, or groups of people. **Attributes** are the characteristics of the system such as color, temperature, speed, maturity, personality, and energy level. The **relationships** are the processes that occur between the parts. The possibilities are innumerable: ionization, metabolism, circulation, communication, and negotiation are examples. The following example illustrates these aspects of a system:

> *A patient care team (system) consists of one registered nurse, one practical nurse, and two unlicensed assistive personnel (components). This team is known for its efficiency and energy (attributes). The team provides dialysis treatment*

| | Traditional Mechanistic Perspective | Open Systems Perspective |
|---|---|---|
| **Table 1–1** | Comparison of Two Perspectives in Leadership and Management | |
| Guiding metaphor | Machine, clock | Organism, ecology |
| Preferred structure | Hierarchical division of labor | Team-based, synthesis of ideas |
| Strategic objective | Operational consistency | Continuous improvement |
| Leadership approach | Command and control | Autonomy for employees Articulate a vision |

*Source:* Data from Petzinger (1999). A new model for the nature of business: It's alive! *Wall Street Journal* (February 26, 1999), pp. B1, B4.

to 25 outpatients daily and reports to the manager of the Dialysis Center (relationships).

Living systems also exhibit a number of other important characteristics: a hierarchical nature, wholeness, openness, energy, growth, patterns, individuality, and sentience.

## Hierarchy of Systems

Systems are nested within systems in multiple levels (Stafford, 1994). Together they are called the **hierarchical order of systems** (Laszlo, 1972). Smaller systems within systems are called **subsystems.** Larger systems may be parts of even more inclusive **suprasystems.** In Table 1–2, the systems are listed from left to right in order of increasing size and complexity. Whatever is outside of the suprasystem is referred to as the **environment.**

A vast difference in size separates the systems in these examples. The choice of where to begin in defining a hierarchy of systems depends on your purpose and interest (Ashby, 1968; Bell & Vogel, 1968). In leadership and management, the individual, the group, the organization, and the community are usually of greatest interest.

## Wholeness

**Regardless of the field one chooses to study, it is essential to remember that one cannot generalize from parts to a whole. For example, studying the members of a group will not provide knowledge about the group.**
—M. E. Rogers, 1994a, p. 247

A system as a whole has characteristics that are different from and greater than the sum of its parts (Rogers, 1970; Von Bertalanffy, 1976). A

| Table 1–2 | Examples of Hierarchical Order of Systems | |
|---|---|---|
| **Subsystems** | **Systems** | **Suprasystems** |
| Cells | Organs | Individuals |
| Individuals | Teams | Agencies |
| Local groups | State organizations | National organizations |

person, for example, is not just a collection of bones, skin, heart, lungs, and intestines, but something quite different: a living, breathing, self-aware organism.

A part of a system by itself does not have the properties of the whole system. For example, a part of a car such as the engine or the tires cannot take you anywhere, but the car as a whole can (Flower, 1992). The following are some other examples:

*An audit committee can be dynamic and productive even if it has one member who sleeps through most of the meetings.*

*Another group can consist of dynamic, high-energy individuals but get nothing done because each member is caught up in competing with the others.*

Although the parts or subsystems do not define the whole system, they do influence the larger system. For instance, in the last example, the fact that the group's members are mature individuals can facilitate the process of developing ways to work together.

**We often think that when we have completed our study of one we know all about two, because "two" is "one and one." We forget that we have still to make a study of "and."**
—Eddington, 1998

The concept of wholeness has many implications. In nursing practice, for example, wholeness emphasizes the importance of assessing the client as a whole being with thoughts, feelings, and beliefs that affect bodily functions, and vice versa. The basis for many complaints about the medical model of health care is that it treats specific organs—for example, lungs, stomachs, or uteri—instead of people. The problems inherent in this model have been well documented:

*If you treat just the cardiovascular system and not the person, the individual may continue smoking, gaining weight, and not exercising, making the situation worse.*

*A stress-related colitis will not stay healed unless you deal with the sources of stress.*

*Performing a mastectomy will not heal the whole person if it leaves the patient feeling she is no longer attractive sexually.*

## Openness

The term **openness** refers to the permeability of a system's boundaries (Mabry, 1999). A system is open if it exchanges matter, energy, or information with its environment (Hall & Fagen, 1968). All living systems are continuously open systems according to Rogers (1994b). They are neither just a little open or sometimes open but continuously open.

The term **closed** is often used somewhat inaccurately to mean that a system has relatively impermeable boundaries, that it resists input and change, or that it lacks the ability to interact effectively with the environment (Mabry, 1999). It is difficult to even imagine a system that is totally impervious to its environment. Even an object as inanimate as a rock is affected by its environment. If you put a cool rock out in the sun, it will become warm. This effect is clearly the result of a change in environment.

The exchange of matter, information, and energy between a human system and its environment is a dynamic relationship. A human being is active, not passive in relationship to the environment. Although the living system is continuously being influenced by its environment, it is also influencing that environment (Bateman & Crant, 1993). The system uses its energies to maintain itself as a system in dynamic interplay with the environment.

An act of leadership involves a particular kind of interpersonal exchange in which one person attempts to influence another. Whenever this exchange between people occurs, at least three elements or systems are involved: the **leader**, the **co-actors** (person or groups to be influenced) (Scheflen, 1982), and the **environment** (surroundings) in which the attempt to influence takes place (Figure 1–1). These categories can be broken down into many more elements, but the leader, the co-actor(s), and the environment are the most essential elements that need to be considered when analyzing a leadership event.

The leader and the co-acting system continually influence each other, even when no action

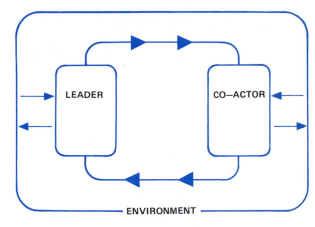

**Figure 1–1**  Elements of a leadership event.

or reaction is apparent. The following example shows how people can influence each other without taking any overt action:

*The team leader enters the conference room to distribute assignments for the team. The rest of the team sit silently as the leader enters. The team is usually noisy and talkative in the conference room, so the leader wonders why they are silent today. Is this silence a respectful hush so that the leader can begin talking, or is it a sullen silence intended to make the leader feel uncomfortable? In either case, the silence has definitely affected the leader.*

The four elements of a management situation, which is simply an extension of the fundamental elements of a leadership situation, are the **manager**, the **staff members**, the **work** to be done, and the **environment** (Figure 1–2). The manager and staff members are equivalent to the leader and co-actors. The environment in a management situation is usually the unit, department, service, or institution in which they work. The work to be done is the added element in a management situation.

## Energy Fields

Martha Rogers (1994c) emphasized that humans and their environments don't just *have* energy fields, they *are* energy fields. Every living system requires energy to maintain life and to grow (Hanchett, 1979). The energy may be in the form

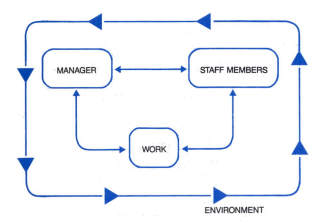

**Figure 1–2** Elements of a management situation.

of matter, including food and oxygen, or it may be an exchange of information, such as how to carry out a procedure. Economic energy in the form of money available to spend is an important source of energy for most organizations. Other kinds of energy include measurable ones such as light, heat, or sound, and the less measurable kinds such as love, hate, fear, caring, or healing.

Energy can be exchanged in small, hard-to-detect amounts or in explosive bursts. It can accumulate, reaching the point of intensive pressure to release it. A balance of positive energies flowing in and out is usually a sign of a healthy system.

When you study a system, you need to look at how it exchanges energy with its environment. You may ask, for example, whether your nursing unit effectively exchanges information with other departments such as pharmacy, dietary, and social services. You may also ask whether the organization as a whole provides sufficient economic energy (budgeted funds) to support its nursing services and to provide adequate salaries for the nurses employed there.

### Growth

The process of growth proceeds **unidirectionally;** it does not reverse itself or regress back in time (Boulding, 1968). Relationships also change unidirectionally over time (Stafford, 1994). Human growth and development reflect an increasing complexity of pattern and organization (Rogers, 1970). People do not go back to being what they were last week, last year, or when they were children. Aging, for example, is not a regression but

a progression to new conditions and behaviors. This principle applies to older coworkers: they continue to have a need to grow and develop despite their older age and years of experience.

To traverse the adult years successfully, an individual must continue to learn and grow developmentally. Many opportunities for learning and growth are found in the work setting, from learning new technical skills to improving ability to work as part of an interdisciplinary team. Work can also contribute to the accomplishment of such developmental tasks as developing a sense of identity or guiding the next generation of healthcare professionals.

A leader or manager who is aware of these needs can organize work in such a way that it contributes substantially to each staff member's learning and growth. The following is an example of how a nurse manager can foster growth:

*A staff nurse has worked in the same position long enough to know the job well. In fact, the nurse knows it so well that it is beginning to get boring. The nurse, however, will not be eligible for a promotion into a more challenging position until she is finished with school.*

*The nurse manager recognizes this problem and assigns the staff nurse to orient new nurses to the team. The staff nurse gets a great deal of satisfaction out of this opportunity to share expertise with others and to gain some recognition. The nurse also has to learn new leadership skills in order to carry out this new assignment effectively.*

It is not only individuals who show evidence of growth and change over time. Teams, groups, organizations, and communities are also open systems that change and evolve over time, either positively or negatively. These larger systems can also be thought of as having life cycles in which they begin as immature systems with poorly defined behavior patterns and gradually develop into mature systems with well-defined, highly functional behavior patterns. Like other living systems, their existence also has an ending.

### Patterns

Any behavior or relationship that recurs at regular intervals reflects a **pattern** of that system. Some patterns vary over short periods; others extend beyond the life span of an individual. The unidirectional and predictable stages of the life cycle are long-interval patterns. Seasonal patterns are recognizable in the occurrence of certain illnesses and some kinds of behavior such as seasonal affective disorder (SAD) or suicide. Seasonal variations also affect hospital admissions and agency workloads. The patterns of our clients' daily lives also affect service delivery: Outpatient clinics have extended services into the evening and weekend hours to better meet the needs of working people.

Patterns with shorter intervals are also significant to leadership and management. For example, many biorhythms are disrupted by rotating shifts, leaving people feeling fatigued and irritable.

Interpersonal relationships also have a rhythmic nature. For example, people with the same or complementary communication patterns usually get along better than those whose patterns are asynchronous. Some people are quite flexible and can adjust to another's rhythms, whereas others can make adjustments only within a narrow range (Chapple, 1979).

These are also patterns in the interpersonal relations within the larger systems. For example, teams whose members work in concert are usually more effective than those whose members work at different rates (Sommers, 1993). Groups may have free-flowing patterns of communication or stilted patterns that discourage spontaneity. Every work group, from a small team to an entire organization, develops patterns of behavior, commonly called **routines.**

> **Self-organization is a universal property of life, creating order in everything from zebra stripes to human brains.**
> —Petzinger, 1999a, pp. 35–36

Without patterns, we would know only chaos. The patterns of a system allow us to anticipate the behavior of that system with some degree of accuracy. The leader who knows the common patterns of the relevant human systems can not only better predict its behavior, but also influence its patterns.

### Individuality

Every system has a unique pattern, organization, and behavior unlike any other system. Do you remember learning in elementary school that no two snowflakes are alike? In the same way, no two people are alike, no two groups are alike, and no two organizations or communities are alike.

Although systems share many common attributes, each one expresses these attributes in a unique way. For example, every person has a need for food and shelter. Just think, however, of the infinite variety of ways in which these common needs can be met. In leadership, we study the common attributes and responses of certain systems, but it is important to stay alert to the uniqueness of each system. For example:

> When something threatens the integrity of an open system (a person, group, organization, or community), you can expect that system to react to the threat. But without an intimate knowledge of that particular system's patterns and attributes, you cannot predict whether the reaction will be to withdraw, to resist the threat, or to attack the source of the threat.

### Sentience

The capacity for thought, abstraction, and feeling is called **sentience.** Sentience brings into play the uniquely human qualities of emotions, values, and personal and cultural meanings. People are not simply aware of the world around them—they are actively involved in trying to make sense out of it and in trying to organize or influence their environment (Boulding, 1968).

In a sense, larger human systems (such as groups) also possess the capacity to think, feel, reflect, and make choices. Evidence of sentience in a group or organization can be seen in comments such as:

> "Our group views this situation as a serious threat to the new program."
> "The community is incensed over the new health department regulation."
> "This agency is proud of its record in delivering the highest-quality care to its clients."

**Systems thinking** seems to be especially helpful in understanding organizations and other large systems. As soon as we try to zero in on a particular aspect of these larger systems, such as the nursing staff of a large medical center, we risk losing sight of the rest of this complex system: the medical staff, administration, dietary department, plant maintenance, security force, laboratory personnel, and so forth. We also have to keep in mind how each of these components interacts with the others. If we do not, we will fail to grasp the dynamic nature of the organization (the medical center) as a whole, the interdependency of its components, and the potential conflicts and synergies that result (Napolitano & Henderson, 1998).

## Individual Factors Affecting Human Behavior

### Assumptions about Human Behavior

Two important assumptions about human behavior are especially relevant for the leader or manager. The first is that *all human behavior has some kind of meaning* (Brown & Fowler, 1971). Although the meaning of a particular action may be obscure to the observer, it is still assumed to have some purpose for the person performing the action. This purpose may be to meet a need for security, to express a feeling, or to cope with a perceived threat. People are not always aware of the purpose of their behavior. In fact, they may not be any more aware of the purpose than their observers are. They do, however, have the potential for developing this awareness.

The second assumption is that *every behavior reflects the person as a whole*—his or her physical as well as emotional state. For example, a person whose energy level is low may have a much weaker response to a major problem than would seem justified by the seriousness of the problem, whereas another person who has been storing up a great deal of tension may seem to overreact to a minor problem.

### Multiple Factors Influencing Behavior

Although it sometimes seems that a single stimulus causes a certain behavior, in truth, multiple factors usually affect the response. For an individual, these factors may include past experience, the present condition of the individual, and the environment in which this interaction takes place. Other factors include the person's cultural background, personal and social values, and social roles. The following example shows not only how multiple factors influence a reaction but also how

important it is for leaders and managers to recognize this complexity.

*Ms. T., a home health aide, walks up the path to a client's home. She stops suddenly when she finds a large dog blocking the path.*

*Her action is influenced by several factors, including the size of the dog, the "Beware of the Dog" sign on the lawn, her fear of dogs, and the way the dog approaches. In Ms. T.'s homeland, dogs are used to guard property and rarely kept as house pets. As a small child, Ms. T. was badly bitten by a guard dog when she put her hand through a fence to feed it. The appearance of the dog threatens Ms. T.'s feeling of safety and security. Unfortunately, at the same time, her startled response excites the dog, who begins barking and runs after her.*

*Ms. T. returns to the agency and refuses to go back to that home. An insensitive supervisor fails to explore the factors that influenced Ms. T.'s refusal and fires her for insubordination.*

A simplistic approach to understanding the responses of human systems fails to appreciate their complexity and is likely to result in inadequate explanations of human behavior.

## Stress, Threatening Situations, and Behavior

According to one survey, 40 percent of workers reported their job was very or extremely stressful (NIOSH, 1999). Some sources of this work-related stress are indicated in the brief quiz in Table 1–2. If you are presently employed, you might want to answer these questions to evaluate how many and what kind of stressors you have at work.

How do people deal with this stress? Actions to reduce stress or deal with a perceived threat may be divided into three categories: reflex actions, nondeliberative mechanisms, and deliberative mechanisms. The importance of examining responses to stress is difficult to overstate. Many illnesses are a response to inadequate or inappropriate coping efforts (Garland & Bush, 1982). These illnesses are not confined to our patients; they can affect us and our colleagues as well.

| Table 1–3 Sources of Work-Related Stress |
|---|

To what extent do each of the following statements describe the way you feel about your job?

| | Disagree | Agree Somewhat | Strongly Agree |
|---|---|---|---|
| I can't say what I really think at work. | 1 | 2 | 3 |
| I have a lot of responsibility but not much authority. | 1 | 2 | 3 |
| I could do a much better job if I had more time. | 1 | 2 | 3 |
| I seldom receive acknowledgment or appreciation at work. | 1 | 2 | 3 |
| I am picked on or discriminated against at work. | 1 | 2 | 3 |
| My workplace is not particularly pleasant or safe. | 1 | 2 | 3 |
| My job interferes with my family obligations and personal needs. | 1 | 2 | 3 |
| I tend to argue often with superiors, coworkers, and patients. | 1 | 2 | 3 |
| I feel that I have little control over my life at work. | 1 | 2 | 3 |

*Source:* American Stress Institute. In Matas, A. (1993) Coping skills are requisite for a shrinking workplace. *Miami Herald* (March 29).

## Reflex Actions

Reflex actions are automatic responses. They occur rapidly and spontaneously, without any conscious effort, but are nevertheless purposeful. Reacting automatically to a sudden loud noise and pulling away from a source of pain are reflex actions. Their purpose is usually protective in some way. People are born with a number of reflexes and acquire others during their lives. Of the three categories of coping behaviors, reflex actions are generally the least likely to be of concern to the leader-manager.

## Nondeliberative Mechanisms

The term **nondeliberative** is used to indicate coping mechanisms that operate primarily below the full awareness of the individual. The description of these nondeliberative mechanisms, which originated with the work of Freud (Schwartz & Schwartz, 1972), has been used to explain behavior even by those who do not use other elements of Freudian psychology. Although their purpose is generally protective, inappropriate or excessive use of any one of them is considered harmful. Because they are below awareness, their connection to a perceived threat or problem is not always apparent. Recalling these mechanisms can help explain the apparently inexplicable behavior of other people.

- *Compensation.* When people believe that they lack a particular ability, they may try to compensate by excelling in another area. For example, a person who has difficulty with technical skills may make up for it by concentrating on developing social skills and becoming popular at work.
- *Repression.* Repression is a complete blocking of certain feelings or thoughts from awareness because they are unacceptable or intolerable in some way. For example, a caregiver may repress anger toward a particular patient (one who was seriously injured in an alcohol or drug-related accident, for example), because anger is an unacceptable response to patients. The result is that the caregiver is unaware of owning these angry feelings but experiences a tension and unease when interacting with this patient.
- *Denial.* Similar to repression, denial involves blocking from awareness something in the environment that is painful or threatening. People can deny problems at work and appear, for example, to believe that everything is going well when they are actually on the verge of being fired.
- *Suppression.* Suppression is a more deliberate form of repression. It is temporarily putting aside disturbing feelings or thoughts until they can be handled. For example, a nurse may suppress emotions and act calmly in an emergency, but notice that his or her hands are shaking afterward.

- *Displacement.*  Displacement occurs when a person holds back or suppresses feelings about a particular person or situation, but later unleashes these feelings in another situation or toward a different person. For example, you might be angry at your boss but afraid to show it. Later, you displace the anger and yell at your friends for leaving coffee cups on your desk.
- *Projection.*  Projection is another way to deal with painful or unacceptable feelings by attributing them to other people. For example, supervisors who feel anxious about instituting a new evaluation procedure may say (and actually believe) that they oppose it because the people they supervise are threatened by it or can't handle it. Another kind of projection that can cause first-line managers some serious problems is when staff members blame others for their own failures.
- *Withdrawal.*  Withdrawal from a threatening situation is sometimes the only solution available to a person facing a problem. However, avoidance does not resolve a problem and, in some instances, may exacerbate it (Lee & Ashforth, 1993).
- *Rationalization.*  Rationalization is the use of an explanation that is logical and reasonable but not the real reason for a behavior. For example, a supervisor may deny a promotion to an eligible employee whom the supervisor dislikes intensely. The supervisor may rationalize the action by claiming the employee "isn't ready to move into that position yet and will be better off staying at this present level for at least another year."
- *Substitution.*  Socially acceptable energy outlets are often substituted for less acceptable but desired outlets. For example, the urge to retaliate against a physician who frequently berates the staff can be replaced by a drive to improve relations with other physicians. The substitute chosen may not always be constructive, however. For example, some people substitute excessive eating or drinking for other desired but unattainable sources of pleasure.
- *Identification.*  Identification involves experiencing the same feelings as another person or behaving the same way. It is often a means of filling a deficit in self-confidence or identity. People frequently identify with others whom they especially admire or with whom

they have something in common. For example, new nurses may identify with a nurse manager they particularly admire and model their behavior after this person.

## Deliberative Mechanisms

The deliberative coping mechanisms that people use to avoid discomfort and reduce tension are even more varied and individual than the nondeliberative mechanisms (Ardell, 1986; Feurerstein, Labbe & Kuczmierczyk, 1986; Menninger, 1963). Most of these mechanisms are helpful, but they too can be misused or overused. The following list suggests a few of the many deliberative mechanisms people use.

- *Seek comfort and reassurance.*  Touching, hugging, and using comforting words can soothe and calm people who are distressed.
- *Sound and rhythm.*  Dancing, listening to music, and other rhythmic activities are a means for expressing feelings and releasing tension.
- *Ventilate feelings.*  Crying, swearing, and laughing, to name only a few, are ways to relieve tension and share feelings with others.
- *Eat.*  Eating can relieve tension and substitute for other needs. When done in the company of others, it can become a time of sharing and support that contributes to well-being.
- *Smoking and stimulants.*  Although not healthful, these substances are often used to ease tension and reduce feelings of fatigue.
- *Relaxation techniques and exercise.*  These nondrug methods are often effective in reducing tension, although they do not solve underlying problems.
- *Discuss a problem.*  Simply talking about a problem with a person who is a good listener often makes the problem seem less intimidating and more manageable.
- *Draw on past experience.*  Having successfully managed a similar experience in the past not only provides clues to action but also confidence in the ability to cope adequately the next time.
- *Take one thing at a time.*  A seemingly unmanageable problem or overwhelming demand may seem less impossible to deal with if it is broken down into manageable parts that are considered and resolved one at a time. This limited focus may help a person get through a time of crisis.

## C A S E   S T U D Y

### Just a Small Change in Procedure

It was not a "big deal," just a small change in procedure. At least that's what the new CEO of the Harborside Home Health Agency thought when she ordered the staff to bring their laptop computers back to the office every evening. "These machines are expensive," the CEO explained, "we cannot continue to let staff take them home because they could be broken, stolen, or used to play games in the evening."

### Questions for Critical Reflection and Analysis

1. How do you think the staff reacted to this change? Explain why they might react as you describe.

2. Adopt an open systems perspective and list as many people as possible who would be affected by this change in procedure. Speculate on the way in which each could be affected.
3. Using the Elements of a Management Situation diagram as a starting point, create a diagram to show the people who would be affected by this change.
4. Did the home health agency's new CEO act primarily as a leader or as a manager in this situation? Explain your choice.
5. What alternative procedures might be implemented to protect the laptop computers?

---

- *Become passive, rigid, or vague.* These behaviors conserve energy temporarily but do not relieve the stress. People using this mechanism tend to internalize their stress.
- *Aggression.* Aggression discharges energy but often exacerbates the problem. Assertiveness, which is a less combative stance, is a more positive response.
- *Take stock of your resources.* This mechanism has both calming and strengthening effects.
- *Sleep.* Not only a means of temporary escape, sleep also restores energy.
- *Rest.* Although it is not the same as sleep, a break in activity can reduce tension and help the body recover from fatigue.
- *Repetitive activity.* Seemingly purposeless and repetitive actions, such as pacing, rocking, grinding teeth, drumming fingers on a table, or swinging a leg, discharge excess energy. It is often seen at meetings or at nursing stations where few other outlets are available.

People sometimes engage in these activities when other behavior would seem more appropriate. The leader or manager who is aware of the meaning of such behaviors can sometimes help the individual solve the problem that led to the need for these coping mechanisms.

## ● SUMMARY

Gaining the skills and knowledge of leadership and management provides healthcare professionals with better understanding and control of what occurs in work situations. More specifically, nurses can learn how to work effectively with other people, advocate for their patients/clients, understand their position within the healthcare system, bring about change, take control of their practice, assume leadership and management responsibilities, and support the nursing profession.

Leadership is defined as influencing and inspiring others to meet their goals. Any member of a group or organization can exercise leadership. Management, on the other hand, is a formal responsibility assigned to individuals who are expected to motivate others to perform and contribute to meeting the employer's goals. Although closely related, leadership is an attained position available to anyone while management is an assigned role.

According to open systems theory, an open system is different from and greater than the sum of its parts (subsystems). Subsystems are related but differentiated parts of the whole. The open human system (which may be an individual, group, organization, or community) interacts mutually and simultaneously with its environment, exchanging energy, matter, and information. An open human system is also characterized by patterns that include growth, which proceeds unidirectionally and sequentially; individuality; and the capacity to think and feel, called sentience.

All human behavior is postulated to have meaning, although the person may not always be conscious of it. It also reflects the present state of the whole individual in relation to the environment and is affected by multiple interacting factors. Automatic reflex actions, nondeliberative coping mechanisms (including compensation, repression, denial, suppression, displacement, projection, withdrawal, rationalization, substitution, and identification), and a large number of deliberative mechanisms are used by people to cope with the everyday challenges and stresses of living and working.

# REFERENCES

Ardell, D.B. (1986). *High level wellness*. Berkeley, CA: Ten Speed Press.

Ashby, W.R. (1968). Principles of the self-organizing system. In W. Buckley (Ed.). *Modern systems research for the behavioral scientist*. Chicago: Aldine Publishing.

Bateman, T.S. & Crant, J.M. (1993). The proactive component of organizational behavior: A measure and correlates. *Journal of Organizational Behavior, 14*(2), 143–158.

Bell, N.W. & Vogel, E.F. (1968). *A modern introduction to the family*. New York: Free Press.

Bennis, W. & Nanus, B. (1985). *Leaders: The strategies for taking charge*. New York: Harper and Row.

Boulding, K.E. (1968). General system theory—The skeleton of science. In W. Buckley (Ed.). *Modern systems research for the behavioral scientist*. Chicago: Aldine Publishing.

Brown, M.M. & Fowler, G.R. (1971). *Psychodynamic nursing: A biosocial orientation*. Philadelphia: W.B. Saunders.

Chapple, E.D. (1979). *The biological foundations of individuality and culture*. Huntington, NY: Robert Krieger.

Chemers, M.M. (1993). An integrative theory of leadership. In M.M. Chemers & R. Ayman (Eds.). *Leadership theory and research*. San Diego, CA: Academic Press.

Drucker, P.F. (1967). *The effective executive*. New York: Harper and Row.

Eddington, A. Quoted in Napolitano, C.S. & Henderson, L.J. (1998). *The leadership odyssey*. San Francisco: Jossey-Bass.

Feuerstein, M., Labbe, E.E. & Kuczmierczyk, A.R. (1986). *Health psychology: A psychological perspective*. New York: Plenum Press.

Flower, J.C. (1992). New tools, new thinking: A conversation with Russel L. Ackoff. *Healthcare Forum Journal, 35*(2), 62–67.

Garland, L.M. & Bush, C.T. (1982). *Coping behaviors and nursing*. Reston, VA: Reston Publishing.

Hall, A.D. & Fagen, R.E. (1968). Definition of system. In W. Buckley (Ed.). *Modern systems research for the behavioral scientist*. Chicago: Aldine Publishing.

Hanchett, E.S. (1979). *Community health assessment: A conceptual tool kit*. New York: John Wiley & Sons.

Kerzner, H. (1998). *Project management: A systems approach to planning, scheduling, and controlling*. New York: Van Nostrand Reinhold.

Kotter, J.P. (1997). What leaders really do. In R.P. Vecchio (Ed.). *Leadership: Understanding the dynamics of power and influence in organizations*. Notre Dame, IN: University of Notre Dame Press, 24–34.

Laszlo, E. (1972). *The systems view of the world*. New York: George Braziller.

Lee, R.T. & Ashforth S.J. (1993). A further examination of managerial burnout: Toward an integrated model. *Journal of Organizational Behavior, 14*(1), 3–20.

Longenecker, J.G. & Pringle, C.D. (1981). *Management*, 5th ed. Columbus, OH: Charles E. Merrill.

Mabry, E. (1999). The systems metaphor in group communication. In L.R. Frey (Ed.) *The handbook of group communication theory & research*. Thousand Oaks, CA: Sage, 71–91.

Matas, A. (1993, March 29). Coping skills are requisite for a shrinking workplace. *Miami Herald*.

McGannon, D.H. Quoted in Fitton, R.A. (1997). *Leadership: Quotations from the world's greatest motivators*. Boulder, CO: Westview Press, 160.

Menninger, K. (1963). *The vital balance: The life process in mental health and illness*. New York: Viking Press.

Morgan, G. (1997). *Imagination: The art of creative management*. Newbury Park: Sage.

Napolitano, C.S. & Henderson, L.J. (1998). *The leadership odyssey*. San Francisco: Jossey-Bass.

NIOSH—Department of Health and Human Services. (1999). *Stress at work*. (DHHS Publication #99–101). Cincinnati, OH: Publications Dissemination, EID, National Institute for Occupational Safety & Health.

Petzinger, T. (1999a). *The new pioneers: The men and women who are transforming the workplace and marketplace*. New York: Simon & Schuster.

Petzinger, T. (1999b). A new model for the nature of business: It's alive! *Wall Street Journal* (February 26, 1999). B1, B4.

Rogers, M.E. (1994a). Nursing: Science of unitary, irreducible, human beings: Update 1990. In V.M. Malinski & E.A.M. Barrett (Eds.). *Martha E. Rogers: Her life and her work*. Philadelphia: F.A. Davis.

Rogers, M.E. (1994b). Nursing: A science of unitary man. In V.M. Malinski & E.A.M. Barrett (Eds.). *Martha E. Rogers: Her life and her work*. Philadelphia: F.A. Davis.

Rogers, M.E. (1994c). Science of unitary human beings. In V.M. Malinski & E.A.M. Barrett (Eds.). *Martha E. Rogers: Her life and her work*. Philadelphia: F.A. Davis.

Rogers, M.E. (1970). *An introduction to the theoretical basis of nursing*. Philadelphia: F.A. Davis.

Scheflen, A.E. (1982). Comments on the significance of interaction rhythms. In M. Dairs (Ed.). *Interaction rhythms: Periodicity in communicative behavior*. New York: Human Sciences Press.

Schwartz, L.H. & Schwartz, J.L. (1972). *The psychodynamics of patient care*. Englewood Cliffs, NJ: Prentice-Hall.

Senge, P. (1999). *The dance of change*. New York: Doubleday.

Sommers, D.I. (1993). Team building in the classroom through rhythm. *Journal of Management Education, 17*(2), 263–268.

Stafford, L. (1994). Tracing the threads of the spider web. In D.J. Canary, & L. Stafford (Eds.). *Communication and relational maintenance*. San Diego, CA: Academic Press.

Tannenbaum, R., Weschler, I.R. & Massarik, F. (1974). Leadership: A frame of reference. In R.S. Cathcart & L.A. Samopvar (Eds.). *Small group communication: A reader*. Dubuque, IA: William C. Brown.

Tichy, N.M. (1997). *The leadership engine: How winning companies build leaders at every level*. New York: Harper Collins.

Von Bertalanffy, L. (1976). Introduction. In H. Werley et al. (Eds.). *Health research: The systems approach*. New York: Springer Publishing.

Williamson, J.N. (1986). *The leader-manager*. New York: John Wiley.

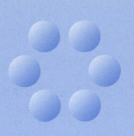

# CHAPTER 2

# Conceptual Base for Leadership and Management

## LEARNING OBJECTIVES

*After completing this chapter, the reader will be able to:*

- Trace the evolution of early leadership and management theories into contemporary theories.
- Distinguish a simplistic leadership or management theory from a comprehensive theory.
- Evaluate the degree to which the major theories include the basic elements of leadership and management situations.

- Compare and contrast the democratic style to the authoritarian and laissez-faire styles; Theory X to Theories Y and Z; task orientation to relationship orientation; and the humanistic approach to the behavioral management approach.
- Discuss the effect of one's choice of theories on the practice of leadership and management.

## TEST YOURSELF

**Whose theory is it?**

*How many of the major leadership and management theorists are familiar to you? See how many of the following theorists listed in the left-hand column (A) you are able to match with the kind of advice the theorist might give to a new leader or manager in the right-hand column (B). Then check your answers.*

**A**
**Theorists**
___ 1. Maslow, *Hierarchy of Needs*
___ 2. Herzberg, *Hygiene & Motivation Factors*
___ 3. McGregor, *Theory X and Y*
___ 4. Taylor, *Scientific Management*
___ 5. Lewin, Lippitt & White, *Leadership Style*
___ 6. Fiedler, *Contingency*
___ 7. House, *Path Goal*
___ 8. Burns, Bass & Avolio, *Transformational Leadership*

**B**
**Statements**
a. Provide safe working conditions to reduce dissatisfaction
b. Share your vision
c. Include staff in decision making as much as possible
d. To increase productivity, pay by the piece
e. Make it clear how accomplishing a particular goal will lead to a specific reward
f. Adapt your style to the situation
g. Provide security and stability *before* working on opportunities for growth
h. Place your trust in the fact that people want to work

*Answers:*

1. G  2. A  3. H  4. D  5. C  6. F  7. E  8. B

An impressive number of leadership and management theories have been developed over the years. All attempt to explain how people influence each other's behavior in work situations. Some are more successful than others.

You will see that some of the earlier leadership theorists tried to explain leadership in terms of a single characteristic or single element of a leadership situation. Some of these theories are so limited that they hardly deserve to be called theories. Despite their limitations, they do have some value and are used more often than you might expect.

The early management theories were also limited in scope. The primary concern at that time was the factory worker, someone whose

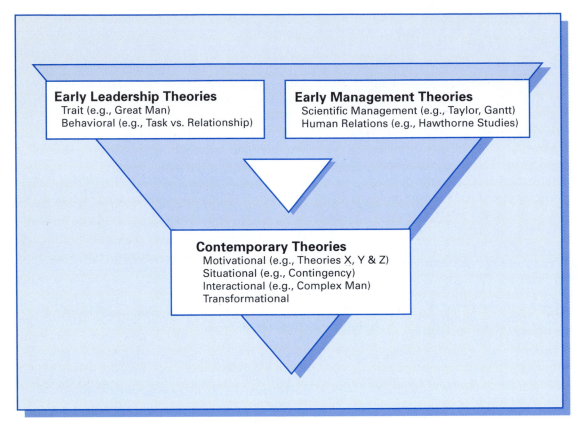

**Figure 2–1**    Diagrammatic representation of the evolution of leadership and management theories.

output could be easily measured in terms of the number of welds completed or objects assembled. Although focused on methods to increase a worker's productivity, the many factors that might affect the worker's skill development and motivation were left out. The output of many workers today, including those in health care, is not so concrete or easy to measure, and the factors that affect their performance are not at all simple.

The later theories are more complex, often combining elements of several earlier theories. They are a little harder to understand but they also explain more. Figure 2–1 is a diagram outlining the interrelationships of the theories discussed in this chapter. You may find it helpful to refer back to this diagram or to the outline at the beginning of the chapter from time to time as you read about these theories.

## ● THEORY
### Why Have a Theory?

Why have a theoretical framework? A brief explanation of the ways in which theory can be used will help you see the purpose of studying different leadership and management theories.

### *Organization*

A theory provides a framework in which to organize your ideas and experiences. Somewhat like desk organizers that have multiple compartments to tuck things into, theories have components or categories into which you can sort your knowledge and observations. In this regard, theories can (1) provide links between separate pieces of information (Waltz, Strickland, & Lenz, 1991), (2) help you detect similarities, differences, and relationships in data, and (3) provide explanations for these patterns.

## Perspective

Theories also provide a perspective, a certain way of looking at things. The particular theory you use can have a great influence on how you interpret what you see. The following is an example:

> *A female physician is observed yelling at a male technician. This woman could be seen by a traditional Freudian analyst as "suffering from penis envy." In contrast, a follower of Thomas Harris and Eric Berne of* I'm OK, You're OK *fame would describe this as an "I'm OK, you're not OK" situation. To someone using an interpersonal relationship perspective the situation represents "a failure to communicate." To a sociologist, it may be seen as an example of "women's liberation." To a practical, nontheoretically oriented union representative, it is a typical example of disrespect for the ordinary worker and a potential grievance.*

Each person in the previous example was looking at the same event from a different perspective. One perspective focused on physical differences between the sexes, another emphasized feelings about self and others, a third was concerned with the prevailing social climate, and so forth. In fact, the Freudian analyst, the sociologist, and the union representative might have difficulty talking to each other about this situation. People who share a common theoretical perspective usually have a greater sense of mutual understanding and ease of communication than those who do not.

### Mental models have awesome power.
—Petzinger, 1999b, p. b1

## Explanation

Theories also provide explanations of events. They provide general statements that help us understand why certain things do or do not happen. Why, for example, does Nurse A work harder than Nurse B? One management theory will say that it is because Nurse A receives a higher salary than Nurse B. Another theory will say that it is because Nurse B is not interested in the type of work that has been assigned. A third theory will say that both factors are operating: Nurse A has interesting, stimulating work and is paid more than Nurse B, who is burned out and underpaid.

## Prediction

A theory may also help you to predict what is likely to happen in a given situation. For example, developmental theory predicts that certain crises occur during adolescence, including conflicts between parents and teenagers. Familiarity with this theory enables a nurse to provide anticipatory guidance to a family with children entering adolescence.

The ability to predict people's behavior enables a leader to anticipate what will happen given a certain set of circumstances. For example, you might expect an experienced nurse to be more interested in being a mentor than one who is still working his or her way up the ladder of success.

## Application

A theory that predicts what is likely to happen also provides some direction regarding what action is to be taken, which is particularly important in a practice profession such as nursing. Leadership and management theories serve as guides to selecting the most effective action, although, as you will see, different theories may suggest different actions.

# Theory Selection

A thorough evaluation of a particular theory is a complex process that is beyond the scope of this book. However, you might want to ask a number of questions (Fawcett, 2000) about the theories that follow that will help you decide whether they will be useful to you in the practice of leadership and management.

- *Is the theory consistent internally?* Are the different parts of the theory congruent with each other? For example, is behavior explained or predicted in a consistent manner?

An inconsistent management theory might claim that people try to avoid work and then suggest that the manager allow staff members to work as independently as possible.

- *Does the theory provide useful guidelines for practice?*  Our primary purpose for studying theories that explain human behavior in work situations is to apply them to practice. Some theories are so broad, however, that it is difficult to apply them to specific situations. Open systems theory, for example, provides little specific advice on how to respond to a particular problem. It does provide a valuable perspective, however, by illustrating the complexity of most work situations, helping us to avoid overly simplistic solutions to complex problems.
- *Has empirical testing yielded evidence in support of the theory?*  Some theories have a natural appeal that tempts us to accept them without sufficient testing. The purpose of subjecting theories to empirical testing is to provide some objective evidence of the theory's ability to explain and predict human behavior. The research examples scattered throughout this book can help you begin this process of evaluation.
- *Is the theory congruent with your values and your philosophy of nursing?*  A management theory that supports the development of the individual employee implies a different set of values from one that supports immediate termination when the employee's skills are no longer needed. You will see such a difference between Miller's behavioral management approach and McGregor's Theory Y later in this chapter.

Shapiro (1997) notes that "profound contradictions" (p. 142) exist among the various theories of leadership and management. Leadership and management are also plagued by theory fads, some of which are new ideas and some simply repackaged old ideas. An intelligent, self-confident leader or manager will critically evaluate these ideas before incorporating them into practice. The lazy, fearful, or overwhelmed will not. Shapiro quotes Henry Ford who once said, "Thinking is the hardest work there is, which is probably why so few engage in it" (p. 143).

*Leadership is one of the most observed and least understood phenomena.*
—James MacGregor Burns, 1997

## EARLY LEADERSHIP THEORIES

### Trait Theories

If you have ever heard the statement that "leaders are born, not made," then you have heard someone expressing the fundamental belief underlying a trait theory of leadership. Trait theories assume that a person must have certain innate abilities, personality traits, or other characteristics in order to be a leader. If this assumption is true, it would mean that some people are naturally better leaders than others.

Because trait theories emphasize given ability over the effects of learning or the development of leadership skills, they lead to the popular conclusion that some people cannot be leaders, no matter how hard they try. This approach also leads to efforts to identify people who have the characteristics of a leader rather than to the development of leadership training programs.

Modern thinking about leadership is that it cannot be reduced to either a set of characteristics or a certain type of behavior (Kim & Mauborgne, 1992). An emerging opposing view reiterates the old idea that leaders really are made, not born, which comes from evolutionary psychology, a controversial viewpoint from the field of psychology (Nicholson, 1998). For more information on the argument behind this theory, see Perspectives . . . Are Some of Us Born to Be Leaders and Others Not?

### Great Man Theory

According to the "*Great Man*" theory of leadership, the tremendous influence of some well-known people has actually determined or changed the course of history. The opposite, **deterministic** viewpoint is that these people happened to be in the right place at the right time and that the events of their time made them great.

## P E R S P E C T I V E S . . .

### Are Some of Us Born to Be Leaders and Others Not?

Human beings today retain the traits that made survival possible in the Stone Age, according to evolutionary psychologists. These traits include fighting ferociously when threatened and trusting one's emotional radar (instincts) over rational analysis. Furthermore, these traits are believed to be programmed in our brains ("hardwired") and to have a permanent and powerful effect on our behavior. We are not all alike, however, according to this theory. Some of us are predisposed to seek risk or to be highly emotional; others of us are not.

If this is true, the consequences for learning and practicing leadership are enormous. Nigel Nicholson, a professor of organizational behavior at the London Business School, begins with the premise that the most important attribute for leadership is the **desire to lead.** He concedes that we can learn managerial skills but does not believe we can consciously develop the passion to dominate or to lead others. "Reluctant leaders," he writes, "can survive as symbolic figureheads but will perform poorly if asked to manage other people" (p. 146). He adds that if a person is not born with the desire to lead, "he or she should do everyone a favor and follow or ally themselves with partners who do" (p. 146).

Nicholson emphasizes that dominance alone is neither sufficient nor necessarily most important in some situations. For example, empathy or negotiating skills might be more urgently needed in some situations. Other traits such as shyness or a low threshold for stress would not necessarily prevent you from becoming a leader but would affect the way in which you lead and, therefore, should affect your choice of leadership positions. For example, if you are sensitive to stress, you might be more effective in a role where you map out strategies for change rather than in a more visible role where you spearhead the change.

From this theoretical viewpoint, then, your efforts to become an effective leader should focus on recognizing your strengths and weaknesses and, instead of trying to change them, seeking situations that call for your strengths and not for those traits in which you are weak.

*Source:* Nicholson, N. (1998, July/August). How hardwired is human behavior? *Harvard Business Review,* 135–146.

Important historical figures, such as Caesar, Alexander the Great, and Hitler have been studied to find the characteristics that made them powerful leaders in their time. Royalty were also of interest to trait theorists. For example, when the characteristics of the rulers of 14 European countries over 500 years were studied, researchers found that the countries were strong when they had a strong ruler but that the conditions in these countries were bad when they had a weak ruler (Gemmill, 1986; Woods, 1913). Proponents of the Great Man theory assumed that the country's condition was due to the influence of the ruler's abilities, ignoring the possibility that the condition of the country could have affected the success of the ruler. The Great Man theory has also failed to recognize the contributions of great women in history.

A modern day version of the Great Man theory is the "hero-leader" or "hero-CEO" (Senge, 1999). This person is usually the chief executive of the organization who is, unrealistically, expected to be able to single-handedly save an organization in trouble and/or lead it into a successful future. Like the original Great Man theory, this modern version fails to recognize the important contributions of the rest of the people who work for the organization.

> *We expect a leader to stand apart . . . be confident . . . act on our behalf . . . protect us . . . take charge . . . be larger than life. It is simply unreasonable to expect that any one individual can bear the burden of leadership in every situation. Hence the need for a new model of leadership in which the leader supports and facilitates the contributions of others.*
> —Napolitano & Henderson, 1998, pp. 4–5

### Individual Characteristics

The search for traits that determine whether a person will be an effective leader has been the focus of many studies. So far, however, no single trait or characteristic has been found in all leaders. In spite of this limitation, the trait approach is often used to choose people for leadership positions.

Many people believe in and try to implement a number of different—and even contradictory—versions of trait theory. Certain physical characteristics are often thought to augment leadership ability. For example, it is commonly believed that tall individuals are better leadership material than short individuals because they seem stronger and more dominating. A tall person can be physically imposing and can literally "look down" on other people. A contradictory but also popular belief is that a person who was always smaller than his or her peers has had to learn how to defend himself or herself and is, therefore, a tougher fighter and potentially stronger leader than most other people (this is sometimes called the "Napoleonic complex").

Many other characteristics and behaviors are associated with leadership ability. For example, the most outspoken person in a group is often assumed to be the leader even when other evidence does not support this assumption. The most intelligent or skilled person in a group may be designated the leader because other group members admire this person. Manipulative people (sometimes called "smooth operators" or "wheeler-dealers") and people who are especially courageous are also thought of as good leadership material.

Despite their limitations and contradictions, these popular versions of the trait theory are often used as the basis for leadership decisions. The most physically imposing or most highly skilled nurse in a group may be chosen for a management position solely on the basis of these particular traits.

## Trait Studies

The beliefs about leadership previously mentioned are clearly subjective in nature. More objective research studies have not been entirely successful in finding any one set of traits that distinguishes leaders from nonleaders (Bryman, 1992). Dozens of different traits have been identified, but so far none have been found that can consistently predict who will be an effective leader and who will not.

Some characteristics, however, were found in a large number of these studies. These are intelli-

gence, skill, initiative, assertiveness, persistence, ability to relate to other people, a strong sense of self, ability to tolerate stress and take the consequences of a decision, originality (creativity), and status within the group. Intelligence and initiative are the two most often cited.

## Comment

By themselves, the trait theories are too limited because they focus on the leader and ignore the other elements of a leadership or management situation (the co-actor, the work, and the environment). Also, they focus on the capacities a leader brings to a situation rather than on what the leader actually does in a situation. They do contribute to our understanding of leadership by indicating those characteristics, especially intelligence and initiative, that are more likely to be found in leaders than nonleaders. Many of the traits associated with leadership may actually be indicators of motivation or desire to lead rather than innate capacities of an individual to lead.

## Behavioral Theories

The behavioral theories, sometimes called the **functional theories** of leadership, still focus on the leader. The primary difference between the trait and behavioral theories is that the behavioral theories are concerned with what a leader *does* rather than who the leader *is*. They are still limited primarily to the leader element in a leadership situation, but they are far more action oriented and do give some consideration to the co-actors. We will consider one theory based on the description of leadership functions and two different approaches to describing leadership styles.

### Authoritarian, Democratic, and Laissez-Faire Styles (Lewin, Lippitt, and White)

A major breakthrough in the development of leadership theories came in the late 1930s. The classic research done by Lewin, Lippitt, and White (White & Lippitt, 1960) on the interaction between leaders and group members indicated that the behavior of the leader could substantially influence the climate and outcomes of the group. The leaders' behaviors were divided into three distinct patterns called **leadership**

## Research Example 2–1    *Leadership Styles*

### Study Design

A classic study of the effects of different leadership styles on groups was done by Lewin, Lippitt, and White in 1938. Twenty 11-year-old boys (described as middle class, Midwestern, and well adjusted) were assigned to groups with autocratic, democratic, or laissez-faire leaders.

The groups met once a week in after-school clubs in which the boys made masks, plaster molds, and other craft items. Each group was exposed to three different leaders and at least two different styles of leadership. Each leader used at least two different styles of leadership to control the effects of differences in skill and personal style of the individual leaders.

The original plan was to test only the autocratic and democratic styles, but it was observed that one of the four leaders in the first series of club meetings was more anarchic than democratic, which had a substantial effect on his group. This leader was then encouraged to assume the laissez-faire style for that series of six meetings, and another leader did the same in the second series of meetings, in order to study the effects of laissez-faire leadership.

The autocratic leaders made all the decisions and expected the boys to obey them. When the groups had democratic leaders, the boys participated in making decisions. The laissez-faire leader avoided making any decisions and allowed the group to work or play without any supervision or direction.

At each club meeting, an observer sat unobtrusively in the corner of the room to record the behavior of both the leader and group members for later analysis. Raw scores and percentages were reported for the behavior observed, such as the number and proportion of friendly, aggressive, or dependent statements made by the boys. The differences were found to be statistically significant at the .05 level of confidence or better.

### Results

The researchers found that the groups behaved very differently under different leadership styles. When the groups had laissez-faire leaders they were less organized, less efficient, and less satisfying for their members. Laissez-faire groups got less work done, spent more time horsing around, and their work was done poorly. When the boys were interviewed later by a neutral party, all of them (100 percent) preferred the democratic leader over the laissez-faire leader.

Autocratic leadership was found to result in much more hostility (in a ratio of 30:1), more demand for attention, more dependence on the leaders, and other more subtle kinds of discontent in the groups. In fact, all four boys who dropped out of the clubs did so when their groups were led by autocratic leaders. It is interesting to note that groups with autocratic leaders were found to be either quite aggressive or quite submissive. The observers thought that less individuality was allowed in the autocratic groups. Motivation to work was clearly lower than it was in the democratically led groups: when the autocratic leader left the room, the work stopped. However, the overall quality of the work done was best under the autocratic leaders.

Democratic groups were more cohesive. They were described as being friendlier and more group-minded. Although they produced somewhat less work than the autocratically led groups, both motivation and originality were found to be higher. Nineteen out of the total of 20 boys expressed a preference for the leader who used the democratic style of leadership.

*Source:* White, R.K. & Lippitt, R. (1960). *Autocracy and democracy: An experimental inquiry.* New York: Harper & Row. (Published after Lewin's death).

styles: authoritarian, democratic, and laissez-faire. More detail on their study can be found in Research Example 2–1. These styles can be thought of as a continuum from a highly controlling and directive type of leadership to a mostly passive, inactive style. (See Table 2–1).

**Table 2–1**    Comparison of Authoritarian, Democratic, and Laissez-Faire Leadership Styles

|  | Authoritarian | Democratic | Laissez-Faire |
|---|---|---|---|
| Degree of freedom | Little freedom | Moderate freedom | Much freedom |
| Degree of control | High control | Moderate control | No control |
| Decision making | By the leader | Leader and group together | By the group or by no one |
| Leader activity level | High | High | Minimal |
| Assumption of responsibility | Primarily the leader | Shared | Abdicated |
| Output of the group | High quantity, good quality | Creative, high quality | Variable, may be poor quality |
| Efficiency | Highly efficient | Less efficient than authoritarian | Inefficient |

The **authoritarian** leader maintains strong control over the people in his or her group. This control may be benevolent and considerate (often called paternalistic leadership) or it may be dictatorial, with complete disregard for the needs and feelings of group members.

Authoritarian leaders give orders and expect group members to obey these orders. Directions are given as commands, not suggestions. Criticism is more common from the authoritarian leader than from the other types, although it is not necessarily a constant occurrence.

Decisions are made by the leader alone, not the group. Some authoritarian leaders try to make decisions congruent with the group's goals, but others make decisions that are directly opposed to the group's needs or goals.

Authoritarian leadership emphasizes the differences in status between leaders and group members. The authoritarian leader clearly dominates the group, making the status of the leader separate from, and higher than, the status of group members. This separation reduces the degree of trust and openness between leader and group members, particularly if the leader tends to be punitive as well.

Procedures and group actions are well defined and usually predictable. This environment reduces frustration and increases group members' feelings of security. Productivity is high but creativity and initiative rarely thrive under this type of leadership. Dependency needs are usually met, but growth and autonomy needs often are not.

Authoritarian leadership is particularly suitable in an emergency situation when clear directions are the highest priority. It is also appropriate when the entire focus is on getting the job done or in large groups when it is difficult to share decision making for some reason. It is often referred to today as a **directive** or controlling style of leadership.

In contrast, democratic leadership is much more participative and far less controlling than authoritarian leadership. It is not passive, however. The democratic leader actively stimulates and guides the group toward fulfillment of the following principles and toward achievement of the group's goals. **Democratic leadership** is based on these principles:

1. Everyone in the organization, department, group, or team is encouraged to participate in decision making.
2. Freedom of belief and action is allowed within reasonable bounds set by society and by the group.
3. Each individual is responsible for himself or herself and for the welfare of the group.
4. Concern and consideration for each group member as a unique individual are expected.

Rather than issuing commands, democratic leaders offer information, ask stimulating questions, and make suggestions to guide the work of the group. They are catalysts rather than controllers, more likely to say "we" rather than "I" or "you" when talking about the group. They set

limits, enforce rules, and encourage productivity. Criticism is meant to be constructive rather than punitive.

Control is shared with group members who are expected to participate to the best of their abilities and experience. The democratic style demands a strong faith in the ability of group members to solve problems and ultimately to make wise choices when setting group goals and deciding how to accomplish those goals. Not every leader or manager finds this leadership style easy.

Because group members participate actively in decision making and have more responsibility for the outcomes of those decisions, dependence on the leader is minimized and independence and originality are encouraged. Participation in goal setting increases the group's commitment to those goals; motivation to get the work done comes from the entire group rather than through pressure from the leader. Group members are usually more satisfied with democratic leadership than with authoritarian or laissez-faire leadership.

Most studies indicate that democratic leadership is not as efficient as authoritarian leadership. While the work done by a democratic group is more creative and the group is more self-motivated, the democratic style is also more cumbersome. First, it takes more time to ensure that everyone in the group has participated in making a decision, which can be frustrating to people who want to get a job done as fast as possible. Second, disagreements are more likely to arise and must be resolved, which can also require much effort.

Democratic leadership is particularly appropriate for groups of people who work together for an extended time; i.e., when interpersonal relationships substantially affect the work of the group. It is also appropriate when a great deal of cooperation and coordination between group members is needed, or when the nature of the work makes close and detailed supervision difficult or impossible. This type of situation is often seen in health care.

Democratic leadership is often called supportive or **participative** leadership today. The degree to which decision making is shared with the group varies, with styles midway between democratic and autocratic. For example, in many cases a leader encourages input from group members and takes their views into consideration.

> *Many employees today did not grow up with authoritarian fathers . . . you've got to transition to a modern style of motivating people.*
> —Ivester in Faust, Smith, & Rochs, 1999, p. 151

The **laissez-faire** leader is generally inactive, passive, and nondirective. The laissez-faire leader leaves virtually all of the control and decision making to the group and provides little or no direction, guidance, or encouragement.

Laissez-faire leaders offer little to the group: few commands, questions, suggestions, or criticism. They are permissive, set almost no limits, and allow almost any behavior. However, many are inconsistent and occasionally become highly directive and command group members to take a particular action. When such an about-face happens, group members often ignore the command or react negatively to this unanticipated attempt to exert leadership.

Some laissez-faire leaders are quite supportive of individual group members and do provide information or suggestions when asked. The more extreme laissez-faire leader, however, turns such a request back to the group. When the laissez-faire style becomes extreme, no leadership exists at all.

In a laissez-faire group, members act independently of each other, often at cross-purposes, because of the lack of cooperation or coordination. In some groups, disinterest and apathy set in; in others, the activity becomes chaotic and frustration rises. In either case, the goals are unclear and procedures are confusing or absent altogether. Neither the task nor the relationship concerns of group members are dealt with satisfactorily.

When all group members are highly self-directed, motivated, and able to coordinate their own activities with others, laissez-faire leadership can give them the freedom they need to be highly creative and productive. In most situations, however, laissez-faire leadership is unproductive, inefficient, and unsatisfactory. Laissez-faire leadership

is often called **permissive** or **nondirective** leadership today.

## Leader Behavior Descriptions (Hemphill; Halpin and Winer)

When attention turned from the qualities of the person who is the leader to the kinds of behavior exhibited by leaders, it became apparent that leadership could be a shared function. For example, each member of a healthcare team may be knowledgeable about some aspect of patient care and have some influence on patient-care decisions made by the team.

Beginning in the 1940s and 1950s, a large number of research studies were done to find out just what these leader functions were (Stogdill & Coons, 1957). The purpose of these studies was to describe and categorize the behaviors of actual leaders. Unlike the subjects of the earlier trait theorists, however, these leaders were not political or historical figures. Instead they were supervisors or leaders of a diverse array of teams, including Air Force crews, school personnel, and more recently, nurses.

More than 1,800 different behaviors were identified in these studies. The behaviors were then organized into nine categories:

1. Integration (increasing cooperation)
2. Communication
3. Production emphasis
4. Representation (speaking for the group)
5. Fraternization
6. Organization
7. Evaluation
8. Initiation
9. Domination

These nine categories developed by Hemphill were later modified, tested, and reduced to two major categories that are still widely used. The first of these categories, called **initiating structure**, includes task-related functions such as:

- Assigns members to particular tasks
- Criticizes poor work

Initiating structure also includes behaviors that clarify roles, organize work, define procedures, and move the group toward its goals.

The second category, **consideration**, includes relationship-oriented functions such as:

- Finds time to listen to team members
- Does personal favors for team members

Consideration also includes behaviors that build trust and show respect for the individual group members.

These two categories have been used in many research studies and in evaluations of leaders by both superiors and subordinates. Both seem to have a significant effect on leadership effectiveness. For example, when leaders are rated high on both initiating structure and consideration, their groups are more cohesive and harmonious. High consideration behavior results in increased satisfaction, lower absenteeism, fewer grievances, and lower employee turnover. High initiating structure seems to improve group productivity.

Leaders who are low in both initiating structure and consideration are usually rated ineffective by both their supervisors and the members of the group. The most effective leader is believed to be high on both initiating structure and consideration.

## Task versus Relationship Orientation (Blake and Mouton)

The concepts of task and relationship orientations are closely related to initiating structure and consideration. The task-oriented leader is concerned with getting the work done and focuses on activities that encourage group productivity. The relationship-oriented leader, on the other hand, is especially concerned with interpersonal relationships and focuses on activities that meet group members' needs.

Unlike the single continuum of authoritarian, democratic, and laissez-faire leadership styles, the task and relationship orientations are on two intersecting axes (Figure 2–2). This interrelationship means that a leader can be high on one scale and low on the other, or vice versa. Blake and Mouton developed what they call a **managerial grid** to show the various combinations of high and low concern for people in the relationship orientation and high and low concern for production in the task orientation

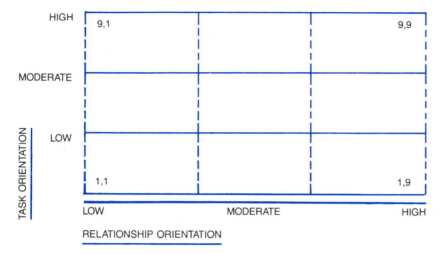

**Figure 2–2** Interrelationship of leader orientation to task and to relationships. Adapted from Blake, Mouton, & Tapper (1981). *Grid approaches for managerial leadership in nursing.* St. Louis: C.V. Mosby.

(Blake & Mouton, 1964; Blake, Mouton & Tapper, 1981). The leader with a 1,1 score is low on both task and relationship concerns, whereas a leader with a 9,9 score is high on both and considered to have the most effective style of leadership.

The leader with a 1,1 score can be described as an inactive and uninvolved leader who does little planning, shows little concern for team members, and rarely takes the initiative to make changes. This style is similar to that of the laissez-faire leader. The high-task, low-relationship (9,1) leader is a controlling, directive leader who closely supervises team members and does most of the planning. Team members are expected to do what they are told, and those who do not may be punished. On the other hand, the low-task, high-relationship leader (1,9) can be described as an accepting, considerate leader who encourages team members and emphasizes good feelings between people but does little planning and allows team members to make many of their own decisions.

The high-task, high-relationship (9,9) leader is an active leader who promotes open communication and team members' participation in setting goals. Leaders using this style also provide constructive (not destructive) criticism, intervene when a conflict arises, and introduce changes after discussing them with team members. This

leader has been found to be the most effective, as was the case with leaders who were high in initiating structure and consideration.

## ● EARLY MANAGEMENT THEORIES

In contrast to the early leadership theories' attention to the leader, the early management theories began with a concern about getting as much work as possible out of each employee. Most of the focus was on blue-collar workers on assembly lines, construction gangs, and similar positions. The two particularly important branches of the early management theories are (1) the forerunners of present management science with its emphasis on quantitative cost and productivity analyses and (2) the behavioral approach to getting the best out of an employee.

### Scientific Management

Almost every management book mentions Frederick Taylor as the founder of management science. Taylor had an engineering background and experience as a machine shop foreman. You can see the influence of this background in the management principles that he developed in the 1890s and 1900s (Lee, 1980; Locke, 1982).

The principles of Taylor and his associates center on ways to increase the efficiency or productivity of each worker. He concentrated on the amount of time an employee took to do a certain task, ways to make the task easier, and ways to get it done in the least amount of time possible so that more work could be done in a day. The elements of the task were analyzed for useless movements that could be eliminated; for workers who seemed to have found the fastest way to do the job and why they were faster; work aids (such as devices for moving heavy objects) that would get the task done faster; and the amount of rest needed to keep workers from becoming too exhausted to work. One incentive Taylor used was paying by the piece, that is, to pay for each item completed rather than by the day or by the hour. Taylor did not expect to create completely satisfied workers; he believed that higher wages would lower, but not eliminate, job dissatisfaction (Howard, 1990). Instead, the focus was on getting more work out of the individual employee and calculating exactly how many employees were needed to do how much work. This practice, by the way, occasionally prompted vigorous protests from workers and their unions (Lee, 1980).

> There is a famous story about Taylor and how he convinced a worker named "Schmidt" to quadruple his output by providing the right incentives. The average worker loaded 12 tons of iron a day and was paid $1.15 per day at a cost of 9 cents per ton to the company. Under Taylor's incentive plan, the legendary "Schmidt" increased his output to 45 tons when offered a raise to $1.85 per day, reducing the company's cost to 4 cents per ton.
>
> Unfortunately, the veracity of Taylor's accounts of his success with "Schmidt" and other workers has been questioned. It is not certain that Taylor actually conducted these experiments, and Taylor himself told many different versions of the same stories. (Lee, 1980)

Despite these questions about the foundations of his principles, the suggestions of Taylor and his associates (such as Gantt, whose famous charts you will see in chapter 16 on Planning) are still in use and were the forerunners of many current business techniques such as inventory control, cost-volume analysis, and other quantitative approaches. In fact, the current reemphasis on cost control, elimination of excess staff, and increasing the productivity of remaining staff is a modern version of Taylor's approach (Lublin, 1992).

In summary, the basic components of early scientific management include:

1. Analysis of the elements of operation
2. Scientific selection of workers
3. Training of workers
4. Proper tools and equipment
5. Proper incentives (Kendall, 1914, p. 123)

Based on these concepts some of the characteristics a follower of the management science school of thought would look for in a first-line manager include:

1. Someone who is well acquainted with the work being done in the department
2. Someone who is a good disciplinarian
3. Someone who is able to get work through and out of the department quickly
4. Someone who is cautious and accurate
5. Someone who is able to keep track of innumerable details (Kendall, 1914)

## Human Relations

The Hawthorne studies of Mayo and his associates may be the most famous set of research studies in all leadership and management literature. In fact, people often use the term **Hawthorne effect** to describe how other people's behavior improves when you give them some kind of extra attention—assuming that "everyone" knows what the Hawthorne effect is. The studies themselves are summarized in Research Example 2–2 and help to clarify what the Hawthorne effect is: the unintended effect of an experimental intervention (Schwartzman, 1993). Actually, these researchers had started out testing some of the concepts of scientific management:

> It is interesting to note that the Hawthorne studies began with the idea that changing simple physical conditions such as the amount of lighting in the work area or the number of breaks during the day could directly affect the

## Research Example 2–2   *The Famous Hawthorne Studies*

A series of evolving research studies, collectively known as the Hawthorne studies, were conducted over many years at the Hawthorne plant of the Western Electric Company, a division of American Telephone and Telegraph, by an interdisciplinary team including people from Harvard University and Western Electric (Landsberger, 1958; Lee, 1980; Roethlisberger & Dickson, 1958). The major studies were done between 1927 and 1932, but the whole series began before and continued after this time.

### Illumination Studies

The preliminary studies, begun in 1924, attempted to determine the effects of increasing and decreasing the level of illumination in several departments. The experimental groups who were given more lighting did produce more than they had previously but, surprisingly, so did those whose lighting level was kept the same or even decreased (until it became almost as dim as moonlight).

### The Relay Assembly Test Room

In the next series, in an attempt to better control the many variables that could affect the workers' output, the researchers selected six women from the relay assembly room and placed them in a separate room where various factors thought to affect output could be tested. The various changes that they tried were as follows:

**Phase I.**    The weekly output of the women was measured for two weeks before they were transferred.

**Phase II.**   The women spent 5 weeks in the test room without any other changes.

**Phase III.**  A separate incentive system for these women was implemented (eight weeks).

**Phase IV.**   Two 5-minute rest pauses (breaks) were added.

**Phase V.**    The breaks were increased to 10 minutes.

**Phase VI.**   Six shorter 5-minute breaks were allowed.

**Phase VII.**  Snacks were provided during the mid-morning and mid-afternoon breaks.

**Phase VIII.** The workday was shortened by a half hour.

**Phase IX.**   The workday was shortened by another half hour.

**Phase X.**    Same as phase VII.

**Phase XI.**   Saturday work was eliminated.

**Phase XII.**  Returned to phases I through III conditions for 12 weeks.

**Phase XIII.** Returned to phases VII and X.

The result was an almost uninterrupted increase in hourly and weekly productivity, especially when they entered phase VII, even though some phases were repeated and the day was lengthened back to its original time in phase XII. The comments of the women seemed to indicate that they had become a "special" group envied by the other workers and were pleased by the way in which they were treated and supervised, especially being consulted about the changes being made.

### Second Relay Assembly Test Series

These women stayed in their departments but were put on a similar special incentive program. This single change also resulted in increased output but only a 13 percent increase compared with the 30 percent increase in the first series. Both rivalry with the first group and the jealousy of other assemblers may have affected these results.

### The Mica Splitting Tests

This series was set up in the same fashion as the first relay assembly tests except that these workers were already being paid for their own individual output and were already on overtime. Each of the five longer phases in this series represented an improvement over previous phases. This group never developed a special identity, and their output increased at first but actually declined in the fourth phase, perhaps due to the worsening employment conditions at the plant (these studies

*(Continued)*

**Research Example 2–2    *The Famous Hawthorne Studies (continued)***

took place over the time of the 1929 Stock Market Crash and the ensuing Depression).

The researchers' conclusions were that the human factors, which had been largely neglected before, especially workers' attitudes and the effect of their informal groups, were an important influence on worker output. They did not suggest, as many assumed, that the human relations factors were the only ones that influenced productivity.

*Sources:* Landsberger, H.A. (1958). *Hawthorne revisited: Management and the worker, its critics and developments in human relations in industry.* Ithaca, NY: Cornell University Press.

Lee, J.A. (1980). *The gold and the garbage in management theories and prescriptions.* Athens, OH: Ohio University Press.

Roethlisberger, F.J. & Dickson, W.J. (1958). Management and the worker. In H.A. Landsberger (Ed.) *Hawthorne revisited: Management and the worker, its critics and developments in human relations in industry.* Ithaca, NY: Cornell University Press.

*workers' output. They were particularly interested in the relationship of working conditions to the degree of fatigue and boredom experienced by the employees. But they soon found that changing physical conditions alone did not explain workers' responses and productivity. There were other important factors that had been previously neglected, in particular, the interpersonal aspects of the situation. (Landsberger, 1958)*

It became evident that employees' attitudes, hopes, fears, personal problems, sensitivity to differences in status within the plant, and ideas about fair treatment had a strong influence on their responses to management. These findings led to the concept that the employee should be viewed as a whole person. (Critics have said that it was still not genuinely holistic because it views the worker only as a producing unit.)

Another important aspect that had been previously neglected was the effect of informal groupings of workers. These groupings are important because they provide employees with the support needed to do such things as resist unwelcome pressure from supervisors, to increase output, or to change routines.

The human relations group called for a different mix of managerial skills: understanding human behavior, counseling, motivating, leading, and communicating with workers. The function of the manager, according to the human relations theorists, is to obtain the cooperation of employees in order to get them to work toward the goals of the organization. Recognizing workers' needs and con-

cerns is necessary to gain their acceptance and cooperation. These studies also documented conflicts between administration and labor and showed that simply being nice was not enough, although some critics of the human relations approach have called its proponents the "happiness boys." Ability to protect workers from the imposition of higher administration's unwelcome changes and pressures is also important (Wren, 1972).

## ● CONTEMPORARY THEORIES

### Motivational Theories

The motivational theories expand upon the co-actor (staff member or follower) element, which was first recognized with the development of the behavioral theories. People's needs and motivations become the central focus and the distinction between leader and manager begins to blur somewhat in these later theories.

The motivational theories have a strong humanistic perspective. Motivational theorists and researchers have concentrated on identifying the specific factors that stimulate satisfaction and productivity and eliminating those factors that inhibit them. From this perspective, the most effective leader or manager is the one who creates an environment in which people are highly motivated and, therefore, highly productive. In addition, rather than focusing on leadership of small groups and teams, motivational theories focus on the larger organizations in which people work. We will consider Maslow's theory of motivation and human needs, McGregor's Theory X and Theory Y, Herzberg's hygiene and motivation factors, Ouchi's Theory Z, and an opposing approach using a stimulus-response perspective.

## Hierarchy of Needs (Maslow)

Maslow (1970) developed a theory of motivation based on the idea that some human needs are more basic or **prepotent** than others. These more basic needs must be at least partially filled before a person has sufficient energy and motivation to work toward gratifying the higher, less prepotent (less powerful or influential) needs. They form a hierarchy beginning with the lowest and most basic physiologic needs, working through needs for safety and security, love and belonging, and esteem, to the highest level, called self-actualization (Figure 2–3).

*Human Needs*    The needs dealt with in Maslow's theory of motivation may be loosely termed *intrin-*

*sic factors,* because they originate primarily from within the individual. You will see, though, that gratification of these needs is certainly influenced by external factors. These needs do not explain all of people's behaviors, but they do provide a useful explanation of the intrinsic motivating forces behind people's behavior.

*Physiologic Needs*    Some physiologic needs are constant and immediate because not meeting them would be life threatening. For example, a person can live only a few minutes without adequate oxygen and blood circulation.

When one of these needs is not sufficiently met, a person is driven only to meet this need and will think of nothing else, focusing all attention and energy on satisfying the need. The following is an example:

> If you began to choke on a piece of steak in a restaurant, you would immediately stop whatever you were doing and try to dislodge that piece of meat. Although ordinarily not consid-

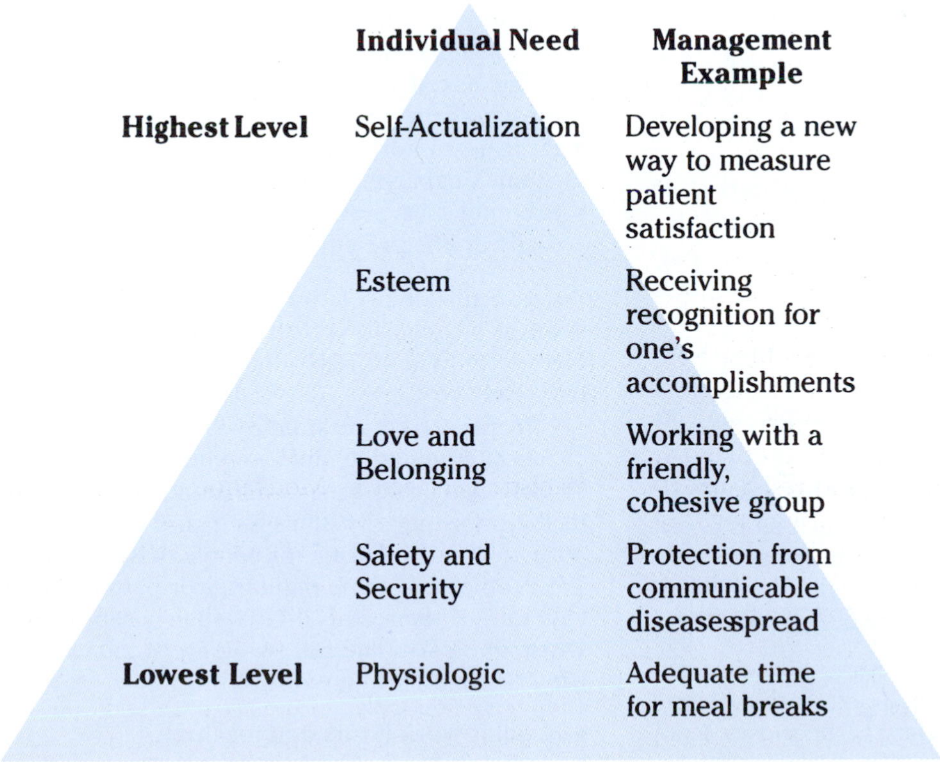

| | Individual Need | Management Example |
|---|---|---|
| **Highest Level** | Self-Actualization | Developing a new way to measure patient satisfaction |
| | Esteem | Receiving recognition for one's accomplishments |
| | Love and Belonging | Working with a friendly, cohesive group |
| | Safety and Security | Protection from communicable diseases spread |
| **Lowest Level** | Physiologic | Adequate time for meal breaks |

**Figure 2–3**    Maslow's hierarchy of human needs applied to leadership and management.

*ered polite, you might put your fingers in your mouth to pull the meat out if necessary. If this action didn't work, you would probably try to get someone's attention to help you with other maneuvers.*

During such an emergency, would you care about the approval of others, your dignity, or your need for independence? Not at all. Staff may have the same response during emergencies on nursing units.

Other less immediate needs that are still necessary to maintain health include normal temperature, adequate sleep, adequate activity and stimulation, freedom from pain, and sexual gratification. These basic needs are important for you to recognize as a leader or manager because people will direct their attention and energy toward meeting these needs and will not be particularly interested in working toward higher-level needs until the basic needs are at least partially met. The following are some examples:

- *Temperature.* If you hold a meeting in a hot, stuffy room, the people at the meeting will concentrate more on staying cool than on the purpose of the meeting.
- *Sleep.* People whose sleep patterns are interrupted because they often have to work overtime or irregular hours will be tired and irritable at work.
- *Activity and stimulation.* Sitting at a desk in the nursing station or in a classroom all day can make a person feel dull and listless. Alternating active and quiet work and allowing time to walk around can provide some stimulation.
- *Pain.* A person who is ill or injured will have difficulty concentrating on work.
- *Sex.* Opportunities to meet people may be provided in a work setting.

The leader who acts to ensure that workers' basic human needs are met (as much as is possible in the work setting) will be helping them to free their energies for work on higher-level needs and to perform their jobs more effectively.

*Safety and Security*  Both actual safety and the feeling of being safe are included in this second level of needs. Physical safety is the most prepotent of these needs, followed by a sense of security, stability, and dependency.

Although work in most healthcare settings is not generally thought of as physically dangerous, some threats to **safety** should be addressed. Many nurses work in high-crime areas. Other threats to safety include exposure to infection, noxious gases, radiation, electric shock, and potentially violent individuals.

Providing **security** is an important and challenging leadership function. Those who feel insecure in their work setting may focus their energy on reducing threats instead of on their work.

Fostering security and trust is a complex task because many potentially threatening situations may arise and people react differently to them. What one person sees as a minor threat may be seen by another as a major one demanding a strong response. The following are examples of situations that may be perceived as threatening:

- Being assigned to a task that one does not feel able to do correctly
- Joining a new group
- Hearing rumors that the new boss is planning to bring in new people and eliminate the current staff
- Instituting evaluation procedures that are inconsistent or subjective
- Being asked to lead a conference or give a presentation
- Hearing rumors that one's unit will be closed or one's department will be eliminated
- Bringing in a more skilled person who could easily do the present employee's job

Because almost any situation can be perceived by some as a threat to security, a leader needs to be alert to individual reactions as well as to group responses.

People need some **stability** in their lives. While change is stimulating and too much constancy can be deadening, too much change at one time can threaten the integrity of a system and create a situation that is too chaotic for people to deal with.

People need some regularity or pattern in the rhythms of their daily lives—their sleep, meals, work, and play. The following are some ways to provide stability in a work setting:

- Regular work hours and mealtimes
- Predictable job expectations
- Clear standards for quality care

- Regular opportunities to give and receive feedback
- Preparation in advance for handling emergencies
- Continuity in patient/client assignments

The leader or manager can do a number of things to ensure some stability in the work setting and free people's energies to address higher-level needs. A completely predictable routine is probably an impossibility in a profession that deals with human behavior and unexpected emergencies daily.

According to Maslow, people also need to be able to ask for help. Of course, healthy adults have fewer **dependency** needs than young children or sick people, but at times they still need assistance from another person. Examples are:

- Learning a new job
- Grieving after a serious loss
- Lifting a heavy object
- Solving a difficult problem
- Carrying out a task that requires more than two hands

The leader or manager's function is to ensure that adequate assistance and support are available to people at work and to create an atmosphere where it is acceptable for an adult to seek help. Asking for help when it is needed is a sign of maturity, not of immaturity.

*Love and Belonging*   People also need love and affection. They need to feel accepted, to give and receive approval, and to be part of a group (such as a family, neighborhood, gang, team, or club) in which they can give and receive affection. They need opportunities for communication and satisfying contact with others. A person whose love and belonging needs are not met will feel lonely, friendless, rejected, or alienated.

The work setting can be an important source of gratification of these needs. For some people, being part of a congenial work group and having the acceptance and approval of this group are major sources of satisfaction from their jobs, particularly when the work itself is monotonous or unsatisfying.

Unfortunately, not every work group is warm and accepting of its members. In fact, interpersonal conflict is a prime source of difficulty in some work settings. It has been said that more people are fired because of interpersonal problems than incompetence.

Some people may question the appropriateness of meeting belonging needs at work. Isn't time wasted when too much socializing is taking place? Shouldn't the leader concentrate on getting the work done? Some leadership theorists raise these questions and conclude that attention to these needs is not important. They believe that people are motivated to work hard in order to avoid such punishments as being reprimanded or fired. But many more, including Maslow, point out that people cannot concentrate their efforts on getting their work done unless their basic needs, including the need for belonging, are met. People put more effort into their work when they are given opportunities to grow and develop on the job. Interpersonal conflicts can paralyze a team to the point where it is nonfunctional. The effective leader-manager will take action to reduce the conflicts so that the team can resume its function. Purely social activities may also be beneficial but need to be kept within limits so that they enhance rather than interfere with the major goal of carrying out professional healthcare functions.

*Esteem*   People need to think well of themselves (self-esteem) and to be well thought of by others (esteem from others). When the more basic physiologic, security, and belonging needs are satisfactorily met, then these esteem needs will emerge and become primary motivators of behavior. The work setting can provide many opportunities for filling esteem needs. Along with the next level of needs (self-actualization needs), esteem needs are frequently important sources of motivation for professionals.

People need to feel that they have an intrinsic worth. This feeling of self-worth is related to a sense of being useful, adequate, competent, independent, and autonomous. The alert reader may note that dependency was listed as one of the safety and security needs while independence and autonomy are listed here as esteem needs. A person can be independent most of the time and yet occasionally need to ask for help. The healthy adult has some dependency needs but, overall, is far more independent than dependent.

Maslow says that a healthier and firmer sense of worth is developed when it is based on who a person really is rather than on a facade or a role. The leader needs to consider the whole person when developing ways to help staff members increase their sense of worth and meet their esteem needs.

The work setting can also provide many opportunities for increasing self-esteem. People feel competent when they are able to use their talents and abilities in their work and when they can do a job well. They feel useful and necessary when they are able to help others. They feel autonomous when they can make their own decisions. These and many other ways in which self-esteem needs can be met at work can be influenced by the actions of the leader or manager.

Respect and recognition from others is another source of esteem. Respect and recognition are more satisfying if they are based on a true appreciation of the real person rather than on a facade or on the opinion of others that is not based on fact. The implication for leadership is that unearned praise is not as effective a motivator as praise that has been earned. Unearned praise may even be counterproductive because it implies that the person is not sufficiently competent to earn it.

People want others to pay attention to them. They want their uniqueness recognized and their need for dignity respected. They need to feel important, to feel that they have some kind of status within their social groups and are able to influence others. Learning and practicing leadership skills is one way to increase esteem.

Expressing recognition or genuine appreciation helps to build esteem. A nurse manager can provide opportunities to meet these needs and increase staff motivation in a number of specific ways:

- Letters of commendation
- Merit raises and promotions
- Positive and frequent evaluative feedback
- Individualized assignments that suit staff members' abilities
- Mentioning a person's positive qualities and accomplishments to that person and to others

Obviously several of the actions (raises, promotions, assignments) are dependent on a manager's authority to grant them.

*Self-Actualization*    Self-actualization is the highest level in the hierarchy of needs. Self-actualization is the growth and development of a person to his or her full potential. Maslow uses many terms to describe his ideal of the fully self-actualized person: perceptive, accepting, spontaneous, natural, autonomous, secure, unselfish, philosophic, creative, flexible, and satisfied.

These terms offer an image of a truly mature and highly functional human being. But self-actualized people are not perfect—they can be lazy, thoughtless, or ill-tempered at times. They are not always happy, either. They can feel sad, guilty, or envious. In other words, although self-actualized people are highly functional, they are not immune from "being human."

If every human being is unique, then what constitutes a person's fullest potential is also unique. Some find expression of their fullest development in artistic ways, others in work with people, and others in work with ideas or material things. The definition of self-actualization may also be influenced by the person's cultural background (Szapocznik et al., 1978).

If you are to be an effective leader, you must seek ways to promote your own self-actualization as well as that of your coworkers. You need to know a great deal about yourself or another person before you can effectively promote self-actualization. People's lower-level needs must be at least partially filled before they are motivated to use their time and energy to work toward self-actualization.

Because of the individual nature of self-actualization, it is difficult to describe exactly what actions will promote it. It would be easier to say what will *not* promote self-actualization. However, the following are some suggestions:

- Encourage innovation
- Include staff members in planning processes and quality improvement initiatives
- Provide opportunities for enhancing skills
- Allow the testing of new ideas in practice
- Include staff in decisions about assignments
- Encourage people to write their own job descriptions and to set their own goals or objectives
- Encourage staff to develop and implement new projects and programs

- Provide resources for continued learning
- Offer challenging work

Maslow's work inspired many other leadership and management scholars and theorists, including McGregor, Drucker, Bennis, and Senge (Petzinger, 1999b), all of whom are quoted in this book. He coined the phrase "enlightened management" and discussed continual improvement and synergy long before contemporary theorists popularized them. He believed that people do their best when they can see the effect of their work. "The only happy people I know are the ones who are working well at something they consider important," he wrote (quoted in Petzinger, 1999a, p. 204).

## Theories X and Y (McGregor)

In his book, *The Human Side of Enterprise,* McGregor (1960) compared two different sets of beliefs about human nature, describing how they led to two different approaches to leadership and management. The first, closer to Taylor's viewpoint approach, he called **Theory X.** The second, more humanistic approach was termed **Theory Y** (Bennis & Schein, 1966).

Theory X is based on a common view of human nature: the ordinary person is lazy, unmotivated, irresponsible, not too intelligent, and prefers to be directed rather than act independently. According to Theory X, most people do not really like to work and do not care about such things as meeting the organization's goals. They work only as hard as they must to keep their jobs, and they avoid taking on additional responsibility. Without specific rules and the threat of punishment, most workers would come in late, goof off most of the day, and produce sloppy, careless work.

Based on this view of people, managers must direct and control people to ensure that the work is done properly. Detailed rules and regulations need to be developed and strictly enforced. People need to be told exactly what to do, and how to do it. Close supervision is necessary to catch mistakes, to make sure people keep working, and to be sure that rules, such as taking only 30 minutes for lunch, are obeyed.

Motivation is supplied by a system of rewards and punishments. Those who do not obey the rules are reprimanded, fined, or fired. Those who do obey the rules are rewarded with continued employment, time off, and pay raises.

According to Theory Y, the behavior described in Theory X is not inherent in human nature but a result of management emphasis on control, direction, reward, and punishment. The passivity, lack of motivation, and avoidance of responsibility are symptoms of poor leadership and indicate that people's needs for belonging, recognition, and self-actualization have not been met.

Theory Y proposes that the work itself can be motivating and rewarding. People can become enthusiastic about their work and will support the team's or organization's goals when these goals also meet their needs. They can be trusted to put forth adequate effort and to complete their work without constant supervision if they are committed to these goals. Under the right conditions, the ordinary person can be imaginative, creative, and productive. Given the Theory Y beliefs, the major function of the leaders and managers would be to provide such conditions. Theory Y leaders and managers remove obstacles, provide guidance, and encourage growth. The extensive external controls of Theory X are not necessary because people can exert self-control and self-direction under Theory Y leadership.

## Hygiene and Motivation Factors (Herzberg)

Herzberg expanded the Theory Y approach by dividing the needs that affect a person's motivation to work into two sets of factors: those that affect dissatisfaction and those that affect satisfaction (Herzberg, 1966; Herzberg, Mausner & Synderman, 1959; and House & Wigdor, 1967). The first set, called **hygiene factors,** meet a person's need to avoid pain, insecurity, and discomfort. If not met, the employee is dissatisfied. The second set, called **motivation factors,** meet the need to grow psychologically; when these needs are met, the employee feels satisfied. These two sets are distinct and independent factors according to Herzberg. Meeting hygiene needs will not increase satisfaction, and meeting motivation needs will not reduce dissatisfaction.

These two sets of factors were derived from yet another set of research studies. Engineers and accountants were asked to describe incidents at work that made them feel especially good or bad. The lists of influential hygiene and motivation factors were derived from the descriptions of these critical incidents. The hygiene factors include:

1. Adequate salary
2. Appropriate supervision
3. Good interpersonal relationships
4. Safe and tolerable working conditions (including reasonable policies and procedures)

The motivation factors include:

1. Satisfying, meaningful work
2. Opportunities for advancement and achievement
3. Appropriate responsibility
4. Adequate recognition

The manager's function is to ensure that both sets of needs are met, some directly and others by providing opportunities to meet them in a conducive work environment.

## Theory Z (Ouchi)

Ouchi (1981) further expanded Theory Y and the democratic approach to leadership to create what he calls **Theory Z.** Like Theory Y, Theory Z has a humanistic viewpoint and focuses on developing better ways to motivate people, assuming that this approach will lead to increased satisfaction and productivity.

Theory Z was developed in part from a study of successful Japanese organizations. It was adapted to the American culture, which is different in some ways but similar in its productivity goals and advanced technology. A number of American organizations known for being well-managed, good places to work have used elements of Theory Z: collective decision making, long-term employment, slower but more predictable promotions, indirect supervision, and a holistic concern for employees.

- *Collective Decision Making.* A democratic, participative mode of decision making is an essential element of Theory Z. This participation is extensive, involving everyone who is af-

fected by the decision. For example, if a decision to provide a new service would affect 70 people, a small team would be assigned to talk with each one of these 70 people to reach a real consensus about offering the new service. If a major change in the plan is made at some point, the team would go back and speak with everyone again. As you can imagine, it is a slow way to get things done.

Everyday problems are also dealt with in a participative manner through problem-solving groups called **quality circles,** in which all members of a team or department are encouraged to identify and resolve problems faced by the group or organization. The emphasis is on keeping everyone fully informed, encouraging active participation, and gaining their commitment to the final decision rather than on making the decision quickly and efficiently. Some critics think that this process stifles innovation and slows decision making too much (Strader, 1987). Others see the use of self-managed teams as a means to reduce cost and improve morale (Lublin, 1992).

- *Long-Term Employment.* Movement within the organization rather than between organizations is encouraged. In the past, most Japanese workers were employed by only one organization for their entire career—reflecting a commitment to employment security unknown in the United States. The drawback in times of economic uncertainty is that it can lead to reluctance to hire new employees who cannot be laid off (Ono & Schlesinger, 1998).

Instead of moving *between* organizations, employees in Theory Z institutions move around *within* the organization, taking on different functions and working in different departments. People who do this become less specialized but more valuable to the Z organization, which is consequently more willing to invest in training its employees and encouraging their growth. In turn, they are better able to understand how a department works, its problems, and its capabilities. This understanding results in better communication and more coordination between departments—an integration of separate units that is almost impossible to achieve when each unit's peculiarities are not understood by people in other groups. Fair treatment also becomes more important when the organization needs to cultivate the commitment and loyalty of this long-term employee. You can see that frequent layoffs and radical downsizing are thoroughly contrary to the principles of Theory Z. The use of temporary workers and layoffs to reduce costs is increasing rapidly in Japan although it is still minimal in comparison with the United States (Weinberg, 1998).

- *Slower Promotions.* Rapid promotions can be illusory; if everyone is promoted rapidly, your relative position in the organization does not really change. It also means that close working relationships within groups do not have time to develop, nor is any incentive present to develop them. Slower but more predictable promotions allow sufficient time to make a thorough evaluation of the individual's long-term contribution to the organization and discourage the kind of game playing that occurs when people try to make themselves look good by undermining others.

- *Indirect Supervision.* Supervision of employees is subtle and indirect rather than direct. Workers become a part of the culture of the organization and are intimately familiar with its working philosophy, values, and goals. In fact, the goals belong to the workers because they are involved in setting them. Decisions are made not only on the basis of what will work but also on the basis of what fits the culture of the organization. A person who is well acquainted with these characteristics of the organization does not need to be told what to do or what decision to make as often as a new, unassimilated employee.

  A similar source of indirect supervision is the influence of the groups in which the employee works. Employees' desire for peer approval motivates group members and supports productive behavior in Theory Z organizations. The result is a well-coordinated, smoothly running team. In this type of environment, however, organizations face a real danger of suppressing creativity and ingenuity.

- *Holistic Concern.* Trust, fair treatment, commitment, and loyalty are all characteristics of the Theory Z organization. These characteristics are part of the overall consideration for each employee as a whole, including concern for the employee's health and well-being, as well as his or her performance as a worker.

## Behavioral Management (Miller)

Although a number of organizations have successfully adapted humanistic approaches, many people believe that these theories are soft-hearted, unproven, and inefficient. Miller's (1978) behavioral management approach is an example of this opposing viewpoint.

Behavioral management is based on the stimulus-response explanation of human behavior, using rewards to influence and control employee behavior. For example, if an employee took too long to complete daily reports, the behavioral management approach to this problem would be to remove any distractions that interfere with the report writing, set reasonable goals for gradually reducing the time it takes to write a report, and reinforce improvement by giving rewards such as intermittent praise. Salary increases, free lunches, and gift items are alternative rewards.

Proponents of this approach believe it is a more suitable approach for a work setting than the humanistic ones, based on the following reasons:

1. Maslow's hierarchy of needs simply means that people are motivated to get what they do not have.
2. Theory Y demands too much of the manager whose main function is to meet production goals, not satisfy human needs.
3. An employer should be interested only in the employee's work performance. Interest in other aspects of the employee's life can be considered an invasion of privacy (Gordon, 1998) and abuse of power (Drucker, in Miller, 1978).
4. Little evidence indicates that training to improve self-awareness or sensitivity to others actually improves leadership effectiveness.
5. Many organizations using Theory X have prospered, so McGregor's analysis of its deficiencies was wrong.

The studies done by Hall and Donnell (1980) in Research Example 2–3 provide an interesting counterpoint to Miller's criticisms.

## Research Example 2–3   *Which Approach Do Successful Managers Use?*

Do successful managers actually use the humanistic theories in their work? A series of five studies called the "Achieving Manager Research Project" was done by Hall and Donnell (1980) to compare a manager's personal success and use of the humanistic, behavioral, and motivational theories of leadership and management. Altogether, 12,000 male managers in more than 50 organizations ranging from drug companies to government and nonprofit agencies were studied. Managers were divided into low-, average-, and high-achieving groups on the basis of their rate of progress toward the top rank of the organization.

**Study I** compared the managers' success with their belief in McGregor's Theory X or Theory Y. Hall and Donnell found a significant (p < .03) negative relationship between belief in Theory X and managerial achievement: low and average achievers had a much stronger belief in Theory X than did the high achievers.

**Study II** compared the managers' preferred work incentives, that is, primary motivating factors derived from Maslow, Herzberg, and others, with their success. Low achievers were found to stress the hygiene and maintenance factors, especially safety and security, and virtually ignored the motivation factors of actualization, belonging, or ego status, which were emphasized by the high achievers. This emphasis on hygiene factors accounted for 77 percent of the variance between the low achievers and the others. Low achievers were also found to be more self-centered, whereas high achievers were more other-centered.

**Study III** focused on the use of the participative management approach. The degree to which managers used the participative style was measured by administering a questionnaire to people who worked for them (not by asking the managers themselves). The difference in use of participative management was dramatic: as a group, the high achievers scored five times higher in participative management than did the lower achievers. The average-achieving group was not much higher than the low-achieving group. Managers with low average success offered their workers few opportunities to participate and used practices that repressed and frustrated the people in their groups. High achievers used the participative style to a much greater extent, with accompanying higher levels of satisfaction in their groups.

**Study IV** measured the extent to which the managers disclosed or shared personal, intellectual, and emotional data about themselves and encouraged others to do the same—called **interpersonal competency** by the researchers. Subordinates, peers, supervisors, and the managers themselves were asked to rate these behaviors. Both self-rating and subordinates' ratings indicated that the high-achieving managers were significantly (p < .001) higher in interpersonal competence measured as disclosure.

**Study V** measured the task and relationship orientations of the managers. Eighteen hundred seventy-eight managers and their subordinates were administered a management style inventory to determine the manager's position on the Blake and Mouton managerial grid. High achievers were found to be using a collaborative, participative, high-task, high-relationship style. The managers' styles seemed to be an overall summary of the individual leader's beliefs, attitudes, and practices.

The studies indicate that the successful managers apply humanistic theories to their practice. The researchers concluded that, when taken together, the results of the five studies suggest that the use of the humanistic, behavioral, and motivational approaches to leadership has implications for career growth. They also hypothesize that, although the data cannot be generalized to women, the same leadership practices would probably distinguish female high and low achievers in management positions.

*Source:* Hall, J. & Donnell, S.M. (1980). Managerial achievement: The personal side of behavior theory. In D. Katz, R.L. Kahn & J.S. Adams (Eds.). *The study of organizations.* San Francisco, CA: Jossey-Bass.

## Comment

Which side is correct? It is possible that one approach to motivation may work better in some situations, and the other in different situations, a concept that is the essence of the situational theories discussed in the next section.

## Situational Theories

The motivational theories were a significant advance over the earlier theories because they included consideration of staff members (the coactors) as well as the leader or manager. However, the fourth element of a leadership situation, the environment, was still barely acknowledged. Leadership and management do not occur in a vacuum. We also need to consider the context in which they take place (McElroy, 1986).

Recognition of the importance of this missing element led to **situational theories.** The contingency and path-goal theories are discussed separately, then other aspects of the environment that have been found to have a considerable influence are described.

### Contingency Theory (Fiedler)

Participative leadership is not necessarily effective in every situation according to situational theorists. Fiedler and Chemers (1974), for example, found that factors such as the nature of the task to be done, the power of the leader, and the favorableness of the situation affect the type of leadership that works best in a situation. In other words, the effectiveness of a certain style of leadership is **contingent** on these other factors.

Fiedler's contingency theory is less straightforward than most discussed so far. The leader's style is reflected in the rating that the leader gives to the **least preferred coworker** (LPC), subordinate or boss, described as the *single worst one the person ever encountered at work*. A low LPC score is interpreted as reflecting frustration with barriers to completing a task; it probably reflects a self-concept based primarily on accomplishment (Ayman, Chemers & Fiedler, 1997). The high-LPC leader is thought of as being predominantly relationship oriented. The low-LPC leader is considered primarily task oriented.

On the basis of more than 200 studies done since the 1950s, the low-LPC, or task-oriented, leader has been found to be most effective in very favorable situations, when the leader has a great deal of power and an excellent relationship with group members, and in very unfavorable situations in which the leader has little power and poor relationships. The low-LPC leader is also more effective when the tasks done by the group are clear and structured.

The high-LPC leader is more effective in moderately favorable situations when the leader's power and authority are weak, the task is not clearly defined, and relationships are good. Generally, Fiedler's research seems to indicate that the most effective leaders overall are those who can adapt their styles to the needs of a particular situation.

### Path-Goal Theory (House)

A different set of situational factors is considered in the path-goal theory developed in the 1970s by House (1971) from earlier work done by Georgopoulas and Vroom. These factors include the scope of the task to be done, role ambiguity, the employee's expectations and perceptions of the task, and ways in which the leader can influence these expectations.

The motivation to perform a certain task is based on a person's expectation that (1) doing this work will result in a desired outcome, and that (2) personal satisfaction or reward will be achieved as a result of this outcome. In other words, people estimate their ability to carry out the task, any obstacles to doing the job, and the amount of support they can expect. They also make some assumptions about what kind of reward (such as recognition from the group or leader or a sense of satisfaction) they can expect after completing the task.

> **People are satisfied with their job if they think that it leads to things that are highly valued, and they work hard if they believe that effort leads to things that are highly valued.**
> —*House & Mitchell, 1997, p. 259*

The leader who can recognize and anticipate these expectations can take such actions as providing support, removing obstacles in the way of completing the task, and pointing out the connection between doing the work and receiving the rewards. The name of this theory comes from this last leader action: the leader clarifies the relationship between the **path** the employees take and the **goal** they want to reach.

House found that when a person has a wide variety of tasks to perform, leader consideration is not as great an influence on satisfaction because the work itself is satisfying. However, he also found that all employees need recognition and other forms of consideration from their leaders. The characteristics of the employees and the number of environmental demands they have to deal with to complete their work also affect the kind of leadership needed to increase motivation.

### Situational Determinants

Both the contingency and path-goal theories emphasized the importance of the task to be done as a situational determinant. Many other determinants have been identified in leadership and management research (Stogdill, 1974; Fiedler, 1979; Ford, 1981; Oldham and Hackman, 1981). The following are a sampling:

- *Group size.* Large groups need more coordination than small groups. Some research also indicates that large groups need more task-oriented leaders than do small groups.
- *Position in group.* Studies of space and territoriality indicate that the leader tends to occupy the head position at a table and that this position reinforces the leader's status. Group members tend to sit opposite the leader rather than next to the leader.
- *Communication networks.* A central position for controlling the sending and receiving of information increases the probability of that person's emerging as the leader of the group.
- *Social status.* People with higher social status usually have more influence on group decisions. (This effect of status may be related to ability and experience.)
- *Interpersonal stress.* The existence of stress and tension between an employee and supervisor reduces the employee's ability to think and

problem-solve creatively. The stress of having a difficult job to do does not seem to affect thinking in the same way.
- *Designation of leadership.* Formal designation of a person as a leader by someone in authority outside the group reinforces that person's position as leader of the group.
- *Organizational structure.* The more formal, hierarchical organization tends to allow less autonomy, identity, feedback, and variety in jobs. In more "organic" organizations, those with more open structures and less emphasis on hierarchy, employees tend to feel more self-confident, more receptive to change, more committed to their work, and less powerless (Morgan, 1997). Organizational structure also affects leader behavior directly. For example, the amount of leader consideration has been found to be negatively related to the size of the organization.

## Interactional Theories

No theory has yet managed to pull together all the influential factors from each of the four elements of a management situation (the leader or manager, co-actors, the work, and the environment) into one coherent, integrated theory of leadership and management.

Many earlier theorists were aware of the need to consider other variables but omitted them when proposing their approaches. Theory Z, for example, is more comprehensive than some of the earlier theories, yet it neglects some apparently influential situational factors, such as the nature of the work to be done. It also assumes that all group members will respond positively to the same approach.

Some theorists have moved in the direction of including the interactions of the four elements of a manager situation. Three examples described are (1) elements of a leader situation, (2) leader-group interaction, and (3) complex man and organizations.

### Elements of a Leader Situation (Hollander)

Hollander (1978) identified three basic elements in a leadership exchange:

1. The **leader,** including the leader's personality, perceptions, and abilities
2. The **followers,** with their personalities, perceptions, and abilities
3. The **situation** or environment within which the leader and followers function, including the norms, size, density, and other characteristics

Leadership is a dynamic, two-way process of influence. Leader and followers are interdependent. Both the leader and followers have other roles outside the leadership situation, and they may both be influenced by environmental factors as well.

Leadership effectiveness requires the use of problem solving, maintenance of group cohesiveness, communication skills, leader fairness, competence, dependability, creativity, and identification within the group.

### Leader-Group Interaction (Schreisheim, Mowby, and Stogdill)

More attention should be paid to the many factors that affect the interrelationships between the leader and the group, according to Schreisheim, Mowby and Stogdill (1977). Group cohesiveness, for example, is affected by leader behavior, but it is also affected by group size, stress, relationships between group members, the nature of the task, and external pressures. Leader behaviors are dynamically interrelated with a group's behavior and characteristics such as cohesiveness and motivation. The productivity of the group, then, is not due to the leader alone but to a mutual and simultaneous interaction of leader and co-actors within an environment. The relationships in this model are complex, yet many others could have been added to it.

### Complex Man and Organizations (Schein)

After reviewing a number of viewpoints on human nature, Schein (1970, 1992) concluded they were all overgeneralized and oversimplified. In their place, he proposed a model of complex man and organizations:

1. People are complex and highly variable. They have multiple motives for doing things, which

vary from one person to another. For example, a pay raise can mean security to one person, recognition to another, and both to a third person.
2. People can develop new motives, and their motives can change over time.
3. Goals can differ in different situations. For example, in a formal group the goal may be to get the work done. In an informal group the goal may be to socialize and whether the work gets done or not is not important to its members.
4. The nature of the task affects people's performance and productivity. Ability, experience, and motivation also affect productivity.
5. Different leadership actions are needed in different situations. No single strategy will be effective in every situation.
6. Multichannel communication systems that can connect everyone within an organization will be essential in the future.
7. Leaders must also take into account the nature and use of time. What, for example, constitutes sufficient time to test a new routine? What would be too long a time?
8. Organization-environment relationships are even more important than usual during times of turbulence.

Use of an open systems framework is implied in these assumptions. Needs, motives, abilities, the nature of the task, the work setting, the type of group, the organizational culture, and the person's past experience and patterns of relating to others all affect the leadership situation. In order to be effective, the leader or manager must be able to diagnose the situation and select the appropriate strategy from a large repertoire of skills.

## Transformational Leadership

Despite years of research and testing of leadership and management theories, something was still missing from these ever more complex models of leadership and management. The missing elements may have been the ability to respond to rapid change cycles and to instill in people a sense of mission that goes beyond their need for positive working relationships or adequate rewards.

Transformational leadership is a response to a contemporary search for meaning and to increasingly rapid and intense change. It reconsiders the characteristics of the leader and manager, reemphasizes the vision that the leader or manager shares with the group, and stresses the importance of preparing people for change. Transformational leadership theory represents an interesting crosscurrent in leadership and management theory. Although transformational leadership did not originate within the nursing discipline, it has struck a responsive chord in many nurses (Barker, 1992; Curtin, 1997; Marriner-Tomey, 1993; Porter-O'Grady, 1992; Smith, 1993).

Drawing on the work of Burns (1978), Bass and Avolio (1993) have concentrated on developing and testing the concepts of transformational leadership. Along with their colleagues, they have collected descriptions of critical incidents associated with effective and ineffective leadership from managers across a wide range of organizations and nations.

The seven primary factors of this leadership model are divided into **transformational, transactional,** and **nonleadership** categories. Using a transactional approach, for example, a manager would explain to employees what is required of them and what compensation they would receive if they fulfill these requirements (Bass, 1997). A transformational leader or manager, in contrast, would appeal to the interests of employees by (1) inspiring them, (2) providing individualized consideration and meeting their emotional needs, (3) providing opportunities for intellectual stimulation, or all three. Transactional leadership is likely to become a "prescription for mediocrity" according to Bass (1997, p. 319), whereas transformational leadership stimulates superior performance.

The seven primary factors are defined below. A quote from a nurse manager is used to illustrate each of these factors after it is defined.

### Transformational Factors

1. *Charisma.*   Charismatic leaders are highly respected by their followers, who view them with a mixture of reverence, dedication, and awe (Bryman, 1992). They set high standards and challenge their staff to go beyond their usual level of effort.

Example: **"We are going to find an innovative way to convince pregnant teenagers that they need early prenatal care."**

2. *Inspirational motivation.*   Transformational leaders share a vision with the staff that appeals to both their emotions and ideals.

Example: **"We will have healthier babies and moms if we solve this problem. We can reduce the infant mortality rate by 25 percent in this county."**

3. *Intellectual stimulation.*   Work can be not only meaningful but also intellectually challenging. This leader challenges followers to question the status quo, to think critically about what they are doing and why.

Example: **"What is wrong with the way we are presently trying to attract pregnant teenagers to the clinic? What could we do to treat them in such a way that they will want to return?"**

4. *Individualized consideration.*   The uniqueness of each employee is recognized and assignments are based on ability and needs, using a facilitative approach.

Example: **"Maria, you've had some success with this group. Would you head the task force on outreach?"**

### Transactional Factors

Transactional factors are less effective than the transformational ones.

5. *Contingent reward.*   Rewards match the employee's achievements. The leader or manager emphasizes mutual agreement on goals.

Example: **"Edith, that analysis was excellent. It will be reflected in your next merit increase."**

6. *Management by exception.*   Those who use management by exception do not react until a problem occurs. They tend to use negative feedback more than positive feedback and are more punitive than facilitative in their approach to staff. An effective manager limits the number of times he or she uses management by exception.

Example: **"Joe, I'm removing you from the outreach task force. Your participation has been minimal, and I am disappointed in you."**

### Nonleadership Factor

7. *Laissez-faire.* Another negative characteristic: the laissez-faire approach can most simply be described as the *absence* of leadership.

> **Example: "Our infant mortality rates aren't any higher than the next county's. It is an insolvable problem. No one has been able to do anything about it."**

As you can see from some of the preceding quotes, first-line managers not only can use transformational leadership approaches but also can play a pivotal role in linking the vision of nurse administrators to direct patient care (Fonville, Killian, & Transbarger, 1998).

Can transformational leadership be learned? Some of the writing about leadership vision and charisma implies that it is primarily an inborn trait possessed by some but not by others. Bass (1997), however, asserts that managers can learn

it through individual guidance and workshops that emphasize identification of exemplary role models, self-evaluation, role play and creation of scenarios that utilize the transformational approach. See Perspectives . . . How *Not* to Be a Transformational Leader.

Transformational leadership hearkens back to some of the earliest leadership theories, including the trait and behavioral theories. Unlike those earlier theories, however, it pulls these pieces together and recognizes the influence of the leader or manager, co-actors, work, and the environment, all of the elements of the leadership and management situations. Research Example 2–4 describes a study that explored some of the concepts of transformational leadership.

A serious criticism of transformational leadership is that its emphasis through related writings and research has been primarily on top-level administrators and on these people as individuals rather than as leaders of teams. A reaction to this limited focus has been what Bryman (1999) calls **dispersed leadership.** The perspective of dispersed leadership is that leaders "develop capacity in others" (Bryman, 1999, p. 33) by providing and supporting opportunities for team members to develop their own leadership capabilities. In this way, leadership is **dispersed** to other members of the group or team rather than centralized within one individual.

We are making some progress toward an integrated model of leadership and management (Chemers, 1993). However, a common set of assumptions about human nature and how people work best, or a complete model that can explain and accurately predict what happens in a leadership or management situation, has not yet been developed.

---

## P E R S P E C T I V E S . . .

### How *Not* to Be a Transformational Leader

Leah Curtin, editor of *Nursing Management,* says she is "utterly mystified" by healthcare administrators' focus on cutting costs when "transforming" their institutions. What's wrong with this approach? Why doesn't it motivate employees? She mentions several flaws in it:

- Cutting costs does not appeal to any higher or more idealistic goal, only to the organization's financial interest.
- This approach does not appeal to employees' self-interest.
- The dollars saved are usually at the employees' expense (e.g., layoffs, salary cuts, fewer raises).

People need a good reason to sacrifice, notes Curtin, "one that taps into their ideals on some level. . . . Getting the costs out may be necessary, but it isn't *leadership,* it's *accounting*," she says (p. 8).

---

*Source:* Curtin, L.L. (1997). How—and how not—to be a transformational leader. *Nursing Management* 28(2), 7–8.

*The world needs fewer parrots and followers of the latest management guru, and more independent thinkers who can offer fresh insights that challenge the existing order of business. Indeed, when theories become enshrined in a particular method, creativity and innovation cease.*

*—Purser & Cabana, 1999, p. XV*

## Research Example 2–4   *Transformational Leadership and Nursing Staff*

How do transformational and transactional leadership styles of immediate supervisors affect nursing staff satisfaction and empowerment?

### Study Design

Morrison, Jones, and Fuller (1997) distributed a self-report questionnaire to all 442 members of the nursing staff of a regional medical center. Of these, 64% were returned; 275 were useable. The questionnaire included Bass's Multifactor Leadership Questionnaire, Speitzer's Psychological Empowerment instrument, and Warr, Cook, and Walls' job satisfaction scale. It is important to note that these researchers defined psychological empowerment as "intrinsic task motivation or self-efficacy," not as having shared power or decision making within the organization.

### Results

A stronger positive relationship was found between transformational leadership style and staff satisfaction than with the transactional style. Within the transactional style, only the contingent reward aspect had a positive relationship to job satisfaction. The use of passive management by exception was negatively related to job satisfaction (i.e., to lower job satisfaction). When the effects of psychological empowerment were taken out statistically, transformational leadership still had a stronger positive relationship to satisfaction than did transactional leadership. Also interesting was the finding that these effects were stronger among the unlicensed assistive personnel who answered the questionnaire than they were among the licensed staff members who responded.

The researchers concluded that use of the transformational leadership style has both direct and indirect effects on staff job satisfaction. The style of immediate supervisors seemed to have more influence on the satisfaction of unlicensed personnel than on the licensed personnel. They speculate that this outcome is related to the nature of the work: licensed personnel probably find greater meaning in their work and have a greater effect on their work environment, particularly on patients and families, than do unlicensed personnel. As a result, unlicensed personnel depend more on their immediate supervisors than do licensed personnel for job satisfaction.

*Source:* Morrison, R.S., Jones, L. & Fuller, B. (1997). The relation between leadership style and empowerment on job satisfaction of nurses. *Journal of Nursing Administration* 27(5), 27–34.

## ● SUMMARY

A number of important theories and models have been developed to describe and predict what makes a person an effective leader or manager and what motivates workers to do their best.

Innate capacity for leadership is the focus of the trait theories. According to the great man theory, important figures who influenced the course of history had innate characteristics that distinguished them from ordinary people. People who adopt popular versions of the trait theory see such characteristics as size, courage, intelligence, or domination as indicators that a person will be an effective leader. Research has shown that traits such as intelligence and initiative are associated with leadership but also that the trait theories alone are too limited to determine effective leadership.

Behavioral theories focus on the behavior or functions of the leader. The authoritarian leader is highly controlling and directive compared to the democratic leader, who encourages participation in goal setting and in planning work. The laissez-faire leader is passive and nondirective.

Early management theories took two different paths. The first path, characterized by the work of Taylor, emphasized the importance of analyzing the details of a particular task in order to figure out how to do it as fast and efficiently as possible. These theories also sought to identify incentives (such as money or rest breaks) that would get more work out of the individual employee. The second path, characterized by the work of Mayo and associates, focused primarily on creating a positive relationship that would increase worker satisfaction and productivity. The emphasis of these humanistic theories was on such factors as understanding human behavior and improving communication.

Similarly, two types of motivational theories developed: those that take a humanistic view and those that oppose it, preferring the view that people are motivated to seek rewards, will avoid additional work or responsibility if possible, and need close supervision and control. McGregor called this opposing view Theory X and proposed a more humanistic Theory Y. Herzberg expanded this concept into two independent sets of influential factors, the hygiene and motivational factors. Theory Z extended this concept further, calling for collective decision making, long-term

---

## C A S E   S T U D Y   I

### Candidate Selection

Consuela Chapman, Vice President for Nursing Service at a large regional medical center, faced a dilemma. The Director of Nursing for Intensive Care and Emergency Services was retiring in 6 months. This director was highly respected within the organization for her fairness, expertise, and sense of humor. The nursing staff's primary concern was that they were losing a good "boss." Several physicians had recently stopped by Consuela's office to express their hope that she would find a replacement as good as the current director. The medical center CEO made it clear she would endorse Consuela's choice, whomever it might be.

Consuela had three promising candidates for the position. Two were nurse managers at the medical center. The third had been a coordinator of emergency services at a smaller community hospital. Each one had excellent references; each one had relevant education and experience. So the question that remained was who would be the best leader.

- CW was a nurse manager in pediatric intensive care. CW was an empathetic listener and a caring nurse. The families loved CW; the staff considered CW their role model. Nurses described CW as a "true clinician" and physicians often sought CW's advice on the feeding and behavioral problems of their young patients.
- TR was a no-nonsense nurse manager in the emergency department. TR was described as the "calm eye in the center of a hurricane" by the staff of this ED but also as a demanding task master. "Shape up or ship out" was TR's favorite expression when staff did not live up to TR's expectations.
- AZ was the outside applicant. AZ appeared to be a sophisticated, scholarly individual. AZ was especially interested in the center's philosophy of care and in the potential for doing collaborative projects with members of other disciplines. AZ appeared to be outgoing and seemed to enjoy the interview process that all three applicant finalists went through.

### Questions for Critical Reflection and Analysis

1. Why do you think Consuela was having difficulty selecting one of the candidates?
2. If you were in Consuela Chapman's place, which candidate would you choose? Outline your reasons for your choice.
3. Review the reasons you gave for your choice and try to match them with one or more of the theories discussed in this chapter.
4. Select two other theories and use them as a framework for critiquing your original selection.
5. How useful are the theories you selected in questions #2 and #3 in terms of guiding a practical decision such as selecting a candidate to fill a vacant position?

## CASE STUDY II

### Who Should Lead?

A number of writers have quoted Napoleon as saying that he preferred having an army of rabbits led by a lion to having an army of lions led by a rabbit (Bass, 1997, p. 8).

### *Questions for Critical Reflection and Analysis*

1. What leadership theory is reflected in this quote attributed to Napoleon?

2. Which "army" would you prefer to have battling disease and injury: an army of "rabbits" led by a "lion" or an army of "lions" led by a "rabbit"? Explain your choice.

3. Create a new version of the quote to describe your ideal "army" of healthcare workers and their leaders.

---

employment, slower promotions, indirect supervision, and holistic concern for people in well-managed organizations. The influence of Maslow's hierarchy of needs is evident in many of these theories.

The fourth element of a leadership situation, the environment, was missing from the preceding theories. The contingency theory, which focuses on how an individual leader rates his or her least preferred coworker, identified the leader's power, relationship with the group, and clarity of the task as determinants of the most effective leadership style. The path-goal theory also focused on the scope of the task as well as the individual's expectations about the difficulties of completing the task and resulting rewards as determinants of motivation. Other factors affecting leader effectiveness directly or indirectly include group size, leader status and position in the group, position in the communication network, social status, interpersonal stress, formal designation as leader, and organizational structure.

None of the preceding leader trait, leader behavior, scientific management, human relations, motivational, or situational theories account for all of the factors involved in the complex and dynamic interactions of a leader-manager situation. The complexity and variability of people and of the work that they do, the use of an open systems framework, inclusion of all four elements of a leader-manager situation, and the interrelationships between these elements were all suggested as the basis for a more complete and integrated interactional theory of effective leadership and management.

Transformational leadership is a combination of the old and the new: charisma, inspirational motivation, intellectual stimulation, individualized consideration, and occasional use of contingent rewards are characteristic of the effective transformational leader, whereas management by exception and a laissez-faire style are not.

## REFERENCES

Ayman, R., Chemers, M.M. & Fiedler, F. (1997). The contingency model of leadership effectiveness: Its levels of analysis. In R.P. Vecchio (Ed.). *Leadership: Understanding the dynamics of power and influence in organizations* (reprint). Notre Dame, IN: University of Notre Dame Press, 351–377.

Barker, A.M. (1992). *Transformational nursing leadership: A vision for the future.* New York: National League for Nursing Press.

Bass, B. (1997). Concepts of leadership. In R.P. Vecchio (Ed.). *Leadership: Understanding the dynamics of power and influence in organizations* (reprint). Notre Dame, IN: University of Notre Dame Press, 3–23.

Bass, B.M. & Avolio, B.J. (1993). Transformational leadership: A response to critiques. In M.M. Chemers & R. Ayman (Eds.). *Leadership theory and research: Perspectives and direction.* San Diego: Academic Press.

Bennis, W.G. & Schein, E.H. (with collaboration of C. McGregor). (1966). *Leadership and motivation: Essays of Douglas McGregor.* Cambridge, MA: MIT Press.

Blake, R.R. & Mouton, J.S. (1964). *The managerial grid.* Houston: Gulf Publishing.

Blake, R.R., Mouton, J.S. & Tapper, M. (1981). *Grid approaches for managerial leadership in nursing.* St. Louis: C.V. Mosby

Bryman, A. (1992). *Charisma and leadership in organizations.* London: Sage.

Burns, J.M. (1978). *Leadership.* New York: Harper & Row.

Burns, J.M. Quoted in Fitton, R.A. (1997). *Leadership: Quotations from the world's greatest motivators.* Boulder, CO: Westview Press.

Chemers, M.M. (1993). An integrative theory of leadership. In M.M. Chemers & R. Ayman (Eds.). *Leadership theory and research: Perspectives and directions.* San Diego: Academic Press.

Curtin, L.L. (1997). How—and how not—to be a transformational leader. *Nursing Management, 28*(2), 7–8.

Drucker, P. (1978). Management: Tasks, responsibilities and practices. In L.M. Miller (Ed.). *Behavior management: The new science of managing people at work.* New York: Harper & Row, 424.

Fawcett, J. (2000). *Analysis and evaluation of contemporary nursing knowledge: Nursing theories and models.* Philadelphia: F.A. Davis.

Fiedler, F.E. (1979). Organizational determinants of managerial incompetence. In J.G. Hunt and L.L. Larson (Eds.). *Crosscurrents in leadership.* Carbondale, IL: Southern Illinois University Press.

Fiedler, F.E. & Chemers, M.M. (1974). *Leadership and effective management.* Glenview, IL: Scott, Foresman.

Fonville, A.M., Killian, F.R. & Transbarger, R.E. (1998). Developing new nurse leaders. *Nursing Economics, 16*(2), 83–87.

Ford, J. (1981). Departmental context and formal structure as constraints on leader behavior. *Academy of Management Journal, 24*(4), 274.

Gemmill, G. (1986). The mythology of the leader role in small groups. *Small Group Behavior, 17*(1), 41–50.

Gordon, J. (1998, November 2). Let daddy help. *Forbes, 162*(10), 68–75.

Hall, J. & Donnell, S.M. (1980). Managerial achievement: The personal side of behavior theory. In D. Katz, R.L. Kahn & J.S. Adams (Eds.). *The study of organizations.* San Francisco: Jossey-Bass.

Herzberg, F. (1966). *Work and the nature of man.* Cleveland: World Publishing.

Herzberg, F., Mausner, B. & Snyderman, B. (1959). *The motivation to work,* 2d ed. New York: John Wiley & Sons.

Hollander, E.P. (1978). *Leadership dynamics: A practical guide to effective relationships.* New York: Free Press.

House, R.J. (1971). A path goal theory of leader effectiveness. *Administrative Science Quarterly, 16*(3), 321.

House, R.J. & Mitchell, T.R. (1997). Path-goal theory of leadership. In R.P. Vecchio (Ed.). *Leadership: Understanding the dynamics of power and influence in organizations* (reprint). Notre Dame, IN: University of Notre Dame Press, 259–273

House, R.J. & Wigdor, L.A. (1967). Herzberg's dual factor theory of job satisfaction and motivation: A review of the evidence and a criticism. *Personnel Psychology, 20*(4), 369.

Howard, R. (1990, December 16). How we got that rundown feeling. *New York Times.*

Ivester, D. quoted in Faust, D., Smith, G. & Rochs, D. (1999, May 3). Man on the spot. *Business Week,* 151.

Kendall, H.P. (1914). Unsystematized, systematized, and scientific management. In C.B. Thompson (Ed.). *Scientific management: A collection of the more significant articles describing the Taylor system of management.* Cambridge, MA: Harvard University Press.

Kim, W.C. & Mauborgne, R.A. (1992). Parables of leadership. *Harvard Business Review, 79*(2), 123–128.

Landsberger, H.A. (1958). *Hawthorne revisited: Management and the worker, its critics and developments in human relations in industry.* Ithaca, NY: Cornell University Press.

Lee, J.A. (1980). *The gold and the garbage in management theories and prescriptions.* Athens, OH: Ohio University Press.

Locke, E.A. (1982). The ideas of Frederick W. Taylor: An evaluation. *Academy of Management Review, 7*(1), 14.

Lublin, J.S. (1992, February 13). Trying to increase worker productivity, more employers alter management style. *Wall Street Journal.*

Marriner-Tomey, A.L. (1993). *Transformational leadership in nursing.* St. Louis: C.V. Mosby.

Maslow, A.H. (1970). *Motivation and personality,* 2d ed. New York: Harper & Row.

McElroy, J.C. (1986). Attribution theories of leadership and network analysis. *Journal of Management, 12,* 351–362.

McGregor, D. (1960). *The human side of enterprise.* New York: McGraw-Hill.

Miller, L.M. (1978). *Behavior management: The new science of managing people at work.* New York: John Wiley & Sons.

Morgan, A. (1997). *Imaginization: The art of creative management.* Newbury Park, CA: Sage.

Morrison, R.S., Jones, L. & Fuller, B. (1997). The relation between leadership style and empowerment on job satisfaction of nurses. *Journal of Nursing Administration, 27*(5), 27–34.

Napolitano, C.S. & Henderson, L.J. (1998). *The leadership odyssey*. San Francisco: Jossey-Bass.

Nicholson, N. (1998, July/August). How hardwired is human behavior? *Harvard Business Review*, 135–146.

Oldham, G.R. & Hackman, J.R. (1981). Relationships between organizational structure and employee reaction: Comparing alternative frameworks. *Administrative Science Quarterly, 26*(1), 66.

Ono, Y. & Schlesinger, J.M. (1998, December 28). Sign of changed times: Japan's jobless rate rises to U.S. level. *Wall Street Journal*, A1, A8.

Ouchi, W.G. (1981). *Theory Z: How American business can meet the Japanese challenge*. Reading, MA: Addison-Wesley.

Petzinger, T. (1999a). *The new pioneers: The men and women who are transforming the workplace and marketplace*. New York: Simon & Schuster.

Petzinger, T. (1999b, February 26). A new model for the nature of business: It's alive! *Wall Street Journal*, B1, B4.

Porter-O'Grady, T. (1992). Transformational leadership in an age of chaos. *Nursing Administration Quarterly, 17*(1), 17–24.

Purser, R.E. & Cabana, S. (1999). *The self-managing organization*. New York: The Free Press (Simon & Schuster, Inc.).

Roethlisberger, F.J. & Dickson, W.J. (1958). Management and the worker. In H.A. Landsberger (Ed.). *Hawthorne revisited: Management and the worker, its critics and developments in human relations in industry*. Ithaca, NY: Cornell University Press.

Schein, E.H. (1970). *Organizational psychology*, 2d ed. Englewood Cliffs, NJ: Prentice-Hall.

Schein, E. (1992). *Organizational culture and leadership*. San Francisco: Jossey-Bass.

Schreisheim, C.A., Mowby, R.T. & Stogdill, R.M. (1977). Crucial dimensions of leader-group interaction. In J.G. Hunt & L.L. Larson (Eds.). *Crosscurrents in leadership*. Carbondale, IL: Southern Illinois University Press.

Schwartzman, H.B. (1993). *Ethnography in organizations*. Newbury Park, CA: Sage.

Senge, P. (1999). *The dance of change*. New York: Doubleday.

Shapiro, E. (1997, March/April). Managing in the age of gurus. *Harvard Business Review*, 142–146.

Smith, M.C. (1993). The contribution of nursing theory to nursing administration practice. *Image, 25*(1), 63–67.

Stogdill, R.M. (1974). *Handbook of leadership: A survey of theory and research*. New York: Free Press.

Stogdill, R.M. & Coons, A.E. (Eds.). (1957). *Leader behavior: Its description and measurement*. (Research monograph 88). Columbus, OH: The Ohio State University, College of Administrative Science.

Strader, M.K. (1987). Adapting Theory Z to nursing management. *Nursing Management, 18*(4), 61–64.

Szapocznik, J. et al. (1978). Cuban value structure: Treatment implications. *Consult Clinical Psychology, 46*, 961.

Waltz, C.F., Strickland, O.L. & Lenz, E.R. (1991). *Measurement in nursing research*. Philadelphia, PA: F.A. Davis.

Weinberg, N. (1998, November 2). Cracks in the iron rice bowl. *Forbes, 162*(10), 310–311.

White, R.K. & Lippitt, R. (1960). *Autocracy and democracy: An experimental inquiry*. New York: Harper & Row. (Published after Lewin's death).

Woods, F.A. (1913). *The influence of monarchs*. New York: Macmillan.

Wren, D.A. (1972). *The evolution of management thought*. New York: Ronald Press.

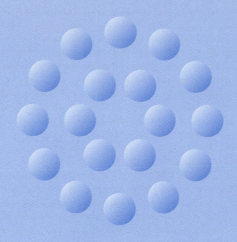

UNIT *II*

# Leadership in Nursing

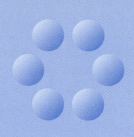

# Components of Effective Leadership

## LEARNING OBJECTIVES

*After completing this chapter, the reader will be able to:*

- Name the components of effective leadership.

- Discuss the importance of each component of effective leadership.

- Evaluate personal leadership effectiveness in terms of the components of effective leadership.

- Evaluate other leaders in terms of the components of effective leadership.

## TEST YOURSELF

**How savvy a leader are you?**

*Leaders can find an abundance of advice out there. Some of it is helpful, some is not. Which of the following typical pieces of advice do you think will be congruent with the components of effective leadership in this chapter? Mark each piece of advice True if you think it is congruent, False if you think it is not. Then check your answers below.*

_____ 1. Visionaries never get anything done.

_____ 2. Admit your mistakes.

_____ 3. Keep your opinions to yourself.

_____ 4. Speak up.

_____ 5. Always trust the facts.

_____ 6. Never share personal feelings with coworkers.

_____ 7. Don't wait for someone else to tell you what to do.

_____ 8. Network, network, network.

_____ 9. Think before acting.

_____ 10. Stay ahead of your group—the further, the better.

*Answers*

1. F  2. T  3. F  4. T  5. F  6. F  7. T  8. T  9. T  10. F

---

What makes a person an effective leader? The answer is found in the components of effective leadership: knowledge, self-awareness, communication, energy, goals, and action (Figure 3–1). Each of these components is explained in this chapter; many are discussed in greater detail in later chapters.

An effective leader is one who is successful in attempts to influence others to work together in a productive and satisfying manner. Occasional failures are inevitable but an effective leader selects the best possible means for influencing others, improving the likelihood of success well beyond what would happen by chance. An effective leader:

1. acquires adequate **knowledge** in leadership and in his or her professional field.
2. possesses **self-awareness**.
3. **communicates** clearly and effectively.
4. mobilizes **energy**.
5. sets meaningful **goals**.
6. takes **action**.

Together these six components summarize the most fundamental concepts of leadership.

The components can also be used to test yourself and others against the ideal of an effective leader. You can use the Leadership Effectiveness Checklist at the end of the chapter to evaluate the

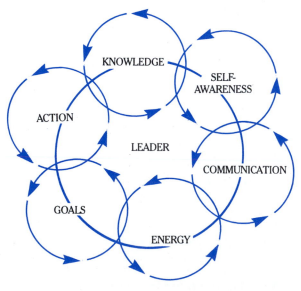

**Figure 3–1** Components of effective leadership.

extent to which you have developed your leadership potential within each of these components and problem areas that require more attention.

## KNOWLEDGE

Knowledge may be classified as declarative (knowing about) or procedural (knowing how) (Squire, 1987). Declarative nursing knowledge is the content component of the discipline; procedural knowledge is the skill component. The same is true for leadership and management content and skills. Both leadership and nursing knowledge are needed by the nurse leader.

Both in leadership situations and in clinical practice, nurses continuously make decisions about the right action to take. These decisions are influenced by two important factors: one's **knowledge** and the **thinking process** applied to that knowledge (NCNR, 1993).

### Leadership Knowledge

What does a person need to know in order to be an effective leader? To answer this question, we can refer to the three basic elements of a leadership event introduced in the first chapter: the leader, co-actor(s), and environment (shown in Figure 1–1).

As a leader, you need to understand human needs and motivation and how they affect behavior. Although many leadership events are one-to-one interactions, others involve far more people (a healthcare team or a client population, for example). How people act and react individually or as a group is the **co-actor** element; it is important information for you as the leader. You also need to be able to relate this knowledge to your own behavior, which is the **leader** element.

Then, the larger system needs consideration. For example, the event can take place in an organization that encourages growth and development of its individual members or in an organization with rigid job descriptions and a dictatorial administrator. An attempt to bring about a change in nursing roles would proceed differently in these two **environments**. In fact, you would approach the change itself differently. The environment of interest may be even larger.

For example, a healthcare organization operating in an economically depressed area may have to control its costs far more than one operating in an economically robust environment.

Specific leadership skills can be learned. Once a situation has been analyzed in terms of the basic elements of a leadership event, an appropriate leadership response can be selected. For example, a leader may use one of several different ways to confront a person or to bring about change. For example, some paradoxical ways to bring about change may appeal to your sense of humor as well as help you become an effective leader.

An emphasis on the importance of knowledge does not deny the value of intuition. In fact, what experienced professionals have been calling **intuition** may really be "reaching into personal experience, racing through patterns and contexts for a match" (Petzinger, 1998, p. B1) so rapidly that they don't realize they are doing it. For example, researcher Gary Klein and associates noted that neonatal nurses "harbored intricate inventories of cues and combinations of cues that signaled the need for action" (Petzinger, 1998, p. B1). Formal knowledge and experience can work together synergistically, resulting in creative solutions to leadership problems. If you let your knowledge and this "intuition" work together, you will draw on more of your inner resources for leadership. For another perspective on the different types of intelligence each of us has, see Perspectives . . . The Six Intelligences.

### Nursing Knowledge

The substantive content and skills of nursing practice are also important to the leader. Planning and organizing patient care are leadership responsibilities of the professional nurse. Doing this requires accurate assessments and diagnoses based on adequate knowledge. Your peers expect you to share your expertise with them; your patients count on you to give skillful nursing care; your assistants look to you for guidance in helping them provide that care.

What can you do to increase your knowledge? First, take responsibility for your own learning. Your basic education provides you with the knowledge to begin practicing nursing.

PERSPECTIVES . . .

## The Six Intelligences

People are intelligent in a variety of ways, but most of us have not learned how to use all of our intelligences, according to Roberts (1999). To be most effective, leaders and managers need to exercise all six different types of intelligences. The first two are relatively easy to exercise, but the last four are often difficult for people to access.

1. *Fiscal intelligence*: The ability to understand and manage the flow of money and other resources.
2. *Social intelligence*: The sensitivity to social issues and ability to handle them effectively. "Leaders don't have the luxury of saying, 'The quality of relationships is not part of my job,' " Roberts says (p. 549).
3. *Noetic intelligence*: The ability to comprehend and reflect upon information. It includes the quest for continual learning, and what we usually refer to as "thinking."
4. *Emotional intelligence*: The ability to detect "inarticulate, suppressed or mistargeted" emotions. This type of intelligence is rare because discussion of emotion is considered inappropriate in many organizations.
5. *Environmental intelligence*: The recognition of the effect of the physical environment in which we work.
6. *Spiritual intelligence*: The valuing and respecting of people as whole beings.

How many of these six intelligences do you use regularly? How could you access more of them?

*Source:* Roberts, C. (1999). Conscious oversight. In P. Senge (Ed.). *The dance of change*. New York: Doubleday.

If you are uncertain about the adequacy of your present store of knowledge, look for extra learning experiences wherever possible. You can study on your own, attend seminars, ask for extra practice time in the laboratory or clinical area, seek out instructors and supervisors for guidance, and let other staff members know you are interested in observing and learning—most of them will welcome your interest. Remember that it takes time to develop expertise. And because new information is added to our store of healthcare knowledge almost daily, the truth is that you can never "finish" learning and improving your skills.

It may surprise you to learn that the leader who is too far ahead of the group can lose them as quickly as the leader who is not as knowledgeable as the group. A leader who knows far more than the group and is not willing to go back to where the group is in terms of knowledge will probably not communicate on the same level as the rest of the group.

> ### *A good leader can't get too far ahead of his followers.*
> —Roosevelt, 1997

A leader who is "not too far ahead" of the group seems to be the most effective leader (Beal, Bohlen & Raudabaugh, 1962). For example:

> *You would not tell a brand new nurse's aide that a child has "acute pharyngitis." Instead, you would say the child has a sore throat and, if the aide were not overwhelmed by new responsibilities, explain the technical term for future reference.*

It is important to adjust your expectations and choice of terminology to the level of the individual or group.

## Critical Thinking

Critical thinking is defined as the rational examination of ideas, assumptions, beliefs, and actions (Bandman & Bandman, 1988; White et al., 1990). Simply accumulating knowledge is not enough. You also need to evaluate the knowledge offered to you. A leader is an active rather than a passive participant in the learning process, a person who maintains a reflective, questioning attitude about the knowledge offered.

Healthcare professionals often fail to question the validity of recommended practices, accepting the statements of authorities without critically evaluating their validity and usefulness in nursing practice. Although we shudder now at the indiscriminate use of bleeding to heal people or shake our heads over the belief that too much learning endangered a woman's health, some of our current practices will probably seem just as irrational 50 years from now.

> *A great many people think they are thinking when they are merely rearranging prejudices.*
>
> —James, 1998

Procedure manuals and standardized care plans typically prescribe practice as if there were only one correct way to provide care (Rodgers, 1991). Predetermined times for baths, medications, diagnostic procedures, and even surgery are based more on tradition than on the rationale of theory or the substantiation of research. Any routine can become a habit in need of critical evaluation. For example:

> *For as long as most nurses can remember, "vital signs" has meant the measurement of blood pressure, pulse, and respirations. But other, newer, noninvasive measures such as pulse oximetry can provide more specific information about an individual's physiological state and may be more useful than pulse or respiration rate in some situations. (Bayne, 1997)*

These routines can be put to the test: nursing research results can be used to guide changes in practice and standards of practice (Silberger, 1998). Wherever possible, decisions should be guided by research results rather than impressions or assumptions about the best way to practice (Hammond, Keeney, & Raiffa, 1998).

Holt said that if we do not maintain a questioning attitude, we face a danger that we will "go stupid" (Holt, 1964; Green, 1973, pp. 5, 80). Experienced staff members can be excellent resources of information, but some of them have "gone stupid" and succumbed to a numbing routine. An alert leader will find many examples of this acting from habit in everyday practice. The following is an example:

> *A nursing assistant developed a time-saving routine for toileting patients in the morning and planned to share this routine with fellow nursing assistants. She systematically worked her way up and down the hall placing each patient,*

*some of them frail and at great risk for developing decubiti, on a bedpan and left them for as long as an hour before returning. The routine had become her main concern; the assistant had made the routine more efficient but, unthinkingly, also made it potentially harmful.*

Even "facts" can be inadequate or proven wrong by new evidence. A few examples:

- Antibiotics were considered miracle drugs when they were first introduced in the 1940s. For some time, people believed that infectious diseases were no longer a threat. Today, however, the combination of microorganisms' remarkable ability to develop resistance and a scarcity of new classes of antimicrobials threatens a "medical disaster" when even minor infections could become lethal due to the lack of an effective drug (Trairs, 1994, p. 360).
- We once thought that premature infants should be given a high concentration of oxygen to assist respiration, but too much oxygen for too long a time is responsible for the occurrence of retrolental fibroplasia in these infants.
- Often thought of as a man's disease, coronary artery disease actually kills more women than men over the age of 65 (Moser, 1997).

What you learn in school or read in journals will also change as new discoveries are made. Even "facts" can be wrong, and leaders must be ready and willing to challenge them.

## ● SELF-AWARENESS

Knowing yourself is the next step in becoming an effective leader (Pagonis, 1992). Self-awareness or self-insight means knowing and understanding yourself as a thinking, feeling being interacting with an ever-changing world. It means being in touch with your aspirations, fears, values, and principles.

> *Learning to lead starts with knowing yourself.*
>
> —Rosen, 1997, p. 304

For example, you probably know the symptoms of anxiety, but can you recognize them in yourself when they occur? If you do, how do you cope with them and with the source of anxiety? Do you recognize your habitual responses to difficult situations? (Grainger, 1993). Are you satisfied with your current ways of coping? Can you recognize and constructively express anger? Can you express feelings of warmth and positive regard for other people?

## Importance of Self-Awareness

Self-insight alone does not solve leadership problems, but it does increase your sensitivity to people's problems, their responses to you, and your responses to them. It does not mean that you will always be satisfied with yourself. People are forever changing and growing, whether in positive or negative directions, and it is natural to experience discomfort and even distress related to changes and the consequences of some of your decisions.

Those who are not self-aware tend to live out their lives in response to other people's expectations. Once you become aware of such influences, it is easier to recognize their "programming" effect and to do something about it, freeing yourself to determine your own direction for the future (Helmstetter, 1982).

It may not have occurred to you before, but some people do not fully recognize their thinking side. On the whole, our society has rewarded cool, clear thinking rather than emotional responses. "Keep emotions out of the workplace" has been the general rule in management thinking (Napolitano & Henderson, 1998, p. 27). Yet some people suppress their thinking side instead, especially women. If you experience a shiver of apprehension when you hear the word "research" or are in the habit of saying "I was never good at math," then you might be suppressing your thinking side along with, or instead of, your feeling side.

Self-awareness helps you to evaluate your abilities realistically. Being objective about your abilities enables you to identify the areas in which you need to improve, and to recognize and build on your strengths. Here is an example:

*It is your first position in school nursing. You quickly realize that most parents are unaware of the many services offered through the school health program. If you are afraid to speak in front of a large group, you would not plan to address the PTA about the school health program. Instead, you could involve students in putting on a health fair for their parents. Still, you also need to work on reducing your fear of talking to large groups because, next time, it may be your most effective strategy. (For one way to work on such a fear, see reframing in Chapter 10).*

Self-insight helps you to develop **empathy**. Although some psychologists suggest that you try to "get into the other person's skin," you cannot actually experience what another person is feeling. You can, however, relate their experiences to your own to develop some empathy for them.

Self-awareness also contributes to the development of effective interpersonal relationships. It helps you to understand the motivations that influence your behavior. Are you, for example, confronting your colleagues about excuses to avoid doing care plans so that they will improve their work? Or are you doing it to even a score with them for pointing out something you forgot to do last week?

Finally, the genuineness of the self-aware person inspires trust. Trust in a work situation is based on two characteristics: character and competency (Gabarro, 1990). People tend to evaluate messages in terms of their feelings about the messenger. Even an obviously true statement may be ignored or discounted if the source is disliked or believed to be lacking in integrity or discretion (Conrad, 1990).

## Increasing Self-Awareness

One way to increase self-awareness is to increase your knowledge of human behavior, especially the effects of emotions, human need, motivation, and coping on behavior.

Observation of people's reactions to your own behavior can give you many clues about your effect on others. You can also seek feedback from others, formally, by asking colleagues to evaluate your performance, or informally, by asking them how they think you are doing. It is also worthwhile to ask your patients whether you have been of any help to them, and if so, how. You may be surprised at some of the responses.

Many people underrate themselves. They dwell on their negative characteristics and downplay their real strengths. If you do the same thing, you may be in for a pleasant surprise when you seek feedback from other people.

**Tape recordings and videotapes** are good sources of objective feedback. We do not hear our voices the same way others do, and the tape recorder can supply another set of ears as well as a record of what you have said. Videotape is even better because nonverbal communication is also picked up. Both of these can be played back several times to allow you to analyze the effect of your behavior. They can also be reviewed in private, which is more comfortable for some people.

Joining a group can be a valuable experience for a developing leader. Because of the many kinds of groups, you will have to evaluate both your own needs and the purpose of a group before joining one. Some groups are formed explicitly for the purpose of increasing self-awareness, but for other groups this goal is secondary. You can learn something from almost any group (even if it is how *not* to conduct a group), but a group that has an open, accepting climate in which you feel comfortable and free to be yourself is one that would be most productive.

## ● COMMUNICATION

Communication is at the heart of leadership. Whether it is a word of praise, a written set of instructions, a frown of displeasure, or an encouraging squeeze of the hand, communication is the means through which leadership is accomplished.

Leadership cannot occur except in relationship to other people, and communication is the means we use to engage and sustain these relationships (Mulholland, 1991). Even refusing to respond to someone sends a message indicating "I will not answer," although it does not tell the other person why you will not respond. We "cannot *not* communicate" is the way that Watzlawick, Beavin, and Jackson (1967, p. 5) so neatly phrased it.

Messages have different levels of meaning, including informational, emotional, and relational levels. The **informational** level is simply the facts or information conveyed in the message. It is usually overt, not hidden. It is at this level that most people attend to a message (Conrad, 1990). The **emotional** level may be partially covert. Emotions are often revealed in the nonverbal portion of the message, sometimes clearly but often subtly. The **relational** level conveys information about the interpersonal relationship between the sender and receiver. This level is usually the most difficult to interpret correctly.

Sometimes what is left unspoken in an exchange is the most important message (Kim & Mauborgne, 1992). Unexpressed complaints, for example, may be the most difficult ones to deal with.

### Active Listening

Active listening is necessary to pick up all three levels of meaning in a communication. Inattention, or "surface" listening, frequently leads to misunderstanding. A person's attitudes can also affect what is heard and how it is interpreted. Psychological "noise," such as high anxiety, can interfere with your ability to fully attend to the other speaker. Other times, the speaker's vagueness makes clarification necessary (Mulholland, 1991).

Guessing is often inaccurate as well as inadequate. You will learn more by asking the right questions and listening to the answer. If someone seems angry about an assignment, you should not change it until you find out why that person is angry. The anger could be unrelated to the assignment—the individual might have gotten a speeding ticket on the way to work. Or the manner in which you gave the assignment, rather than the work involved, may have caused the anger.

### Encouraging a Flow of Information

An adequate flow of information between people who are working together (a primary nurse and associate nurses, for example) is necessary for smooth operation in any setting. Without it, many misunderstandings and omissions can occur, especially in community settings where some members of the healthcare team never actually see each other. For example:

> Operating without adequate communication, the nurse care manager may be gathering resources for an older woman to return home from the hospital while the social worker is checking out suitable nursing homes for her. The patient and her family, of course, would be in a state of confusion until someone realized what was happening and improved communication between all the people involved.

People are more likely to assume that the exchange of information is adequate when they see each other every day. However, people may literally be only seeing each other and not actively listening at all.

A leader uses available channels of communication and creates new ones when they are needed. A leader also encourages others to do the same. In the previous example, for instance:

> The nurse care manager could arrange to meet with the social worker, the older woman, and her family to discuss discharge plans. In fact, similar meetings should be held with all patients preparing for discharge. Some home health agencies have scheduled regular meetings with hospital discharge planning staff in order to create a new channel of much needed communication.

Think about all of the people who can be involved in one patient's care. You can see why adequate communication is so important in managing the care of many different patients or clients.

## Assertiveness

Frequent, clear, direct communication is vital for leadership effectiveness. Indirect, tentative messages or, worse, failure to send any message, should be avoided. You cannot assume that others will understand what is expected of them. For example, imagine the following being said in a hesitant manner:

> You know, I'm sure, that it is possible to do some harm, or at least no good anyway, not to listen to a patient's complaint that something

is wrong. Now, I do know that you really don't have much time, you're so busy and we've been so short-handed today, but if it's at all possible, if you could find time somehow in your schedule . . . ?

Do you know what this team leader wants? Hasn't this leader wasted time talking around the subject instead of making the simple but apparently necessary request to pay attention to a patient's complaint? If you tend to be this tentative in your statements, you may need to practice getting to the point directly.

Some type of insecurity is usually related to this tentative manner. People joining a new team, for example, are often uncertain about their role on the team at first and so will try to avoid making statements that might antagonize other team members or make them seem out of place on the team.

## Seeking and Providing Feedback

Some people avoid giving any negative feedback because they fear that other people are fragile and may "fall apart" if they are not careful, particularly if they say something negative (Satir, 1967, p. 15). In reality, people are quite resilient. Negative feedback can be expressed clearly and constructively, without harm to either person involved in the exchange. Remember, avoiding negative responses can do more harm than good in the long run because it denies that person an opportunity to change.

Negative feedback should be communicated without placing blame or attacking the person. The focus of the communication is on a specific behavior. For example:

> If you found an orderly feeding a patient the wrong diet, you would not say, "Hey, stupid! The patient can't eat that!" Instead, you could say, "This patient is on a low-purine diet and cannot eat these chicken livers. Let's get the patient something else to eat."

The second response is specific but not insulting. It allows for open dialogue that can lead to a solution of the problem (a simple one in this case) instead of provoking a defensive response. It provides an opportunity for learning rather than for feeling bad.

Respecting the rights and dignity of your co-workers is as important as respecting the rights and dignity of your patients. Except in an urgent situation when the correction must be made immediately, look for a way to speak to the person privately. Yelling is not acceptable behavior, and yelling in public creates bad feelings for everyone concerned. You may have witnessed such an incident at some time in school or at work. Such behavior embarrasses people, increases anger, builds defensiveness, and closes off communication.

Feedback from the group can help you evaluate your effectiveness and serve as a guide for improving your leadership skills. Here is an example of its usefulness:

*Suppose that your team members are not showing up for team conferences. By yourself, you could probably come up with 100 possible reasons why they are absent, each reason suggesting a different solution. But how could you decide which of these solutions is the right one? Ask team members how they see the situation. State the problem and then say to them something such as "To prevent this from happening again, I need to know why people are not coming to the team conference."*

If you lack self-confidence, an assessment of your strengths is a good starting point. Assertiveness training is helpful for many people, including those who are insecure behind their aggressive fronts. Leadership skills are helpful in building self-esteem because they can provide a genuine sense of personal power (empowerment) to the individual who uses them correctly.

Team members need feedback for the same reasons that a leader needs feedback: to increase self-awareness, to avoid operating on the basis of erroneous assumptions about other people's behavior, and to serve as a guide for growth and change.

## Linking

Linking is a concept that may be less familiar to you than the communication strategies discussed so far. Linking involves seeing and then expressing a connection between two separate ideas. For example, when people in a group make separate, unconnected statements at a meeting, the group is likely to go in several directions at once unless the leader intervenes. When someone assumes leadership and provides the link between unconnected statements, the discussion begins to flow in one direction, building up energy as each statement is connected to the main flow of the discussion (Lifton, 1972). The following is an example:

*A group member suggests providing a television for a bored long-term rehab patient. The next person to speak follows this suggestion with an unrelated comment on the terrible weather. The leader then connects the two by commenting that if the weather were better, the bored patient could go outside every day, but in the meantime, what else could people suggest to alleviate the patient's boredom in addition to getting the patient a TV?*

You can create links between people's ideas even when they are not physically together:

*A home health nurse complains about the number of clients whom she is seeing who have had their food stamp allocations reduced. You can answer, "A social worker in our agency has also expressed concern about the situation. We may have a problem here."*

Finding such links can be a creative endeavor and a catalyst for action in many leadership situations.

## Networking

Whereas linking is done to develop connections between ideas, networking is done to develop connections between people. A leader actively networks with other people. Why? Once a relationship of trust and professional respect has been developed with another person, that individual will have a bias toward agreeing to your reasonable request rather than refusing it. This type of relationship makes it possible to get things done without numerous bureaucratic barriers and delays. For example:

*If you have developed connections with social service staff, it will probably be easier to rush a special request for placement of a client with an urgent need or to have something done late on a Friday afternoon when they would ordinarily say, "You will have to wait until Monday."*

Networking also opens up channels of important information. Opportunities to share new ideas with colleagues are not only stimulating but may provide information needed to get ahead at work or to discover new job opportunities. Some of the most interesting and challenging positions are never advertised because they are filled with people from within the organization or with people known to those who are doing the hiring.

People like to talk about the "old-boy" networks of men in positions of power who share information and opportunities among themselves but prevent others from gaining access to these valuable resources (Christy, 1987). Whether nurses should set up their own exclusive networks and how they would operate is an open question. What is clear is that a leader should be aware of the value of networking, develop his or her own networks, and work on gaining access to existing networks. The sharing of information and opportunities with fellow professionals has a synergistic effect: we can increase our energy supply of information and influence by sharing it.

## ● ENERGY

If you have ever had an exhausting exchange with a difficult patient, then you probably have experienced the meaning of the phrase "feeling drained" (McNeese-Smith, 1993). That entity of which you felt drained is human energy. At times people feel "bursting with energy" as if they had an overflowing supply. Other times they are so low that they feel as if they are suffering an energy deficit. Although we know that a person can feel high or low in energy, scientists cannot yet define exactly what this energy is or measure it accurately (Howard, 1990). From a holistic point of view, we need to be careful about separating the person from the amount of energy he or she has. Rogers (1994) emphasizes that humans don't just *have* energy fields, we *are* energy fields.

## Neural and Emotional Energy

Human energy seems to be more than a purely physical phenomenon because our emotional states have a great effect on the amount of available energy we have. Consider, for example, how hard it is for a depressed person just to get out of bed in the morning. Compare this situation to a manic state of excitement in which a person can be active for hours and even days on end without pause. Although usually described as being either physical or emotional, they are probably manifestations of the same energy field.

It is possible that some kind of energy transformation takes place in people, changing the neural (electrochemical) energy of the nervous system to emotional energy. Some time ago, Gruen (1979) conducted an interesting test of this idea:

> *In a random sample of heart attack patients, the experimental group of patients who had psychotherapy during their hospital stay had shorter hospital stays, a feeling of increased vigor, and participated in more activity with less anxiety four months after the heart attack than did the control group of patients who did not have psychotherapy. The conclusion was that an increase in available energy resulted from the change in self-concept that occurred during therapy.*

Gruen theorized that the person-to-person interaction of the therapy helped release energy so that the patients could do more and felt more energetic—a release and transformation of energy.

## Energy and Leadership Effectiveness

We all have energy, but some of us use it more productively than do others. Ineffective use of energy is to waste it on negative activities such as resisting inevitable changes or getting caught up in internal politics. Using energy to solve problems and meet new challenges is more effective. As Tichy wrote, "positive energy produces positive results" (1997, p. 130).

Some people have difficulty using their energy to its best advantage. They waste it doing things the hard way or in a disorganized fashion.

An energy squanderer will do ten things to solve a single problem where one action would do just as well. Using effective leadership techniques can reduce the number of draining experiences.

A high energy level can increase your effectiveness as a leader. As you interact with other people, your energy level will have an influence on their response to you (Chemers, 1993). One person's enthusiasm for a project can be infectious in the positive sense of the term. For example:

*A group of nurses and assistants decided at their team meeting that one of their long-term rehab patients needed more social stimulation and would enjoy being with friends down the hall. The idea involved shifting several patients' units. Having to move beds around usually provokes tired groans and much procrastination, but before the meeting was over, one of the nurses went out and checked with the patients involved. The nurse came back saying, "Yes, they want to do it." Before the chairs in the conference room were put back in place, units were wiped down and a convoy of beds rolled down the hall. In 30 minutes, everyone was settled in their new rooms and the glow of accomplishment was visible on the staff members' faces.*

Something happens when an idea catches fire in this manner. The people involved in the interaction seem to recharge from each other's enthusiasm, and the level of available energy in the group rises dramatically. This surge of energy that results when people exchange positive energy with each other is called **synergic power** (Claus & Bailey, 1977; Craig & Craig, 1975).

### *Nothing great was ever achieved without enthusiasm.*
*—Emerson, 1997*

You can share your energy with people in many ways. Information is a form of energy that can be used and exchanged. It is the "fuel" that fires the imagination and provides the impetus to bring about changes in health care. A lack of energy and enthusiasm will work in the opposite direction. If no one believes an idea will work, then it probably will not:

*A favorite phrase on students' patient care plans is the direction to "spend time with the patient." If you give such an assignment with little enthusiasm (knowing it won't be done) and do not check later to see that it was done, it will probably not be done. But if you emphasize spending time with the patient, citing why it is needed by this particular patient and explaining what is meant by "spending more time," in other words, if you make it clear that you are interested in the results of the interaction, you are far more likely to see it done.*

## Energy Flow and Reserves

Most people are at least subliminally aware when their energy reserves are low. They feel listless and weary and realize that they need to recharge. How people recharge seems to be an individual matter—the same experience can be restorative (positive) for one person and draining (negative) for someone else, as in the following example:

*Some people love horror movies—the more terrifying the better. Others get frightened and have bad dreams for days afterward. The enjoyment recharges one person in a positive manner, but has a negative effect on the other person that is released in bad dreams. A companion of these two is just plain bored by horror movies and would not be recharged by going to the movies, but loves tennis and feels exhilarated after a good match.*

Some activities, like a tennis match, seem to be both discharging and recharging activities. Tichy (1997) suggests that even demanding work can be recharging if it is work we are doing not just because we have to but because we find it rewarding and enjoy doing it. He compares it to children who have fun playing "house" and do their "work" with evident enjoyment. This whole concept of human energy and its positive and negative aspects needs further research.

The availability of human energy may be related to states of health and illness. Indications are that the differences in energy levels between the sick and well person may be measurable. Consider, too, the growing notion that every human being has resources of personal power and energy that have hardly been tapped. Even if we cannot actually use our psychic energy to move objects across the room (and who knows for sure that we cannot?), the sharing of the energy that is within each of us has a tremendous potential for impact on people.

## Energy Inventory

You might try making an inventory of your energy reserves, discharges, and recharges to see where your energy is going. List all of your activities for a day. Be sure you include the little things such as receiving a word of thanks from someone and routine things such as meals. Mark them as sources of either positive (+) or negative (−) energy and rate the amount of energy involved on a scale of 1 to 5 with 1 being low, 3 moderate, and 5 high amounts. A tremendously recharging activity would be +5 and an especially draining experience would be −5. Your total would indicate a positive or negative balance for the day.

Do you find yourself with a deficit at the end of the day? Which negative sources could you reduce or eliminate? What positive sources could you add or increase? Are you satisfied with the way in which you use your energy?

You may also want to look at your energy cycles and note the daily and weekly patterns of highs and lows (Haynes, 1991; Moshowitz, 1993). Do you work better in the morning? Or late at night? When is your peak? When do you reach your low point of the day? Is the first part of the week better for you than the end of the week, or vice versa? Figure 3–2 illustrates a personal energy cycle for one day.

## ● GOALS

Goals are the desired end results or outcomes; they are the reason for performing various tasks and activities. The relationship between the leader or manager and staff exists primarily for the purpose of getting some kind of work done (Gabarro, 1990). Achievement of the work is the **goal** of the team or department. A leader aligns his or her own efforts and the efforts of others in such a way that their goals and those of the organization can be met (Benton, 1997).

## Goal Levels

It is unusual to find an individual who has just one goal. It is even rarer to find a group with a single, agreed-upon goal. In most instances, three levels of goals are of particular interest to leadership: individual, group, and environmental (Tannenbaum, Weschler, & Massarik, 1974). Table 3–1 illustrates these different goal levels.

Individual goals, or **personal goals,** are those of a particular person. For any number of reasons, a person may or may not want to achieve something. The following is an example:

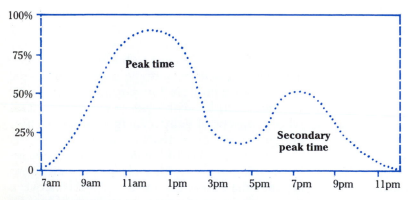

**Figure 3–2**   Example of a personal energy cycle.
*Source:* Adapted from Haynes, M.E. (1991). *Practical time management.* Los Altos, CA: Crisp Publications.

**Table 3–1** Levels of Goals within a Group

| Goal Levels | Examples |
| --- | --- |
| *Organizational goals* | Organization wants to please accrediting agency |
| *Group goals* | Have a coffee break |
| *Individual goals* | |
| Personal goals of members | Contribute to group achievement; show that conferences are a waste of time |
| Personal goals of leader | Help patient; demonstrate leadership ability |

*You have invited several other nurses to a care plan review focused on a patient whose depression seems to be increasing. Your primary goal is to come up with better ways to help this patient. But you are organizing this conference for additional reasons: you are hoping to interest the other nurses in holding regular reviews on all patients and you also want to show them how well you can lead one of these conferences.*

All the goals just mentioned would be your individual goals as leader of the group.

Every person in a group has personal goals. What makes this complicated is that some of these goals may be quite different from or even in conflict with your personal goals as leader. For example:

*Some of the nurses invited to the meeting want to contribute to solving the problem. Others, however, believe that they have more important work to do and want to rush through the meeting. Some do not want to come at all. One group member, for example, believes that meetings are a waste of time. This group member's goal is seeing to it that your meeting turns out exactly the way this nurse predicts—a complete waste of time.*

Despite their number, the goals mentioned in the example are only a few of the many possible goals that individual members of a group might have.

The second level of goals comes from the group as a whole. As you may recall from chapter 2, the characteristics of the group as a whole, including its goals, are different from those of its individual members. For example:

*When you get the group together for a team meeting at 10 A.M., it is also time for a coffee break. The group as a whole may be more interested in relaxing for a few moments than in discussing a depressed patient.*

If the group prefers (or needs) a break rather than a serious discussion, then the goal of the group as a whole conflicts with your goal as the group leader.

The third level of goals that needs to be considered is the environmental level. What constitutes the environment is defined in terms of the particular situation. The most influential part of the environment may be the climate of a particular department or team, the economic health of the organization, or the attitude of an entire community. Referring back to the meeting example:

*In this particular case, the environment that concerns you is the organization in which you and the rest of the group work. Because your employing organization is anticipating the visit of surveyors from a national accrediting agency, patient care plan reviews are being encouraged.*

As this example indicates, the environmental level may reach as far as the national or even international level.

Goals within and between the different levels are numerous, different, and sometimes in conflict. It is important that the leader try to identify the varying goals at the three different levels.

## Meaningful Goals

The goals you set need to be meaningful to the group. You will be a more effective leader if the group sees you as someone who identifies with them and has their best interests in mind (Hollander, 1974). Another way to say it is that you need to "begin where the group is." For example, if the group senses that your main interest in calling a meeting is to meet your personal goal of demonstrating leadership ability rather than the group goal of helping the patient, their response is likely to be resistant and resentful.

## Communicating a Vision

Sharing a vision for the future has a tremendous power to inspire and excite team members and rally their support for organizational goals (Bass, 1997). Vision was absent from earlier leadership formulations but has become increasingly emphasized, particularly in transformational leadership (explained in Chapter 2).

A vision should communicate an innovative, ambitious, far-reaching goal for the work group in a few words. The leader's vision of where the group is going adds meaning to the work, focuses attention on the core task of the group, increases motivation, and boosts team spirit. Most important, it provides direction and excitement to the work (Bryman, 1992).

## Clarity and Congruence

Your goals also need to be clear to and congruent with those of your followers. Sufficient agreement about goals will help the entire group, including the leader, to move in the same direction. Looking back at the various goal levels in Table 3–1, you can see that the leader's personal goals and the organizational goals both favor the idea of a conference although the goals themselves are not identical. The group goal and the goals of some individual members, however, are in serious conflict with the leader's goals. If the leader cannot change this situation, the conference probably will not succeed.

You cannot be sure that goals are actually congruent until they have been articulated. People often assume that everyone agrees without checking out the validity of their assumption. For example, you often hear a comment such as, "Everyone knows why we're here, let's get on with the job," at the beginning of a meeting (Beal, Bohlen, & Raudabaugh, 1962, p. 130). Group members can honestly believe that they share a common goal and yet actually have diverse goals. The following is an example:

*A group called the "Committee to Improve Patient Care" might seem to have an obvious and self-explanatory goal. However, one member, a physician, thinks the committee's goal is to increase the hospital's medical staff. An adminis-*

*trator on the Committee expects the committee to endorse the building program that the administrator proposed. The third member, the nurse executive, expects more nurses to be hired as a result of the committee's recommendations.*

A patient representative on the committee may not agree with any of these opinions. Every committee member interpreted the committee's goal from his or her own perspective and needs. A clear and complete statement of each of the group's goals would include:

1. **Who:** The people who will be involved or who "own" the goal
2. **What:** The target of the goal, which may be people or objects
3. **Why:** The outcome or end result desired, stated in observable terms (Mager & Beach, 1975)

In a working group such as this committee, it is important to state the end result in observable terms so that everyone can see whether each goal has been met. Try to use an action verb to begin every statement, as you would when writing objectives. The statement of a group's goals should not include how you are going to achieve the results—actions should be decided after the goal is clarified. Using the committee example:

*A lot of discussion may be required to clarify and improve the congruence of the goals of members of the Committee to Improve Patient Care. Fulfilling the first criterion (Who) is easy in this case. The people who "own" the goal will be the three committee members—the physician, the administrator, and the nurse executive—and perhaps the groups each one represents: the medical staff, the administration, and the nursing department.*

*Although the overall target population (What) for the committee was all patients who received care in their institution, once the committee selected its specific objectives, the target could be stated more specifically. The target populations could be the outpatients using the emergency department, patients receiving radiation therapy, or patients anticipating discharge.*

*To please all three members, the committee might finally decide on three specific outcomes (Why) to work toward simultaneously. These outcomes include the following:*

**Research Example 3–1** *The Importance of Shared Goals*

How important are shared goals? Do they affect employee commitment or job satisfaction? A great deal of emphasis has been placed on purpose, goals, and objectives in the leadership and management literature. Haas and Syphen (1992) studied the degree to which the clarity, means of communication, and degree of consensus about group goals affected job satisfaction and organizational commitment in a public agency.

The sample in this study consisted of all 21 paid professional staff of an agency, 10 members of the board of directors (25 percent of the board), and 8 members of the agency's 5 advisory councils (24 percent of council membership). Subjects were asked several questions about the goals of the organization (what they were, how clear they were, and how they were communicated), how satisfied they were, and how committed to the organization they were.

A high degree of agreement about the goals of the organization was found in these groups.

Eight ways to communicate goals were reported: meetings, newsletters, reports, information from supervisors, self-discovery, the agency's annual retreat, and conversations with staff members. Actually, many were not really sure how they had learned of the agency's goals. A strong relationship between job satisfaction and the perception that goals were shared was found.

The researchers concluded that the goals of an organization are likely to be ambiguously stated. They believe this ambiguity is not necessarily a problem and may be not only inevitable but helpful in creating a sense of sharing. They suggest that clear goals (i.e., how explicitly they are articulated) are not as important as is the *perception that they are shared* and that people feel they are working together for a common purpose.

*Source:* Haas, J.W. & Syphen, B.D. (1992). Do shared goals really make a difference? *Management Quarterly, 6*(2), 166–179.

- *Provide 24-hour physician coverage in the emergency department.*
- *Renovate the radiation therapy building.*
- *Supplement the work of the present home care coordinator to include transitional care.*

To be sure that everyone agrees on the goals, they should be articulated clearly and specifically. For example, the committee will need to determine such things as how many patients the transitional care program should accommodate.

After the goals are clearly stated and accepted by the group, the committee can proceed to discuss how they will achieve them.

*Now the committee can proceed to a discussion of how they will go about achieving their goals. They may decide to hire advanced practice nurses to supplement the work of the present home care coordinator. They may also decide to hire more physicians to provide 24-hour medical coverage in the emergency room.*

How important is it for an entire healthcare organization to have clearly articulated goals? Research Example 3–1 indicates that the perception of having shared organizational goals may be more important than the actual clarity of the goals.

How do you increase goal congruence? Suppose you do not agree with the group's goals, or you believe that their goals are unrealistic? When the problem is lack of information or understanding, supplying information may be sufficient to change the group's goals. When the issue is a difference of opinion, interest in others' points of view will encourage open discussion of goals that can lead to finding some areas of agreement with which the group may be willing to begin.

How willing you are to compromise your own goals is going to depend on you, the gravity of the situation, and the kind of compromise you would need to make. If compromising your goals is going to mean violating your own personal set of values, then you must ask yourself what you will gain by doing so. Although showing some flexibility is usually productive, yielding too much is often ineffective.

When the actions mentioned (supplying information, expressing an interest in the other point of view, seeking a common ground among diverse goals, and sometimes negotiating a redefinition of the goal) do not reduce differences enough to make the goals congruent, you will need to apply change strategies (see chapter 10) to bring them into congruence. When the goals are congruent, you and your group have a starting point from which you can proceed to work together.

## ● ACTION

The effective leader is decisive and action oriented (Quillen, 1988). All of the components that came before this one—knowledge, self-awareness, communication, energy, and goals—are of value in leadership only if they are put to use.

By now, you have probably noticed some connections between the components. More examples follow, and by the time you reach the end of this book, you probably will have found many new connections between these aspects of leadership. You may also want to think about the type of leadership that was displayed by the plant manager in Perspectives . . . The Bus Ride.

### Working with Others

A leader **guides** others, sharing his or her knowledge and experience with them when helpful. The amount of guidance and direction varies according to the needs that arise in particular situations. For example, a new nurse needs a lot of guidance in comparison to an experienced nurse, but even the most experienced nurses benefit from some direction and from an exchange of ideas. In addition, frequent exchanges of ideas help to prevent individuals, groups, and even organizations from "going stupid." It is not a one-way exchange: an effective leader is also open to suggestions from others and eager to learn from others' knowledge and experience.

A leader **evaluates** the actions of himself or herself and of others. Nursing audits and peer

## PERSPECTIVES . . .

### The Bus Ride

In *The Leadership Engine,* Noel Tichy describes a creative approach to a serious leadership problem. Employees of the Appliance Division of General Electric faced a bleak future. Sales were down, employees had been laid off, and more layoffs were feared. They were being trounced by the competition.

Forty employees ranging from engineers to shop workers boarded a bus in Louisville, headed for the annual Kitchen and Bath show in Atlanta. The plant manager, Tom Teller, described the bus trip as both a signal that the situation was serious and the beginning of their search for a solution. "There was a deep sense," said Teller, "of 'We've got to do something. We've got to do it fast . . . and we're going to do it.' " (Tichy, 1997, p. 129).

They did do it. Three new products were designed, produced, and marketed, and the plant went from a $10 million loss in 1992 to a $35 million profit in 1994.

Can you think of a parallel in nursing?

*Source:* Tichy, N.M. (1997). *The leadership engine: How winning companies build leaders at every level.* New York: Harper Business.

review are formal evaluation procedures that are becoming established parts of nursing practice. Informal evaluation should take place constantly. Is your nursing care helping the patient recover or is it adding to the patient's distress? Has your leadership made it possible for your team members to work well together or has it resulted in disruptive behavior? An evaluation of what behavior has been productive and what behavior has not provides a guide for selecting strategies in the future. Evaluation done well can be a source of increased insight and a stimulus for growth and development.

A leader **calls meetings** of all kinds. The meetings should have a specific purpose. Examples would be to discuss plans or progress, organize work, work out solutions to problems, ventilate feelings, or share information. Getting people together as a group rather than dealing with them individually has several advantages. First, you can get the same message to everyone with less chance of the message being changed as it is transmitted. Second, you may also benefit from the tremendous effect of joint action, the synergic power that can develop within a group. Communication with everyone at once improves coordination, saves time, and often has better results.

A leader **mobilizes support systems.** You are not expected to do all of these things alone. In fact, many things cannot be accomplished single-handedly. There are two kinds of support: actual assistance with a task and psychological support. Your healthcare team usually provides the actual assistance with the work that needs to be done. Psychological support can come from a number of additional sources, including administrative backing of your activities, colleagues who say, "I'm with you on this," and your patients who appreciate your skilled care. Support can also come from outside work and, last but not least, from yourself.

A leader **empowers** others. Empowerment is the sense that one is not only capable of acting, but expected and encouraged to act. Empowered staff members feel free to make appropriate decisions and to act on those decisions. Administrative support for empowering others is essential but not always forthcoming (Argyris, 1998). Without it, staff members who show initiative will feel abandoned. Even worse is the situation in which the staff members are punished for their initiative. The result is a powerless, over-cautious, or apathetic staff.

## Initiating Action

A leader **initiates** action. Ideas, suggestions, and plans must be implemented in order to be effective. A good idea has no influence if it remains only in your head. Furthermore, even the best plan does little good if it remains only a plan. Many worthwhile proposals die of neglect because no one puts any energy behind the proposals to bring them into action. For example:

> *You may hear a colleague say, "Whatever happened to that idea we had about getting a mobile health unit?" In response, everyone shrugs and looks around at the others. Someone had made a good suggestion, but no one had taken the initiative to pursue it any further.*

A leader **confronts** himself and others. Confrontation is a powerful strategy used to present people with the way others perceive their actions. It should be a thoughtful reaction, not a thoughtless one that degenerates into telling each other off. The ways in which you can confront an individual or group range from gentle to strong.

A leader does not sit back and watch a power struggle destroy working relationships or a client being put off by one agency after another. A leader confronts the issue and takes action to solve these problems. Sometimes it is necessary to wait for the right opportunity to initiate action. What happens much more often, however, is that people delay too long before initiating action.

A leader **takes risks.** Every leadership action has some risk attached to it. It takes courage to stand up and speak out, to correct people when they are wrong, and to volunteer to take charge. A leader is not afraid to risk confrontation; a leader is willing to make direct statements, question decisions, and sometimes break rules. Leaders choose their battles; they do not get trapped in them. Leaders decide for themselves when to take risks after weighing the consequences of doing so.

Some people find risk taking easy, having been accustomed to speaking up and taking charge, perhaps even taking over. The need to risk holding back and trusting others to take responsibility may be hard for these leaders. They may need to practice weighing consequences and choosing their battles in order to avoid scattering their energies.

Others may quake at the thought of confronting people and standing up for their rights. These individuals may need extra practice in leadership techniques such as assertiveness and confrontation to build up confidence and get into the habit of speaking out. Having backup support and concentrating on personal strengths before acting makes risk taking easier. When you think about it, you probably take many small risks every day without thinking about it. Sometimes the action is so necessary that you do not even stop to think about the risk to yourself until it is all over.

Remember, whether you choose to act or not to act, you have made a decision. When you choose to lead, you are choosing to risk criticism, confrontation, and challenges to your leadership. But choosing not to lead also has its risks: a loss of autonomy, reduced opportunities to achieve self-actualization, and a loss of self-esteem. Confronting the risks of leadership is a choice to open up opportunities for more satisfying person-to-person interactions, greater rewards in your personal life, and greater career rewards.

## Decision Making

An effective leader thinks before acting. For example, leaders **problem solve** when confronted with difficult situations. Problem solving is a systematic process that assists the leader in the analysis of a situation and choice of actions. It consists of a series of steps (collect data, define the problem, select strategies, take action, evaluate results) that serves as a guide to dealing with a problem or difficult task.

> *. . . nurses need the space to think creatively when problem solving.*
> —Benton, 1997, p. 18

Leaders **plan** and **organize** activities. Planning and organizing contribute a great deal to the efficiency and effectiveness of an endeavor. Without them, people waste time and energy. An important job may be done twice or not at all, and this is a frustrating experience for everyone involved. Poorly planned meetings are also time wasters.

Project and strategic planning are primarily managerial responsibilities and will be discussed further in the components of effective management.

## Professional Activities

A leader **develops** the structure of his or her own practice. Leaders do not wait for someone else to tell them what to do. For example, a professional nurse should not wait for a physician's order before doing some health teaching, yet some nurses still wait. Consider the following examples of ways in which nurses develop the structure of their roles:

> *A school nurse seeks opportunities for intervention; the nurse does not sit in the office hoping that teachers and students will remember that he or she is there.*
>
> *An infection control nurse visits the units, checks patients' charts, collects data, evaluates the data, talks with personnel, and institutes changes in procedures as necessary; he or she does not wait to be called in when a problem occurs.*

In order to do these things, a nurse must have both leadership ability and a clear idea of what nursing is. Although many written definitions of nursing are available, it is suggested that you formulate a personal definition to live by, one that you can use when someone asks you what nurses really do or why nurses should have more autonomy, more authority, or a salary increase.

Although nurses need to recognize the contributions of other members of the health team, they do not need to do so by diminishing their own contribution. For example:

> *Some nurses call in a psychologist to counsel a patient for a minor problem before they try to help the patient deal with the problem. They also call in "experts" to diagnose a patient's response to a health problem, run a clinic, lead team conferences, and so forth. Yet nurses can do all of these things and more.*

Although it is appropriate to call on experts when they are needed, nurse leaders need a strong sense of professional identity and confidence in their abilities.

> **To survive and thrive in a capitated health system, we need to articulate our positive impact on health care resources and clinical results. We must communicate why we are essential leaders in health care and demonstrate our clinical experience.**
> —Hansten & Washburn, 1998, p. 45

A leader **interprets** the role of the professional nurse to others: coworkers, clients, and the public. Developing structure emphasizes actual practice, whereas interpreting the role emphasizes telling people about it. If you listen closely, you will find plenty of opportunities to inform people about what nurses can do. Here are just two examples:

> *You might notice that teachers call on the school nurse to deal with head lice problems, but not with family problems that are keeping a child out of school.*
>
> *After hearing a community group bemoaning their difficulty in getting someone to do camp physicals, you could take the opportunity to say, "A nurse can do that."*

Does a leader **seek recognition?** Some people question whether seeking recognition is an appropriate leader action. A willingness to speak out in support of yourself, your group, and your profession is part of being a leader. But anyone who is obviously on an ego trip and has only personal interests in mind is unlikely to be effective.

## ● LEADERSHIP EFFECTIVENESS CHECKLIST

Now that you have read the chapter, think of a current or past leadership situation and analyze your actions in terms of the components of effective leadership. The Leadership Effectiveness Checklist (Figure 3–3) is not one of those quick checklists where you add up your score and find out if you are "superior," "above average," or "fair." It is meant as a guide to serious analysis of your leadership ability. This checklist does not tell you how effective or ineffective you are; effectiveness is better measured in terms of the results you have been getting. Rather, its purpose is to help you identify the strengths you can build on and use to your best advantage and to indicate where you need to make some changes or develop more skill to become a more effective leader. As you were reading the chapter, you probably thought of times you had taken the actions described and times when you forgot or avoided them. Using the checklist will help you to be more systematic and thorough in your self-analysis.

Every reader will find areas of personal strength and weakness within the components of effective leadership. You may find, for example, that you are usually direct in your approach to people, but that you often fail to consider what they are trying to get out of a situation (their goals). Or, you may find that you are usually sensitive to the needs and goals of others, but tend to be too indirect in your approach. The possible combinations number as many as the readers of this book. You may want to return to this checklist after you have finished the book to reevaluate your effectiveness.

## ● SUMMARY

The six components of effective leadership are adequate knowledge, self-awareness, communication, energy, goals, and action.

The effective leader has adequate knowledge of leadership and of his or her own profession. A thorough understanding of leadership makes it possible to analyze all three aspects of a leadership situation—the leader, co-actors, and environment—and then choose the most effective strategy. A questioning, open-minded attitude enables the leader to critically evaluate information and to avoid the pitfall of "going stupid."

Through increased sensitivity to yourself and others, you can become more flexible and accepting of yourself and others. Self-awareness can also improve your ability to develop close relationships with other people and to understand their behavior. As you learn more about your own unique characteristics, you can select the most appropriate leadership techniques and generally improve your effectiveness in interpersonal relationships.

Adequate communication is at the core of effective leadership. Active listening, directness, checking out perceptions, giving feedback, linking, networking, and sharing a vision are all elements of good communication for effective leadership.

Energy can be shared with people as information, help, enthusiasm, and motivation. Its influence is increased through synergic power. An adequate energy reserve is needed to be prepared to act.

An effective leader ensures that goals are clear, congruent, and meaningful to the group. Sharing a vision for the future has a positive effect on others' motivation and willingness to commit their energies to the work at hand.

## The Leadership Effectiveness Checklist

| A. Knowledge | Very Much | Somewhat | Not At All |
|---|:---:|:---:|:---:|
| 1. Do you have as much or more knowledge as the rest of your group? | ☐ | ☐ | ☐ |
| 2. Do you feel confident of your knowledge in this situation? | ☐ | ☐ | ☐ |
| 3. Are you able to speak to the group on their level? | ☐ | ☐ | ☐ |
| 4. Have you identified the needs and motives of the people in the group? | ☐ | ☐ | ☐ |
| 5. Have you identified the sources of power and authority in the situation? | ☐ | ☐ | ☐ |
| 6. Have you critically analyzed the situation, including the leader, co-actor(s), and environment? | ☐ | ☐ | ☐ |
| 7. Have you kept an open mind about the situation? | ☐ | ☐ | ☐ |
| **B. Self-Awareness** | | | |
| 1. Do you know what your own needs are? | ☐ | ☐ | ☐ |
| Have you found ways to meet these needs? | ☐ | ☐ | ☐ |
| 2. Do you know what you expect to gain from this situation? | ☐ | ☐ | ☐ |
| 3. Are you able to empathize with the people in the group? | ☐ | ☐ | ☐ |
| 4. Do you think of yourself as a leader? | ☐ | ☐ | ☐ |
| **C. Communication** | | | |
| 1. Do you know what channels of communication are usually used? | ☐ | ☐ | ☐ |
| Are you using them? | ☐ | ☐ | ☐ |
| 2. Is there an adequate flow of information? | ☐ | ☐ | ☐ |
| 3. Have you created any new channels of communication? | ☐ | ☐ | ☐ |
| 4. Are your communications open and direct? | ☐ | ☐ | ☐ |
| 5. Do you attend and respond (listen actively) to what others are saying? | ☐ | ☐ | ☐ |
| 6. Do you check out your perceptions of the situation with other people? | ☐ | ☐ | ☐ |
| 7. Do you see and point out connections (links) between the statements of different people? | ☐ | ☐ | ☐ |
| 8. Have you deliberately increased and strengthened your network(s)? | ☐ | ☐ | ☐ |
| 9. Do you have a vision for the group? | ☐ | ☐ | ☐ |
| Have you shared it with the group? | ☐ | ☐ | ☐ |
| **D. Energy** | | | |
| 1. Are you interested in the work of the group? | ☐ | ☐ | ☐ |
| 2. Have you shared your interest and enthusiasm with the group? | ☐ | ☐ | ☐ |
| 3. Do you monitor your energy level? | ☐ | ☐ | ☐ |
| 4. Do you monitor the energy level of the group? | ☐ | ☐ | ☐ |
| 5. Do you have enough energy for the task? | ☐ | ☐ | ☐ |

**Figure 3–3**  Test your leadership effectiveness.

| E. Goals | Very Much | Somewhat | Not At All |
|---|:---:|:---:|:---:|
| 1. Have you identified: | ☐ | ☐ | ☐ |
| Your personal goals? | ☐ | ☐ | ☐ |
| Group members' personal goals? | ☐ | ☐ | ☐ |
| The organization's goals? | ☐ | ☐ | ☐ |
| The larger system's goals? | ☐ | ☐ | ☐ |
| 2. Are your goals congruent with the group's goals? | ☐ | ☐ | ☐ |
| 3. Do you identify with the group? | ☐ | ☐ | ☐ |
| Do you use "we" instead of "I" and "you"? | ☐ | ☐ | ☐ |
| 4. Do members of the group see you as identifying with the group? | ☐ | ☐ | ☐ |
| 5. Have you clearly and specifically stated the group's goals, including: | | | |
| The people involved? | ☐ | ☐ | ☐ |
| The target? | ☐ | ☐ | ☐ |
| The expected outcomes? | ☐ | ☐ | ☐ |

| F. Action | Very Much | Somewhat | Not At All |
|---|:---:|:---:|:---:|
| 1. Have you defined your nursing role and communicated this to the group? | ☐ | ☐ | ☐ |
| 2. Have you developed a plan for getting the work done? | ☐ | ☐ | ☐ |
| 3. Have you organized the work efficiently? | ☐ | ☐ | ☐ |
| 4. Do you share your ideas with the others? | ☐ | ☐ | ☐ |
| 5. Do you call the group together often enough? | ☐ | ☐ | ☐ |
| 6. Do you use the authority you have? | ☐ | ☐ | ☐ |
| Do you delegate it? | ☐ | ☐ | ☐ |
| Have you tried to increase it? | ☐ | ☐ | ☐ |
| Have you tried to empower your group? | ☐ | ☐ | ☐ |
| 7. Have you mobilized support systems? | ☐ | ☐ | ☐ |
| 8. Are you willing to take risks? | ☐ | ☐ | ☐ |
| Have you taken any risks? | ☐ | ☐ | ☐ |
| 9. Do you confront when it is needed? | ☐ | ☐ | ☐ |
| 10. Do you initiate action when it is needed? | ☐ | ☐ | ☐ |
| Without delay? | ☐ | ☐ | ☐ |
| 11. Do you seek feedback? | ☐ | ☐ | ☐ |
| Informally? | ☐ | ☐ | ☐ |
| Formally? | ☐ | ☐ | ☐ |
| 12. Do you provide feedback? | ☐ | ☐ | ☐ |
| Informally? | ☐ | ☐ | ☐ |
| Formally? | ☐ | ☐ | ☐ |
| 13. Have you tried to improve your leadership effectiveness? | ☐ | ☐ | ☐ |

**Figure 3–3** *(continued)*

---

## C A S E   S T U D Y

### Leadership Effectiveness

Laurel's best friend was recently killed in a car accident. The other passengers survived because they had been wearing seat belts. Laurel could not stop thinking about her friend and wondering why she had not been wearing a seat belt. For weeks, she turned this question over and over in her mind.

The idea for the Seat Belt Project occurred to Laurel on her way to work. She could not help her friend, but she could help to prevent similar tragedies. Why not launch a safety campaign in her community?

Laurel's fellow nurses were sympathetic. They agreed to help her put up posters and distribute bumper stickers around the hospital. Laurel also appeared in several public service announcements about seat belt use on local radio and television stations. Her colleagues were excited about her being a "celebrity" and praised her efforts, calling them a "worthy memorial to your good friend."

However, when Laurel asked the nurses to help her distribute pamphlets at local shopping malls on their days off, the nurses began making excuses. They were too busy, would be away that weekend, etc. Finally, when Laurel tried to organize a safety fair for the hospital, the nurses told her they had to concentrate on their patient care responsibilities and could not help her with the fair.

### Questions for Critical Reflection and Analysis

1. In what ways did Laurel display leadership in this situation?
2. Why did the nurses agree to help Laurel at first and then refuse later on?
3. Use each of the components of effective leadership to evaluate the effectiveness of Laurel's leadership. On which components did she excel? On which did she fall short?
4. What could Laurel have done to keep the nurses interested in the Seat Belt Project?

---

Action is the sixth component of effective leadership. Leaders develop the structure of their practice and interpret their professional role to others. They also initiate actions of many kinds, including planning and organizing work, guiding and evaluating others, calling meetings, mobilizing support systems, empowering others, taking risks, and confronting themselves and others. Leaders use the basic skills of problem solving, critical thinking, and communication to carry out these actions.

## REFERENCES

Argyris, C. (1998, May/June). Empowerment: The emperor's new clothes. *Harvard Business Review*, 98–105.

Bandman, E.L. & Bandman, B. (1988). *Critical thinking in nursing*. Norwalk, CT: Appleton & Lange.

Bass, B.M. (1997). From transactional to transformational leadership: Learning to share the vision. In R.P. Vecchio (Ed.). *Leadership: Understanding the dynamics of power and influence in organizations*. Notre Dame, IN: University of Notre Press.

Bayne, C.G. (1997). Vital signs: Are we monitoring the right parameters? *Nursing Management, 28*(5), 74–76.

Beal, G.M., Bohlen, J.M. & Raudabaugh, J.N. (1962). *Leadership and dynamic group action*. Ames, IA: Iowa State University Press, 130.

Benton, D. (1997). The leadership challenge in nursing. *Nursing Management (London), 4*(2), 18–21.

Bryman, A. (1992). *Charisma and leadership in organizations*. London: Sage.

Chemers, M.M. (1993). An integrative theory of leadership. In M.M. Chemers & R. Ayman (Eds.). *Leadership theory and research: Perspectives and direction*. San Diego: Academic Press.

Christy, K.A. (1987). Networks: Forming "old girl" connections among nurses. *Nursing Management, 18*(4), 73–75.

Claus, K.E. & Bailey, J.T. (1977). *Power and influence in health care*. St. Louis: C.V. Mosby.

Conrad, C. (1990). *Strategic organizational communication: An integrated perspective.* Ft. Worth: Holt, Rinehart & Winston.

Craig, J.H. & Craig, M. (1975). *Synergic power: Beyond domination and permissiveness.* Berkeley: Pro-Active Press.

Emerson, R.W. Quoted in Fitton, R.A. (1997). *Leadership: Quotations from the world's greatest motivators.* Boulder, CO: Westview Press.

Gabarro, J.J. (1990). Development of working relationships. In J. Galegher, R.E. Kraut, & C. Egido (Eds.). *Intellectual teamwork: Social and technological foundations of cooperative work.* Hillsdale, NJ: Lawrence Erlbaum.

Grainger, R.D. (1993). Choosing mental health. *American Journal of Nursing, 93*(1), 18.

Green, M. (1973). *Teacher as stranger.* Belmont, CA: Wadsworth, 5, 80.

Gruen, W. (1979). Energy in group therapy: Implications for the therapist of energy transformation and generation as a negentropic system. *Small Group Behavior, 10*(1), 23.

Haas, J.W. & Syphen, B.D. (1992). Do shared goals really make a difference? *Management Communication Quarterly, 6*(2), 166–179.

Hammond, J.S., Keeney, R.L. & Raiffa, H. (1998, September/October). The hidden traps in decision making. *Harvard Business Review,* 47–58.

Hansten, R. & Washburn, N.J. (1998). Professional practice: Facts and impact. *American Journal of Nursing, 98*(3), 42–45.

Haynes, M.E. (1991). *Practical time management.* Los Altos, CA: Crisp Publications.

Helmstetter, S. (1982). *What to say when you talk to yourself.* New York: Simon & Schuster.

Hollander, E.P. (1974). Leader effectiveness and the influence process. In R.S. Cathcart & L.A. Samovar (Eds.). *Group processes.* New York: Academic Press.

Holt, J. (1964). How children fail. New York: Pitman. In M. Greene (1973) *Teacher as stranger.* Belmont, CA: Wadsworth.

Howard, R. (1990, December 16). How we got that rundown feeling. *New York Times.*

James, W. Quoted in Napolitano, C.S. & Henderson, L.J. (1998). *The leadership odyssey: A self-development guide to new skills for new times.* San Francisco: Jossey-Bass.

Kim, W.C. & Mauborgne, R. (1992). Parables of leadership. *Harvard Business Review, 70*(2), 123–128.

Lifton, W.M. (1972). *Groups: Facilitating individual growth and societal change.* New York: John Wiley & Sons.

Mager, R.F. & Beach, K.M. (1975). *Developing vocational instruction,* 2d ed. Palo Alto, CA: Fearon.

McNeese-Smith, D. (1993). Leadership behavior and employee effectiveness. *Nursing Management, 24*(5), 38–39.

Moser, D.K. (1997). Correcting misconceptions about women and heart disease. *American Journal of Nursing, 97*(4), 26–33.

Moshowitz, R. (1993). *How to organize your work and your life.* New York: Doubleday.

Mulholland, J. (1991). *The language of negotiation: A handbook of practical strategies.* London: Routledge.

Napolitano, C.S. & Henderson, L.J. (1998). *The leadership odyssey: A self-development guide to new skills for new times.* San Francisco: Jossey-Bass.

NCNR Priority Expert Panel on Nursing Informatics. (1993). *Nursing informatics: Enhancing patient care.* Bethesda, MD: National Center for Nursing Research.

Pagonis, W.G. (1992). The work of the leader. *Harvard Business Review, 70*(6), 118–126.

Petzinger, T. (1998/August 7). Gary Klein studies how our minds dictate those "gut feelings." *Wall Street Journal,* B1.

Quillen, T. (1988). The ideal boss. *Response, 1*(7), 5.

Roberts, C. (1999). Conscious oversight. In P. Senge (Ed.). *The dance of change.* New York: Doubleday.

Rodgers, B.L. (1991). Deconstructing the dogma in nursing knowledge and practice. *Image, 23*(3), 177–181.

Rogers, M.E. (1994). Science of unitary human beings. In V.M. Malinski & E.A.M. Barrett (Eds.). *Martha E. Rogers: Her life and her work.* Philadelphia: F.A. Davis.

Roosevelt, F.D. Quoted in R.A. Fitton (1997). *Leadership: Quotations from the world's greatest motivators.* Boulder, CO: Westview Press.

Satir, V. (1967). *Conjoint family therapy.* Palo Alto, CA: Science and Behavior Books, 15.

Silberger, M.R. (1998). Tracing our rituals. *Nursing Leadership Forum, 3*(1), 80–12.

Squire, L.R. (1987). *Memory and brain.* New York: Oxford University Press.

Tannenbaum, R., Weschler, I.R. & Massarik, F. (1974). Leadership: A frame of reference. In R.S. Cathcart & L.A. Samovar (Eds.). *Small group communication: A reader,* 2d ed. Dubuque, IA: William C. Brown.

Tichy, N.M. (1997). *The leadership engine: How winning companies build leaders at every level.* New York: Harper Business.

Trairs, J. (1994). Reviving the antibiotic miracle? *Science, 264*(5), 360–362.

Watzlawick, P., Beavin, J.H. & Jackson, D.D. (1967). *Pragmatics of human communication.* New York: W.W. Norton, 5.

White, N.E., Beardslee, N.Q., Paters, D. & Supples, J.M. (1990). Promoting critical thinking skills. *Nurse Educator, 15*(5), 16–19.

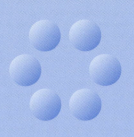

*CHAPTER* **4**

# Advanced Communication Skills: Conflict and Negotiation

## LEARNING OBJECTIVES

*After completing this chapter, the reader will be able to:*

• List common sources of conflict in a work situation.
• Discuss strategies for creating a climate in which conflicts can be more readily resolved.
• Identify situations in which negotiation would be useful.

• Use confrontation techniques appropriately.
• Apply the informal negotiation process to everyday work situations.
• Participate in formal negotiations in the workplace.

## TEST YOURSELF

**Do you know how to handle conflict?**

*Can you successfully complete a negotiation? Mark each of the following below* True *or* False, *and then check your answers.*

_____ 1. There's no such thing as a healthy disagreement.

_____ 2. When confronting another person, emphasize "you" not "me" in your confrontational statements.

_____ 3. Most people can handle confrontation most of the time.

_____ 4. If you confront a coworker about a problem at work, you need to be prepared to be confronted in return.

_____ 5. Open a negotiation with a soft, easy-going statement emphasizing your willingness to compromise.

_____ 6. If you make a threat, be sure you can carry it out.

_____ 7. The ideal outcome of negotiation is win-win i.e., both sides feel satisfied.

_____ 8. Anger is often a secondary response to a primary reaction of fear, embarrassment, or disappointment.

_____ 9. Little or no risk is involved in confronting one's boss.

_____ 10. Most negotiation processes are unemotional.

*Answers*

1. F  2. F  3. T  4. T  5. F  6. T  7. T  8. T  9. F  10. F

---

Conflict is inevitable. Attempting to prevent it from occurring and avoiding situations that might lead to conflict are not only futile but may actually reduce the quality of the work done. Conflict in a work situation can be either good or bad, constructive or destructive. Leonard and Strauss call the healthy kind of conflict "creative abrasion" (1997, p. 112), pointing out that having different people with different thinking styles on a team may occasionally make us uncomfortable but will ultimately make the team more innovative and productive. The unhealthy type of conflict can be corrosive, making people feel cut off from each other and draining energy (Tannen, 1998). The challenge for the leader-manager is to prevent the degeneration of healthy conflict into dysfunctional disagreements that lead to frustration, anxiety, and anger (Eisenhardt, Kahwajy & Bourgeois, 1997).

In this chapter, we consider the typical sources of conflict within a work site, informal conflict resolution for everyday disagreements, and the use of confrontation and negotiation in the resolution of serious conflicts.

*Management teams whose members challenge one another's thinking develop a more complete understanding of the choices, create a richer range of options, and ultimately make the kinds of effective decisions necessary in today's competitive environments.*

—Eisenhardt, Kahwajy & Bourgeois, 1997

## ● SOURCES OF CONFLICT

Conflict can arise from any number of sources. The most common sources in a work situation are the following:

- **Disputes over allocation of resources, especially scarce resources such as money, equipment, space, power and recognition**

    *Example:* Both Jean and Jonathan applied for a new assistant nurse manager position. Because they were almost equal in education, experience, and skill level, their ability to demonstrate high staff and patient satisfaction ratings could be the critical factor in the choice made. Attempting to get these high ratings, the two began to compete for the best assignments, arguing with their manager and with each other almost daily about the division of work on their units.

- **Perceived personal threat**

    *Example:* A consultant hired to evaluate the work systems on various inpatient units of a large medical center wanted to "shadow" several unlicensed assistive personnel (UAPs) in order to understand their role in patient care. The UAPs were so afraid that the consultant might report mistakes they made that most them called in sick on the scheduled "shadowing" days. Those who did come to work refused to be "shadowed," angrily declaring that they did not want to be "spied on" as they worked.

- **Perceived threats to the organization**

    *Example:* When a large medical group renovated its building, it added an on-site pharmacy to the services offered by the group. Elderly patients and parents of sick children appreciated the one-stop convenience of the new pharmacy but local pharmacy owners vehemently protested the "unfair competition" and threatened to refuse to fill any prescriptions written by members of this medical group.

- **Personal, social, and cultural differences, including differing concepts of work and responsibility, employer-employee expectations and relations, productivity, absenteeism, and appropriate behavior work**

    *Example:* J.P. came from a family that placed a high value on work and defined success in terms of promotions and salary increases. J.P. was described by coworkers as "hard-driving and ambitious." T.W., who worked for J.C., came from a family that placed a high value on family, defining a good person as one who put their family's needs ahead of their own. T.W. was described by coworkers as "laid back, easy going, and relaxed." When T.W.'s niece was hospitalized, T.W. called in sick, explaining "I'm the only nurse in the family, and they need me."

    J.P. threatened to fire T.W. T.W. was shocked that J.P. could be so "unreasonable and heartless." T.W. complained to the director of nursing for their division. J.P. retaliated by giving T.W. the hardest assignments and worst time schedules. Each considered the other impossible to work with.

Feuding departments, unhappy unions, dissatisfied patients, angry trustees: all of these conflict situations can occur in a healthcare organization (Pape, 1999; Sherer, 1994). An individual team member or the group as a whole can become involved in a conflict in an attempt to remove a perceived threat. Conflicts may arise over who can change treatment orders, who tells the patient the diagnosis, who teaches the patient how to manage problems, who counsels the patient, who orders the laboratory tests needed, and so forth.

## ● PREVENTIVE MEASURES

Even before conflict arises, the leader or manager can take certain actions to create an environment in which conflict is more readily resolved. It is especially helpful to create a climate in which individual differences are considered natural and acceptable. Although fostering such an atmosphere does not sound difficult, strong pressures for conformity are often present in work environments, especially in immature groups or autocratic organizations. Encouraging open communication and developing skills in confrontation and negotiation prepares the group to handle conflict constructively. Leader and group efforts to confront problems and meet the needs of team members help to reduce the occurrence of conflicts (Glaser, 1994; Pape, 1999).

The existence of a conflict within a group should not be interpreted as a symptom of serious malfunction but rather as a sign of a problem that needs to be resolved. It is helpful to maintain a realistically optimistic attitude that the conflict can be resolved. When group members refuse to accept the fact that a conflict exists, either because they cannot handle it or because of norms that support suppressing conflict, it delays conflict resolution.

Once the group has accepted the existence of the conflict, the situation should be analyzed to determine the source and who is involved. If the source is not clear or tension is too high to move into problem solving, confrontation and issue-focused meetings are needed first. During this whole process, a high level of leadership skill is essential to keep the conflict from escalating.

The next step is to discuss areas of agreement. This discussion helps to reduce the gap between the opposing sides in the conflict and also serves to make the conflict appear smaller and more manageable than it did when the focus was on the areas of disagreement. When the areas of agreement have been mapped out, the core conflict or key issue is more apparent and may actually be different from what it first appeared to be. Once the core conflict is evident, the group can generate alternative solutions. If the conflict is a serious one, it may take a great deal of confrontation and negotiation to finally arrive at an acceptable resolution.

## ● CONFRONTATION

At times, staff members, colleagues, or supervisors will not readily participate in free and open discussion and negotiation for any number of reasons: defensiveness is high, trust or empathy is limited, the problem-solving process gets bogged down, and so forth. As leader you may face these situations fairly often. They are difficult to handle, but a group of communication skills known as confrontation techniques (Tappen, 1978) will help break up these common interactional log jams.

Confrontation is an act that challenges others, directs them to reflect on their behavior, and as a result, change that behavior. Walton (1969) defined confrontation as the "process in which the parties directly engage each other and focus on the conflict between them." It is not just "telling someone off," as some people assume. In fact, it is preferable not to do it when either party is angry, but after they have calmed down (Jones, 1993).

Anyone in a group or organization can confront another individual or group. The nursing staff of a unit can confront the pharmacy over medication distribution problems or the dietary department about the adequacy of nutrition edu-

cation for their patients. Aides may confront nurses, the medical staff may confront administration, and so on. One organization may also confront another organization. For example, a state nurses' association may confront a hospital on employment issues or another professional organization on encroachment into nursing functions.

## Avoidance of Confrontation

Avoiding a problem that is impeding progress is usually an unproductive strategy because many problems grow larger and more serious if you avoid dealing with them. People often think to themselves, "If I leave it alone, maybe it will resolve itself." Although this strategy sometimes works, more often minor disagreements become major conflicts when ignored, and small misunderstandings become serious communication blocks when they are not resolved. In addition, silence in the face of a conflict may be interpreted as acceptance of the status quo. The manager should move quickly to intervene when a conflict arises or progress toward a goal ceases.

Usually, misunderstandings continue unless you confront what is happening. The following story is an illustration of what can be lost if you fail to confront a problem:

*A student in a community health nursing course visited a young mother (15 years old) every week to see how she and her infant were progressing. Every week the mother undressed the baby and every week the student did a complete physical assessment of the infant's condition. At the end of the semester, the student would no longer be visiting the young mother and informed her of this fact. The mother then asked if the student had found her care of the infant satisfactory. This question led to a more open discussion than had occurred before and some surprising discoveries.*

*The young mother thought the student was coming to check the infant for signs of neglect and abuse because the student had been sent by a government agency, the public health department. The student thought that the mother wanted the infant checked every week to see if the infant was all right. The mother feared that any negative evaluation from the student would result in the baby being taken away from her. The student had been aware of the lack of trust between them but failed to confront the problem until the client did so at this last meeting. What a loss for both of them that the misperception of each other's motives wasn't dealt with sooner.*

Many writers have been critical of nurses' tendency in the past to avoid confrontation. Nurses, they said, lack assertiveness. They prefer to keep the peace rather than to stimulate change (Jones, 1993), and they nurture and protect people when they should confront and challenge them. This tendency is attributed to a humanitarian set of values and also to the habit of overclassifying people as "sick" and in

---

# PERSPECTIVES . . .

## Assertiveness on Behalf of One's Patients

Elizabeth Peart, a nurse and administrator of a cerebral palsy center, had to fight for the rights of one of her center's residents. "Gino" was hospitalized and ventilator dependent. The hospital wanted him taken off life support. The center staff felt this decision was based primarily on the fact that Gino was profoundly mentally retarded. "Our response," wrote Peart, "was that they needed to give Gino a chance, as he was a fighter but needed extra time to rally" (p. 7).

Center staff petitioned the court for a guardian to look out for Gino's interests and held many meetings with the hospital staff to explain their philosophy of care for the developmentally disabled. Although hospital staff had said that Gino could not survive the nosocomial infections or be weaned from the ventilator, he has done both (he was not entirely weaned when she wrote this story).

Peart concludes that Gino demonstrated "strength, courage and determination." So did his caregivers in fighting for his right to be treated as well as any other human being.

*Source:* Peart, E. (1997, December 9). I'm a real person, too. *Vital Signs,* 6–7.

need of help rather than as well and able to handle a confrontation (Smoyak, 1974). This situation is changing rapidly as nurses become more assertive and confrontational. (See Perspectives . . . Assertiveness on Behalf of One's Patients.)

Your colleagues can handle an objective and appropriate confrontation. So can your employer. In fact, if you go too far in being protective of them, you may violate your own rights and inhibit the growth of others. The following is an example:

*Imagine that your employer has refused to consider your request for a salary increase and tells you how much the agency would like to give you a raise but cannot because of its terrible financial troubles. If you are really unassertive, you might find yourself reassuring your employer you understand the problem. A more appropriate response would be to describe your accomplishments and your value to the organization.*

Some people avoid confrontation because they fear retaliation. This fear is not always unreasonable and may be realistic in some instances. Bennis (1976) provided an example:

*Samuel Goldwyn (the movie producer) was a notorious martinet. He called his top staff together after a particularly bad box-office flop and said, "Look, you guys, I want you to tell me exactly what's wrong with this operation and my leadership—even if it means losing your jobs."*

If you are unfortunate enough to work for a "notorious martinet," you have to consider retaliation a possibility. In most cases, however, a confrontation done well is much more likely to improve your work situation than remove you from it.

## Confronting Another Person

Bradford and Cohen (1998) suggest a graduated or stepped approach to confrontation. In their approach, confrontation begins with sharing information about the effect of the person's behavior on you; continuing with statements about the effect of that behavior on the person himself or herself, including what it does and what it costs; and, finally, asking the other person how you might be contributing to the conflict. The following are examples of each of these steps:

1. Tell the other how you are experiencing the situation.
   *Examples:*
   I am overwhelmed when all of the patients on monitors are assigned to me.
   I feel devalued when someone else gets credit for my suggestions.
2. Point out what the other person's behavior does for him or her.
   *Examples:*
   Interrupting other people makes you appear impatient.
   Coming late makes it seem as if you think the meeting is not important.
3. Point out what the person's behavior costs him or her in the long run.
   *Examples:*
   People listen when you raise your voice, but they are reluctant to make suggestions for fear you will yell at them.
   It's true you get a lot of work done by being so tough on employees, but no one wants to work for you and several have requested transfers to other departments.
4. Ask the other person how you have contributed to the problem.
   *Examples:*
   Every time we talk about this project, we seem to end up arguing about it. Is there something I'm doing or saying to contribute to this tension between us?
   You have expressed unhappiness with your assignments several times. Is there something about the way I'm distributing assignments that distresses you?

## Cautions

Confrontation is used to draw attention to a problem area and to open the subject to discussion. It is a "wake-up call" to individuals or groups that have been ignoring a problem or, in some cases, are unaware that the problem exists or how serious it is.

The first move in a graduated confrontation is usually delivered as an "I" message (Clark, 1994; Gordon, 1970). It is an honest and direct communication of the way you are experiencing a situation. The purpose is to stimulate a reciprocal open response to your communication in order to improve the interpersonal relationship. It is an indirect challenge to the other person. The following are examples of "I" messages:

> *"I was embarrassed that the lounge was dirty when our visitors came through today."*
> *"I have been assigned the last-minute tasks every day this week."*
> *"I'm afraid that we're not going to get done on time."*

Several cautions are important to keep in mind. First, do not make the confrontation message a put-down of the other person. Messages that begin with "you" instead of "I" tend to put all the blame on the other guy. For example:

> *"You didn't clean up the lounge after your break."*
> *"You've been picking on me, giving me all the last-minute tasks every day this week."*
> *"You're running late again today."*

These "you" message usually provoke defensive responses such as:

> *"If it's so important, why didn't you clean it up?"*
> *"I couldn't help it."*
> *"No, I'm not!"*

The fact that a message begins with "I" is not enough if a put-down or blame message is hidden in the confrontation. For example, "I am really disappointed in you" is full of blame even though it looks like an "I" message. A little more subtle but still negative is, "I feel that you have been careless." You can be sure that these lightly disguised blaming messages will be recognized for what they are by the person receiving them.

A second caution is to avoid the temptation to attack the other person. Examples are "You are so lazy" or "You never get your work done." It is also important to focus on the behavior, not your interpretation of that behavior, which is likely to provoke a defensive response. Some examples:

> *"You have trouble relating to patients because you're always on an ego trip."*
> *"Your insecurity is at the root of all your problems here."*
> *"Your hostility is showing."*

Think a moment how you would feel if someone said those things to you. How would you react?

Direct challenges to shape up also provoke defensive responses. Some direct challenges are:

> *"Why don't you pay more attention?"*
> *"Pull yourself together."*

All the nonrecommended forms of confrontation show more concern for the confronter than for the confronted and a lack of faith in the confronted person's or group's ability to make constructive decisions to change. Direct challenges are usually stronger than they need to be.

> **Many people have trouble distinguishing between criticism of specific performance and general disapproval or dislike of the person.**
> —*Bradford & Cohen, 1998*

Inappropriate confrontations often contain a ready-made solution devised by the confronter. Inappropriate confrontations also are frequently done in anger. Gordon (1970) noted that anger is a secondary response following a primary reaction of fright, embarrassment, or disappointment. For example, anger at a coworker's rough handling of a patient with multiple myeloma is the secondary result of your fear that the patient will be hurt. Similarly, anger at a friend who reveals a confidence may be secondary to the embarrassment you feel. Of course, it is the primary reaction you should express in a confrontation, not the secondary anger.

It is possible for a confrontation through information to be ignored, most often when you have understated your own feelings regarding the situation. If it does happen, you can tell the other person how you feel about being ignored—this kind of expression usually gets through to the other person.

Finally, when you confront someone, be prepared to be confronted in return. In fact, a whole lot of issues may arise as a result of a confrontation, issues that had not been confronted in the past and so were left to grow more serious. This multiplication of issues is called **issue proliferation**. Frequent use of confrontation through information and the fostering of open communication can prevent issue proliferation.

Sometimes all that is needed to resolve a conflict is to raise the issue through confrontation and to resolve it in the discussion that follows. When this process is not sufficient, then negotiation becomes necessary.

## ● RESPONDING TO CONFLICT

When responding to conflict situations, three aspects of the conflict need to be considered: your own views, the other party's (person or group) views, and the emotional valence of the situation (positive, neutral, or negative). **Assertive** behavior attends to your view but not the other person's view. Assertive approaches usually employ a calm and positive manner. **Aggressive** behavior, which is more often hostile or defensive in tone, has a very different emotional valence. An **accommodating** approach attends only to the other person's view. **Avoidance** is ineffective because no one's view is considered and no interaction regarding the conflict occurs, leaving it unresolved.

A **consolidating** approach is considered preferable. When a consolidating approach is used, both parties' views are attended to in a nondisruptive manner. Respect for each other's opinions is evident, and efforts are directed toward finding a solution that works best for both sides in the conflict (Nicotera, 1993).

## ● NEGOTIATION

Negotiation is a give and take between individuals or groups during which the parties involved try to come up with a resolution of their problems that is acceptable to all concerned. Contrary to popular opinion, it is not a form of verbal combat. Instead, negotiation is an everyday process that can occur in minute-long conversations as well as in lengthy meetings (*Business Week*, n.d.).

Negotiation is needed to resolve complex problems, especially conflicts, once they have been identified and explored. Much more has been written about facilitating open communication than about negotiation, as if it is assumed that once you have an agreement with the other person or group on what the problem is, you will also agree on the solution. Such an assumption is frequently mistaken.

Many questions can arise during the negotiation. Should you compromise? If you are willing to concede something, should you do it immediately or wait until the negotiations get bogged down? Should you start out tough or try to sound reasonable? Who wins? Much of the negotiation literature concerns union-management relations, but negotiation is necessary in any interpersonal relationship and is discussed here in a more general sense. Collective bargaining is discussed in Chapter 21.

## Setting the Stage

Several conditions set the stage for negotiation (Rubin & Brown, 1975). First, recognition of **conflict of interest or incompatibility** is necessary between the people or groups involved. Those involved in the negotiation must be prepared, often by using some form of confrontation, to enter into the exchange of offers and counteroffers that constitutes the negotiation process.

Second, the relationship must be **voluntary**; the people involved must not only want the relationship to continue, but have the option to withdraw from it. In fact, it is the existence of this option to withdraw that motivates both sides to seek a resolution that will allow the relationship to continue. In an employment relationship, for example, the employee has the option (however reluctantly it might be exercised) to quit, and the employer has the option (again, however reluctantly) to fire the employee.

Third, negotiation should end in an agreement that satisfies everyone involved. Negotiation should be a **win-win** proposition; neither side should feel as if they have lost or even compromised something that was important to them. Realistically, however, some negotiations will turn out to be win-lose situations in which at least one party has to compromise. A reluctant compromise is more likely to occur when the distribution of power is unequal.

## Key Issues

The key issues need to be identified at the beginning of the negotiation. They are the issues that are of primary concern to the people involved in the negotiation. The key issues may be divided into two categories: emotional issues and substantive issues. **Emotional** issues may revolve around feelings such as desire for recognition or status, fear of rejection, anxiety, or personal need deprivation. **Substantive** issues are those concerned with such things as policies, rules and regulations, differing concepts of roles, role invasion, salary, and other questions about the work being done and the way it is organized (Walton, 1969).

It is important to find out as much as possible about the other side's position on the key issues and to uncover any underlying emotional issues that may be disguised as substantive ones during these discussions. Any situation that has created enough conflict to require negotiation usually has a mixture of both emotional and substantive issues. Separating the issues into emotional and substantive ones helps to identify all the major issues and determine which ones are primary in a given situation.

We will consider two different approaches to negotiating resolution of a conflict. The first is an informal, incremental approach using continuous mild confrontation and open discussion. The second is a more direct and formal approach that is usually necessary for resolution of a major conflict.

## ● INFORMAL NEGOTIATIONS

Boden (1995) described informal negotiations as "an interactional dance whose steps and stages are paced across many meetings and telephone calls, rather than in a single or formal negotiation" (p. 85). Highly confrontational tactics are often unnecessary when a conflict is of the everyday variety (Tannen, 1998). In this low-key type of negotiation, statements can be quite mild in tone. The following is an example from an analysis of the way in which informal negotiation takes place in real life:

> *. . . you're not actually saying you DON'T want a shorter working week if I'm right, you're just saying that you can't afford one at this particular time. (Walker, 1995, p. 134)*

## Opening Move

Informal negotiations usually take place in short conversations. The opportunity to begin an informal negotiation may be a chance meeting at the elevator, a coffee break, or a rare quiet moment at the nurses' station (*Business Week*, n.d.). Your goal in making this opening move is simply to get the other person involved in a dialogue. You may, for example, ask your counterpart if the two of you can meet to talk about the subject at another time, or if you both agree that some concern needs to be discussed. Your goal at this point is to engage the other person in dialogue, to find some areas on which to agree (even if it's just agreeing to talk), and to keep moving, however slowly, toward your goal.

## Continuing the Negotiation

Continue the informal negotiation with open-ended questions that seek more information about your counterpart's needs and viewpoint. Objections are not necessarily harmful—they provide opportunities to further explore differences and seek areas of agreement. At the same time, keep testing gently for agreement.

## Reaching Agreement

At some point in the series of small agreements that constitute informal conflict resolution, you will sense that you and your counterpart are approaching common ground. Some common ground can almost always be found between participants, no matter how serious the conflict (Anderson, 1993). At this stage, you continue to push, but gently, seeking agreement but open to discussion of any remaining areas of disagreement or conflict. For example:

> *It seems as if we could both be comfortable with a change in staff scheduling that allows people to be responsible for finding their own substitutes once the schedule is posted. Shall we try it for a month and see how it works?*

Remember, a poor compromise leads to one or both sides feeling they have lost something in the negotiation. A good agreement results when both sides feel they have gained something important to them. It has the added benefit of leading to improved working relationships in the future.

## ● FORMAL NEGOTIATION
### Opening Move

In a more formal negotiation, the opening move is considered a decisive point because it sets the tone for the rest of the negotiation. "Extreme but not ridiculous" seems to be the best description of the general rule for making your opening move. In other words, you should begin the negotiation phase by informing the other person or group of the upper limit of what you want. Here is an example:

> *Let's say that you are negotiating for a new position. If you think $54,000 is a reasonable beginning salary but really want $59,000, then begin the negotiations by asking for the upper limit of your expectations, which in this instance is $59,000. If you begin by asking for $54,000, you have little chance of getting $59,000 and in the negotiation you are likely to come down a little in your demands.*

Beginning with the upper limit of your wishes makes you more likely to get what you think is reasonable. Do not worry too much about seeming unreasonable—you will have an opportunity to demonstrate your reasonableness later in the negotiation. To reiterate, avoid the absurd demand, but inform the other party of the upper limit of what you want from the negotiation during the crucial opening move.

It is harder to escalate your demands later than it is to moderate them. In addition, moderating your demands in a later move makes you

## Research Example 4–1 *A Simulated Negotiation*

Is a tough initial stance more effective than a soft one in the opening move of a negotiation? What effect does mediation or arbitration have on the course and the outcome of negotiations?

A simulated collective bargaining game was used by Bigoness (1980) to compare the effects of taking a hard or soft initial position and to test the effects of anticipating mediation, voluntary arbitration, or compulsory arbitration on a negotiation. In order to provide some incentive to bargain seriously, game players were paid on the basis of their success in bargaining for wages, fringe benefits, and cost-of-living increases.

Game players were divided into pairs: one of the pair represented management, the other represented the union. Each was instructed to take a hard or soft initial position. For example, a soft management position was to offer a 6-cent increase whereas the tough position was to offer a 2-cent increase. On the other side, the soft union position was to demand 10 cents more, and the tough position was an opening demand for a 20-cent increase. Pairs of players who were assigned to mediation or arbitration were told to accept a 10-cent increase for either if they had not reached an agreement on their own after 15 minutes of play.

When analyzed, the results showed that the total amount eventually conceded by "management" was significantly less under a tough initial stance than under a soft one. The difference was not significant for the "union" side. However, fewer issues were left unresolved at the end of the game when management began with a soft stance.

The least number of issues were left unresolved when straight bargaining without mediation or arbitration was done. Compulsory arbitration left fewer issues unresolved than mediation or voluntary arbitration. Mediation was not usually successful. The researcher found that the players were most likely to reach a successful agreement when they could not anticipate having any outside assistance. Straight bargaining was the most successful when management took a tough initial stance, but arbitration was more effective when a soft stance was taken. Parties who entered into negotiations with less distance between their initial positions were most successful in reaching an agreement. It was concluded that the threat of outside intervention may facilitate agreement under low-conflict conditions but may be detrimental under high-conflict conditions.

*Source:* Bigoness, W. (1980). The impact of initial bargaining position and alternative modes of third party intervention in resolving bargaining impasses. In D. Katz, R.L. Kahn & J.S. Adams (Eds.). *The study of organizations*. San Francisco: Jossey-Bass. Reprinted from *Organizational Behavior and Human Performance* (1976), 17, 185.

---

seem more cooperative. The extreme but within reason opening move sets the tone of the negotiation. It allows you room to negotiate without having to compromise your needs and gives you time and space to maneuver and to find out more about the other person's or group's preferences and intentions. It also communicates that you will not allow yourself to be exploited, which may be even more important. Assertive positions have proven to be the most effective way to begin negotiations. At least one research study indicated that it is by far the most influential factor deciding the outcome of negotiations. The extreme opening move followed by gradual

concessions results in far more satisfaction with the outcome than a moderate stance held firmly (Rubin & Brown, 1975).

The commonly recommended pattern for a negotiation, then, is a tough opening move followed by willingness to make some concessions, but not to give in on the basic needs that led you into the negotiation process in the first place. The effect of a strong opening move in collective bargaining was tested in the experiment described in Research Example 4–1.

With a second point of view about the opening move, Bazerman and Neale (1992) recommend neither a tough nor a soft opening but a rational one. Too tough an opening stance may create an impasse in which any compromise makes the individual feel as if he or she is caving into the other side. A more rational approach is to determine the range, called the **bargaining zone,** you can both agree with and determine the best alternative for both of you.

## Continuing the Negotiation

After the opening moves of a formal negotiation, a series of offers, counteroffers, and elaborations of each side's position continues until an agreement is reached. Too many concessions made too quickly weaken your ability to get any concessions from the other side. Because negotiations proceed most effectively under conditions of relatively equal power, making concessions too quickly could result in giving too much of your power to the other side. It is more effective to pace your concessions in order to appear cooperative but firm.

As the negotiation process proceeds, each party tries to do several things. Each party will be seeking to find out the real preferences of the other side. They will also be attempting to communicate their own positions more clearly. Most important, each side will be trying to influence the outcome of the negotiation. To show how events lead up to this point and then proceed to a series of offers, counteroffers, and elaborations, an example of a common staffing problem is used:

*A group of staff nurses confronted their nurse manager because they were dissatisfied with the organization of nursing care on their unit. As a result of their confrontation meeting with the nurse manager, the group concluded that the main conflict was over the fact that each nurse was assigned a different set of patients daily. The result of this assignment procedure was that continuity of care on the unit was minimal; the satisfaction that results from continuity had been drastically reduced. The staff nurses felt that they had no autonomy, and the nurse manager felt that the staff had been uncooperative.*

*In their opening move, the staff nurses declared that they should be allowed to choose their own patients and be assigned the same patients every day. The nurse manager responded that this arrangement was impossible. Suppose some patients were not chosen? How will they provide for continuity on their days off?*

Elaborations of positions follow:

*The nurse manager said he must assure that the patients receive the best nursing care possible and that he is responsible for the care given to all patients. The staff nurses agreed but pointed out that the present system was not doing this well.*

## Reaching Agreement

In formal negotiations, the positions and differences between each side are usually directly articulated. If a competitive or hostile atmosphere prevails, both sides can become entrenched in their positions. Both can refuse to budge and the negotiations would then be likely to be concluded with a power play from either side:

*The nurse manager could declare the staff nurses' plan unworkable, assert managerial authority, and insist that they continue with the old assignment method. The staff nurses, on the other hand, could refuse to work until their proposal is accepted.*

However, if a cooperative mood prevails, either side can suggest a workable alternative:

*Either the nurse manager or staff nurses could suggest a workable way to provide better continuity of care and increased satisfaction for the staff while ensuring quality care for all patients. The group could then proceed with suggestions from both sides and further elaborations of exactly what each one wants and why certain conditions are particularly important to them.*

*For instance, a set of criteria to be used by the nurse manager in making patient assignments could be agreed on by the group so that it would satisfy everyone, including the patients. The nurse manager would retain his authority to assign staff as well as gain increasing continuity in care and staff cooperation. The staff would also gain increased satisfaction in their work and empowerment from having had input into the way they were assigned.*

## Strategies to Influence the Process

A number of factors can influence the course of a negotiation and its outcome (Bigoness, 1980). Most of the research studies on the subject indicate that a cooperative orientation results in more satisfactory outcomes than a competitive orientation. It is usually worthwhile to try to establish a cooperative climate and to encourage cooperative efforts. This attempt does not mean, however, that a lot of concessions or compromises should be made. In fact, some evidence indicates that the cooperative stance, if carried too far, can be interpreted as weakness by an aggressive opponent (Williams, 1993).

One strategy for influencing the negotiation process is to emphasize the similarity between your demands and theirs, pointing out that you really want the same thing or have the same concerns as occurred in the previous example of the staff nurses, or that you have a common enemy. The latter is a popular political strategy, by the way. You can also supply information that supports your proposal as the nurse manager in the example did by pointing out the need to account for days off in making patient assignments.

Appeals to fair play are often persuasive. For example, the nurse manager in the example could point out everyone's responsibility to provide quality care to every patient, not just those selected by individual staff members, whereas the staff nurses could point out that an arbitrary method of making assignments does not divide the work fairly.

Promising some kind of reward, if you can provide one, is another way to influence the outcome. In the example, neither side had much capability for providing tangible rewards. However, the nurse manager could write favorable evaluations or grant time off, and the staff nurses could make the work climate more agreeable if they were satisfied with the work assignments. Both could provide general satisfaction for each other from a job well done, but this type of satisfaction is really an outcome of the process, not a specific reward that one side could promise the other.

If overdone, promises make you seem too eager to concede. They can appear to be bribes, in which case the other side may begin to de-

mand these rewards in subsequent negotiations. Used sparingly, promises can increase the cooperative climate of the negotiation. If used too often, they weaken your position.

**Threats** do just the opposite of rewards: they increase the competitive climate of the negotiating process. If the threat is too small, it may be interpreted as an insult. If it is too large, it increases hostility to the point where effective negotiation is not possible. To return once more to the example, the nurse manager could have threatened to fire the nurses, and the nurses could have threatened to walk off the job, either of which would have increased the tensions tremendously.

Even if it is left unspoken, both sides are aware that the other has these weapons, such as the ability to quit or fire. Any statement regarding this kind of ultimate weapon is going to be perceived as a threat. When the problem is solvable by other means, the threat is better left unstated.

Some occasions will arise in which a person or group refuses to enter into cooperative negotiations despite confrontation and attempts to engage them in the negotiation process. Such cases offer two choices: to concede or use the more powerful political strategies that are discussed in Chapter 21.

## ● SUMMARY

Healthy conflict stimulates creativity and innovation, but unhealthy conflict eventually has a corrosive effect on individuals, work groups, and sometimes entire organizations. Sources of conflict include disputes over allocation of resources, perceived threats and differences in beliefs, values, and norms. A climate in which such differences are acceptable not only reduces the number of conflicts that arise but also supports resolution of those that do arise.

Once a conflict occurs, a consolidating approach that respects the views of both parties is most conducive to resolution. Identification of key issues, both emotional and substantive, is necessary. Sometimes confrontation of the issues is needed to get the negotiation process started. Confrontation challenges by telling the other

# C A S E   S T U D Y

## Conflict

St. Luke's Nursing Home was located in a poor neighborhood of a large midwestern city. Originally constructed 50 years prior as an "old folks' home," St. Luke's patient population changed dramatically in the last 10 years. Most now were people discharged from city hospitals in physically unstable condition. Virtually all of St. Luke's patients were on Medicaid. Renovation and refurbishing of this old facility were sorely needed. Incredibly, some units still had beds that had to be cranked up and down by hand! Wall suction and oxygen, more sophisticated monitoring systems, and better utility rooms were needed, but little money was available. The board of trustees announced that they recognized the need to renovate but due to limited funds would have to modernize the building in phases over the next 10 years.

The second-floor units had already gotten electric beds and some other equipment, but the nurse manager wanted the unit redecorated as well. On hearing this, the third-floor nurse manager told the CEO, "I need new medicine carts, electric beds, and better monitors. You should review the back injury rates on our units. We really need these things to do our job."

Three weeks later, the third-floor nurse manager was back in the CEO's office. She was nearly apoplectic because she had heard through the staff grapevine that the second-floor nurse manager was lobbying members of the board of trustees to redecorate her unit first. Even worse, she'd heard that the second-floor nurse manager's lobbying would be successful. "If this happens, half of my staff will resign," she declared. "In fact, I might quit with them." She did not wait for an answer but walked out without saying another word.

### Questions for Critical Reflection and Analysis

1. How did this conflict begin? What is the primary cause?
2. By the time they reach fever pitch, conflicts usually have several causes. List the various parties (people) involved in this situation and describe their contribution to the escalation of this conflict.
3. Now, look at each party again and suggest how he or she could initiate a resolution of this conflict.
4. Create a different scenario in which the nurse managers negotiate a resolution of their conflict that would leave all parties satisfied with the solution.

how you experience the problem, pointing out the effect of the other party's behavior and its cost, and asking how you contribute to the problem. When confronting others, it is important to use "I" messages and avoid blaming others.

Both an informal, mildly confrontational form and a more direct form of negotiation were described. The opening move is considered to be a crucial point in formal negotiation. This opening is then followed by a series of offers, counteroffers, and elaborations of each side's positions. A cooperative atmosphere, emphasizing the similarity of each side's demands, supplying information, and appealing to fair play positively influence the negotiation process. Threats and competitiveness generally have a negative influence. The best outcome is one that leaves both parties satisfied and inclined to be cooperative in the future.

## REFERENCES

Anderson, K. (1993). *Getting what you want*. New York: Dutton.

Bazerman, H.H. & Neale, M.A. (1992). *Negotiating rationally*. New York: Free Press.

Bennis, W.G. (1976). Post-bureaucratic leadership. In W.P. Lassey & R.R. Fernandez (Eds.). *Leadership and social change*. LaJolla, CA: University Associates.

Bigoness, W. (1980). The impact of initial bargaining position and alternative modes of third party intervention in resolving bargaining impasses. In D. Katz, R.L. Kahn & J.S. Adams (Eds.). *The study of organizations*. San Francisco: Jossey-Bass. [Reprinted from *Organizational Behavior and Human Performance*, (1976), 17, 185].

Boden, D. (1995). Agendas and arrangements: Everyday negotiations in meetings. In A. Firth (Ed.). *The discourse of negotiation: Studies of language in the workplace*. Oxford, UK: Elsevier Science Ltd.

Bradford, D.L. & Cohen, A.R. (1998). *Power-up: Transforming organizations through shared leadership*. New York: John Wiley & Sons.

*Business Week* (n.d.). Negotiating to win. Adapted from Steensma, C.A. (1987). *ACCEL's negotiating to win*. New York: Communications, Inc.

Clark, C.C. (1994). *The nurse as group leader*. New York: Springer.

Eisenhardt, K.M., Kahwajy, J.L. & Bourgeois, L.J. (1997, July/August). How management teams can have a good fight. *Harvard Business Review*, 77–85.

Glaser, S.R. (1994). Teamwork and communication. *Management Communication Quarterly*, 7(3), 282–296.

Gordon, T. (1970). *Parent effectiveness training*. New York: New American Library.

Jones, K. (1993). Confrontation: Methods and skills. *Nursing Management*, 24(5), 68–70.

Leonard, D. & Strauss, S. (1997, July/August). Putting your company's whole brain to work. *Harvard Business Review*, 111–121.

Nicotera, A.M. (1993). Beyond two dimensions: A grounded theory model of conflict-handling behavior. *Management Communication Quarterly*, 6(3), 282–306.

Pape, T. (1999). A systems approach to resolving OR conflict. *AORN Journal*, 69(3), 551–561.

Peart, E. (1997, December 9). I'm a real person, too. *Vital Signs*, 6–7.

Rubin, J.Z. & Brown, B.R. (1975). *The social psychology of bargaining and negotiation*. New York: Academic Press.

Sherer, J.L. (1994, April 20). Resolving conflict the right way. *Hospitals and Health Networks*, 52–55.

Smoyak, S.A. (1974). The confrontation process. *American Journal of Nursing*, 74, 1632.

Tannen, D. (1998). *The argument culture*. New York: Random House.

Tappen, R.M. (1978). Strategies for dealing with conflict: Using confrontation. *Journal of Nursing Education*, 17, 47.

Walker, E. (1995). Formulations in union/management negotiations. In A. Firth (Ed.). *The discourse of negotiation: Studies of language in the workplace*. Oxford, UK: Elsevier Science Ltd.

Walton, R.F. (1969). *Interpersonal peacemaking: Confrontation and third-party consultation*. Reading, MA: Addison-Wesley.

Williams, G.R. (1993). Style and effectiveness in negotiation. In L. Hall (Ed.). *Negotiation: Strategies for mutual gain*. London: Routledge.

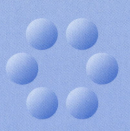

*CHAPTER* **5**

# Dynamics of Working Groups and Teams

## LEARNING OBJECTIVES

*After completing this chapter, the reader will be able to:*

- Define *group* and describe characteristics of groups as open systems.
- List the five stages of group development and describe the group climate, individual and group tasks, and appropriate leader actions for each stage.
- Identify hidden agendas and dysfunctional interactions in small groups.

- Use the seven dimensions of group process to analyze a work group's dynamics.
- Build an effective nursing or interdisciplinary healthcare team.
- Discuss the advantages and disadvantages of teamwork.

## TEST YOURSELF

**Attitude check**

*Do you like working on teams? Have your experiences with groups been positive ones? Circle* agree *or* disagree *for each of the following statements.*

| | | |
|---|---|---|
| 1. The most effective committee has three members, two of whom are absent. | *agree* | *disagree* |
| 2. A team is a group of unqualified people selected by the unwilling to do the unneccessary. | *agree* | *disagree* |
| 3. "Interesting meeting" is an oxymoron. | *agree* | *disagree* |
| 4. A camel is a horse put together by a committee. | *agree* | *disagree* |
| 5. A team is people sitting around talking about what they should be doing. | *agree* | *disagree* |

*Scoring: If you* disagree *with the statements, you have a* positive *attitude; if you* agree *with the statements, you have a* negative *attitude toward teams and groups.*

*Source:* Adapted from Riley, J.B. (1997). *Instant tools for healthcare teams.* St. Louis: Mosby.

---

T he challenge of leading and managing various individuals in a work setting is compounded when they come together in a group. Effective leaders need to think in terms of the group or team as a whole as well as about individual team members (Shonk, 1996). One pair of authors on the subject of working groups and teams waggishly remarked, "Teams are trouble, because they're made of people, and people are trouble" (Robbins & Finley, 1995, p. 219). Much of what drives groups to act the way they do is below the surface, invisible to the untrained eye (Krebs, 1992). These unconscious, often irrational, forces are at least as important as the conscious and rational forces in a group (Gillette & McCollom, 1990). A surface explanation of what is driving a group is almost always inadequate and sometimes dead wrong. The information included in this chapter will help you see below the surface of the groups in which you are a member, leader, or manager.

## ● SMALL GROUPS

A **group** is an open system composed of three or more people who are held together by a common bond or interest. The individuals who make up the group are its subsystems. Only when three or more people make up the system does the complex set of relationships develop that characterizes a group. Then interactions are affected by the presence of other people and a group climate in which the exchange takes place (Sapir, 1973).

### Common Bonds

The common bond that holds people together as a group may be either physical proximity, a shared purpose, a special meaning that has been attached to the group, or a combination of these.

Sharing the same physical space is one common bond that can bring people together as a group. Five people who get caught in a sudden rain shower and huddle together under an awning to keep dry form a temporary group. If they had not been caught by the rain, they would not have become a group but remained an **aggregate** with nothing to hold them together, even temporarily. People in a group have developed some kind of connection with one another; people in an aggregate have not. Working in the same physical space increases the number of contacts between people and the likelihood of their developing additional common bonds over time.

For most groups in the work setting, **a shared purpose** is the strongest bond. The shared purpose of a work group might be to provide nursing care for a given number of patients. Other work groups, such as task forces and committees, are formed to accomplish more limited goals. Committees may, for example, be formed to develop a new protocol for patient-controlled analgesia, to evaluate research utilization across the organization, or to carry out a quality improvement project. The following story, reported in a column of a national newspaper, illustrates the power of shared purpose in bringing people together and motivating them to work hard to achieve a particular goal.

> When a cancer patient succumbed to vancomycin-resistant enterococci (VRE) and even the light switches and blood pressure cuffs were found to be contaminated with these organisms, the staff of a Chicago hospital used an interdisciplinary team approach to attack the problem.
>
> Regular Monday morning meetings were instituted to track the outbreak and resolve the problem. Physicians, pharmacists, nurses, equipment technicians, admissions personnel, and even maintenance officials eventually joined the team. The sense of urgency created by loss of patients to VRE broke down many of the usual barriers to communication across rank and discipline. Open dialogue was essential in resolving this serious problem. At first, some staff members were offended when questioned about their infection control practices but information about the seriousness of VRE usually changed their attitudes. Hospital administration also responded well, including monetarily: funding a new lab that speeded up detection of potential problems, ripping out drinking fountains to install more sinks, and changing building plans to put staff-only sinks inside patient rooms. All of this effort paid off. Over three years, the hospital's nosocomial infection rate dropped 22 percent, saving $4.2 million in healthcare costs and uncounted numbers of lives. (Petzinger, 1998)

Why did this team effort succeed? The experience, expertise, and involvement of people from many departments was vital to the design of an effective response. The seriousness of the situation broke down communication barriers, opened administration's purses, and rallied staff, raising motivation to extraordinarily high levels. People really *wanted* to be part of this team because they wanted to solve the problem. This situation was unique, one that you neither could nor would want to create to have an effective team, but it does illustrate how well a team can solve a problem that a single individual could not have solved at all. It illustrates the extent to which teamwork can unleash the potential of team members (Ling, 1996).

Some groups are formed primarily because of the special meaning they have for their members. This kind of group holds some special significance or meets some basic need of its members. Community groups often begin this way. They may be formed on the basis of shared religious beliefs, a common ethnic background, or a shared concern or community need, such as groups of bereaved parents or families of AIDS patients.

Groups originally formed to accomplish a specific purpose may develop a shared meaning for its members over time. For example:

> *Membership on the Professional Practice Committee may become a desirable position because of the power of the committee and the qualifications for membership. The committee then becomes a symbol of power and prestige to its members.*
>
> *A team that was formed to provide transtelephonic defibrillation for a hospital's cardiac patients may become a source of satisfaction for its members when patient lives are saved by the team. It may also develop social significance if team members find that they enjoy spending time together during and after work.*

## Groups as Open Systems

For many people, looking at the group as a whole is a totally new perspective, one that requires a real change in perspective. The group as a whole has its own unique characteristics that are different from the characteristics of the individual members. It has its own identity, its own rhythms, its own growth patterns, and its own interactions with the environment. The behavior of a group cannot be accurately predicted from an assessment of the individual members (Burggraf & Sillars, 1987; Glisson, 1986). One group theorist pointed out that a group can act completely irrationally even though its members are rational people (Bion, 1961). It is also interesting to note that people act differently in different groups.

In leadership and management, we are interested in several levels of interaction within work groups. The first is the **intrapersonal,** that is, what occurs within the individual. The second is the **interpersonal** level, the person-to-person interactions. Next is the group level, which is the primary focus of this chapter. Finally, there are the **intergroup** (between groups), **organizational,** and **interorganizational** levels, which are the subjects of later chapters (Wells, 1990). Both the patterns of interaction that characterize the group as a whole and the patterns exhibited by people when they are acting as members of a group are important.

A group's boundary serves both to define it and provide its structure. By identifying its boundaries, one is able to determine its physical, spatial, temporal, and psychological form. Boundaries are permeable. If a group's boundary is not permeable enough, it may starve for information or resources; if it is too permeable, on the other hand, it may be overwhelmed by outside forces (McCollom, 1990).

Groups have common patterns of behavior that can be identified, analyzed, and influenced by the leader. The way in which a group responds to its members, makes decisions, and handles conflicts are just a few examples of these patterns. Some of these patterns promote group development, others are indications of group disharmony, and still others are downright destructive.

A regular and predictable sequence is also evident in the development of a group. Although not every group completes this sequence successfully, those that are able to do so will proceed through identifiable stages in their evolution. Distinct differences can be observed between an immature group in the early stages of development and the mature group that has progressed to the later stages of development.

These differences are discussed in the next section of this chapter.

A group may take action to change its environment, or it may make a decision based on the expectations or demands of people outside the system. Environmental influences may be as subtle as the effects of spatial arrangements or as obvious as a directive from the administration. This influence is not a one-way exchange—the group may also make demands of the administrator. The group's very existence can subtly affect those who are not members and see themselves as "outsiders."

## ● STAGES OF GROUP DEVELOPMENT

Years of observation by group theorists as well as a number of research studies indicate that groups generally go through identifiable developmental stages in the course of their existence from an immature form to a mature stage of development.

Of course, not every group achieves maturity, just as not every individual successfully fulfills the developmental tasks of each stage of life. Also, like individuals, groups may proceed to the next stage without completing the tasks of the earlier ones and may need to go back to complete them later. They may also terminate before they have progressed through all of these stages. Tuckman and Jensen (1977) and Lacoursier (1980) called these five stages of group development **forming, storming, norming, performing,** and **adjourning.**

Groups first go through a formation stage characterized by the uncertainty felt by group members about their place in the group. This stage is followed by a stormy period in which conflict is prevalent and emotions are high. The group must find a way to deal with these conflicts and develop a functional pattern of interaction. If it succeeds, the group then matures into a highly functional system abundantly able to perform its tasks and meet the relationship needs of its members. At some point, the group finishes its task or is no longer of use to its members or to the organization and thus ceases to exist. The course of the group's development is affected by the purpose of the group and the setting in which it functions as well as by the internal dynamics of the group (Bennis & Shepard, 1978; Braaten, 1974–1975; Bradford, 1978; Brill, 1984; Hill, Lippitt & Serkownek, 1979; McCollom, 1990; Nielsen, 1978; Robbins & Finley, 1995).

## Forming

This first stage has two phases: expectation and interaction. Future group members will come with a number of **expectations** about what a group will be like, how they will fit into the group, and what the group expects of them. These expectations will be unknown to the leader unless he or she asks people to talk about their expectations.

**Interaction** begins when the group meets. At this formative stage, the group develops a sense of self and defines a boundary between itself and the environment. People in the group will be able to say who is and who is not a member of the group but will not yet know exactly what being a member entails.

In this first stage, the group is immature. Its members have just begun to identify their common bonds and have not yet formed any relationships within the group. Group members will have differing perceptions of the purpose and goals of the group and will be uncertain about their position within the group.

### Individual Tasks

The first task of individual group members is to learn about the group and to find out what roles and responsibilities they will be fulfilling in a particular group. They also need to deal with their feelings about entering a new group: uncertainty, curiosity, high hopes, mistrust, or anxiety related to the unknowns of the group. The amount of stress varies according to the demands of the situation and individual response to these demands. For example, joining a group similar to one you have enjoyed working in before would be much less stressful than joining a group in which you will be asked to carry out an entirely new task for which you do not feel prepared.

### Group Tasks

The group as a whole has two tasks to accomplish in the forming stage, establishing its identity as a group and providing support for group members. Establishing identity is done by defining who is and who is not a member of the group and talking about what members of the group have in common with each other (for example, all are new in their jobs, have the same problem, have the same goal). A third way is to give the group a name and to decide on a time and place to meet again, which extends the existence of the group beyond the initial encounter.

Providing support is difficult for the immature group. Introductions and discussion of potential commonalities help. Avoiding conflict and confrontation are also a temporary means of providing support. As the group matures, it is more capable of meeting its members' needs and can therefore allow more open communication and confrontation.

## Climate and Behavior

Uncertainty and insecurity characterize the forming state. Members' needs for security and belonging have not yet been met within the group, so much of their behavior is aimed at meeting these needs: gaining acceptance, avoiding rejection, increasing feelings of comfort, reducing anxiety, reducing ambiguity, and attempting to clarify roles and expectations.

Because members of a forming group do not know whether they will be accepted by the group, they are cautious in their behavior. For some people, this uncertainty and anxiety can become so intolerable that they literally flee from the group.

The level of trust within the group is low at this stage (Gibb & Gibb, 1978). Coupled with unmet needs for security and belonging, this results in attempts to bring some order and structure to the group and in guarded, nonconfronting, nonrevealing communications. Typically, conversation is somewhat formal and polite. People talk about safe, familiar subjects (such as the weather, the traffic, or a current item of general interest) and try to conceal their concerns.

A new group lacks form and organization. It has not had time yet to develop regular patterns of interaction, so it is quite unpredictable, even to its members. The politeness and formality used for self-concealment also serve to structure and pattern communication.

Another way the group can increase structure and predictability is to set limits on each

other's behavior. For example, members will control participation by having each one take a turn to speak or by interrupting those who stray beyond the limits set, saying, "Let's stick to the subject." They may also set an agenda for the meeting and designate not only a specific time and place for the next meeting but also a specific duration and restrictions on who is welcome to attend.

Forming groups often get stuck on minor points, sometimes spending the whole meeting squabbling about them, so that the group does not have to deal with its major task. What may appear to be progress is actually motion without movement (Berg & Smith, 1990). The group is going around in circles rather than moving ahead to explore new territory. This "stuckness" can occur at any stage but is most common in the earlier stages of group development. Another group may take a different approach and try to rush through too many decisions at the first meeting in order to reduce tension. With a rushed approach, it is usually necessary to return to the issues later and resolve the issues in a more mature manner.

Despite these limitations, an underlying tone of optimism usually prevails. People who enter a new group usually bring with them the expectation that the group will somehow be able to accomplish its purpose. While it does need to be kept within realistic bounds, this optimism helps to keep the group together through its difficult early stages.

## Leadership

A newly formed working group needs a leader who can provide support and structure without encouraging dependence. It is important to be alert to the individual needs of group members. For example, some people may prefer to remain silent at this stage; you can encourage the group to allow them to "skip their turn for now." Others may need recognition to feel comfortable in the group and the leader can supply some of this recognition.

You may experience some of the same feelings of ambiguity the group does. Recognizing that they are related to the formation of the group can help you deal with them constructively. You can also be a role model for mature group behavior by engaging in more open communication than the rest of the group. Your openness encourages others to speak more freely. Only indirect, low-pressure kinds of confrontation should be used at this stage.

You can also help the group develop its identity and structure and begin to clarify its purpose. Simply using the word "we" in referring to the group helps to promote a group identity. Giving the group a name, using this name, and distinguishing it from other groups also reinforce the group's identity.

Although some structure is needed, it should be flexible enough to allow growth. Rigidity retards further development. The following illustrates the difference:

*Flexible: Encourage the group to discuss when they want to meet next time and to decide what they want to do or discuss.*

*Rigid: Ask the group to make a list of each item to be discussed at the next meeting; allow no deviation from that list.*

A general statement about the reason why people are getting together as a group is appropriate and reduces ambiguity to a more manageable level. Firmly set goals would be premature and probably have to be renegotiated later on. Group members can also be assigned responsibilities such as taking minutes, thinking about the group's goals, and bringing some information or ideas with them to the next meeting.

**EXAMPLE**   No substitute could replace the real group experience in which you can actually be involved in the interactions and feel the tensions rise and fall as the group moves through the stages of development. The following example illustrates the way in which a group changes from stage to stage.

*An outbreak of meningitis in a grade school upset many parents in the district. Three parents met with the school superintendent to express their concern and demand that action be taken to improve school health services. The superintendent suggested that they meet with the district coordinator of special services who was responsible for health services.*

*The following evening, the three parents and the coordinator met at the grade school.*

*The coordinator expected that the blame for inadequate health services would fall on her and was apprehensive about the meeting. Each of the parents was eager to see some action taken and had a list of suggested actions. Each list was different from the others.*

*After everyone arrived and had been introduced to everyone else, the coordinator read a long report (originally written for the school board) to the parents. When she finally finished, the parents took turns asking questions about the way the outbreak had been discovered and handled. They gradually realized that the person who had been most actively dealing with the outbreak was a nurse from the health department. Someone suggested they speak with the nurse. One parent offered to call the nurse and ask the nurse to meet the group at the same time next week. At that point, the meeting ended.*

Not a single item on any of the three parents' lists was accomplished at this meeting. The coordinator was expected to attend another meeting despite the coordinator's hope that the parents would be satisfied by the report and drop the whole thing. You may have noted that only the coordinator felt any real anxiety about the formation of the group in this particular example. The maneuver of reading the long report succeeded in protecting the coordinator from attack but did not help the group make any progress toward a goal. A real leader has not yet emerged in this group. The example will be continued at the end of the discussion of the second stage, storming.

## Storming

It would seem that after the uneasiness of the first stage, the group would move into a calmer phase, but it does not. Although group members usually feel a little more comfortable by the end of the first stage, the second stage is characterized by an increase in tension and conflict. This stage is difficult but the tension has some value because it pushes the group to work on resolving the problems and issues that were evaded in the first stage.

### Individual Tasks

As the group reorganizes itself throughout this stage, the main task of the individual member is to find a position in the group. This task includes defining what one is able to contribute to the group, the degree to which one can fulfill group expectations, and a decision as to whether that individual member will remain a part of the group.

To do these things, the group member needs to develop more connections with other group members and some idea of the purpose of the group and its probable objectives. Group members frequently test several different roles and options available to them before the conclusion of this stage.

## Group Tasks

The group's tasks in this second stage are to resolve the conflicts that emerge and to begin reorganizing itself into a more functional whole. Conflicts that were avoided in the first stage now emerge and demand much of the energy of the group to resolve them.

In order to successfully reorganize, the group must develop more common bonds between its members and further develop its identity. The minimal structure developed in the first stage is usually challenged and often reworked. While the purpose of the group becomes clearer, specific objectives are usually established in the next (norming) stage.

## Climate and Behavior

As the name of this stage implies, the climate of the group is unstable and emotional. When previously hidden conflicts emerge, the tension level rises rapidly. Trust is still low and the group is clearly still immature, although struggling to mature.

People who are not familiar with group dynamics are often surprised that decisions made in the first stage are either ignored or completely changed in the second stage. This seemingly irrational behavior is necessary if the decisions were based on a superficial consensus that concealed substantial disagreement.

In some groups, communications become openly hostile in the second stage. Angry individuals may stomp out of a meeting when they do not get their way. The noise level can rise dramatically, and shouting matches may occur. In other groups, communication is more restrained, particularly in work settings where open expression of anger and other negative feelings are frowned upon. Hostility is more covert but still evident to the alert observer and is still felt by members of the group. People who fear open hostility may withdraw from the group, temporarily or permanently, physically or emotionally.

The conflicts that arise in the group may stem from such trivial matters as the way to pay for refreshments or from serious issues such as the purpose of the group. Personal conflicts are also common. For example, one group member may become irritated by another's mannerisms; another may become upset or sulky when criticized. When a group focuses too long on a trivial disagreement, it is usually because it is unable to deal with more substantial issues.

A work group with an assigned task may have difficulty defining its purpose for any of several reasons. First, the task may not have been clearly defined by administration or by the leader. Second, the task may be surrounded by conflict; investigation into potential malpractice or financial misdeeds would be examples of conflict-producing tasks. Finally, the group may not be up to the task. Group members' capabilities may not match the demands of the assigned task.

Differences between individual members become much more apparent than they were in the first stage. As they appear, individual members begin to develop affiliations with those who share their interests. **Subgroups** or factions may form out of these affiliations. Within the subgroups, members begin to show more interest and concern for one another than had been shown earlier.

As these subgroups form, people begin to take sides on issues and to support those who agree with them against those who disagree. The conflicts between these subgroups can escalate into serious battles. The group may even seem ready to split into two or more separate groups, which occasionally happens.

**Power struggles** may erupt as people try to maneuver themselves into favorable positions within the group. For example, two or more people may try to designate themselves as leader of the group or they may try to remove the already-designated leader by calling for a vote, by constantly challenging the leader's actions, or by simply taking over. Power struggles also develop over control of group functions. For example, a group member might try to impose a set of rules on the group, and in response, a second member will demand that the group accept his or her own completely different rules. The struggle over whose rules will be accepted can turn into a shouting match or become an endless argument unless someone intervenes.

## Leadership

The group leader helps the group channel its energies into constructive activity by using confrontation and negotiation, linking, testing for consensus, encouraging, and reinforcement.

Confrontation and negotiation are appropriate at this stage. They can be used to get things moving again when the group gets stuck on a trivial matter and to resolve the conflicts and power struggles that emerge in this stage.

When using confrontation, however, it is important to lay down ground rules for communication. It means using "I" messages and not attacking the person. Group members can be encouraged to listen carefully, attend to different points of view, try to see things as others do, and show a willingness to change. They can also be encouraged to express dissent, that is, to question evidence, express doubt, and discuss their points of view so members can learn from each other (Howard & Barton, 1992). Group members may also need to learn how to accept constructive criticism from each other (Glaser, 1994). Frankness, objectivity, and respect for other people's viewpoints are essential to group function. These ground rules may need to be repeated and violations pointed out until the group becomes accustomed to following them. Their purpose is not to suppress expression of feelings but to keep these expressions from feeding the tension that already exists, to avoid provoking more hostility, and to avoid driving anxious or angry members away from the group. They help to keep emotions and tensions within reasonable bounds.

The leader can also point out the commonalities that exist between individuals and subgroups. This linking function, you may recall, is a component of effective leadership (discussed in Chapter 3). **Linking** can strengthen group identity, assist people in making connections with each other, and clarify the purpose of the group.

Also important in clarifying the purpose of the group is encouraging free discussion and then testing for consensus. Once some commonalities have been found, the leader can ask, "Do we all agree that . . . ?" When dealing with disagreements, testing for consensus may be used to identify what commonalities do exist.

During the second stage, the group may not be ready to come to consensus on some of the questions raised and may have to vote on some issues. The problem with voting is that the minority will lose to the majority, and this result can polarize the group even further. Voting is preferable, however, to autocratic decisions by the leader or pressure from a few members of the group. On some points, it may be necessary for group members to agree to disagree to avoid splitting the group permanently.

The leader can encourage and reinforce positive individual and group action in several different ways. The leader can point out to the group that it usually takes a long time to get organized and to get to the planning stage. This realization can restore sinking optimism. The leader can also reinforce positive action by recognizing contributions and pointing out ways in which individual members have been helpful to the group. Considerable evidence from research on group leadership supports the idea that rewarding group members for their contributions increases participation while punishing them in any way decreases participation (Pavitt, 1999). Humor can also be used to reduce tension and promote cohesiveness provided it does not contain elements that embarrass or attack others (Keyton, 1999).

EXAMPLE    Let us return to the group of three concerned parents and the coordinator of special services as they come together for their second meeting and enter the second stage—storming:

*As group members sat down around a table, the parent who had offered to call the nurse was asked when the nurse was coming. "The nurse couldn't come this week because of a previously scheduled conference. The nurse will be here next week." The other group members looked annoyed, "Why didn't you tell us! We wasted our time coming tonight." The first parent responded that they could use the time to decide what questions to ask the nurse.*

*Although everyone thought they had agreed on the questions, when people began bringing up their questions, each one was different. One parent wanted to ask how meningitis spread, but another one said they knew that already. When the third parent suggested that they ask the nurse how the problem could be handled better next time, the coordinator took offense and said, "No one said it was badly handled this time." Almost in a chorus, three parents said, "But that's why we're here! Our children were dangerously exposed." Again, the coordinator said that everything possible had been done, and anyway, the coordinator didn't think that parents should get involved in administrative decisions. While saying this, the coordinator started to put papers away as if getting ready to leave.*

*As the coordinator finished packing up the papers, a parent said coldly, "If you don't want to cooperate, we'll be happy to inform the superintendent," and the other parents nodded in agreement. The coordinator backed down from the aggressive stance and said, "Well, I do want to be cooperative." The first parent said, "I know you're concerned; we all want the children to be healthy."*

*The group then decided that each person could ask the nurse questions that kept to the subject. Everyone agreed to return the next week.*

The first parent (who called the nurse) is emerging as the leader of the group. At one point the parents sided together against the coordinator, and the group nearly split apart. But the meeting ended with a positive although vague agreement that they were all concerned about the children's health. The group now has a defined purpose, even though it still has no specific objectives.

## Norming

In the norming stage, the group experiences some relief from the anxieties and tensions of the first two stages. Positions and responsibilities are defined, plans are made, actions are more productive. The group establishes more predictable patterns that will be carried over into the next stage.

The group is more relaxed in the norming stage and participation in the group is less stressful than it was in the first two stages. By the end of this stage, group members feel a sense of belonging and of progress. The group is clearly maturing.

### Individual Tasks

By this stage, the individual has made a decision to remain a member of the group (to the extent that a choice is allowed in a work situation) and has begun the task of defining a position for himself or herself in the group. In the norming stage, members can test and refine their positions and begin functioning as an integral part of the group as a whole.

Interactions with others in the group are more purposeful and constructive now. The individual member can disagree and collaborate within this more predictable group. He or she should be contributing to the accomplishment of the group's task and offering support to other group members by now.

### Group Tasks

A major task of the group is to decide on the specific goals or objectives that it will carry out in the next stage. If the purpose was not clearly defined during the second stage, it needs to be defined now in order to develop objectives. The group also needs to decide what has to be done and who will do it, in other words, determine and assign tasks.

Two other tasks are to develop cohesiveness as a group and to establish functional patterns of behavior. The group also needs to work out its own constructive ways to resolve conflicts and to meet individual members' needs.

### Climate and Behavior

This third stage is characterized by a gradually increasing feeling of progress, openness, and relatedness. This change in group climate is not quite as radical as it may seem. Although unnoticed because of the tension and conflict of the second stage, some positive steps were being taken then that finally bear fruit in the third stage. Instances of mutual support and developing connections between subgroup members are common in the second stage. These relationships are now extended to the rest of the group.

As connections develop, group members feel less isolated. People are more likely to share individual concerns than they were before. When they do, the group is more likely to respond with support and helpful suggestions.

Responses from the group are now more predictable. Predictability does not, however, mean that people do or say the same thing over and over again. It means that if a group member offers a constructive suggestion, someone will at least acknowledge the contribution. Or, if someone makes an insulting remark, this violation of the ground rules will be pointed out in some way, usually constructively. In neither case will people be either completely ignored or attacked as they might have been in the storming stage. Discussion turns away from trivial matters. As it proceeds, the group is finally able to agree on how it will carry out its purpose.

The group becomes more autonomous and less likely to look to the leader for assistance. As each member of the group learns more about effectively influencing other group members, the leader becomes more like just another member of the group.

Decisions are made in a more democratic manner now. Reaching consensus on an issue is not only possible but happens more frequently. Voting is much less common, and autocratic decisions are no longer acceptable to the group.

Cautious optimism about the contributions of the group replaces frustration and discouragement. The group has finally proven that it can get something done, but it has not yet proven its ability to carry the plan to completion.

## Leadership

As the leader, you can help to guide the group through the planning process by keeping the group from getting sidetracked, testing the feasibility of suggestions, and encouraging the use of consensus in making decisions. The group should assume much of the responsibility for planning

its work so that it will own the final plan and be more committed to it.

It is still helpful to encourage debate on issues that arise, to test for consensus, and to use confrontation and negotiation when necessary. Members show less need for support or enforcement of the ground rules for confrontation except for an occasional reminder.

At this point, the reader might enjoy looking at the list in Box 5–1 of what *not* to do when leading a group.

**EXAMPLE**   At the third meeting, the three parents and coordinator meet with the nurse from the health department to discuss the meningitis outbreak:

*Each group member brought a list of questions to ask the nurse and was surprised that the others had done so as well. Most of the questions were about the handling of the meningitis outbreak. The discussion flowed freely. The coordinator seemed less defensive and more relaxed than at the second meeting. The parents were attentive and impressed with the nurse's thorough knowledge of the situation and the way the nurse had dealt with the problem.*

*As they neared the end of their questions, one of the parents said, "I guess we were fortunate to have you on hand when this hap-*

---

**Box 5–1   How *NOT* to Lead a Group**

Be unpredictable.
Be absent as much as possible.
Use threats and bluffs.
Secretly pursue your own goals.
Volunteer to be the record keeper.
Assume the role of a joker.
Come on strong and stay that way.
Demonstrate your contempt of the group.
Contribute as little as possible.
Follow the rest of the crowd.
When you do contribute, do it incompletely.

*Source:* Fisher, B.A. & Ellis, D.G. (1990). *Small group decision making: Communication and the group process.* New York: McGraw-Hill. Used with permission.

*pened." "Yes, it was very fortunate because I only visit the school once a month," said the nurse. The parents gasped and asked the nurse to explain. The nurse described the way in which nurses were assigned to schools in the district. The nurse was able to provide only minimal services to the school because that was all the district contracted for.*

*Another parent asked the nurse what services should be available, and the discussion of this subject took up the rest of the meeting time. When it was time to end the meeting, the first parent thanked the nurse for coming and said that the nurse had given them something to think about. The others agreed and asked if the nurse could return to consult with their committee in the future. The nurse agreed.*

*At the next meeting, the group discussed the nurse's suggestions for a comprehensive health service. The coordinator pointed out that such services would be expensive. The parents agreed but said it would be worth the cost.*

*By the end of the meeting, the group had decided to propose an improved health program for the district but also agreed that they needed more information. The coordinator was asked to look into the costs and feasibility of improved services. The first parent volunteered to speak with other health department officials, and the other two parents offered to do some library research. Each member would bring their information back to the group in two weeks.*

Not every group progresses as rapidly or successfully through the stages of development as this one. It may take many weeks for some groups to even enter the second stage. The group in the example has matured substantially; note how differently the coordinator's disagreement was handled at this stage.

## Performing

The performing stage is the most productive and enjoyable part of the life cycle of a group. By this stage, the group has clearly defined its purpose, agreed on its objectives, and has a plan or system in place for achieving them. Each member feels a part

of the group, knows what behaviors are expected, and knows what to expect from other members of the group. The group has reached maturity. Its members are now able to work in concert, performing their tasks smoothly and efficiently most of the time (Frigon & Jackson, 1996).

> **The hammers must be swung in cadence, when more than one is hammering the iron.**
> —G. Bruno, c. 1548–1600, in Eigen & Siegel, 1989, p. 467)

### Individual Tasks

Individual members carry out the roles and responsibilities that were defined over the last three stages. The first task of every individual member is to carry out their share of the work. Efforts are usually made during earlier stages, but it is not until this stage that group members have sufficient energy free to fully concentrate on performing the work of the group.

The second task is to relate effectively to both the group as a whole and to individual members. Group members now address their messages to the group as a whole as well as to the other individuals. For example, a characteristic of the mature group is the degree to which a group member who is unhappy about a group action discusses that displeasure with the group (mature group behavior) rather than with another person outside the group (immature group behavior). Although a need to have subgroups within the group may still remain in order to divide up complex tasks, communication between these subgroups should flow freely and openly.

### Group Tasks

Like the individual tasks, the tasks of the group at this stage are to move toward its goals by engaging in productive behavior and to maintain effective relationships within the group and with the environment. The needs and goals of the group as a whole are much more congruent with those of the individual members now.

To fulfill these tasks, the group must now function as a whole whose members are functionally interrelated. The following description of a group exercise may help to illustrate this functional interrelatedness:

*Six or seven volunteers are asked to stand together in a group and link arms with each other. Then each person is asked to select a point somewhere in the room and move toward it. After each person indicates that they have decided on a point in the room, they are told to move toward that point.*

*Of course, with their arms linked, everyone finds themselves pulling against the others and the group goes nowhere. The people in the group become frustrated. Finally, they realize that they can't all reach their different points at once and begin to move together from point to point in the room until each person's point has been reached. As they move in concert, the people in the group usually begin to smile and laugh with pleasure at their accomplishment. You can see the climate change as the group moves from unproductive to functional behavior.*

## Climate and Behavior

The climate of the group at this stage is generally open, pleasant, and relaxed. Most behavior is purposeful and constructive. The level of trust among group members is high, and each member has a sense of involvement in the group. Cooperation has replaced conflict as the primary operational mode.

This new level of cooperation does not mean that differences among group members no longer exist. They simply are handled in a different manner. In fact, the leader should be suspicious of a group that claims it never has to deal with differences or disagreements among its members. When a group presents a totally harmonious, unanimous front, it *may* mean that it has set up rigid norms that prohibit disagreement. Beneath this surface agreement, members may be concealing concerns and opinions for fear of rejection by the group. The harmony is an illusion; those who believe in it are deceiving themselves.

In contrast, the mature group recognizes that each member is a unique individual who is likely to disagree with some of the things that are said or done. The mature group can tolerate individuality and disagreement; it is capable of openly confronting conflicts that may arise from disagreements and of negotiating their resolution. Each member's abilities are recognized and used. Individuality is appreciated rather than suppressed.

Table 5–1 compares the characteristics of mature and immature groups (Bion, 1961).

## Leadership

The effective leader acts as a group facilitator in the performing stage. Even more than in the last stage, group members can assume many of the early stage leader functions although they still benefit from guidance during this stage.

| Table 5–1 | Characteristics of Mature and Immature Groups |
| --- | --- |

| Mature* | Immature |
| --- | --- |
| Definite boundary | Indefinite, shifting boundary |
| Defined purpose | Vague purpose |
| Common, shared goals | Conflicting or absence of goals |
| Strong identity as a whole | Uncertain identity threatened by gain or loss of members |
| Relaxed, informal | Rigid, formal, or chaotic |
| Open, confronting communications | Closed, concealing communications |
| Accepting | Rejecting, indifferent, or hostile |
| Tolerates differences | Suppresses or is disrupted by differences |
| Flexible, predictable norms | Inflexible or inconsistent norms |
| Cohesiveness | Few connections between members |
| Deals with both tasks and relationships | Over-focused on either tasks or relationships |
| Recognizes and responds to members' input and needs | Fails to recognize or respond to its members |
| Feedback is constructive | Feedback is minimal, destructive, or both |

*A group that has achieved all of these characteristics of maturity may not be perfect, but it is far more functional and effective than the immature group.

The leader is still a valuable resource for the group. The group still needs to be refocused on objectives when they are sidetracked and to receive feedback on their progress, support when they face a particularly difficult task, and guidance for such things as how to delegate responsibility, make assignments, and revise their plans when necessary.

Working out any problems that arise contributes to the cohesiveness of the group and to its general development. An overly helpful leader could actually inhibit the group's continued development.

**EXAMPLE**    The school health committee, composed of three parents and the coordinator of special services, met again after gathering some data:

> *Committee members shared their findings with the rest of the group. As they discussed their proposal for improving health services again, they began to realize how many people would be affected by this change and decided that they needed more input. They decided to survey not only school and health department officials but also the students, parents, and teachers in the entire school system.*
>
> *At the same time, they also planned to find out how other school systems designed and financed their health services. To accomplish these tasks, they formed two subcommittees. Two additional parents and a school principal joined the committee.*
>
> *The group as a whole met regularly to discuss their progress and share the results. Some of the ideas presented were too ambitious; others were too limited. Many disagreements arose as discussions progressed. Finally, the committee worked out a realistic proposal that satisfied each member and was feasible financially.*
>
> *The survey activities had generated much community support for the proposal by the time the committee presented it to the school board. The school board conducted public hearings on the proposal and finally approved it after making some minor changes.*

In this example the group completed its work successfully, but not every group is able to do so. Some fail to progress this far in their development as a group and either abandon their objectives or work ineffectively on them. Even those groups that do reach this stage may find their project cannot be completed or will not be accepted for some reason that was not apparent when they began their work. Then the group has to decide whether to give up its objectives or revise its work plan and continue on.

## Adjourning

Some working groups continue indefinitely; others have a specific time-limited purpose and are disbanded once the purpose is accomplished. In this fifth and last stage, the group comes to some kind of closure and ends. Closure should include a summary of events that took place over the life of the group and an evaluation of both the group process and the degree to which the group fulfilled its purpose. The evaluation of the relationship aspects of the group process is often omitted, which may be due to its potentially threatening nature and/or a failure to appreciate its value. When a group fails to complete closure, its members are left with an unsatisfied, unfinished feeling.

### Individual Tasks

The task of the individual member in this stage is to evaluate both the process and the outcome of the group. All members give and receive feedback on their own roles, other members' roles, and the group as a whole. Group process, achievement of the group objectives, individual members' contributions, productive and unproductive behaviors, and ways in which all of these could be done better in the future may be included in the evaluation.

### Group Tasks

The group's tasks at this last stage are to support a thorough evaluation of the group's processes and outcome, to continue to foster an open climate in which the evaluation can take place, and to obtain or provide some recognition of the group's work and achievements. This recognition can be in the form of an announcement of the group's success, a recounting of what has been attempted and accomplished, or a celebration of some kind.

## Climate and Behavior

This stage is characterized by mixed emotions; relief that the work is done, satisfaction from a job well done, sadness that the group is coming to an end. Not every group succeeds, but even if it does not, its members can get some satisfaction from having at least attempted to reach their objective. They can also evaluate how well they worked together and how they would do it differently in the future.

Evaluation can make the group more aware of how it has changed since its first meeting, something people often will not realize unless it is pointed out to them. It can also raise self-awareness as people receive feedback on how they have influenced others.

## Leadership

As a member of the group, the leader should expect to both give and receive feedback. An important function of the leader at this stage is to encourage this sharing. Because many are reluctant to do this kind of assessment, the leader can initiate the process by asking the others to evaluate the leader's role. Another method is to ask group members to fill out questionnaires or checklists and then share the results with the group. For example, the leader could give group members the list of characteristics of mature and immature groups and ask them to rate the maturity of the group on each characteristic. As with other confrontations, the leader sets the ground rules for constructive rather than destructive feedback if needed.

The leader can also challenge the group to face the reality that it is coming to an end. The group can be encouraged to recognize and validate members' contributions to the process and to the achievement of goals. Some expression of appreciation of the group's efforts and a celebration of the group's accomplishments are important so that members can leave the group with some satisfaction from having completed what they and their fellow group members set out to do.

**EXAMPLE** With the acceptance of their proposal by the school board, the school health committee had met its primary objective:

*All seven members of the committee gathered after the school board meeting and a reporter took a picture for the local newspaper. They decided to celebrate their success by meeting for lunch at a favorite restaurant.*

*Over lunch the next day, committee members reminisced about all the meetings they had had and the work they had done. The newer members expressed surprise over the difficulties the committee had in getting started. One of the parents from the original group said to the coordinator, "You seemed to think we were out to get you at first." The coordinator responded, "Yes, it did seem that way. None of you realized how little money we had to work with. I thought I was doing the best I could." The other parents agreed and shared how angry they had felt about the poor health services and how their feelings changed as they began to work on ways to improve the services offered.*

*At the end of lunch, one of the newer members expressed some regret that the committee would no longer meet. "We could meet once in a while to check on the progress of the proposal," said this parent. "No, it's up to the school board now. It's our job as individual citizens and parents to check their progress," said the parent who had been the informal leader of the group. The others agreed somewhat reluctantly, congratulated each other on a job well done, and left the restaurant.*

## Different Perspectives on Group Stages

The linearity of this sequence troubles some theorists. Some prefer to describe groups as moving along a spiraling path from initiation to completion. When a suggestion is accepted by the group, it becomes an anchor point from which the group can reach for new ideas, test them, and, if they are accepted, make them the new anchor point, and so on as illustrated in Figure 5–1. The process is both progressive and cumulative, with modifications and remodifications continuing to completion of the task (Fisher & Ellis, 1990). Other theorists believe that groups go through more or somewhat different stages than those already described. Still others are more concerned about the assumption that a group moves forward only when its conflicts are resolved. Instead, they prefer

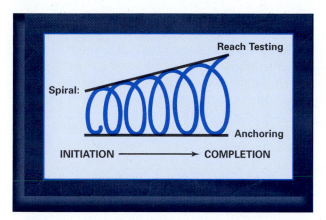

**Figure 5–1** Alternative models of group development. *Source:* Adapted from Fisher, B.A. & Ellis, D.G. (1990). *Small group decision making: Communication and the group process.* New York: McGraw-Hill, with permission, using data from Tuckman (1977) and Lacoursier (1980).

---

**Box 5–2   Seven Dimensions of Group Process**

Authority Relationships
Caretaking Functions
External and Internal Communications
Management of Conflict
Management of Intimacy
Provision of Security
Getting the Work Done

*Source:* Adapted from McCollom, M. (1990). Group formation: Boundaries, leadership, and culture. In J. Gillette & M. McCollom (Eds.). *Groups in Context: A New Perspective to Social Identity.* Reading, MA: Addison-Wesley. Used with permission.

---

to define progress as a willingness to work on these conflicts (Keyton, 1999).

An additional concern is that frankness, openness, and honesty are not necessarily risk-free actions. In organizations where such risks are a reality, the leader needs to carefully consider the consequences of frank discussions that are repeated outside the group. Despite these valid concerns, the forming-storming-norming-performing-adjourning sequence is easy to learn and is still useful if you keep its limitations in mind.

## DIMENSIONS OF GROUP PROCESS

As you can see, a number of different processes occur simultaneously within any work group or team. Another approach to analyzing a work group's dynamics at any stage of development is to look at the way it handles each of the following (McCollom, 1990):

- *Authority relationships.* Are member relations collegial? Or does the group defer to those with the greatest power and authority?
- *Caretaking functions.* How does the group meet the needs of its members? Does it provide for its members' comfort and convenience or does it leave them uncomfortable and inconvenienced?

- *External and internal communication.* How is the exchange of information within the group and with other groups maintained and controlled? Does communication flow freely or is it stilted, guarded, or rigidly controlled?
- *Management of conflict.* Is conflict avoided? Is it dealt with openly? Can group members disagree without retaliation?
- *Management of intimacy.* Does the group encourage the development of close, collaborative, positive relationships among its members and between members and the group itself? Does it prevent or punish closeness and personal revelation? (Gillette, 1990)
- *Provision of security.* How does the group handle anxiety? Does it protect its members from internal or external retribution or does it expose them to it?
- *Getting the work done.* Does the group complete its work efficiently and effectively? Does it emphasize task over relationship, or vice versa? (See Box 5–2.)

## HIDDEN AGENDAS

As they form and begin to operate, working groups develop purposes for meeting. These purposes are called the public, or official, agenda. Below the surface, however, other goals may be operating that influence the group process even though they are not openly acknowledged. These unannounced, underlying goals are called the hidden agenda (Bradford, 1978). Unless called to the group's attention, hidden agendas usually continue to operate below the surface of the group's awareness.

Despite the fact that their existence is not recognized, hidden agendas can be strongly felt by group members and can greatly influence the outcome of the group process. The following is an example:

*A task force was formed to develop a peer review procedure for a community health agency. However, the staff members appointed to the task force found peer review threatening. As a result of these feelings, a hidden agenda of avoiding the implementation of peer review developed and operated below the surface of this group.*

*While this hidden agenda operated, the task force employed an astonishing variety of delay tactics in the course of its discussion of peer review. At the end of an entire year of meetings, the task force was still unable to find or develop a working definition of peer review that satisfied everyone in the group.*

Either the leader of this group or the manager who created the task force should have intervened long before a year had passed. Nonproductive hidden agendas can prevent a group from making any progress at all if they are not dealt with in some way.

## Sources

An individual group member, several group members together, the leader, or the group as a whole can have a hidden agenda. Sometimes people are aware of having a hidden agenda, but more often it is outside the awareness even of those who are its source.

Some hidden agendas arise from individual needs that are not met within the group. For example, individual group members may feel that their position in the organization is threatened by something that is happening in the group.

Preconceived ideas about how the group should function are a common source of hidden agendas. For example, people may come to the group with a ready-made solution to the problem the group is trying to solve. Their hidden agenda would be to convince the group to accept their solution and to block acceptance of any other solution.

A similar kind of hidden agenda occurs when one or more group members have a special interest or a strong loyalty to another group. Either of these can influence behavior in the group. For example:

*Two nurses were appointed to an interdisciplinary committee that was responsible for screening research studies proposed in their institution. Both worked on the unstated goal (hidden agenda) of assuring that all proposals submitted by nurses would be approved.*

Leaders may also bring hidden agendas to the group. They too have individual needs and conflicting loyalties. More often, they find themselves wanting to present the group with ready-made solutions. Even if they resist the temptation to share their solution with the group, it can be difficult to keep it from operating as a hidden agenda. Some enjoy being dominant or having others dependent on them and unwittingly encourage dependence, even though they say publicly that they want group members to be independent and assertive.

Groups often give lip service to a goal that they do not genuinely accept. This lack of acceptance may be due to the fact that the goal was imposed on the group by the leader or by an outside authority; the group may have chosen a goal that sounded good, but really was not important; or the group may be working on a goal that is no longer relevant to it.

Another kind of hidden agenda found in groups is the unspoken agreement to behave in a certain way. You may recall that immature groups frequently have an unspoken agreement that members will be polite and nonconfrontational. This "rule" is not discussed, but it is understood by group members. Groups may also have an unspoken agreement to ignore certain behaviors (such as the acting out of a particular member), or they may agree to attack certain behaviors.

Another hidden agenda in groups may be to avoid discussing certain subjects. Ross and Roberts (1999) call these hidden agendas "sleeping dogs." Most groups or teams have three types of concerns:

- "Barking Dogs": important, urgent concerns that are readily discussed by the group
- "Nonbarking Dogs": also important but not urgent
- "Sleeping Dogs": the undiscussable issues, concerns that no one is willing to raise but need to be raised

These undiscussable "sleeping dogs" should not be allowed to continue to sleep (Ross & Roberts, 1999).

### Leader Response

The first and most important leader action is to recognize the existence of a hidden agenda. Once identified, the leader must then decide how to deal with it. Hidden agendas are not entirely negative. Some of them reflect attempts to meet real needs that have been ignored in the public agenda. When these situations exist, finding a more direct way to meet these needs is generally preferable to confronting the individual or group about the hidden agenda. When the hidden agenda seems to reflect the real goals of the group or to be a sign that the group cannot or will not work on the publicly stated goal, an open discussion of both public and hidden goals is usually appropriate.

The leader needs to judge how much confrontation the group is ready to handle. A mature group accustomed to evaluating its own processes would be able to handle a confrontation about the hidden agenda. However, making a direct statement that a hidden agenda is operating is likely to provoke a defensive response even from a mature group. A more acceptable form of confrontation would be to present the information without interpretation. For example, if the group is avoiding dealing with staffing changes that have to be made, you could say either of the following:

> *"We have been talking more about problems on units than about the coming staffing changes."*
>
> *"What kinds of problems do you think these staffing changes will cause on your units?"*

You will also find that it is helpful to recognize the legitimacy of the needs or problems reflected by the hidden agendas and to avoid implying that anyone should feel bad or guilty about their existence. The achievement of congruent, acceptable goals can have a dramatic effect on the group's ability to progress toward maturity and work on fulfilling its objectives.

## ● DYSFUNCTIONAL GROUP INTERACTIONS

The power of a group's dynamics is rarely felt so keenly as when it turns ugly. A group's interactions may develop into one of several destructive patterns. In their mildest forms, they are simply another challenge to one's leadership. In their most virulent form, however, they can be harmful and require an all-out effort to eradicate them.

### Social Loafing

One of the positive aspects of working in small groups is the synergic effect that results from sharing enthusiasm and energy. Responsibility is also shared among group members. The downside is that it can reduce the amount of responsibility each individual feels. It also makes it more difficult for the manager to identify the individuals responsible when work is not done. Some evidence indicates that individual effort decreases as the size of the group increases (Hogg, 1992). Inaction may seem to be a safe alternative, especially to group members with little motivation or with some anxiety regarding the outcome of planned action.

A positive leader response to the intrusion of social loafing into a work group is to make the work itself appear challenging and attractive. Encouraging friendly competition with other groups is also helpful. In particular, the leader-manager needs to foster norms that support hard work and high productivity.

### Groupthink

Groupthink is an interesting but potentially dangerous phenomenon that occurs when group members either abandon or suppress their own views, and uncritically accept the prevailing attitude or over-identify with either the leader or the group. Groupthink is not dangerous when a group makes a noncritical decision such its next meeting place or the annual picnic. It is dangerous, however, when the group is making a decision about life-or-death matters in patient care. Groupthink can, for example, lead to failure to recognize a serious deficiency in operating room procedures or failure to recognize the patient's best interests in making a decision about terminating life support.

Prevention of groupthink may be the best intervention. Promotion of a collegial environment, support of people who dare to disagree, and encouragement of critically reflective thinking are all preventive measures. Once groupthink occurs, the leader may have to challenge the dominant decision makers and the group's norms regarding acceptance of their opinions.

## Polarization

Like groupthink, polarization is a symptom of deficient group decision making. It occurs when the group makes a decision that is more extreme than the initial opinions of its members (Fisher & Ellis, 1990). It is most likely to happen when the group becomes incensed about a particular issue or when dominant members pressure the remainder to support their extreme position.

As with groupthink, supporting the person who disagrees, encouraging critical analysis, and challenging the extreme position may be necessary to reduce the polarization that has occurred.

## Scapegoating

Scapegoating represents a particularly cruel behavior because the group singles out one individual on whom all its guilt, anger, and hostility are poured (Wells, 1990). It begins with an enormous sense of frustration or futility on the part of the group, usually over a situation the groups feels helpless to improve. Instead of constructive criticism, the group chooses (perhaps unconsciously as well as irrationally) someone to blame. Often, the target is someone who stands out in some way, the silent one in an otherwise noisy group or

the opinionated one who continually attracts attention to himself or herself. The group then isolates this person, destroys him or her, and ejects him or her from the group. The final phase is denial: group members deny that they created a scapegoat and further deny that they had any responsibility whatsoever for their failure to improve the situation. For example:

*A local interdenominational organization wanted to expand their community service program. While discussing their options, one group member, Ms. B., said she knew of a group that had started a feeding program for the homeless. "That's what we should do," exclaimed the group leader. Group members joined in and unanimously selected Ms. B. to run the program over her protests that she did not have time and did not know the first thing about running a feeding program.*

*Despite her protests, Ms. B. did a fine job organizing the program. It was an immediate success. They were soon feeding 150 people a day, many of them homeless families with small children. Ms. B. wanted the group to hire a program administrator, but they said, "No, you are doing a fine job. Keep up the good work. We can use the money to feed more people."*

*The program became too successful. The number fed daily jumped from 150 to 250. Some of the people began to hang around the building after the meal. Soon they brought their few belongings and slept under the awnings or under the trees. Group members began to complain about the "derelicts" hanging around their building. Neighbors complained about spillover onto their lawns and driveways. The city threatened fines if the group did not keep its beneficiaries off the neighbors' property.*

*Group members were furious. At their next meeting, they insisted that Ms. B. control the homeless, keep their number to under 100, and get them to leave as soon as they ate. "I can't do that," she protested. "Then resign your position. Clearly, you cannot handle this responsibility." "I never wanted it in the first place. I've devoted all my time to it. I've taken time off from work to run your program," protested Ms. B. Did the group express its appreciation of Ms. B.? No, they voted to censure her and to close down the feeding program. The publicly stated reason they gave was that they were unable to find a capable administrator. Ms. B. left the group. The group used the remainder of the considerable amount of money that had been set aside for the feeding program to redecorate the meeting rooms in their building.*

Another viewpoint on the importance of treating every member of the team well is illustrated in Perspectives . . . Respect.

---

## PERSPECTIVES . . .

### Respect

Every member of every working group or team, no matter how high or low they are in the organizational hierarchy, desires recognition and respect.

Noel Tichy (1997) tells the story of Phil Myers, a former janitor. Myers says he knows what it feels like to be ignored so he makes a point of recognizing every employee as he passes them in the hallway because it makes them feel valued. He also defends them ferociously if anyone treats them badly. For example, he stormed into the office of the surgery department director and threatened to pull his 21 employees out because the director had used "foul language" and "talked to them like dogs." "If you've got a problem, you yell at me," he said. "Don't yell at them. No one deserves to be talked to that way" (p. 136).

Consider the effect that this type of attention to recognition and respect would have on team morale.

---

*Source:* Tichy, N.M. (1997). *The leadership engine: How winning companies build leaders at every level.* New York: HarperCollins.

---

## ● TEAM BUILDING

To be considered a team, a work group must have some stability of membership and a common purpose. The people who are members of an effective team work interdependently, as in-

terrelated parts of the whole. People who work independently of each other, with little communication, coordination, or shared responsibility, are not working as a team.

Effective teams do not just happen. Many people are simply not well prepared to function as part of a team. Some of the problems that occur within teams are due to lack of understanding of team processes (Holbeche, 1998). See Box 5–3 for a list of reasons why teams fail. In this section, leader actions to build a team into an effective functioning unit are explained.

*Many teams fall into the trap of operating like totalitarian regimes, which demand conformity rather than spirited dialogue and debate, forcing individuals to abide by "group norms" and policing deviant members who threaten to rock the boat.*
—Purser & Cabana, 1999, p. 35

### Select Team Members

The composition of the team is critical to its success. Although you may not be free to choose the people who are on your team, you will often have an opportunity to influence the selection. Ability to contribute to both the task and to the relationship aspects of team functioning is important. Neither one alone is sufficient. Technical or professional competence is the primary consideration for the task aspect. Ability to work well in collaboration with others and to communicate effectively are primary considerations for the relationship aspect. Don't select team members on the basis of friendship or family relationship, however tempting that might be (Frigon & Jackson, 1996).

A third consideration in selecting team members is an appropriate mix of skills on the team. For example, some nurses are especially good at responding quickly but calmly in emergencies, whereas others have more skill in gaining the trust of a new client. Or you might find that your team needs a bilingual member in order to communicate more effectively with some of the clients served by the team. Some stability of membership is important in maintaining the team. If too many team members are lost, it becomes a new team and further team building must be done (Cound, 1992).

## Set Goals

The need to clearly define your purpose is a component of effective leadership and a common theme throughout this book. Many teams are formed with only the vaguest idea of what they are actually expected to do. In fact, teams are often formed to deal with a problem that has not been effectively handled in the past and for which no solution has yet been found. Unfortunately, the group's purpose is often not clearly spelled out and the team flounders, trying to resolve the problem before it has been analyzed and the solution has been worked out.

Even when the purpose is self-evident, as would be the case with a surgical team or a home care team, a lack of agreement on specific objectives of the team or on the way the team is expected to meet these objectives hampers the group's efforts. The following is an example:

*The home care team has obviously been formed to provide health care in the client's home. However, many questions about carrying out the team's objectives arose when it was first formed. Is the purpose of the home visit to enable the person to stay in the home rather than be hospitalized or is it to encourage hospitalization for a serious illness? Will the team meet only physical needs or will it also provide psychosocial support and counseling? Will the team help a client with housework and repairs, or make referrals to meet these needs, or not deal with these needs at all?*

You can imagine the inefficiency and potential for conflicts that will result if these questions are not answered before the team begins to provide home care.

## Define Roles

As with the purpose and objectives of the team, the roles of individual team members are often not clearly defined. This ambiguity can lead to conflicts, especially on an interdisciplinary team, which provides even more opportunities for misunderstandings about others' roles than does a single-discipline team.

Role clarification is essential to smooth team function. Definition of roles is related to the purpose and objectives of the team. For example:

> *A question arose at a planning meeting for the home care team: Will the physician and dentist on the team visit people in their homes or will the team's clients have to travel to the hospital for medical and dental care? Because most physicians and dentists do not make home visits, some team members assumed that their clients would travel to the hospital for these services. However, if an objective is to reduce the necessity of travel as much as possible for their home-bound clients, then the physician and dentist should also be expected to provide as many of their services in the home as possible.*

It is difficult to overstate the importance of clarifying such role expectations. Conflicts over differing expectations can immobilize a team and even contribute to its demise.

Even when the team's objectives are clearly spelled out, role negotiation among team members may be necessary if more than one team member can and wants to do a specific task or fill a certain role. Many overlaps exist between the functions of people in different healthcare professions. Nurses, social workers, psychologists, psychiatrists, and chaplains may all see themselves as counselors or group therapists. Physicians, physicians' assistants, pharmacists, and nurses are all likely to consider themselves prepared to develop and dispense information about medications to their patients. When this type of situation occurs, a decision must be made whether to share the task, divide it, or designate who will do it. This decision needs to be made in such a way that it does not become a power struggle and that each person's ability is recognized and fully utilized by the team.

## Develop Team Identity and Cohesiveness

The team needs to develop both a sense of itself as a functioning whole and cohesion so that its members will engage in the sharing and support functions of the team. The leader can take a number of actions right from the formation of the team to build identity and cohesion.

### Definition

The team first needs to be defined. The more team members know about their team and its functions, the more they can identify with the team. They need to know who is and who is not a member of the team. If the team has not been given a name, you can do it or encourage team members to come up with a name that reflects the purpose of the team. Using "we" to refer to team members and yourself emphasizes the team as a functioning whole.

### Territory

A new team needs to stake out its territory; an established team holds and often expands its territory. This territory is not only geographic but also functional and psychological.

The influence of geography on a team should not be underestimated. The team needs a place to meet, one that is sufficiently quiet, comfortable, and private so that team matters can be discussed freely. Also, if the work spaces of team members (offices, examining rooms, or patient rooms) are physically close together, more opportunities for informal exchanges can occur during the course of the workday.

The team needs to acquire a functional and psychological space as well, and other healthcare providers must also recognize and accept the functions and purposes of the team. To develop and maintain its identity and cohesiveness, a team needs people outside itself to respect its territory. Here is an example:

> *If you were the director of staff education, you would want your team (department) to be involved in the development of all the educational programs given within your organization. You would not necessarily insist that members of your team actually conduct every program or seminar, but if you are to hold on to your territory, you would want all of them to be coordinated through your department.*

## Connections

Cohesiveness is also built by increasing the number of connections (links) among the team members. Simply holding team meetings increases these connections. In a truly cohesive team, the whole team shares a sense of accomplishment when one member achieves success (Glaser, 1994).

A leader can carry out this linking function in many other ways. For example, whenever something exciting happens, the leader can make sure the experience is shared with the rest of the team. When someone on the team needs help solving a problem or getting work done on time, the leader can ask another team member to offer help. When a job is done well by the team, the leader can point out how cooperation between team members contributed to its successful completion. Each of these actions builds positive connections among team members and increases team cohesiveness.

> *The really successful teams we have seen have almost all been marked by a sincere spirit of wanting the best for one another.*
>
> —*Robbins & Finley, 1995*

## Esprit de Corps

Esprit de corps is a shared feeling of enthusiasm that characterizes the team as a whole. The leader's own energy and enthusiasm can suffuse the entire team. Setting some worthwhile but fairly easy goals helps to develop an esprit de corps. Success increases the team's motivation. Even failure can be used by the resourceful leader to show how team members need to work together in order to overcome the failure in line with that famous saying "We must hang together or we will all hang separately." Competition between teams can be used the same way. Remember that team members may not have been given a choice as to whether they would join your team. For those who would have preferred not to, it's not surprising if they join the team with some negative attitudes (Brown & Neal, 1997).

## Guide Decision Making

The different ways in which decisions are made by a group include default, authority, minority, majority vote, consensus, and unanimous consent (Schein, 1969).

## Default

Decision by default is the result of a group's failure to reach a decision. Silence or lack of response from the team is taken to mean consent.

An idea is proposed to the group. When no opposition to the idea is expressed, it is assumed that everyone accepts it. This assumption is often false—team members may actually be strongly opposed to the idea but, for some reason, have not expressed their opinion. It is usually a sign of withdrawal or apathy on the part of team members and a symptom of serious problems in team relationships. A team in which people feel restrained from speaking or are too apathetic to speak cannot function effectively.

## Authority

A decision by authority is made by a single person who has some authority, usually the leader. This method is faster than having the whole team make the decision but fails to use the expertise of other team members in making the decision. It also fails to encourage the professional growth of individual team members or the maturing of the team as a group. It may reduce the team's motivation to carry out the decision.

Sometimes, however, decision by authority is the most appropriate method. In an emergency situation, for example, the speed and accuracy with which the decision is made is more important than either the team's growth or motivation. Also, some administrative decisions, such as the firing of an employee, are more appropriately done by someone in authority rather than by a team.

## Minority

Decisions made by a minority are those made by a small number of people on the team, usually a dominant subgroup. This kind of decision making occurs when the rest of the team either feels powerless to oppose the subgroup or has succumbed to withdrawal, passivity, and apathy. When a decision is "railroaded" this way by a small number of people, it is often resented by the rest of the group. An effective leader or manager tries to prevent this from happening.

On some occasions the team may decide to designate a subgroup to make certain decisions. Subgroup decisions would be appropriate when only the people in the subgroup are affected by the decisions or they are the only ones with sufficient information to make the decision. However, when the decision affects the whole team it is preferable to at least present a summary of the information with recommendations to the whole team and ask for a final decision.

## Majority Vote

Decisions made by taking a poll of the entire team are acceptable to most people. Voting has the advantage of soliciting everyone's opinion on an issue and of recognizing the desire of the majority of the group. However, it may leave the minority who voted for the losing side feeling dissatisfied even though they usually accept the decision.

Although voting has the advantage of fairness, it sets up a win-lose situation in which the majority wins but the minority loses. It can lead to some serious battles to gain the majority vote, which can be divisive if opponents begin attacking each other. Voting is appropriate in a large group where it is difficult to give everyone a chance to speak on every issue or in an immature group that is not ready to come to a consensus on an issue.

## Consensus

Decisions made by consensus are those in which the team seeks to gain every member's agreement on an issue. Decision by consensus is based on a prior understanding that everyone will go along with the final decision even if they are not completely satisfied with it. Members of a mature group are willing to participate in consensus building because it is also understood that the team will attempt to resolve any differences of opinion in order to come as close as possible to a decision that satisfies every team member.

Decision by consensus recognizes both the right to disagree and the necessity of having some basic agreements in order to work well together. It avoids setting up a win-lose situation and makes the achievement of a win-win situation possible. True consensus decisions demand that all members be willing to openly express their opinion and to negotiate their position when disagreement exists. To achieve this on a difficult issue requires substantial maturity on the part of the group.

## Unanimous Consent

Unanimous consent is the genuine agreement of every team member on an issue. Although usually a sign of a mature group, it can be achieved on less controversial questions even by immature groups. However, when unanimous consent is reached too easily, the agreement may be a superficial one concealing underlying disagreement. For this reason, the leader should test the unanimity of a decision. Unanimity is not always possible on an issue. It is preferable to agree to disagree and to try to resolve these differences enough to work together rather than to press for unanimous consent and force team members into hiding their disagreement.

## Selection of a Decision-Making Mode

Although each of these six ways to reach a decision are used by teams, some are more appropriate than others. Consensus and unanimity on a difficult issue require more maturity than voting does. Decisions by authority may be necessary, but decisions by default should be avoided as much as possible. Minority decisions are occasionally appropriate but often cause problems when the decision affects the team as a whole.

The type of decision, maturity of the group, and the effect on the team of the particular mode of decision making should be considered when guiding your team in regard to their choice of decision-making method. Most teams will not actually discuss their choice of decision-making method unless the leader brings up the subject, so you will probably have to initiate the discussion when a decision is about to be made rather than wait to be asked about it.

# Influence Group Norms

Norms are those unwritten rules that prescribe acceptable behavior in the group. Because they are often unspoken, these norms can develop in a team virtually unnoticed, yet their influence on what happens within the group is significant. Norms that support creativity and flexibility rather than rigidity and resistance affect the way the team responds to a new assignment. Norms supporting open communication rather than the suppression of feelings and disagreements affect the way conflicts are handled. Norms can support arriving at work on time, working at a steady pace, and getting finished on time, or they can support arriving late, doing the least amount of work possible, and leaving early.

Once a norm is established within the group, it can be difficult to change. The following is an example:

*When the IV team was first established, team members often finished their work early and were allowed to leave at 3 o'clock although their workday actually ended at 3:30. Over the next year their workload increased gradually, but team members were still able to finish by 3 o'clock. The team coordinator usually stayed until 3:30 to provide coverage until the evening shift came in and thought that the team would appreciate his allowing them to leave early. He had not verbalized any of his thoughts to the team.*

*The team's work increased more rapidly the next winter and team members worked harder to be finished by 3 o'clock. One Friday, the team had a particularly heavy workload and twice the usual number of emergency calls. By 3 o'clock, the emergencies were over but much of the routine work had not been finished. When team members began putting on their coats at 2:55, the coordinator asked them what they were doing. They responded that it was time for them to leave. The coordinator pointed out that there was a lot of work left, and a team member said, "Well, you usually do the leftover work because you work later than we do." The coordinator told them it was too much for one person to finish and that they would have to stay. The same team member said, "Sorry, but we leave at three," and the entire team walked out, leaving an angry coordinator with several hours of work to complete because the evening shift team was a small group that could barely handle its own work.*

In this example, the norm had developed to the point that team members actually believed they had the right to leave at 3 o'clock and felt that the coordinator's request was unreasonable. As you can imagine, a great deal of tension existed between the coordinator and the team the following week until the differences in expectations were clarified and the norm was changed.

The leader who is alert to the development of norms within the team can reinforce those norms that support effective working relationships and challenge those that would reduce effectiveness, preferably before the latter become well established. Effective norms are supported by pointing out their positive effects, by encouraging and rewarding their use, and by role modeling them. If these actions fail to change an established norm that is interfering with team function, stronger measures, including confrontation, negotiation, and change strategies, would be needed to modify the troublesome norm.

## Encourage Frequent and Open Communication

Busy people often neglect the communication aspects of team building (Bolton et al., 1993). A lack of communication greatly increases the likelihood of failure within the team. Open communication is essential to the development of effective working relationships within the team and with outside groups. It leads to the kind of understanding that promotes positive relationships and is the means by which purposes and objectives are clarified, roles defined and negotiated, conflicts dealt with, and decisions made.

> *. . . we are mistaken if we regard relationship building as something separate from our real work instead of recognizing that it provides the means by which we can get more and better things done.*
> —Napolitano & Henderson, 1998, p. 97

Well-run team meetings are worth every minute spent on them because they can prevent so many misunderstandings, duplication of effort, and omission of important tasks. Rounds are an-

### Research Example 5–1    *Characteristics of Troubled Work Groups*

Seago surveyed 115 members of the Association of Nurse Executives (AONE) and ONE-California during their meetings in 1995. She asked respondents to check off characteristics of troubled work groups from a list of 25 descriptors. Respondents could add descriptors if they wished and were also asked about the strategies they used to manage a troubled or conflicted work group.

The most frequently checked characteristics were: poor attitudes, a high level of anger, difficulty with change, stressful environment, reputation for "eating their young," and a complex and/or heavy work load. Some of the terms respondents used to describe members of these troubled work groups were rebellious, judgmental, subversive. Team leaders or managers were described as inconsistent and unclear on goals. The strategies suggested for managing a troubled work group included improved communication, increased staff governance, and setting clear expectations.

The researcher commented that less emphasis on poor leadership or high absenteeism than had been expected was observed and that the strategies suggested were hardly novel but had been repeated often in the literature.

*Source:* Seago, J.A. (1996). Culture of troubled work groups. *Journal of Nursing Administration, 26*(9), 41–46.

other effective way to exchange information, develop mutually agreed upon goals with patients, and plan and evaluate care. Interdisciplinary rounds can also reduce the rigidity of hierarchical relationships across disciplines and ranks (McHugh et al., 1996) and thereby contribute to the development of effective interdisciplinary teams.

Written communications are also important, especially when team members are not in frequent personal contact with each other. They need to be direct, clear, concise, and free of jargon and abbreviations likely to be misunderstood by people with different backgrounds, education, and experience. If written communications are to serve any purpose, they must also be read by other team members, which you cannot assume will happen.

### Manage Conflicts

Conflicts within a team are inevitable and even necessary sometimes. As a general rule, conflict is neither to be avoided nor stimulated, but managed. Too much conflict or unresolved conflicts reduce the team's effectiveness and eventually immobilize the team. On the other hand, suppressed conflict continues to grow underground and is more difficult to resolve when it eventually surfaces because people have had time to harden their position on issues and to become increasingly bitter or angry about the continuing conflict. The following is an example of the way in which a team leader handled a team problem through a relatively mild confrontation.

> *"A couple of people have told me that some team members are taking long breaks," said the leader to the team.*
>
> *"It's important that everyone comes back from breaks on time so that others can take their breaks," said a team member.*
>
> *"Yeah, that's only fair," added another team member.*
>
> *The team leader noticed several heads nodding in agreement. "Ok, let's all work on getting back from our breaks on time. I know it's hard sometimes but we all have to get our work done." (Adapted from Barker, 1999, p. 142)*

Too many confrontations at once can overstress team members, so it is sometimes necessary to wait until the most immediate problems are taken care of, restoring energy to deal with the remaining conflicts. (See Research Example 5–1 related to conflicted work groups.)

### Communication with Other Teams

Although the focus has been on what happens within the team, teams operate within a given environment and have to deal with other individuals and groups within that environment. Relationships between teams can be cooperative and productive, or they can be full of conflict, even hostile. Teams often have overlapping areas of responsibility, a frequent source of conflict. When concerns are discussed openly, the potential for understanding each other and developing cordial working relationships is increased. The team needs to know what type of work is being done by other teams to prevent the problems of duplication of effort and working at cross-purposes, both of which are even more likely to occur between teams than within a single team. Teams with similar or overlapping functions can be widely separated and isolated from each other, so the leader may have to plan meetings between the teams. Stronger measures may also be necessary when conflicts with other teams arise. See Perspectives . . . When Teamwork Failed for some additional reasons why teams fail.

## ADVANTAGES OF TEAMWORK

Using teams presents a number of challenges as well as benefits (Francis & Young, 1979; Parker, 1972; Wise et al., 1974). Although some people prefer to work independently rather than interdependently, many types of health care can be delivered effectively only by well-functioning teams. The following are some of the advantages of using teamwork.

- *Best use of skills.* When people with complementary skills are brought together on a team, each is able to contribute his or her own special skill, experience, and viewpoint to the task at hand. With the right combination of skills, a highly functional team can manage more complex situations, provide more comprehensive care, and produce more creative ideas than any individual could alone. Teams also allow greater use of paraprofessionals by providing close supervision from the professionals on the team.
- *Coordination.* Teamwork demands that team members communicate with one another about the work they are doing. It reduces duplication of effort and the possibility that people are

working at cross-purposes. For example, clients who receive uncoordinated health care may be

## PERSPECTIVES . . .

### When Teamwork Failed

Concerns about cost, the monotony of the work, and the incidence of repetitive-stress injuries that resulted from doing a single task all day such as setting in pockets or stitching belt loops led jeans maker Levi Strauss to introduce teams into their factories across the United States. Under the old system, a factory worker was paid on the basis of the number of pieces he or she completed. Under the new system, empowered teams of 10 to 35 employees were paid on the basis of the total number of jeans finished by the team as a whole.

What happened when the team approach was implemented? Efficiency plummeted. A pair of jeans that had cost $4.00 to assemble under the old system now cost $7.50 to assemble. Morale plummeted as well. Fights broke out. Shouting became commonplace and friendships were destroyed. Team members even started checking the amount of time a coworker took to use the bathroom or visit the nurse's station. They were described as "merciless" with injured coworkers. Output decreased.

Why did the new system fail? Employees had been prepared with team-building and problem-solving seminars as well as cross-training on unfamiliar machines. But many felt they needed to know more about managing work flow and dealing with work quality problems. Team members who worked faster than others felt cheated when their paychecks were smaller as a result of having slower coworkers on their team. This dissatisfaction led to acrimonious exchanges, intense peer pressure, even expulsion of slower or injured members by their teams. Supervisors were not prepared to implement or deal with the new system successfully or to respond effectively to challenges to their authority. Many improvised; others abdicated.

One factory worker summed up the general feeling about the new team-based system neatly: "I hate teams."

*Source:* King, R.T. (1998, May 20). Levi's factory workers are assigned to teams, and morale takes a hit. *Wall Street Journal.*

given conflicting advice from their caregivers: one advises more rest, another advises more exercise, and clients do not know what to do.

- *Synergy.* Combining energies to complete a task has a synergic effect in which each team member stimulates and reinforces the others. This synergy contributes to the development of a highly motivated group of people committed to producing high-quality work.
- *Flexibility.* With its combination of talents and skills a team is able to handle a greater variety of situations competently. Team members are also able to help one another and to substitute for each other in an emergency so that the team is more flexible and responsive than individual workers can be.
- *Support.* Team members can also provide emotional support for each other. Effective teams can help manage the stresses and tensions that build up in many healthcare situations. Teams are also a source of collective strength, supplying a small power base and political support when needed.
- *Increased commitment.* When team members have been involved in setting the team's objectives and deciding how they will be met, they are usually more committed to the successful completion of these objectives. Team synergy and support reinforce this commitment.
- *Evaluative feedback.* When people work together on a team, the quality of their performance is more apparent and fellow team members can serve as valuable sources of feedback.
- *Opportunity for growth.* In addition to being a valuable source of feedback, the team provides other opportunities for growth. Because people work more closely together and share more of their experience with other team members, team members can expand their knowledge and skills in areas outside their specialities.

## ● DISADVANTAGES OF TEAMWORK

Many of the advantages of teamwork occur only when the team functions well. Likewise, many, though not all, of the disadvantages arise primarily when the team functions poorly. Many people are simply not well prepared to function as part of a team. Some of the problems that occur within teams are due to lack of understanding of team processes (Holbeche, 1998).

- *Demands interpersonal skills.* People often assume that you can simply put people together and they will function as a team. Of course, it does not happen quite so simply. Effective teamwork requires a considerable amount of interpersonal skill from team members as well as the leader. Without these skills, teamwork can be frustrating, discouraging, and energy-consuming. Also, people who prefer to work by themselves may find the continued interaction and demands for sharing among team members quite wearying.

*We are by nature a tribal people.*
—L. Ellerbee in Eigen & Siegel, 1989, p. 468

*I don't like to work in a group. I don't get along well with other people.*
—J. Breslin, in Eigen & Siegel, 1989, p. 467

- *Conflicts.* Differences in personality, culture, professional experience, norms, education, skills, status, and pay are all potential sources of conflict among team members. If you consider the fact that many healthcare teams work together 8 hours a day, you can see why tensions and conflicts can build up to an intolerable level if not dealt with effectively.
- *Time demands.* Even the most ardent supporters of participative management cannot claim that it is the fastest way to make decisions. An autocratic leader can make an immediate decision and communicate it to the group. It takes more time to bring team members together and ask for their input.
- *Reduced autonomy.* The person who values independence and autonomy over opportunities for feedback, support, and sharing of experiences may feel a sense of loss when assigned to a team. Some caregivers find it difficult to "share" their clients with others and prefer to think of themselves as able to provide all the care needed. Others find it difficult to compromise or to go along with the team's decision when it is not in agreement with their own opinion.

> *Teamwork is consciously espoused but unwittingly shunned by most people in business because they are deathly afraid of it. They think it will render them anonymous, invisible.*
>
> —S. Blotnick in Eigen & Siegel, 1989, pp. 466–467

- *Conformity.* An overly cohesive, authoritarian group may pressure its members to adhere to group norms. This rigidity can have serious consequences when complex healthcare demands flexibility and a great deal of professional judgment.
- *Increased scrutiny.* A person who works alone can hide mistakes and inadequacies better than the person who works on a team. Being put in a position where these flaws will be revealed can be threatening to many people, especially to professionals who feel they should be perfect.
- *Diffusion of responsibility.* Because of the differences and uniqueness of each team member, teamwork demands flexibility and tolerance about the way work will be done by different team members. This variety of individual styles can frustrate people who have a great need for structure and predictability. Also, when responsibility for patient care outcomes is shared by

all team members, each member has to be able to trust the skill and judgment of other team members.

For most members of the healthcare professions, work is increasingly being done by teams. The ability to work with a wide variety of people as part of a team is an essential skill for the nurse leader-manager.

## SUMMARY

A group is an open system consisting of three or more people joined together by either physical proximity, a shared purpose, a special meaning, or a combination of these common bonds. As open systems, groups have their own characteristics and identifiable patterns, are open to and exchange energy with their environments, and may grow and evolve over time.

The evolution of a group can be divided into five stages: forming, storming, norming, performing, and adjourning. Each of these stages has a characteristic emotional climate, group behaviors, and specific group and individual developmental tasks. Different leader actions are appropriate for each of these stages. The group reaches maturity by the fourth, or performing, stage, and is a

---

### C A S E   S T U D Y

#### Women and Teams

Do women have more difficulty working as part of a team than men do? Antai-Otong (1997) claims that, because the majority of nurses today are women between the ages of 35 and 50 and have had little or no experience with team sports, they are at a distinct disadvantage when called upon to lead or participate in teams.

#### Questions for Critical Reflection and Analysis

1. What was your first response to Antai-Otong's claim? Do you think it's a commonly accepted idea?

2. Is experience in team sports helpful? In what way?
3. In what ways other than team sports can a person develop his or her team skills?
4. How would you respond to an administrator who said that he or she would never name a woman as leader of an emergency response team "because women don't know how to be team players"?

far more functional and effective system at this point than it was in the earlier stages, during which it was likely to be disorganized, inflexible, unresponsive, and uncertain of its purpose or goals. During the fifth stage, the group reaches closure by reviewing prior events, evaluating both the process and achievements, and celebrating its achievements.

Hidden agendas are unacknowledged goals that operate below the surface but exert an enormous influence on the group. Dysfunctional patterns such as social loafing, groupthink, polarization, or scapegoating may develop unless the leader intervenes.

Teams are groups of people who work together for a common purpose over a given period of time. Team members should be selected on the basis of their ability to contribute to the team. The team's purpose and objectives and team members' roles need to be clearly defined, often through negotiation. The team needs to define itself, stake out its territory, develop connections, and build a team spirit to achieve identity and cohesiveness. The leader guides the team in decision making, influences the establishment of norms, encourages effective communication, and manages the resolution of conflicts within the team and with other teams.

Advantages of teamwork include the best use of skills, improved coordination, synergy, flexibility, support for members, increased commitment, availability of evaluative feedback, and opportunities for growth. Disadvantages include the increased demand for interpersonal skills, conflicts, time demands, reduced autonomy, conformity, increased scrutiny, and diffusion of responsibility.

# REFERENCES

Antai-Otong, D. (1997). Team building in a health care setting. *American Journal of Nursing, 97*(7), 48–51.

Barker, J.R. (1999). *The discipline of teamwork.* Thousand Oaks, CA: Sage.

Bennis, W.G. & Shepard, H. (1978). A theory of group development. In L.P. Bradford (Ed.). *Group development.* La Jolla, CA: University Associates.

Berg, D.N. & Smith, K.K. (1990). Paradox and groups. In J. Gillette & M. McCollom (Eds.). *Groups in context: A new perspective on group dynamics.* Reading, MA: Addison-Wesley.

Bion, W.R. (1961). *Experiences in groups and other papers.* New York: Basic Books.

Bolton, L.B., Ayden, C., Popolow, G. & Ramseyer, J. (1993). Ten steps for managing organizational change. *Journal of Nursing Administration, 22*(6), 14–22.

Braaten, L.J. (1974–1975). Development phases of encounter groups and related intensive groups: A critical review of models and a new proposal. *Interpersonal Development, 5,* 112–129.

Bradford, L.P. (1978). *Group development.* La Jolla, CA: University Associates.

Brill, N. (1984). *Teamwork: Working together in the human services.* Philadelphia: J.B. Lippincott.

Brown, N.L. & Neal, L.J. (1997). Development of a managed-care team in a traditional home healthcare agency. *Journal of Nursing Administration, 27*(10), 43–48.

Burggraf, C.S. & Sillars, A.L. (1987). A critical examination of sex differences in marital communication. *Communication Monographs, 54*(3), 276–294.

Cound, D.M. (1992). *A leader's journey to quality.* Milwaukee: ASQC Press.

Eigen, L.D. & Siegel, J.P. (1989). *The manager's book of quotations.* New York: American Management Association.

Fisher, B.A. & Ellis, D.G. (1990). *Small group decision making: Communication and the group process.* New York: McGraw-Hill.

Francis, D. & Young, D. (1979). *Improving work groups: A practical manual for team building.* La Jolla, CA: University Associates.

Frigon, N.L. & Jackson, H.K. (1996). *The leader: Developing the skills and personal qualities you need to lead effectively.* New York: American Management Association.

Fry, R.E., Lech, B.A. & Rubin, I. (1974). Working with the primary care team: The first intervention. In H. Wise, R. Beckhard, I. Rubin & A.L. Kyte (Eds.). *Making health teams work.* Cambridge, MA: Ballinger Publishing.

Gibb, J.R. & Gibb, L.M. (1978). The group as a growing organism. In L.P. Bradford (Ed.). *Group development.* La Jolla, CA: University Associates.

Gillette, J. (1990). Intimacy in work groups: Looking from the inside out. In J. Gillette & M. McCollom (Eds.). *Groups in context: A new perspective to social identity.* Reading, MA: Addison-Wesley.

Gillette, J. & McCollom, M. (1990). *Groups in context: A new perspective on group dynamics.* Reading, MA: Addison-Wesley.

Glaser, S.R. (1994). Teamwork and communication. *Management Communication Quarterly, 7*(3), 282–296.

Glisson, C. (1986). The group versus the individual as the unit of analysis in small group research. *Social Work with Groups, 9*(13), 15–30.

Hill, B., Lippitt, L. & Serkownek, K. (1979). The emotional dimensions of the problem-solving process. *Group and Organization Studies, 4*(1), 93.

Hogg, M.A. (1992). *The social psychology of group cohesiveness: From attraction to social identity.* New York: William Morrow.

Holbeche, W. (1998). *Motivating people in lean organizations.* Oxford: Butterworth-Heinemann.

Horak, B.J., Guarino, J.H., Knight, C.C. & Kweder, S.L. (1992). Building a team on a medical floor. *Health Care Management, 16*(2), 65–71.

Howard, V.A. & Barton, J.H. (1992). *Thinking together: Making meetings work.* New York: William Morrow.

Keyton, J. (1999). Relational communication in groups. In L.R. Frey (Ed.). *The handbook of group communication theory and research.* Thousand Oaks, CA: Sage, 192–222.

King, R.T. (1998, May 20). Levi's factory workers are assigned to teams and morale takes a hit. *Wall Street Journal.*

Krebs, V. (1992). Measuring how your organization really works. *Health Forum Journal, 35*(1), 34–39.

Lacoursier, R.B. (1980). *The life cycle of groups: Group developmental stage theory.* New York: Human Sciences Press.

Ling, C. (1996). Performance of a self-directed work team in a home healthcare agency. *Journal of Nursing Administration, 29*(9), 36–40.

McCollom, M. (1990). Group formation: Boundaries, leadership, and culture. In J. Gillette & M. McCollom (Eds.). *Groups in context: A new perspective to social identity.* Reading, MA: Addison-Wesley.

McHugh, M., West, P., Assatly, C., Duprat, L., Howard, L., Neloff, J., Waldo, K., Wandel, J. & Cliffora, J. (1996). Establishing an interdisciplinary patient care team: Collaboration at the bedside and beyond. *Journal of Nursing Administration, 26*(4), 21–27.

Napolitano, C.S. & Henderson, L.J. (1998). *The leadership odyssey.* San Francisco: Jossey-Bass.

Nielsen, E.H. (1978). Applying a group development model to managing a class. In L.P. Bradford (Ed.). *Group development.* La Jolla, CA: University Associates.

Parker, A.W. (1972). *The team approach to primary health care.* Berkeley: University of California, University Extension.

Pavitt, C. (1999). Theorizing about the group: Communication-leadership relationship. In L.R. Frey (Ed.). *The handbook of group communication theory and research.* Thousand Oaks, CA: Sage.

Petzinger, T. (1998, May 8). A hospital applies teamwork to thwart an insidious enemy. *Wall Street Journal.*

Purser, R.E. & Cabana, S. (1999). *The self-managing organization.* New York: The Free Press (Simon & Schuster, Inc.).

Riley, J.B. (1997). *Instant tools for healthcare teams.* St. Louis: Mosby.

Robbins, H. & Finley, M. (1995). *Why teams don't work: What went wrong and how to make it right.* Princeton, NJ: Peterson's/Pacesetter Books.

Ross, R. & Roberts, C. (1999). *Barking and nonbarking dogs.* In P. Senge (Ed.). *The dance of change.* New York: Doubleday, 87–91.

Sapir, E. (1973). Group. *Group Process, 5*(2), 105.

Schein, J.E. (1969). *Process consultation.* Reading, MA: Addison-Wesley.

Scherer, J.J. (1979). Can team building increase productivity or can something that feels so good not be worthwhile? *Group and Organizational Studies, 4*(3), 335.

Seago, J.A. (1996). Culture of troubled work groups. *Journal of Nursing Administration, 26*(9), 41–46.

Shonk, J.H. (1996). *Team-based organizations: Developing a successful team environment.* Chicago: Irwin Professional Publishing.

Tichy, N.M. (1997). *The leadership engine: How winning companies build leaders at every level.* New York: HarperCollins.

Tuckman, B.W. & Jensen, M.A.C. (1977). Stages of small group development revisited. *Group and Organization Studies, 2*(4), 419.

Wells, L. (1990). The group as a whole: Systematic socioanalytic perspective on interpersonal and group relations. In J. Gillette & M. McCollom (Eds.). *Groups in context: A new perspective on group dynamics.* Reading, MA: Addison-Wesley.

Wise, H., Beckhard, R., Rubin, I. & Kyte, A.L. (1974). *Making health teams work.* Cambridge, MA: Ballinger Publishing.

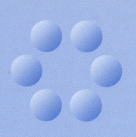

CHAPTER **6**

# Leading Workplace Meetings

## LEARNING OBJECTIVES

*After completing this chapter, the reader will be able to:*

- Discuss the various purposes of workplace meetings.
- Distinguish between functional and nonfunctional group roles at meetings.
- Identify communication patterns within small groups.

- Lead informational, problem-solving, and issue-focused meetings.
- Participate in meetings in a constructive manner.

## TEST YOURSELF

*Part I. Some people love meetings; others hate them. All of us have had good and bad experiences with meetings. This exercise will focus your attention on the way meetings affect people. You can work on both lists at the same time. When you finish, compare your "best" and "worst" with the guidelines for leading meetings found in this chapter.*

| The BEST meeting I ever attended was . . . | The WORST meeting I ever attended was . . . |
| --- | --- |
| | |

*Part II. Most people are not fully aware of their effect on others in a meeting. Try matching each statement with the effect (i.e., the role played by the person) on group process.*

_____ 1. Blocker      A. I have more important things to do than to sit here talking about something that's done and gone.

_____ 2. Playboy      B. We're getting off the track. Let's get back to the subject under discussion.

_____ 3. Expresser    C. I'll go along with whatever the group decides.

_____ 4. Follower     D. That's the dumbest idea I ever heard!

_____ 5. Aggressor    E. That reminds me of a great joke I heard.

_____ 6. Leader       F. I have been concerned about this situation for quite a while. I believe some of my colleagues share my concern.

*Answers*

1.A  2.E  3.F  4.C  5.D  6.B

"**I** hate meetings!" How often have you said that? Or heard others say it? Yet whenever a problem arises in a work setting, someone invariably says, "We'd better have a meeting about that."

Why do so many of us have this love-hate relationship with meetings? In an effective meeting, the knowledge, skill, and experience of everyone in the group can be combined in a synergic manner impossible to achieve in one-on-one discussions. The solutions generated can be powerfully creative and successful. On the other hand, the experience of attending an ineffective meeting can be almost physically painful: whether boring and tedious or tense and acrimonious, ineffective meetings rarely produce anything useful and often do harm to productivity and morale.

In this chapter, we will consider some of the do's and don'ts of effective workplace meetings for both leaders and participants. Because a workplace meeting is really a variant of working in groups or teams, the information on the dynamics of small groups presented in Chapter 5 pertains here as well. Additional information on the dynamics of small groups that focuses on a single coming together of people for the purpose of face-to-face talk, whether for a one-time meeting or a regular meeting of a work group or teams, is presented in this chapter.

## ● PURPOSE OF WORKPLACE MEETINGS

Three primary reasons to have a meeting are to (1) share information with others, (2) discuss important issues, and (3) solve problems.

### Informational Meetings

The need to exchange information and learn more about one's job is almost continuous in healthcare settings. This ongoing education ranges from simple, straightforward reports to formal classes, courses, or conferences.

The most common mistake made in sharing information with coworkers is to treat them as if they were school children in a classroom, rather than adults with vast life and work experience. The second most common is to underestimate their potential motivation to learn. The following are some tips to keep in mind when you are the leader of a meeting held for the purpose of sharing information with other adults:

- Adults want to know why they should learn something.
- Motivation is increased when adults see that what they are learning will help them perform a task or solve a problem.
- Negative self-concept, the pressure of other responsibilities, and poorly designed communications block learning (Knowles, 1984).
- Past experiences in classrooms (good or bad) can affect present responses; in some cases they may even lead to resistance to returning to any "class" at all. For others, calling a meeting a "class" may make it less threatening. Know your audience!
- Adults can be self-directed. They do not have to be "spoon-fed" information. Information that requires little or no explanation or discussion can be shared via e-mail or printed materials so people can read it at their own pace.
- Adults' life experiences can be a rich resource if they are encouraged to share them.

*I hear and I forget; I see and I remember; I do and I understand.*
—Confucius

### Problem-Solving Meetings

The term **problem** is used here in the broad sense to mean any kind of difficulty, dilemma, or complex situation in which thought and planning are needed to work out the best way to approach the situation. The problems can be minor ones dealt with in a few minutes, or they can be major ones that require a series of meetings for their resolution. They may be related to patient care, or they may be related to the operation of the team, unit, or organization.

When the subject is not a particularly emotion-laden one, the group usually can be quickly engaged in the steps of the problem solving process (see Chapter 9). A clear description of the problem sets the stage for the rest of the meeting. Once that step is completed, the leader's role is to do the following:

- Keep the group focused on the subject of the meeting.
- Encourage creative suggestions.
- Minimize criticism but encourage critical thinking.
- Discourage nonfunctional behaviors and recognize functional ones (described in the group roles section of this chapter).
- Ensure that the group tests its commitment to a decision because a superficial agreement will fall apart after the meeting (Howard & Barton, 1992).
- Summarize the decisions made at the meeting.
- Do not close the meeting until a mechanism for actual implementation of the solution is agreed upon or another meeting time to continue the work has been set.

How can you judge whether a problem-solving session was worthwhile? If the group ends the meeting (or series of meetings in some cases) with a well-conceived solution and is committed to carrying it out, then the meeting was worthwhile. If not, you need to reflect on the process, the behaviors of attendees at the meeting, and your role in leading the meeting to determine what went wrong. This evaluative process will be discussed in greater detail later in this chapter.

## Issue-Focused Meetings

When emotions are high, a situation is so complex and chaotic that it is difficult to identify what the problem really is, or when a group or team needs to work on morale and solidarity, issue-focused meetings are appropriate. Most of these issue-focused meetings call for the highest level of leadership skill of all.

The leader's most critical responsibility during this type of meeting is to foster open communication within a nonthreatening environment. This task is much less difficult within an environment that generally allows open communication; in one that does not, the leader is faced with the considerable challenge of developing sufficient trust within the group to allow open discussion of a potentially sensitive subject.

It may be necessary to specify the ground rules for this kind of discussion. A statement at the beginning of the meeting that all group members should recognize and respect the personal and subjective nature of the opinions expressed will help to establish an accepting climate within the group.

The leader can confront any nonfunctional behavior. For example, someone who is monopolizing the conversation can be asked to give someone else a chance to speak. Confrontation is also appropriate if the group evades the issue or denies having any problem when it is evident that a problem exists (the "sleeping dog" referred to in Chapter 5).

At the end of this chapter, you will find the complete script from a meeting of nursing staff on an extended care unit. This meeting was held to encourage the staff to express their feelings about caring for a particular patient and to critically evaluate that care in order to improve in the future.

> *The subject of the meeting was how the staff felt about caring for patients like Mr. C. Mr. C. was an older man who had been on the unit several months before he died. (His death occurred one week before the meeting.) Mr. C. had an extensively gangrenous foot that was horribly decayed but could not be treated surgically because he was considered an extremely poor surgical risk.*
>
> *Mr. C. also had many decubiti, was contracted into a fetal position, and was unable to care for himself at all. He did not respond verbally to the staff, and his level of awareness fluctuated. Most members of the staff found it distasteful to care for him because of the odor, the horrible condition of his foot, and his complete dependence. The team leader had observed several staff members expressing their distaste in Mr. C.'s presence. The team leader also noticed that they spent as little time as possible in his room although he had been there a long time and had few visitors.*

When Mr. C. died, the staff felt a mixture of relief from the horror of his physical condition and guilt for the feelings they'd had about caring for him. The meeting could have focused on the staff's feelings about his death, but the team leader who planned it believed that it was more important to deal with their feelings about giving care to patients in this condition in the future.

If you have looked ahead to the script, you may have noticed that the leader of the meeting about Mr. C. did not directly confront the staff with their attitudes or behavior toward this patient. Based on knowledge of the staff, the leader judged that such a strong confrontation would have been difficult for some of them to handle. Instead, the leader took a less direct, more general approach and encouraged the staff to discuss their experiences with Mr. C. and how they felt about caring for him. If the members of the group had not brought up some of these issues, however, the leader probably would have had to introduce them in order to achieve the purpose of the meeting.

The leader of the problem discussion about Mr. C. prepared and used the following list of questions to bring out important issues during the meeting:

1. How did you feel about Mr. C.? How did you feel about caring for him? About the condition he was in?
2. Do you think that he was suffering?
3. Toward the end, was he conscious of anything?
4. Put yourself in this patient's place. How would you feel if you were in the same state as Mr. C. was?
5. How do you deal with suffering? Is it difficult?
6. Can nurses become desensitized to others' pain? How can desensitization be counteracted?
7. Was it worthwhile to speak to Mr. C.?
8. What was the likelihood that Mr. C. could still hear you and understand how you felt about him?
9. How should we deal with patients who are suffering like Mr. C., who are comatose part of the time and aware some of time?
10. How well did we take care of Mr. C.? What could we have done better? What can we do in the future to give better care to patients like Mr. C.?

While you may want to look at the script now, you will need to know more about group roles, communication patterns, and other small group phenomena before you can analyze the effectiveness of the meeting.

## GROUP ROLES

What people say and do during a meeting (and sometimes what they do not say or do) has an effect on the group as a whole and on the outcome of the meeting. A comprehensive list of these effects, called **group roles,** was devised by Bradford a number of years ago (1978). Using this list, you can sort out the helpful from the nonhelpful behaviors of yourself and others during a meeting.

These group roles are descriptions of the behavior of individual group members in terms of their effect on the group. With this definition in mind, the various roles can be divided into two categories: functional and nonfunctional roles. Behaviors that contribute to the completion of a group task are called **task roles;** those that support group function and meet members' social or relational needs (Fisher & Ellis, 1990) are called **group-building roles.** Both task and group-building roles are functional roles to play within a group.

Roles that meet the needs of the individual member, but not of the group, are called **individual roles.** Usually these roles are nonfunctional or at best neutral in terms of group progress.

Each time a person interacts within a group, that member is playing at least one and sometimes several roles. Some people will restrict themselves to one or two roles, whereas others may play many different roles. Although some relationship between personality and the roles a person plays in a group is obvious, remember that when you describe the roles played, you are not describing the person or the person's intent, but rather the effect the person's behavior is having on the group process (Trujillo, 1986). For example, a person's objections to a decision may be blocking group progress but personal objections do not mean this person is always a blocker or even deliberately being a blocker. Even more important, the objector may be correct.

The functional task roles are listed first, then the group-building roles, and finally the nonfunctional roles (Bradford, 1978). Examples of these roles are found in the script at the end of the chapter.

## Functional Task Roles

The following roles contribute to the completion of a group task.

- *Initiator/Contributor:* Makes suggestions, proposes new ideas to the group. The suggestions may be ways to solve a problem, a new way to approach a problem, or a new way for the group to proceed in its work.
- *Information Giver:* Offers pertinent information that might help a group in its deliberations.
- *Information Seeker:* Asks for pertinent information or clarification of facts or suggestions.
- *Opinion Giver:* Offers opinions, judgments, or feelings; may comment on their appropriateness in terms of a particular set of values.
- *Opinion Seeker:* Asks for opinions, judgments, or feelings of other group members; seeks clarification of values.
- *Disagreer:* Points out errors in information given or takes a different point of view.
- *Coordinator:* Points out relationships (links) between different suggestions or statements that have been made.
- *Elaborator:* Expands on suggestions or ideas made and offers examples or rationale.
- *Energizer:* Stimulates the group; encourages activity and movement toward group goals.
- *Summarizer:* Pulls together the ideas or suggestions from the group; briefly outlines what the group has accomplished.
- *Procedural Technician:* Performs needed mechanical tasks such as setting up chairs, running the video camera, passing out papers, or serving refreshments.
- *Recorder:* Writes down ideas, suggestions, or decisions made by the group; may also diagram group interactions.

## Functional Group-Building Roles

The following roles support group development and meet relational needs.

- *Encourager:* Responds to others warmly; accepts and sometimes praises contributions of others.

- *Standard Setter:* Expresses standards or guidelines for the group to use in its deliberations.
- *Gatekeeper:* Elicits contributions from other members; sometimes suggests limits or ways to make sure everyone has a chance to speak.
- *Consensus Taker:* Tests group opinions and decisions by stating them and asking whether members agree.
- *Diagnoser:* Identifies and points out blocks to group progress.
- *Expresser:* Describes feelings, reactions, and responses of self and others; expresses feelings of the group.
- *Tension Reliever:* Provides an outlet for tensions in the group by using humor, conciliation, and mediation.
- *Follower:* Accepts group decisions; goes along with the group without taking other active roles.

## Nonfunctional Roles

The following roles are played to satisfy individual needs rather than to promote group progress.

- *Aggressor:* Makes hostile, attacking remarks; criticizes others; is overly assertive.
- *Recognition Seeker:* Does things to call attention to himself or herself; uses the group as personal audience.
- *Monopolizer:* Talks so often or so long that others do not get a chance to speak.
- *Dominator/Usurper:* Tries to take over leadership of the group; wants to have his or her own way and tells the group what to do.
- *Blocker:* Obstructs progress of the group by making unconstructive remarks, being negative, and resisting beyond a reasonable point.
- *Playboy:* Makes irrelevant and silly comments; whispers; plays around; does not take the group task seriously.
- *Zipper-Mouth:* Does not participate even in a nonverbal manner; demonstrates no acceptance of the group (as follower does); may sulk.

How many "playboys" and "zipper-mouths" did you notice at the last meeting you attended? Were more of these nonfunctional roles played than the functional ones such as "gatekeeper" or "consensus-taker"? Identifying the group roles played by individuals attending a meeting is a useful way to describe what is happening during the meeting. When you are able to recognize the effects of these behaviors, you can take action to encourage the functional ones and discourage the nonfunctional ones. A high proportion of nonfunctional roles is indicative of such problems as low morale, lack of cohesion, poorly defined tasks, or inadequate leadership in a group.

## ● COMMUNICATION PATTERNS

Although each meeting will have a unique combination of people and behaviors, there are five common patterns to which communication during the meeting can be compared.

These common patterns range from formal one-way communication to the completely chaotic patterns found in some disorganized groups. Between these extremes are the stilted, limited, and open patterns of verbal communication (Bion, 1961). Diagrams illustrating the flow of communications in these different patterns are shown in Figure 6–1.

## One-Way

Verbal communication moves in only one direction in this pattern: from the speaker to the rest of the group. The formal lecture is the best-known example of this pattern. This pattern can be compared to a live performance in a theater in the sense that the speaker is performing and the rest of the group acts as the audience.

The one-way pattern is a highly organized form of communication controlled primarily by the leader or speaker. Although the leader appears to have total control in this kind of group, it is important to note that the group has allowed this control.

The extreme form of one-way communication allows no verbal feedback from the group, but the nonverbal responses from the group can have surprising power. Boos, hisses, laughter, and clapping from an audience obviously tell the performer how well he or she is doing. The more subtle smiles and nods of agreement from a group listening to a lecture positively reinforce the speaker, whereas frowns, yawns,

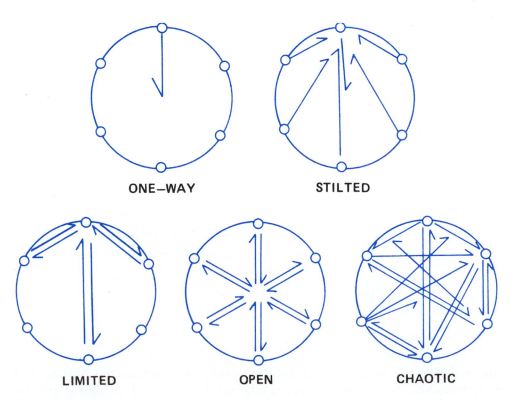

**Figure 6–1**  Patterns of verbal communication in groups.

or restlessness can discourage the speaker. Despite the highly controlled nature of this communication pattern, the principle that you cannot *not* communicate still holds true.

In less extreme forms of this pattern the speaker recognizes people in the group and lets them ask questions or make comments. The speaker responds to these questions and comments but retains control of participation. This type of exchange allows for some clarification and disagreement, which the extreme form does not.

The one-way pattern is appropriate for a performance or for rapidly transmitting information to a group. It sets the leader apart from the group and allows little or no group interaction. It is an efficient way to communicate information to a large number of people in a short time, but it is not necessarily the best way to facilitate discussion or learning. It is not appropriate for group problem solving, decision making, clarifying issues, confrontation, evaluation, and other processes in which people need to reflect on and respond to each other's input. A group cannot mature when a one-way pattern is continued.

## Stilted

Verbal communication flows in both directions in the stilted pattern, but the pattern is still somewhat formal. The most familiar version is one in which each member takes a turn to speak, usually going around the circle or up and down rows in order. In the most stilted version, all communication is directed at the leader. In the less formal version, communications may also be addressed to the group as a whole.

Although less controlling than the one-way pattern, the stilted pattern still imposes a great deal of structure on the group's interaction. Discussion is not likely to be relaxed or lively while the stilted pattern continues.

The stilted pattern is common in new groups and can be helpful as a temporary way to impose some order or to make sure that everyone has a chance to speak. Insistence on continuing this pattern would retard the development of the group. It is also used for introductions and for "show-and-tell" types of presentations, even with adults. Its use may be due to the authoritarian style of the leader or because group members are not yet comfortable with each other. Members can simply be asked to talk to the whole group to make the pattern less stilted, but it usually takes more than a simple request for members to relax enough to move from this pattern into a more open pattern of communication.

## Limited

In the limited pattern of communication, some group members communicate with the leader and with each other, but others do not. When these interactions are animated, it may seem to the casual observer that the group has an open pattern of communication, but careful observation or recording of the interaction reveals that the communications are limited to some members of the group and that other members are not taking part.

This limited pattern can be the result of increasing dominance of a subgroup. It may also be due to the leader's and group's inability to prevent some members from monopolizing the discussion. Monopolizers are not always seeking dominance—some people mask anxiety by hyperactivity, whereas others may withdraw and become isolated.

The silent members in the group must also be considered. Their silence may indicate disapproval of the group's actions, feelings of discomfort or disinterest, or they may be interested followers who simply need some encouragement to participate more actively. Leader intervention should be directed at diagnosing the reasons for the pattern and promoting group progress toward maturity.

> *If one thinks of business meetings as a series of speeches which are simultaneously composed, rehearsed, and delivered by several persons at once, one begins to understand the complexity and inherent weakness of the meeting process.*
> —Mosvick & Nelson, 1996

## Open

The open pattern is characterized by free and easy exchange between all members of the group, including the leader. Each member of the group has an opportunity to speak, to be heard, and to receive some kind of response. The leadership style is usually democratic, but it could be laissez-faire. This pattern is usually found in mature groups.

An open pattern of communication is flexibly organized but predictable in the sense that members know what they can expect of each other. This underlying order may be hard for an observer to detect in an open pattern.

Open communication is appropriate for most group interactions. However, it is not the most efficient pattern for completing a simple task or the fastest way to make a decision.

## Chaotic

The chaotic pattern goes beyond the free and easy exchange of the open pattern to disorganized, unpredictable, and uncontrollable interaction. Side conversations between two members are common. Group members interrupt each other, ignore each other, or talk at the same time, sometimes shouting to be heard. The group may be as relaxed as people at a party, or it may be tense, with openly warring factions. The leadership is usually laissez-faire and lacking in control.

The open pattern may seem to approach chaos at times, but closer observation reveals the predictability and organization that the chaotic pattern lacks, somewhat like the difference between a three-ring circus and a rioting mob.

The chaotic pattern is not appropriate for a group that has a task to accomplish. Anything accomplished by a group with a chaotic pattern of communication has happened by accident. Leader intervention should be aimed at bringing some order into the communication pattern and then increasing group maturity.

These patterns are best identified by observing and recording who speaks to whom in each interaction during a group meeting. While casual observation will pick up the extreme patterns of communication, a written, audiotape, or videotape recording of group interaction is more complete and will pick up the less extreme patterns.

## ● LEADING MEETINGS

Some of the many things to consider when you are leading a meeting (often referred to as **chairing** a meeting) include the pre-meeting preparation, opening a meeting, guiding the discussion and bringing the meeting to a conclusion, and following-up on any decisions that were made.

### Pre-Meeting Preparation

Thorough preparation increases the likelihood of having a more effective meeting and making the best use of everyone's time and input. Once you have an agenda for the meeting you can select an appropriate time and place and invite the appropriate people. You can also decide whether refreshments, staff coverage, publicity for the meeting, and other details need to be taken care of before this particular meeting.

#### *Agenda*

It is time to be concerned about the value of a meeting if, when asked why they are attending a meeting you called, your colleagues give answers such as the following:

"I don't know. My boss just told me to be here!"

"We meet every third Wednesday of the month, don't we?"

"You asked me to come."

Albert (1996) estimated that a one-hour meeting costs $150 in terms of the amount of other people's time that is used. This estimate is probably a conservative one. If you add up the hourly wage of each person who attends the meeting, the total will give you an idea why emphasis must be placed on making the best use of everyone's time during a meeting.

Preparing and distributing an agenda before the meeting accomplishes several things. First, it forces you to articulate the purpose of the meeting and what you hope to accomplish. Second, it communicates your goals for the meeting to the other participants. Third, it serves as a reminder to everyone who is expected at the meeting. Fourth, it helps keep everyone on track during the meeting. An agenda alone will not prevent digressions but the group's attention can be directed

**Research Example 6–1    *Stand-Up versus Sit-Down Meetings***

Three researchers from the Department of Management at the University of Missouri randomly assigned 555 management students to 111 five-person groups to compare the effectiveness of stand-up and traditional sit-down meetings. During the meetings, participants were given a task to do as a group. It involved ranking 15 pieces of equipment on their importance for survival. The length of the meeting, quality of the decisions made, and satisfaction with the meeting were measured.

As hypothesized, the sit-down meetings on average were 34 percent longer than the stand-up meetings. However, the quality of the group's de-

cisions were no different despite the researchers had expectation that the sit-down meetings to produce better decisions. On the other hand, participants in sit-down meetings were more satisfied with the meeting. While sit-down groups used more information in making their decisions, they did not use it more effectively.

The researchers concluded that stand-up meetings can be both efficient and effective ways to deal with well-defined nonroutine problems.

*Source:* Bluedorn, A.C., Turban, D.B. & Love, M.S. (1999). The effects of stand-up and sit-down meeting formats on meeting outcomes. *Journal of Applied Psychology, 84*(2), 277–285.

back to it when the discussion strays. At times, of course, an urgent issue arises after the agenda has been distributed, in which case the agenda can be changed.

*I know of a staff meeting that goes from 2:00 to 7:00 each week. Problem: no agenda. It's just a free-for-all . . .*
—Albert, 1996

### Time

Your first consideration will be to select a day and time that is convenient for meeting attendees. In some cases, however, the nature of the meeting will dictate the day and time. For example, if a patient committed suicide, the nurse manager would call a meeting within hours to deal with the emotions aroused by such a traumatic event, rather than wait for the most convenient time.

### Place

A minimum of time and effort should be required to get to a meeting in most instances. However, it is occasionally important to take people away from their usual meeting place to reduce interruptions or to better accommodate the activities that will occur during the meeting. For example, if the group needs to meet for several hours to complete the department budget, a cramped staff

lounge that becomes crowded during meal and break times is a poor choice for a task that requires concentration. Instead, look for a quiet, comfortable room with adequate lighting, seating, and work space for the group. It may not be a good idea to make people too comfortable, however. One research study showed that meetings where people remained standing were 34 percent shorter in time but produced the same quality decisions on well-defined tasks (See Research Example 6–1, Stand-Up vs. Sit-Down Meetings).

### Participants

Do not invite anyone who does not have to be at the meeting. On the other hand, be sure you will have all the input you need to deal with the agenda. For example, if your team is meeting to discuss a problem with timely delivery of patient meals, then you will want to invite the person who coordinates meal deliveries not only because this person should know the system well, but also because this person is likely to be able to make the changes necessary to improve the system.

### Additional Factors to Consider

Each situation, each meeting, is different in some ways. The following factors will be relevant in some cases but not in others.

• *Refreshments.* Serving food may actually distract people from the task they are supposed to be doing. On the other hand, people who have time for *either* lunch *or* your meeting but not both would greatly appreciate meeting in the room next to the cafeteria or a plate of sandwiches brought in during the meeting. Sometimes refreshments are used to attract attendees:

> *Health Care, Inc., was known in medical circles for the lush lobster and shrimp platters served at medical board meetings. Their medical board had the highest attendance rate of any medical board in the city.*

• *Coverage.* Unless meetings are held before or after the usual workday, staff members must be assured that their responsibilities are being taken care of while they attend the meeting. This may necessitate having someone answer the telephone or having several staff members remain on the unit in order to provide adequate care. Unless this coverage is provided, staff members will not be able to focus their full attention on the subject of the meeting. Even worse, they may have to run in and out of the meeting to attend to other responsibilities, which is distracting.

• *Publicity.* A team meeting rarely needs publicity. At most, you may have to remind people, particularly if the time or day is not consistent. However, attendance at educational offerings and community meetings is often dependent on getting the word out to those who would be interested in attending.

• *Pre-Meeting Politicking.* Are you confronting a hot issue at the meeting? One that faces strong opposition? Do you need more support than you already have? If yes, you may need to talk with people before the meeting, in some cases to persuade them to support your side. Be careful when you use this strategy: an inept approach could alienate potential supporters. You might also find that those opposed to your point of view are correct, so it is important to hear both sides before you make up your mind.

• *Help People Feel Comfortable.* A meeting can represent a welcome break from demanding intense work or an unwelcome confrontation with an upsetting or threatening situation.

Knowing the situation and the people involved will help you anticipate the extent to which participants might be uncomfortable at the meeting and how to put them at ease.

People in low status positions, such as unlicensed assistive personnel, may be uncomfortable when asked to give their opinions in front of the professionals on the healthcare team. Professionals with poor communication skills could be uncomfortable revealing their inadequacies in a group of peers. Both of these groups need to trust that others will be accepting, not critical of their contributions. Others may be uncomfortable when they are *not* leading the group. Some people have a great need to be in control and may try to usurp your leadership to fulfill this need, which may require firm leadership to prevent.

• *Presentation.* If the type of meeting planned requires a lengthy presentation, you need to be well prepared. Consider using visuals: transparencies, blackboards, or flip charts are inexpensive, portable, and flexible. It is said that the use of visuals can shorten meetings by as much as 28 percent. They not only help to reduce lengthy monologues from meeting participants but also can enhance your image as a well-prepared, more persuasive leader (Albert, 1996).

An entirely different approach to planning a meeting is described in Perspectives . . . A Different Way to Conduct Meetings.

## Implementation

Mosvick and Nelson (1996) say that most meetings are unplanned, disorganized, and poorly run. In surveys of more than 1,600 managers and professionals done between 1981 and 1995, they found that the top five problems with meetings were (1) the discussion got off track; (2) meetings were too long; (3) no goal or agenda was set ahead of time; (4) no decision or follow-up occurred after the meeting; and (5) the leadership of the meeting was ineffective. It was especially interesting, they said, that the problems listed did not emphasize interpersonal dynamics. Instead, it seemed that people got particularly frustrated with meetings when nothing was accomplished.

## PERSPECTIVES . . .

### A Different Way to Conduct Meetings

Michael Jones and John Shibley (1998) are jazz musicians as well as organizational consultants. They point out that musicians practice continually while most organizations seem to expect perfection on the first try.

What would happen if organizations adapted the practice orientation? Jones and Shibley (1998) suggest that we would conduct meetings in the following manner:

- Call a meeting *without* an agenda. Meetings with a preset agenda are often boring and produce unimaginative results. One way to stimulate creativity would be to review mistakes made in the past and talk freely about the lessons learned from them.
- Open the meeting with a "check-in." During the check-in, everyone gets a chance to say whatever is presently on his or her mind.
- Practice your "piece" before the meeting. People can become more articulate by listening to the way they speak and practicing ahead of time.
- Improvise. Both the context (environment) and group members will change. All will be better prepared for change if they have practiced improvising.

Would you prefer attending the type of meeting described by Jones and Shibley? Do you think most people would?

*Source:* Jones, M. & Shibley, J. (1999). Practicing relevance. In P. Senge (Ed.). *The dance of change.* New York: Doubleday, 190–192.

### Opening the Meeting

1. *Timing.*   Begin the meeting on time. Some attendees may have left work undone to get there on time and will resent being kept waiting; next time they may come late. Those who want to socialize can do so at the end of the meeting when others are free to leave. Starting late was the #6 problem in the surveys reported in Mosvick and Nelson (1996).

2. *Welcome.*   Greet people by name as they arrive. Even "important" people like to feel welcome so do not skip them. Saying "Thank you for coming" when you open the meeting recognizes the value of participants' time and attendance.

3. *Orientation.*   Following the brief welcome, it is essential to restate the purpose of the meeting. It provides a structure for the meeting and shared understanding of what should be covered and how it should be covered during the meeting (Mosvick & Nelson, 1996). For some meetings, a little more detail as to the nature of the problem and ground rules for proceeding with the discussion may be necessary, particularly when the meeting has been called to discuss a patient problem or a difficult issue.

### Guiding the Discussion

1. *Staying on track.*   Both the agenda and the statement of purpose at the beginning of the meeting communicated the intended structure to the participants. Now it is the leader's responsibility to help the group stay on track and accomplish these goals during the meeting. Reminders of the purpose of the meeting may be necessary when the group gets off track. Usually, questions pertaining to the subject of the meeting bring the group back on track, but sometimes confrontation is necessary, particularly when the group is struggling with the topic of the meeting.

2. *Dealing with nonfunctional behavior.*   **Monopolizers** can be asked directly to give someone else a chance to speak. Thank the person for his or her contribution and then say that you would like to hear other people's opinions as well. **Nonparticipants** can be encouraged nonverbally by looking at them (eye contact) when you ask a question and positive recognition of others' contributions. You can also ask people if they have anything to add, giving them the opportunity to accept or decline your invitation to participate. **Aggressive** behavior will sometimes end if it is ignored but usually requires confrontation. Remember that any hostility expressed is not necessarily due to your leadership or even the purpose of the meeting. It may be related to individual prob-

lems or situational difficulties that need to be resolved at a time or in a manner other than during the meeting. **Usurpation** of your leadership may be a power play that you can confront or counter with a stronger power play. Or it may be due to weak leadership on your part, leaving a gap that others try to fill. In either case, assertive behavior on the part of the leader is necessary to maintain leadership of the group. Remember, the participative leader shares leadership with the group but does not abdicate the leadership role.

3. *Encouraging open communication.*  The leader's evident interest acts as a primary stimulus to group interaction. Open-ended questions encourage participant response. Nonverbal nods, smiles, positive voice tones, eye contact, and verbal expressions of valuing others provide recognition and encouragement to contributors. If necessary, cut off any personal attacks immediately and point out the difference between constructive and destructive criticism.

4. *Stimulate creative problem solving.*  A climate of acceptance encourages creative suggestions. Every suggestion should be responded to in some way to encourage additional ones. Listing them on a blackboard or flip chart is one form of acknowledgment. If the group gets stuck, suggest trying brainstorming. If necessary, stress that contributions should not be attacked or labeled as a "wrong" feeling or "wrong" thought. Instead, contributions should be explored, discussed, and eventually accepted, rejected, or blended with others' suggestions. Recognition that every issue has at least two sides can help people remain open-minded (Perloff, 1993).

5. *Identify hidden agendas.*  As indicated in the previous chapter, hidden agendas can have an enormous impact on any group. Without realizing it, people, including the leader, often bring hidden agendas to a meeting. When a group gets stuck for no apparent reason, consider the possibility that a hidden agenda may be operating.

## Concluding a Meeting

Don't skip this step. If time is limited, then make your concluding statements brief. Be sure to include the following:

- Summary of what was decided during the meeting and how these decisions would be followed up
- Time and place of the next meeting (if appropriate)
- Expression of thanks to everyone for their contributions to the meeting

Finally, end the meeting on time. If additional time is needed, decide with the group whether another meeting should be scheduled or if the meeting should continue. Be specific: does the group need another 10 minutes or will it take an hour to complete the work? This information will help the group choose the best alternative.

## Follow-up

### Communicate Results of Meeting

A written summary or minutes of a meeting has several purposes: (1) to permanently record what occurred for future reference, (2) to remind attendees of what was decided, and (3) to communicate what occurred to those who did not attend. It is often appropriate to also communicate the results of a meeting to a manager or administrator, not only for informational purposes but also to obtain support for the group's decisions and recognition of their efforts.

### Implement Decisions

What is the point of having a meeting if no follow-through action is taken on the decisions made? Have you ever attended a meeting or workshop where some really creative ideas were generated only to find that nothing was ever done with them? That the group or team went back to its usual routine afterward? That nothing had changed? If follow-up fails to happen too often, participants will soon stop taking such gatherings seriously.

For this reason, the responsibility of both leader and participants extends beyond the meeting. Even when a group appears to be highly motivated, you cannot assume that decisions will be implemented without follow-up. If they are not, the time and effort spent on the meeting are wasted and future meetings are likely to be viewed with disinterest or even resistance.

> **Nothing so convinces people of the value of participating as seeing the input they offer get results.**
>
> —Napolitano & Henderson, 1998, p. 86

According to Napolitano and Henderson, if a group recommendation cannot be implemented, a reasonable explanation should be provided. Good communication on organizational issues, say Frigon and Jackson, is essential to understanding an individual's particular role and how they fit into the larger picture.

## Evaluation

Both the process and the content of the meeting should be evaluated in some way. Often, it is done informally. "That was a good meeting" and "We really accomplished a lot today" are the types of comments you will hear after a well-run meeting. "We really got off track today" or "What a waste of time" may be heard after a poorly run meeting.

Both content (the decisions made, issues clarified, information gained, etc.) and process (everyone contributed, the group stayed on track, etc.) can be evaluated more formally as well. Although such evaluations can become quite lengthy and complex, a short, simple form is often sufficient. An example of such a form that takes a minute to fill out may be found in Figure 6–2.

## ● ATTENDING MEETINGS

The individuals who attend a meeting are equally responsible for its outcomes. Remember that effective leadership can be displayed not

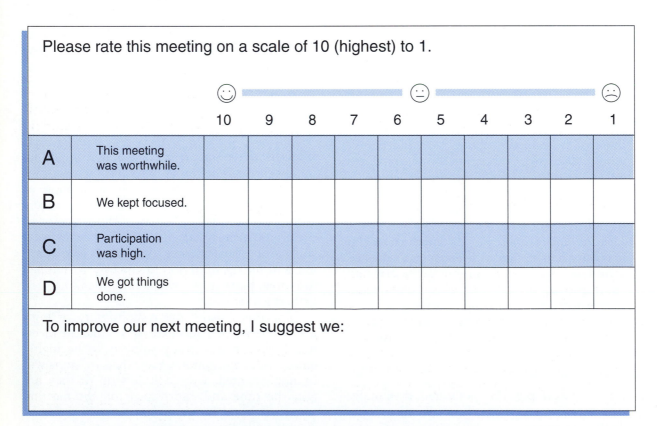

**Figure 6–2**  Brief meeting evaluation form. *Source:* Albert, B. (1996). *Fat free meetings.* Princeton, NJ: Peterson's.

only by the designated leader (or chair of the meeting, in this case) but by members of the group as well. Because many of the do's and don'ts for effective participation in meetings parallel those for the leader, they will be summarized in the same order as was followed for leading meetings.

## Pre-Meeting Preparation

It may only take a few minutes of thought to prepare for a meeting or it may take some serious homework on your part. You need to know what will be expected of you at the meeting, what the leader hopes to accomplish, and how you can contribute to accomplishing that goal. In some cases, you may have to speak to the person who called the meeting to obtain answers to your questions. Don't hesitate to communicate. Most leaders will be pleased to know that you are taking your role as meeting participant seriously. You may also save yourself the embarrassment of being entirely unprepared when you are unexpectedly called on to make a report to the group or provide expertise during the meeting.

## Implementation

### Opening the Meeting

Arrive on time and plan to stay for the entire meeting. People who pop in and out or come late and leave early are disruptive. They may also miss the most important information shared at a meeting or fail to provide important input because they were distracted or unavailable.

### Participating in the Discussion

1. *Staying on track:* You can help to keep the group on track by avoiding making distracting comments and by reminding others when they stray from the agenda.
2. *Nonfunctional behavior:* Review the lists of functional and nonfunctional behaviors and identify the roles you are playing during a meeting. Are you having a positive effect on the group? Are you contributing in a constructive manner? You do not have to agree with everyone to be constructive. In fact, when "groupthink" is a threat, your best contribution could be to confront what is happening.

On the other hand, be sure that you are not disagreeing just to get a rise out of people or to keep the meeting interesting. When you contribute your best in a meeting, it will be noted and appreciated by the leader and other participants.

3. *Identify hidden agendas:* Did you bring any hidden agendas with you to the meeting? Are you sure? Perhaps you think that you could do a better job leading the meeting or that you really have more important things to do than attend this meeting. These feelings will affect your behavior if you do not attend to them.
4. *Stimulate creative problem solving:* Accept others' suggestions as well as provide your own. Think about how you feel if one of your suggestions is ignored or is immediately rejected as "that would never work" or "what a dumb idea!" and you will treat others' suggestions as if they were your own.

> *. . . many individuals contribute to the ineffectiveness of information processing through poor listening habits, weak critical thinking skills, and communication anxiety.*
>
> —Mosvick & Nelson, 1996, p. 33

5. *Communicate openly:* Imagine what a meeting of all zipper-mouths or blockers would be like! The group needs your contributions and your honest opinion. Do consider carefully, however, the way in which you communicate them.

### Concluding a Meeting

Stay until the meeting is ended. Add to the summary if something was missed and ask about the scheduling of the next meeting if it is not mentioned.

## Follow-Up

Participate in the implementation of any decisions that were made and in any requested evaluations. A brief comment on how the meeting went from your perspective as a participant can be of great value to the leader.

Just imagine for a moment a meeting that has only a leader and no participants and you will understand the importance of your role as a participant in a meeting at work.

## ● SCRIPT

The following transcription of a real meeting shows group members playing many of the group roles discussed earlier. It also shows the leader carrying out some of the actions discussed but omitting others. You should be able to identify these actions as well as the overall pattern of communication that characterized this meeting. Comments about the leader's actions and the individual roles played are given alongside the script. An analysis of the dynamics of this meeting and its outcomes follows the script. You will note flaws in the way the meeting proceeded—these are to be expected in a real meeting.

● ● ● ● ● **PROBLEM DISCUSSION SCRIPT** ● ● ● ● ●

| Script | Comments and Roles Played |
|---|---|
| **Leader:** I'm really happy that you're all taking time out to do this today, 'cause I know it's time out of your really busy schedules. We've been talking a little about what an issue-focused meeting is. That is when you take a subject and examine your own feelings about it and share with others your feelings and perhaps things that influence your thoughts—maybe something to do with nursing. And hopefully, the goal of this is to understand your fellow team members and to promote communication. The end result is better patient care. | **Role:** Initiator <br> The leader sounds uncertain about staff members' interest in attending the meeting. The leader could have been more positive and assertive about the value of their spending time at this meeting. |
| This is the ideal. Would you like to try this for the next 15 minutes? (Pause) OK. I would like to talk about Mr. C. Even though he passed away about a week ago, I thought we might still discuss him because we might have patients now who are like him. Or in the future, you'll most likely run into patients like him again. | The words by themselves do not convey the non-verbal interest in the meeting evident in the leader's voice, which had staff members nodding their heads at this point. |
| Would someone briefly like to run over his problems, what his condition was? | Here the leader looked at the primary nurse, encouraging this individual's participation and showing a willingness to share leadership of the meeting. |
| **Primary Nurse:** Mr. C. was a cardiac patient. His problem was that he was such a poor surgical risk that he was not operated on. He had gangrene of the foot, and it got worse. He had contractures of both arms and legs; in fact, he was almost in the fetal position. At first he was unable to speak to us. | **Roles:** Information Giver, Contributor |
| **Leader:** How many people here came in contact with him or cared for him? | **Role:** Information Seeker |

*(continued)*

## PROBLEM DISCUSSION SCRIPT *(continued)*

| Script | Comments and Roles Played |
|---|---|
| **Nurse 2:** I think all of us did at one time or another. | **Role:** Information Giver |
| **Leader:** How did you feel about him? About caring for him? About the condition he was in? | Note how every other exchange is spoken by the leader here. This is a stilted pattern that gradually changes as the conference progresses. |
| **Primary Nurse:** Sorry for him. So sorry that someone would have to suffer like that. | **Role:** Expresser |
| **Leader:** Do you feel that he was suffering? | |
| **Licensed Practical Nurse (LPN) 2:** Oh yes, because he knew what was going on for a long time. Like, when you were doing anything to him, when he'd had enough, he'd pat you on the arm. That was it for a long time. Well, toward the end it was like he wasn't a person. I mean, he was a person, but it was like he was already dead but still alive. | **Roles:** Information Giver, Expresser |
| **Leader:** So, toward the end, do you think he was conscious of anything? | Not an open-ended question. Note the response. |
| **LPN 2:** Yes. | |
| **Leader:** Why do you think so? | |
| **LPN 2:** Because I still think Mr. C. responded to pain. When you did his dressing, he certainly indicated his discomfort. When you spoke to him and managed to get through his subconscious, I think he sort of acknowledged the fact that you were there. The response of his eyes. But even the last days it seemed he was aware. | **Roles:** Information Giver, Opinion Giver |
| **Leader:** How did you feel when you cared for him? Was it something you liked doing because he was suffering, or was it distasteful to you? | |
| **LPN 2:** I found it unpleasant. With Mr. C., I just felt like I could pick him up and hold him. You just felt empathy and I never minded being assigned Mr. C. I mean it was distasteful, yes. But he was just so dear. When he was himself he used to squeeze your hand and his eyes would just twinkle. And I think when you remember these things about a patient . . . when you had a patient for so many weeks, I don't think anybody could enjoy doing the dressings because it was an almost insurmountable task. Sometimes, we ended up with the dressing looking less than desirable. It was a difficult chore. Speaking for | **Role:** Expresser |

*(continued)*

**PROBLEM DISCUSSION SCRIPT** *(continued)*

| Script | Comments and Roles Played |
|---|---|
| myself, I never minded doing Mr. C. I just thought he was the sweetest thing. | |
| **Nurse 3:** I feel pretty much the way LPN 2 did. I have my own personal problem with odors. I had to leave the room many times and come back because I really got kind of nauseated at times. I'd walk away for a minute, but I came back. But I just felt he was a patient who needed a lot of care, the basic needs. I think he was very much aware that you were taking care of him—that we did care, that we'd do anything we could to keep him comfortable. I do feel he had pain, and more could have been done in that area. We could have stressed that he should have had something for pain, which he did not have. He was a real challenge to do, but I think he was very much aware of what was happening in his room, and who came and went. | **Roles:** Expresser, Elaborator, Contributor<br><br>This group member is openly sharing a reaction to the patient, which is what the leader had hoped to elicit from the group. |
| **Leader:** How do you deal with a patient who's suffering? Someone like Mr. C. who is semicomatose some of the time, aware some of the time? | **Roles:** Information Seeker, Gatekeeper |
| **LPN 2:** I don't think Mr. C. was ever what you'd call "comatose." He was, I think deep in sleep quite a bit, but we could always manage to reach his subconscious. | At this point, the leader had to decide whether to clarify these terms for the LPN or to continue the focus on feelings—a difficult decision. |
| **Leader:** Do you think it was worthwhile to speak with him, to him? | **Role:** Opinion Seeker<br><br>Again, not an open-ended question. Could have discouraged discussion, but it did not. |
| **LPN 2:** To him, yes. | |
| **Nurse 3:** Oh, definitely, yes. Because he was aware that we were in the room. They don't have TVs, they don't have radios, and I think a lot of the patients really look forward to whatever reason we come in. That's a couple of minutes they can talk to somebody. Because I think it's extremely lonesome for these patients and I really think that's a very important part of our nursing care, that you do talk about the weather or what's in the headlines. To talk to them—some kind of interaction—it keeps them in touch with reality. | **Roles:** Elaborator, Contributor |
| **LPN 2:** I know in orientation classes, they tell us that we are to keep a patient in contact with time and place, and even though the patient is | **Role:** Information Giver |

*(continued)*

## PROBLEM DISCUSSION SCRIPT *(continued)*

| Script | Comments and Roles Played |
|---|---|
| unable to respond to you, you should still treat the patient as somebody with a mind that is still functioning whether we're aware of it or not. No matter how comatose a patient is, that's always the proper thing to do. | |

**Nurse 2:** I had what would be termed, I suppose, a real awakening. I know when I was at another hospital we had a young man, not Mr. C., but I think it is a good simile. This young man had been in a motorcycle accident. He was only married about three months. I think he was about age 25. He was on a Stryker frame, fully paralyzed, totally unresponsive, with a tracheostomy tube, foley catheter, and the whole bit. And yet his wife—it was almost eerie, and it sent shudders up and down your spine to walk past the room and hear her—day after day, reciting her marriage vows, for richer and poorer, in sickness and health. She and his whole family came in and would tell him what happened in church today, and do you know that boy came around. He walked out of that hospital and went home. And I think it's because his family kept his brain alive. As a matter of fact, even when he had the tracheostomy, we had to caution his wife against feeding him whole pieces of turkey that she had prepared at home and we'd end up suctioning him. But I mean, they would not give up on him. And I'm glad they didn't. I'm not going to say that his mind was as healthy as we would have liked it to have been; he was rather juvenile. But at least he was a functional human being. So we can't ever say that they don't hear you and that it's not going to be worth the effort.

**Roles:** Elaborator, Recognition Seeker

The example given here generally supports the idea that it's important to give good care to a comatose patient but is getting off the track and could divert the group from the subject of the meeting.

**Leader:** So you feel even if they can't respond to you in some big way that they still can hear you and understand you and get your vibes and feel how you're feeling.

**Role:** Consensus Taker

The leader is bringing the discussion back to the subject.

**Role:** Information Giver

**Nurse 2:** Hearing is supposed to be one of the very last senses to leave the body. And this is something we have to caution our visitors about repeatedly. Visitors will come in and they'll even talk about funeral arrangements right over a patient. And we always have to caution them, "You know, the patient may not be talking to you but he is listening to us."

*(continued)*

**PROBLEM DISCUSSION SCRIPT** *(continued)*

| Script | Comments and Roles Played |
|---|---|
| **LPN 3:** Some things, even to say, "Gee, he must be so uncomfortable"—at least that person may hear what you're saying and at least know that you're trying to understand he's uncomfortable. Those things, I feel are right to be said. It's a real situation to them, it's a real situation to us. And I think we should be factual, and if he's uncomfortable, let's do something about it. | **Role:** Opinion Giver |
| **Leader:** When you're caring for a patient who is in very sad condition, like Mr. C., or someone who really wins your heart, do you feel sorry for those patients, do you ever put yourself in their place? | **Role:** Opinion Seeker |
| **LPN 2:** I think that's a good idea, to put yourself in another's place, because then you would be gentler with them. And you wouldn't want somebody to be rough with you if you were a patient. | **Roles:** Encourager (accepting another's idea), Opinion Giver |
| **Leader:** Is it difficult to deal with suffering? | Again, this question could have elicited a discussion-stopping "yes" or "no" answer but the group is moving along well enough that it did not have this effect. |
| | **Roles:** Information Giver, Contributor |
| **LPN 2:** Yes, it always is if you have compassion for someone. We had a nursing arts instructor who told us whenever we enter a room we are to consider a patient's age. And if the patient is 25 years old and you are 24, you can consider this could be your husband, brother, sister, or whatever the case may be. If the patient's twice your age you can say, "this could well be my father or mother, and I intend to take care of the patient as I would for my own parents and so forth." I think this is something everybody should do. Aside from putting yourself in that person's position, just to think in terms of this person belonging to you in some relationship. | |
| **LPN 3.** Just in terms of interaction between one human being and another, if you were very ill, and some stranger came in to care for you, you'd hope that stranger would treat you like a human being. The family concept I was also taught—person to person, stranger to stranger. You walk into that room and consider how you'd like to be cared for by a stranger. | **Role:** Elaborator |

*(continued)*

| Script | Comments and Roles Played |
|---|---|
| **Leader:** Do you feel that a nurse can be desensitized to pain? Can you be bombarded with people who are suffering so much that you might forget? | **Role:** Consensus Taker |
| **Nurse 3:** I think you can be too busy sometimes, for the moment, to stop and think, but I don't think you could ever be really desensitized. | **Role:** Opinion Giver |
| **Nurse 2:** You build up certain protections for yourself, because you are around them so much. You have to protect yourself—we'd be drained, thoroughly drained, if we didn't. But myself, no, I would never be completely desensitized. | **Roles:** Elaborator, Opinion Giver |
| **Leader:** So, summing up, if we were to walk into a patient's room who couldn't communicate with us, or else that patient's communication was minimal, and it was evident that the patient was suffering a great deal—and needed total care—and you had to give the patient a bed bath, what kinds of things would you consider or should do or think of while you were caring for the patient, knowing that the patient is suffering? | **Roles:** Coordinator and Information Seeker (not Summarizer)<br><br>The leader is not really summarizing as stated but is guiding the group toward moving on to the second purpose of the conference, which was to critically evaluate the care they give. |
| **LPN 3:** Be gentle, don't take too long, just straighten the patient out, wash, turn, and position the patient. Just remember the patient's a human being. Every patient's different and you see so much suffering. And I really felt terrible for Mr. C.—it was terrible to see someone have to die like that, and see that gangrene every day. And then we had a Mr. H. here and I found that very bad. That was enough to break your heart, watching that man suffer. | **Roles:** Contributor, Expresser |
| **LPN 2:** They both had the problem, too, of loose bowels. I know I will certainly admit to being guilty of saying, just after getting Mr. C. repositioned and dressed, "Oh, no, not again!" I would voice what crossed my mind because all of a sudden it was running all over and we had to begin from scratch again. | **Roles:** Information Giver, Expresser |
| **LPN 3:** What could you talk to the patient about when you were going to give the patient a bath? If you had to move him into the portatub? | **Roles:** Information Seeker, Gatekeeper<br><br>Nonverbally, the LPN looked around the group while saying this. |
| **Nurse 2:** You're supposed to tell your patient, "Now, Mr. C., we have to move you, and pick | **Roles:** Information Giver, Opinion Giver |

(continued)

## PROBLEM DISCUSSION SCRIPT *(continued)*

| Script | Comments and Roles Played |
|---|---|
| you up. It's going to hurt." Let them know what's being done. You're not supposed to pick the patient up and just suddenly put the patient in the middle of the air even though they're supported by strong arms. They should know where they're going and why. | |
| **LPN 2:**  I don't think any of us do that. We all talk to them—we all say, "OK, you're going to get a bath and have to roll over." We all talk to them. That would be scary . . . | You can see that the meeting has become much less stilted here. This pattern is common as people relax and become more involved in the discussion. |
| **Nurse 3:**  Even a patient that you're not sure what they're hearing and seeing or how much they're aware of, if we say our name to them, "I'm S.T., and I'm going to take care of you and give you a bath," a voice and a name. They remember good things and bad things, so, if they're waiting for that one person, it must drive them crazy when we don't say our name! Even though they can't say, "Good morning, I'm Mr. C.," we should still say, "Good morning, I'm S.T." | **Role:**  Elaborator |
| **LPN 1:**  He didn't want to be touched. He just wanted you to leave him alone and let him die. | **Role:**  Blocker<br><br>The tone of voice and body language strongly communicated negative feelings from this group member who only spoke once. If it were not for this nonverbal negativism, the role would have been disagreer. |
| **LPN 2:**  I know, especially when you were doing his mouth and suctioning and so forth, he just sort of looked up annoyed. I think sometimes they just wish you wouldn't show up on the scene when they're bubbling froth and so forth. I got that impression. | **Role:**  Elaborator |
| **Nurse 2:**  I think we were with him the last day, and LPN 2, you were doing him up and we rolled him over. He ceased breathing. We suctioned him and he went on for another 12 hours. | **Role:**  Information Giver<br><br>This group member is getting off the track again. |
| **Leader:**  But you felt he communicated with his eyes. | Again, the leader is bringing the group back on the track by restating what LPN 2 had said. This tactic is also a good way to support what people have said. |
| **Nurse 2:**  I think he certainly did, and with his hand, too. There would be pressure from his hand. When I spoke to him and asked if he could hear me, it was like he was really trying to | **Roles:**  Expresser, Information Giver, Opinion Giver<br><br>Note that this response is back on the track.<br><br>*(continued)* |

**PROBLEM DISCUSSION SCRIPT** (continued)

| Script | Comments and Roles Played |
|---|---|
| communicate. The reason we knew he was in pain, too, because when you were dressing him, and he was turned to his side, his arms were extremely long and he had 7-inch fingers, and he'd be doing this, trying to grasp your bottom or your waist or your back, just to let you know that you were hurting him. I mean I don't think it was any other sense, it was just his way of reacting. You don't often see, thank goodness, challenges quite like Mr. C. Most of them never get to that stage. He was an elderly man, but he had an extremely strong heart. He had pneumonia three times while he was here. | |
| Leader:  Is there anything else anyone would like to say? | Role:  Gatekeeper |
| Leader:  Well, thank you all very much for taking time out. I really am very appreciative of it. | The summary belongs here but was omitted by the leader. |
| LPN 2:  Thanks a lot. I learned a lot from you. | Role:  Encourager |

## ● SCRIPT ANALYSIS

### Sociogram

A sociogram (Beal, Bohlen & Raudabaugh, 1962) is simply a diagram that illustrates the seating arrangement of the group, the number of contributions and side comments each member made, and to whom they were directed. It can be drawn during the meeting, or it can be done afterward from a videotape of the meeting. The leader of the group is usually too involved in other activities to make a sociogram during the meeting.

Begin with an outline of the room and a schematic representation of the furniture arrangement. As people take their seats, their names are placed on the diagram. When the meeting begins, the recorder draws a line from one group member to another to indicate who spoke to whom. An arrow to the center of the diagram indicates a comment made to the group as a whole. The slashes on these lines indicate how many times a message was sent in this same direction. Each uninterrupted comment from a participant is considered a unit of communication for which a line is drawn (Fisher & Ellis, 1990).

When it is done, the sociogram tells you who the most active contributors were, who was the recipient of most of the comments, and who did not participate. The pattern of interaction can be seen from the lines and direction of the arrows. It may also show how the seating arrangement influenced the interaction. The sociogram cannot tell you what the climate of the group was, what roles were played by group members, or the value of the contributions made. For example, Figure 6–3 shows the sociogram drawn for the issue-focused meeting relating to Mr. C.'s care. You can see that the leader spoke much more often than anyone else and that none of the nurse's aides spoke at all. Note also that Nurse Aide 1 was positioned outside the group. LPN 1 spoke only once, but the other two LPNs were more active contributors. Nurse 2 directed comments to several different people as well as to the group. This active role would lead you to look at the script to see whether Nurse 2 dominated the group, which did not happen.

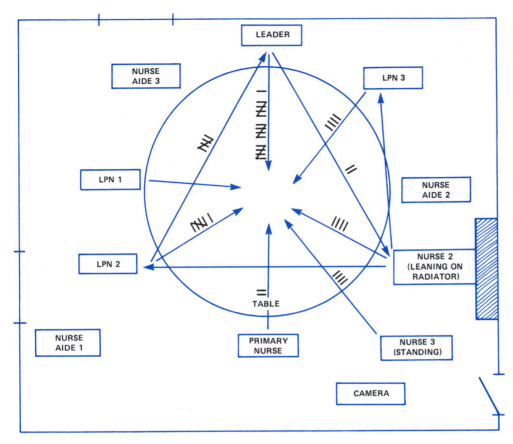

**Figure 6–3**    Sociogram drawn during a problem discussion.

## Seating Arrangement

The number of chairs available was inadequate, leaving two people standing throughout the meeting. One of the people standing began shifting from one foot to another as though tired of standing.

The arrangement of the chairs was an informal circle that allowed each member to make eye contact with everyone else who sat in a circle. Those who stood and the aide who moved to sit in the corner could not make eye contact as well as the others.

## Communication Pattern

Both the sociogram and the script indicate that the overall communication pattern was somewhat stilted, especially at the beginning of the meeting when every other contribution came from the leader. Later in the meeting, the spontaneity of the group increased considerably.

## Roles Played by Group Members

The majority of roles played by group members were functional ones. Note that nonverbal behavior, which cannot be communicated well in either the script or the sociogram, is an important component of the role played.

1. The primary nurse played the roles of **information giver, contributor, expresser,** and **follower.** At the beginning of the conference, the primary nurse reviewed Mr. C.'s situation. This summary served as the basis for further discussion. Throughout the rest of the meeting the primary nurse remained silent, not a disinterested or sulky silence, but one that communicated an attentive attitude as this member

looked at each speaker with an expression of interest. The primary nurse also indirectly encouraged others to feel free to say what they felt by having done so early in the conference.

2. Nurse 2 played the roles of **information giver, recognition seeker, elaborator,** and **opinion giver.** Nurse 2 played a nonfunctional role once. Nurse 2's contributions got off the track twice but overall were supportive of the purpose of the meeting and of other people's comments. Due to the lack of chairs, this group member stood leaning against the radiator through the whole meeting.

3. Nurse 3 played only functional roles: **elaborator, contributor, opinion giver,** and **expresser.** Nurse 3 shared feelings near the beginning of the meeting about caring for Mr. C. and finding odors offensive. This member's overall contribution was positive, and with frequent participation, Nurse 3 helped to keep the discussion moving along. This group member also stood through the whole meeting and appeared to be tired near the end.

4. LPN 1, in contrast, played only nonfunctional roles. LPN 1 was a **blocker** and a **zipper-mouth.** Except for one comment, which was negative, this member sat silently throughout the conference, looking around the room, not making eye contact with any of the speakers. A slight scowl and peeved expression was evident on this member's face.

   Apparently, LPN 1 came to the meeting because this member felt pressured to attend after being invited by both the leader and the primary nurse, not due to a desire to attend. Before the meeting LPN 1 said, "I can't be in two places at one time. Someone has to stay on the floor!" in an angry voice. During the meeting, LPN 1 sulked and LPN 1's overall contribution was negative because this member's behavior could only have had a dampening effect on the group.

5. LPN 2 was an **information giver, opinion giver, expresser, contributor, elaborator,** and **encourager.** The roles LPN 2 played were as functional and positive as those played by Nurse 3, except that some of what LPN 2 said was not entirely accurate. LPN 2 sat at the table actively listening and making eye contact with each speaker, sometimes frowning with concern when Mr. C.'s suffering was mentioned. LPN 2's contributions and voice were warm and friendly in tone, which indicated this member's willingness to support the stated purpose of the meeting.

6. LPN 3 played the roles of **opinion giver, elaborator, contributor, expresser, information seeker,** and **gatekeeper.** LPN 3 responded positively to other people's contributions and expressed some feelings about Mr. C. This group member sat at the table and remained silent at the beginning of the meeting, seeming to need time to warm up.

7. Nurse Aide 1 played only the role of the **zipper-mouth.** Nurse Aide 1 did not say one word during the conference but sat in a corner, removed from the group physically as well as interactionally. This member seemed completely inattentive, looking down frequently, and had a bored facial expression. This member's yawns seemed to be an indication of lack of interest. Nurse Aide 1 enjoyed the refreshments and seemed to regard the conference as a chance to sit down and get away from the unit for a while. This group member's effect on the meeting was neutral to negative. Nurse Aide 1's presence was barely felt.

8. Nurse Aide 2 acted as **follower.** Although Nurse Aide 2 did not say a single word, this member sat up straight and made eye contact with each speaker, occasionally nodding in agreement. Nurse Aide 2's contribution to the group was positive in the sense that this member nonverbally supported the others when they spoke.

9. Nurse Aide 3 was also a **follower** during the meeting. Nurse Aide 3 sat at the table near the leader and watched with wide-eyed curiosity. This group member had never attended a problem discussion before and was attentive throughout the meeting. Nurse Aide 3's contribution was positive in the sense that this member acted as an attentive audience.

## Maturity of the Group

The somewhat stilted communication pattern is one indication that the group did not achieve maturity. Much of the discussion had an air of politeness and restraint (noted also nonverbally), and no group-generated confrontations took place except from the leader. Several group members were quite open about their reactions to Mr. C., but others seemed to hold back. Still others contributed nothing, and the group made no attempt to include them, which would have been another sign of a mature group.

This group was composed of people from the same patient care unit. They work together on a regular basis but evidently have not achieved the performing stage of group development. It is likely that they are working on some of the tasks of the norming stage of group development.

## Course of the Discussion, Decision Making, and Outcome

Only two minor instances of members of the group getting off the track were observed. With these exceptions, the discussion remained focused on the subject introduced by the leader.

Although the discussion became less stilted and a little more relaxed as it continued, little change characterized the way in which group members dealt with the subject. Not much more sharing happened at the end of the meeting than at the beginning, nor did the depth or strength of the feelings shared or the emotions aroused during the meeting increase at all. This neutral atmosphere indicates that an unspoken agreement—that no group member would confront another member about their feelings or about the care they gave to Mr. C.—was probably operating as a hidden agenda. In spite of this hidden agenda, the group had some discussion of the ways in which patients such as Mr. C. should be cared for, which was something the leader had hoped to accomplish.

It is interesting to note that all of the nurses and most of the LPNs participated verbally in the discussion but the aides did not. The reasons for their lack of verbal participation need to be explored before the next problem discussion. The aides could have been uncomfortable with the subject of the meeting, with expressing negative feelings in a group that contains people who have some authority over them, or both. Because the aides did not participate verbally, any decision made by this group would not have been a true consensus.

The group did come to some agreement on the fact that a patient such as Mr. C. can suffer terribly, can understand and respond to their communications, and is greatly in need of good nursing care. The meeting did increase the staff's awareness of the needs of patients such as Mr. C. and supported those who tried to give them good care. However, the group did not confront the fact that their care of Mr. C. had been lacking in several respects or that they needed to improve in the future for patients with similar conditions, which was the leader's hoped-for outcome of the meeting. Additional meetings with a deeper exploration of the issues could eventually lead to such a commitment from the entire group.

To summarize, the first purpose of this meeting, to encourage a sharing of feelings about caring for Mr. C., was fairly well accomplished, although the depth of the sharing could have been greater. The second purpose, to critically evaluate the care they gave, was partially met. The hoped-for commitment to improve care in the future was not achieved.

## Leadership Style and Effectiveness

The leader's style during the meeting was clearly participative, although the leader had been more directive in the preparation of the meeting, having chosen the subject without input from the group. The choice itself was appropriate, however.

The leader's preparation for the meeting was thorough in some respects but not in others. Everyone invited to the meeting was given adequate notice of the date, time, and place, and they all knew what the subject of the meeting would be. Everyone who was invited attended, although one did so under protest and this member's needs were clearly not met by the leader or the group. The meeting started and ended on time. The seating was inadequate, a problem that clearly could have been avoided. The leader prepared some helpful questions and comments ahead, but the opening remarks did not explain the ground rules clearly. Apparently, the leader did not take notes or have anyone record comments during the meeting to use as a summary at the end.

Regarding the effectiveness of the leader's actions, the leader's questions, though not always open-ended, were pertinent and helped to keep the discussion moving along in the right direction. The group was kept on track most of the time, which is not always easy to do, and did share some feelings. The leader's verbal and nonverbal behavior was supportive, encouraging, and nonjudgmental throughout the meeting, which is especially important during an issue-focused meeting.

No meeting or conference is perfect. The flaws pointed out in this analysis do not reflect any serious errors on the part of the leader. Instead, they reflect the ordinary ups and downs of leading meetings that you can expect to encounter in the practice of leadership and management.

## ● SUMMARY

Three types of workplace meetings are discussed. The information meeting is held primarily for the purpose of sharing information in the form of reports and/or in a teaching format. It is particularly important when leading this type of meeting to remember that the participants are adult learners. The problem-solving meeting utilizes the problem-solving process in group format. Issue-focused meetings are most useful when the topic is emotion-laden or the purpose is primarily team-building.

Several patterns of interaction were discussed. On the individual level, group members may play functional or nonfunctional roles. Functional task roles include initiator/contributor, elaborator, energizer, summarizer, procedural technician, and recorder. Functional group-building roles are encourager, standard setter, gatekeeper, consensus taker, diagnoser, expresser, tension reliever, and follower. Nonfunctional roles are aggressor, recognition seeker, monopolizer, dominator/usurper, blocker, playboy, and zipper-mouth. On the group level, patterns of communication may be one-way, stilted, limited, open, or chaotic.

The leader or chair of a meeting should set an agenda, time, and place for the meeting well in advance in most cases. Selection of participants, a decision about offering refreshments, providing

---

## C A S E   S T U D Y

### Meetings: An Administrative Point of View

Read the meeting script once more. This time, pretend you are the nurse manager of the unit on which the meeting was held. The nurse who led the meeting is a new graduate who will be sitting down with you shortly for a three-month evaluation.

### Questions for Critical Reflection and Analysis

Based on the script, re-evaluate the meeting as follows:

1. What did this meeting cost in dollar terms? (To simplify your calculations, assume that the meeting took ½ hour and that all aides earn the same salary, as do all licensed practical nurses and all registered nurses on your unit).

2. From your perspective as the nurse manager, what did your staff accomplish at this meeting? What will result from this meeting? Will teamwork be enhanced? Will patient care improve? Be sure to explain how you arrived at your answers.

3. Was any harm done at the meeting? Would you expect teamwork or patient care to suffer in any way as a result of the meeting? Again, be sure to explain how you arrived at your answers.

4. Evaluate the leadership capability of this new graduate. What strengths did you identify? What weaknesses? What recommendations for further development of leadership skills would you make?

5. Would you encourage the nurse who led the meeting to hold follow-up meetings on the same subject? Why or why not? What should occur at a follow-up meeting if one were to be held?

staff coverage, publicizing the meeting, politicking beforehand, helping people feel comfortable, and preparing a presentation may also have to be done. Meetings should begin on time with a welcome and reiteration of the purpose of the meeting. Once underway, the leader's responsibilities are to keep the discussion on track, discourage nonfunctional behavior, encourage open communication, stimulate creative thinking, and deal with any hidden agendas that interfere with the group's progress. Equally essential is a well thought-out conclusion to the meeting and thorough follow-up on any decisions made during the meeting.

Meeting participants are urged to be prepared to respond to the purpose of the meeting, to arrive on time, and to contribute to the discussion. Without their contributions, a meeting would be purposeless. Participants can share responsibility for guiding the meeting, bringing it to a successful conclusion, and following up on any decisions made at the meeting.

The script of an actual problem discussion meeting was included, followed by a detailed analysis of the group dynamics and the leader's actions.

## REFERENCES

Albert, B. (1996). *Fat free meetings*. Princeton, NJ: Peterson's.

Beal, G.M., Bohlen, J.M. & Raudabaugh, J.N. (1962). *Leadership and dynamic group action*. Ames, IA: Iowa State University Press.

Bion, W.R. (1961). *Experiences in groups and other papers*. New York: Basic Books.

Bluedorn, A.C., Turban, D.D. & Love, M.S. (1999). The effects of stand-up and sit-down meeting formats on meeting outcomes. *Journal of Applied Psychology, 84*(2), 277–285.

Bradford, L.P. (1978). *Group development*. La Jolla, CA: University Associates.

Fisher, B.A. & Ellis, D.G. (1990). *Small group decision making: Communication and the group process*. New York: McGraw-Hill.

Fitton, R.A. (Ed.). (1997). *Leadership: Quotations from the world's greatest motivators*. Boulder, CO: Westview Press, 280.

Frigon, N.L. & Jackson, H.K. (1996). *The leader: Developing the skills and personal qualities you need to lead effectively*. New York: American Management Association.

Howard, V.A. & Barton, J.H. (1992). *Thinking together: Making meetings work*. New York: William Morrow.

Jones, M. & Shibley, J. (1999). Practicing relevance. In P. Senge (Ed.). *The dance of change*. New York: Doubleday, 190–192.

Knowles, M. (1984). *The adult learner: A neglected species*. Houston: Gulf Publishing.

Mosvick, R.K. & Nelson, R.B. (1996). *We've got to start meeting like this!* Indianapolis, IN: Park Avenue Productions.

Napolitano, C.S. & Henderson, L.J. (1998). *The leadership odyssey*. San Francisco: Jossey-Bass.

Perloff, R.M. (1993). *The dynamics of persuasion*. Hillsdale, NJ: Lawrence Erlbaum.

Trujillo, N. (1986). Toward a taxonomy of small group interaction-coding systems. *Small Group Behavior, 17*(4), 371–390.

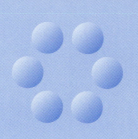

CHAPTER *7*

# Diversity in the Workplace

## LEARNING OBJECTIVES

*After completing this chapter, the reader will be able to:*

- Describe trends in diversity in the nursing workforce.
- Discuss the importance of sensitivity to differences across diverse groups in the workplace.

- Identify cultural influence on beliefs, values, and behavior.
- Critique approaches to increasing sensitivity.
- Suggest strategies to improve working relationships among people from diverse groups.

## TEST YOURSELF

**Feeling "different"**

*Think of a recent experience you have had where you felt you were being treated as though you were "different" from others and not recognized as a unique person, or were being stereotyped. It could be an experience at school, at work, or anywhere.*

*When you have finished, score your experience for its intensity of differentness.*

1. Describe what happened.

2. What did you think at the time? What did you do? How did you feel?

3. What did the others do? What do you believe the others were thinking? Feeling?

4. What was the outcome of the situation?

|  | Circle the Number That Applies | | |
|---|---|---|---|
| **1.** How important was the situation to you? | 0<br>Relatively unimportant | 1<br>Important | 2<br>Critical |
| **2.** How different were you? | 0<br>Little difference | 1<br>Some difference | 2<br>Great difference |
| **3.** Were these differences visible to others? | 0<br>No | 1<br>A little | 2<br>Obvious |
| **4.** Were there power differences? | 0<br>I was one-up, in charge | 1<br>Equal | 2<br>I was one-down |
| **5.** Were you isolated from others similar to you? | 0<br>I had several others like me for support | 1<br>One other supportive | 2<br>I was alone |
| **6.** Were you stereotyped? | 0<br>I was treated as a unique individual | 1<br>I felt stereo-typed | 2<br>There was direct evidence of stereotyping |
| **7.** Did the situation cause you to react emotionally? | 0<br>No emotional reaction | 1<br>Slightly upset | 2<br>Strong emotional reaction |

Add the numbers circled to get your total intensity of differentness score: _____

*Source:* Kolb, D.A., Oslund, J.S. & Rubin, I.M. (1995). *Organizational behavior: An experiential approach.* Englewood Cliffs, NJ: Prentice-Hall. Used with permission.

Look around you in class, at work, in your clinical setting. Do you see a mix of ages, genders, or ethnic groups among the people you see? The diversity you see is expected to increase in the next decade. Although they are still referred to as the "majority," white male workers now constitute only 45 percent of the U.S. workforce. This proportion is expected to decrease: 85 percent of new entrants into the workforce will be women and minorities and 25 percent will have come from the so-called Third World countries (Andrews, 1998; Trossman, 1998). Workforce diversity in terms of age, gender, culture, ethnicity, race, primary language, physical capabilities, and lifestyle present a great challenge to effective leadership and management.

What are some of these challenges? The following are some examples:

*A new pediatric care center was established by a group of pediatricians and pediatric nurse practitioners who had worked together for* many years at the County Children's Hospital. The practice ran smoothly when it was new and small but as it grew and new employees were brought in, nurse-physician relationships deteriorated into power struggles. The new employees had brought in an entirely different set of attitudes and beliefs (i.e., a different culture) about nurse-physician relationships.

A long-term care facility operated by a Protestant church-affiliated organization had drawn most of its residents and employees from the surrounding community. With increasing immigration of people from Puerto Rico and the Phillippines, the community changed from the original German and Scandinavian population to a primarily Catholic Spanish- and Tagalog-speaking population. Disagreements between employees and residents of the facility increased as language and other culture-based barriers to mutual understanding developed. Complaints from unhappy family members and threats to withdraw residents from the facility increased.

In an effort to reduce costs by combining support and administrative services, two hospitals located in a small southwestern city merged. They soon found that merging services was more difficult than was anticipated. One hospital's organizational culture was aggressive and efficiency oriented. The other hospital's organizational culture was meditative and family centered. Disagreements were turning into serious conflicts and costs were increasing rather than decreasing after the merger.

In this chapter, we briefly consider how diversity in nursing compares to diversity in the general population and the importance of developing sensitivity to both differences and similarities across diverse individuals and groups. A classic model for understanding differences in shared meaning across cultures and some additional factors and issues related to these differences are then discussed. The chapter ends with some suggestions for effectively leading and managing a diverse work group.

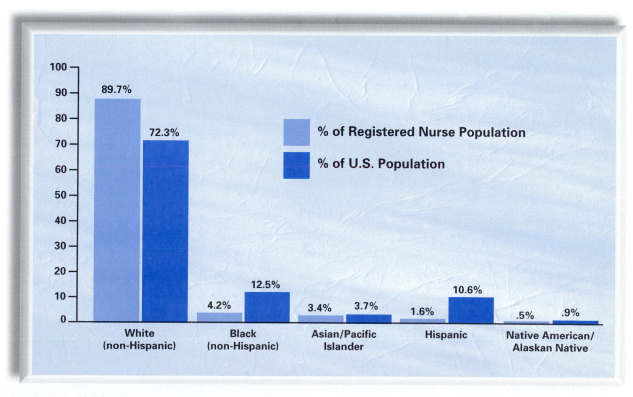

**Figure 7–1** Distribution by racial/ethnic group.

## ● DIVERSITY IN NURSING

### In the Past

The nursing profession has not been immune to the discriminatory practices that existed in the United States at the beginning of the twentieth century (Carnegie, 1995). Men were not granted membership in the American Nurses Association (ANA) until 1930. In the early twentieth century, most schools of nursing were segregated, separating students on the basis of race. Black nurses originally formed the National Association of Colored Graduate Nurses because they had been prohibited from joining some of the state nurses' associations. This separate professional organization was dissolved in 1951 when the membership was assured that the ANA was committed to all nurses (Malone, 1998).

### Today

In the past 10 years, the number of males in the nursing profession has grown steadily. However, the proportion of Hispanic, Asian American, Native American, and African American nurses has not increased substantially (Malone, 1998).

The proportion of minorities in the registered nurse population today is less than the proportion in the U.S. population as a whole (see Figure 7–1). Even though only 72 percent of the U.S. population is white, 90 percent of all registered nurses are white. Only 5.4 percent of the registered nurse population are men, many of whom report that the discrimination they still face in nursing is "almost too subtle to name, yet the effects are still quite real" (Burtt, 1998, p. 64). The number of minority nurses has increased, doubling since 1980, but it has not kept up with the much greater increase in the population as a whole (Trossman, 1998).

## ● NEED FOR SENSITIVITY

### Identification of a Problem

Acting as if people are all alike is a form of denial of the diversity that characterizes both our co-workers and our patients. Recognizing differences and developing enough flexibility to respect and accommodate both differences and similari-

ties promote more effective management (Kavanagh & Kennedy, 1992). The effective management of a culturally diverse workforce has a synergic effect. Not only does it enhance the morale and productivity of the minority groups within the organization, it also enriches the entire organization, bringing new perspectives to the thinking and problem solving that occur daily, as well as more complex and creative solutions.

> *Culture influences the manner in which administration, staff and patients perceive, identify, define and solve problems.*
> —Andrews, 1998, p. 30

Are increased sensitivity and responsiveness to the needs of a culturally diverse workforce needed on your team? In your organization? Some examples of signs that they are needed:

- A greater proportion of lower-level jobs are filled by minorities or women than are higher-level jobs.
- Minorities and women experience lower career mobility and higher turnover rates.
- Acceptance or even approval of insensitivity and unfairness is present (Malone, 1993).

You may also want to observe interaction patterns, such as where people sit in the cafeteria or how they cluster during coffee breaks: are they mixing freely? Or can you see divisions by sex, race, language, or status in the organization? (Moch & Bartunek, 1990; Ward, 1992) Your observations can be graphically illustrated.

> *For example, imagine that you regularly attend an organizationwide risk prevention meeting. The meeting is led by the risk manager, who is a woman. Every department and patient unit is represented and discussions are usually lively. After attending several meetings, however, you begin to notice what you think may be a division within the group.*

In order to check out this hunch, you can draw a sociogram of the patterns of interaction at the next meeting. Using circles for female attendees and squares for the males, you produced a diagram similar to Diagram B in Figure 7–2. You can see that the male members of the group

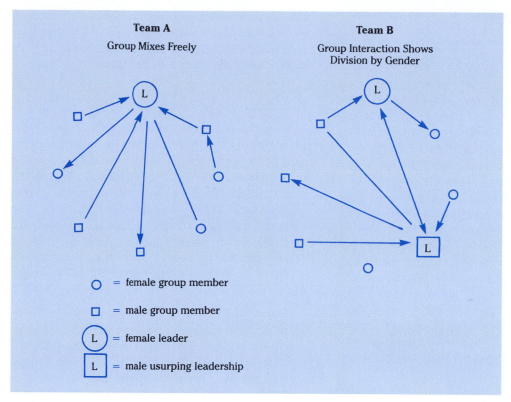

**Team A**

**Group Mixes Freely**

**Team B**

**Group Interaction Shows Division by Gender**

○  = female group member

□  = male group member

Ⓛ  = female leader

□L  = male usurping leadership

**Figure 7–2**  Sociogram illustrating interaction pattern.

are directing more of their comments to another male in the group, not to the group leader. Compare this observation with the pattern in Diagram A, which does not seem to be gender oriented.

Creating sociograms like these can assist you in your analysis and produce objective data to share with others if appropriate (Krebs, 1992).

## Culture and Nursing

Culture includes all the beliefs, values, and behavior patterns common to a particular group of people (Leininger, 1986). Even the way in which the profession of nursing is perceived and valued differs across cultures and ethnic groups. It has been considered a calling by some African and Hispanic groups or a religious vocation by some Catholic groups (Irish, for example). In contrast, some Arab groups think of nursing as a low-class job (the Kuwaitis and Saudi Arabians, for example) (Andrews, 1998). Such patterns of culturally based beliefs are shared by the group

but usually differ in the degree to which the patterns are evident in the attitudes and behavior of individuals. (See Perspectives . . . Nurse-Physician Relationships.)

Because these patterns are learned, not intrinsic, they can differ widely from one group to another. These differences are of concern to leaders and managers because they may result in misunderstandings and conflicts between people from different cultures.

## ● UNDERSTANDING DIFFERENCES IN SHARED MEANING

It is important to remember that all of the differences discussed in the following sections are **group tendencies,** not descriptions or predictors of the behavior of any particular individual (Scarborough, 1998). For example, it is often pointed out that women tend to use a more participative style of

# PERSPECTIVES . . .

## Nurse-Physician Relationships

How are nurses and doctors getting along these days? Florida doctors and nurses were asked to comment on each other's roles, strengths, and weaknesses. The doctors described nurses as the "eyes and ears of the physician" and noted their importance in coordinating care and providing round-the-clock care within a safe environment. They criticized the lack of continuity across shifts and examples of poor judgment regarding patient condition. Nurses, on the other hand, described doctors as the leaders of the patient care team and praised them when they put patient care ahead of other considerations. But they criticized physicians' impersonality, arrogance, and failure to think holistically. Of particular interest were the nurses' comments that the increased number of female physicians has had a positive effect and the physicians' comments that the reduced number of registered nurses on staff has had a negative impact on patient care.

Both old and new aspects of nurse-physician relationships are reflected in these responses. The relationships are changing as more nurses become APNs (advanced practice nurses) with expertise in a specialty area and physicians are increasingly affected by managed care. The surveyors commented that both "must have respect and trust not only for the other profession but in themselves as individual professionals" (p. 17).

*Source:* Pavlovich-Davis, S., Forman, H. & Smek, P.P. (1998, March 9). Nurse-physician relationship: Can it be saved? *Nursing Spectrum, 6,* 7, 16.

management than do men but this generalization does not mean that men never use a participative style or that women always do. In other words, you cannot predict the style of an individual manager on the basis of the person's gender. In the same way, you cannot predict the behavior, beliefs, or values of a particular African American or Chinese American person on the basis of their group identity. Group identity is just one of many factors—albeit an important factor—that affects a person's beliefs, values, and behavior. Judging a person solely based on group identity leads to stereotyp-

ing. In reviewing the results of their research on this subject, Blank and Slipp (1994) report that members of minority groups repeatedly said, "Tell your readers we are not all the same" (p. 6).

## Kluckhohn's Model

One of the classic ways of describing how people of various cultures differ in beliefs, values, and behavior patterns is the model developed by Kluckhohn (1976). According to this model, every culture develops a set of meanings in five fundamental areas, shared by members of that culture (see Figure 7–3). These differences are general, rather than specific. They provide a framework for considering the fundamental differences in shared meaning that can be found across cultures.

1. *Innate Goodness or Evil:* Are people thought to be basically good, evil, or neither? The Puritan ancestors of Anglo-Americans believed that people were inherently evil but that it was possible for them to overcome their evil nature. Managers who held onto this perspective would emphasize discipline and control. An alternative view, more common today, is that people have the potential to be either good or bad. Some humanists believe that

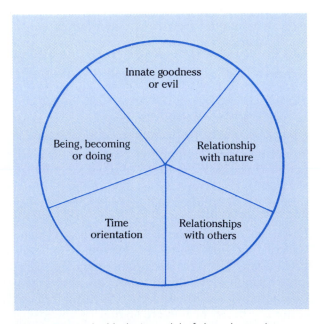

**Figure 7–3** Kluckhohn's model of shared meanings.

people are inherently good and that their "badness" is due to environmental influences. This belief is the basis of some motivational theories of leadership (see Chapter 2).

2. *Relationship with Nature:* Do people dominate natural forces or are they dominated by them? Those who believe that people dominate nature are likely to put a great deal of energy into altering their environment, whereas those who believe that nature dominates them tend to accept their environment as it is. The latter group would accept a harsh work environment—inadequate heat or air conditioning, for example—as a given, whereas the former group would protest its harshness and try to change or control it.

3. *Time Orientation:* Are people most focused on the past, present, or future? Some cultural groups have a great deal of respect for tradition and are likely to see change as a threat to those traditions. The rapid changes in the healthcare system and in relationships between healthcare professions and patients would be particularly unsettling to people with this perspective. Other cultures are oriented primarily to the present and consider the future too unpredictable to plan for. People with this perspective could have some difficulty with the assumptions behind strategic planning or the use of critical pathways. Conversely, an orientation to the future leads to an emphasis on planning ahead. People with a future orientation are more likely to see their present job as a stepping-stone to better positions. They are also more likely to be interested in career planning.

   Another way in which time orientations can differ is the definition of being "on time." For people of some cultural groups, a 2 o'clock appointment means that they will expect to enter your office at precisely 2 o'clock, or even better, a minute or two early. For people from other cultures, however, a 2 o'clock appointment means that they expect to see you at 2:45 or so, depending on what else is happening at the time. They might not expect you to be upset with them unless they arrived well past 3 o'clock.

4. *Being, Becoming, or Doing:* Which aspect is given the most attention—what a person *is*, what the person *can be*, or what that person *does*? People of cultures with a "being"

orientation focus on development of the self as a whole (for example, becoming more knowledgeable, aware, or creative). The third orientation ("doing") focuses on action and accomplishment. In terms of leadership and management, people with this orientation would emphasize an individual's contribution to productivity and profit as measures of success. Those with a becoming orientation would be more likely to look at individuals in terms of what they are learning or how they are developing, and how this process contributes to the purposes of the group or organization.

5. *Relationships with Others:* In some societies, the vertical or lineal relationships, that is, who a person's parents and ancestors were, are of great importance. In others, the focus is on lateral relationships, that is, the members of the groups a person belongs to, including the extended family. This orientation usually includes emphasis on being concerned about others and a mutual dependency on others. For people with this lateral orientation, group goals take priority over individual goals. A third orientation, often found in American organizations, emphasizes the independence and autonomy of the individual. For people with this orientation, dependence has negative connotations, and individual goals are usually expected to take priority over group goals.

   The differences between collective and individualistic orientations may be one of the most important in a work setting (Triandis, 1993). People with an individualistic orientation are likely to have more difficulty working as members of a group or team than those with a lateral orientation. They are also more likely to be competitive rather than cooperative. On the other hand, people with a collective orientation may have difficulty with assignments for which they have individual responsibility.

## Additional Important Differences

A number of other differences in beliefs, values, and behaviors across cultures are significant for leadership and management. They include differences in (1) relationship to people in authority, (2) interpersonal space, (3) the use of eye contact, (4) expressiveness, (5) language and communication, (6) modes of thinking, (7) preferred leadership and management style, and (8) use of evidence (Axtell, 1991; Hall & Whyte, 1976; Sue, 1981).

1. *Relationship to people in authority.*    People in some cultural groups, Asian Americans, for example, may show their respect for those in authority by remaining silent. They expect communication with people in authority to be primarily one way, that is, from the supervisor to the employee. This respectful silence can be misinterpreted as rudeness or lack of intelligence by people from cultural groups that expect an employee to engage in two-way communication and relate to the supervisor on an equal or near-equal basis.

2. *Interpersonal space.*    The amount of space that feels comfortable between people in conversation varies across cultures. Anglo-Americans prefer to keep at least two feet between them during a conversation with a colleague, but Hispanic Americans or African Americans consider this distance too great and try to move closer, which makes many Anglo-Americans feel uncomfortable. The person moving away may be thought of as cold, distant, and indifferent whereas the person moving closer may be thought of as pushy or inappropriately intimate.

3. *Eye contact.*   Generally speaking, Anglo-Americans use eye contact to indicate that they are listening but look away frequently when they are speaking. African Americans make greater eye contact when they are speaking, which may be misinterpreted as glaring by Anglo-Americans. In contrast, Hispanics and Japanese Americans may avoid eye contact to show respect.

4. *Expressiveness.*    People from traditional Chinese, Japanese, and Native American cultural groups value restraint in the expression of strong feelings or discussion of personal matters, whereas people from the Middle East are likely to be louder and more exuberant in expressing their feelings. Somewhere in between is the North American.

5. *Language.*    When people speak different languages, the communication problem is obvious. However, when they speak the same language, they may not be aware that they speak different versions of that language. Here are three examples (Kenton & Valentine, 1997):

- If you **table** an item at a meeting in the United States it means you are postponing discussion but if you **table** an item in Britain, you are going to discuss it during that meeting.
- A **billion** in the United States and Canada is a thousand million (1,000,000,000) but a million million (1,000,000,000,000) in England.
- When an American says "quite good" he or she probably means "very good" but an Englishman or woman probably means "less than good."

The use of nonstandard English and regional differences in the use of some words can also lead to misinterpretations and misunderstandings. In healthcare organizations, the frequent use of abbreviations and shortened words can be mystifying to new employees who assumed they spoke the same language.

Differences in communication style are also critical to mutual understanding. A few examples:

- When a Japanese listener says "yes" it means "I am paying attention," not necessarily "I agree with you." Indications of a negative response are subtle: changing the subject, apologizing, or asking a question (Kenton & Valentine, 1997).
- When an Anglo woman says "I'm sorry" it means she regrets that something happened but it does not mean she is apologizing, but an Anglo man may interpret her "I'm sorry" as an apology.

6. *Modes of thinking.*    A number of differences are present in modes of thinking among cultural groups. Some emphasize the intuitive and creative approach to knowing; others emphasize the objective, logical, and scientific method. Some people make a clear distinction between physical and mental health (a distinction that is evident in the structure of our healthcare system); others do not. Some people are familiar with abstract thought, such as the use of theories and principles, and are comfortable with ambiguity, whereas others prefer a concrete, structured mode that uses examples and offers specific directions. Each of these differences affects exchanges between people from different cultures.

## RESEARCH EXAMPLE 7–1   *A Comparison of Two Ethnic Groups*

Two thousand Hispanics and 1,000 African Americans from across the United States were interviewed both by telephone and face-to-face by Market Segment Research, Inc., a market research firm in Florida, to determine their attitudes and values. The results of this survey found substantial differences within each ethnic group as well as across groups.

The majority of the Hispanics interviewed spoke Spanish at home. A small proportion spoke only English. People in the Hispanic group were less likely to have health insurance than were people in the African American group. Some other in-teresting findings from the comparison of attitudes and values are shown in the accompanying table.

It is important to note that the reported margin of error for these results ranged from plus or minus 2.2 to 9.8 percent for the data about the different cities and that substantial differences were noted within groups as well as among groups.

*Source:* Based on Arrarte, A.M. & Barciela, S. (1993, February 22). Study discovers vast differences within racial and ethnic groups. *Miami Herald*.

|  | Percent Who Agreed with Statement | | | | | | | |
|  | African Americans | | | | Hispanics | | | |
|  | Chicago | LA | NY | Miami | Chicago | LA | NY | Miami |
|---|---|---|---|---|---|---|---|---|
| A woman can have a career and still be a good mother. | 71 | 56 | 77 | 77 | 60 | 68 | 67 | 64 |
| Financial security is very important. | 57 | 47 | 64 | 54 | 65 | 60 | 58 | 70 |
| I am better off now economically than five years ago. | 33 | 32 | 44 | 47 | 31 | 31 | 34 | 41 |
| I resent being called a minority. | 32 | 41 | 34 | 28 | 24 | 49 | 24 | 44 |
| I try to keep up with changes in style and fashion. | 19 | 21 | 32 | 35 | 14 | 19 | 24 | 23 |

Some research also shows gender differences in preferred modes of thinking (Arnst, 1999). Fisher (1999) suggests that women are big picture "web" thinkers while men are more likely to be focused "step" thinkers. Women seem to pay more attention to multiple sources of information, nonverbal cues, and the broader context of an issue. Men compartmentalize and ignore extraneous information more readily than women.

7. *Use of evidence.* Regard for the scientific method has been found to be higher in developed countries. Developing countries, in general, allow more subjective (intuitive, emotional) factors in decision making. These differences may cause difficulty in adaptation for people who are new to the United States, which is a significant concern for the health-care field and its employees from many different cultural backgrounds (Negandhi, 1985).

8. *Preferred leadership and management style.* A number of cross-cultural and cross-national research studies have identified cultural differences in leadership and management styles. Organizations in Brazil, for example, generally have fewer levels within their hierarchies and typically call fewer meetings than do American organizations. A Brazilian manager would be surprised at how many types of authorization an American manager needs to get something done. On the other hand, an American worker would probably find Peru's managers to be formal and authoritarian (Albert, 1992).

Some additional cross-cultural comparisons may be found in Research Example 7–1.

These cultural differences should not be overemphasized because you can find almost as many differences within a culture as between cultures. They are generalizations, meant to heighten your awareness of the differences and the ways they can affect behavior. They are also intended to increase your sensitivity to ways in which misunderstandings can develop between people from different cultures. Many of these differences are subtle and easily overlooked by the leader who is not alert for them.

● WORKING WITH PEOPLE
OF DIVERSE CULTURES

The healthcare field attracts people from many different cultures. You may work with people from your own culture or with people from a culture that is entirely new and unfamiliar to you. In some situations, you may find yourself a part of the majority. In others you may find yourself a part of the minority culture, which is generally a more uncomfortable position and can be a source of considerable stress for some people (Mai-Dalton, 1993).

> **America is not a melting pot but a great mosaic where all the nationalities of the world have come to lend their hues and tints.**
> —*Preston, 1991, p. X*

When you are a part of the majority culture, it will be especially important for you to show respect and consideration for people from different cultural groups. If you are in the minority, you may have to demand this respect and consideration from others. In either case, knowledge of both your own cultural patterns and those of other cultures is an essential first step in developing effective working relationships among people of different cultures.

No shortcut can be taken to reach cultural awareness and effectiveness. Working with people of different cultures requires some insight into your own feelings about those who are different in some way, as well as time to learn about these differences and develop your ability to rec-

ognize them. The following suggestions can help you move in this direction:

1. *Learn more about cultural beliefs, values, and practices.* Knowledge comes before understanding. Learning about your own culture may actually be more difficult than learning about another culture, because it is so much a part of you that it is below your awareness until you begin studying it or are exposed to other cultures.

> **We're not tasters of the diversity stew; we're ingredients.**
> —*Stewart,* The American Nurse, *January/February 1998, p. 1*

2. *Resist seeing everyone in a particular culture as being alike.* If you read about your own culture, you will probably find that some of the descriptions fit you personally, while others do not. The same is true for people from other cultures.

3. *Interpret behavior on the basis of its meaning to the other person and that person's culture.* Try not to interpret the behavior of people from a different culture on the basis of your own culture. The difference in the interpretation of direct eye contact is an example. For some people, it communicates interest and openness; for others, it communicates rudeness and insubordination.

4. *Observe different cultural patterns in behavior.* If you watch the ways in which people from different cultural groups interact, you can begin to get a feeling for the customary distance they maintain between people, the degree of expressiveness, eye contact, and so forth. It both increases your awareness and helps you to feel more comfortable with different patterns.

5. *Adjust your own patterns somewhat to reduce the difference between your own and other people's patterns.* This suggestion does not mean that you must give up your culture and become the same as the people with whom you work. It does mean that you can make some accommodations, such as speaking a little softer or louder, moving a little closer or farther away, or using more abstract or concrete expressions, in order to facilitate com-

munication and develop more comfortable working relationships.

6. *Distinguish between behavior that needs to be changed and behavior that can be accommodated.* This distinction is especially important. Some behaviors do need to be changed. In some jobs, for example, it is necessary for an employee to arrive at exactly the agreed-on time so that people on the previous shift can turn their patients' care over to the next shift and go home. It is also necessary to learn enough of your clients' languages to be able to communicate with them, especially to counsel them. Other behaviors can be accommodated. For example, a wide variation in such differences as preferred personal distance, expressiveness, and responses to people in authority can be tolerated in most work situations.

## ● LEADING AND MANAGING A DIVERSE WORKFORCE

### Basic Do's and Don'ts

Effective management of cultural diversity requires considerable time and energy. Superficial "window-dressing" efforts are usually unsuccessful (see Table 7–1).

### Don'ts

A misguided attempt to increase understanding may be worse than doing nothing. It can provoke frustration, defensiveness, scapegoating, and deep disillusionment that is difficult to reverse (Lynch, 1992). Expecting the management of diversity to be easy and looking for ready-made solutions are common mistakes. Other mistakes include:

- Lowering performance and promotion standards for women and minorities
- Failing to provide good role models and mentors
- Expecting assimilation into the prevailing cultural group
- Expecting change from, or paying attention to, only one segment of the workforce, either the minority group or the majority group (Mai-Dalton, 1993)

Research Example 7–2 describes the results of a survey of American workers' perceptions about discrimination in the workplace.

### Do's

Actions that facilitate movement toward increased sensitivity and responsiveness to the needs of a diverse workforce include the following:

- Raise cultural awareness
- Take steps to increase contact among groups

---

**Table 7–1**  Do's and Don'ts for Managing Diversity

| **Do...** | **Don't...** |
|---|---|
| Recognize diversity. | Pretend everyone is alike. |
| Value diversity. | Expect everyone to conform to the prevailing culture. |
| Develop informal supports. | Seek only the quick, easy solution. |
| Ensure fairness. | Develop different standards of performance. |
| Support diversity as an integral part of the organization's philosophy. | Expect one workshop guest speaker or training film to solve the problem. |

**RESEARCH EXAMPLE 7–2   *A Changing Workforce: What Does It Mean?***

The Families and Work Institute conducted an extensive national study of hourly and salaried workers (Shellenbarger, 1993). In-depth telephone interviews were conducted with 2,598 workers for this national study of the changing workforce supported by 15 private corporations and foundations.

**Diversity and Discrimination**

About half of the employees surveyed said that they still preferred to work with people of the same race, gender, and education. Most of their contact with people of a different race or ethnic group occurred at work. Respondents agreed that minority workers still had fewer opportunities for advancement. The "grass looked greener on the other side of the fence" for many of the respondents: minority men, minority women, and white women rated white men's opportunities for advancement higher than the white men themselves did.

One fifth of the minority respondents said that they had experienced discrimination on the job. This experience correlated with a tendency to feel burned out. Female managers also rated their opportunities for advancement much lower than men did. Respondents did not see much difference in the way male and female managers functioned.

**Work-Family Conflicts**

When conflicts between work and family responsibilities occurred, the respondents reported that they were three times more likely to give up time with their family than to reduce their work time. Two thirds of those who had children said that the time they had to spend with their families was inadequate, that they wanted to spend the time but came home exhausted.

*Source:* Shellenbarger, S. (1993, September 3). Work-force study finds loyalty is weak, divisions of race and gender are deep. *Wall Street Journal.*

- Create informal support systems and networks
- Institute policies and procedures that require fairness and prohibit discrimination

Each of these do's is explained further in the next section of this chapter.

## Cultural Awareness

Workshops, seminars, role playing, and skill building all help to increase cross-cultural understanding. Mai-Dalton (1993) suggests emphasizing the similarities (we all have families of some kind; we all seek love and respect) as well as teaching staff about the differences (our definitions of family are unique; we may express love and respect in different ways) (Kavanagh & Kennedy, 1992).

Adoption and implementation of an organizational philosophy valuing diversity is essential to the institutionalization of these changes. Otherwise, the organization risks the danger that people will begin the process of change in these

sessions but abandon it when returning to their usual routines.

*We know that racism, sexism, and all kinds of other ism's exist and that bigotry and prejudice are facts of life. But we also believe that many people want to be open-minded but are simply not aware of the effect of their words and behavior on others.*

—*Blank & Slipp, 1994*

## Increasing Contact between Groups

Long-term, genuine contact that is clearly valued by those in authority may be needed to increase understanding. Groups composed of culturally and ethnically diverse people may experience more conflict (overt or covert) and take more time to become mature groups. Time, effort, and commitment to the goal of becoming a truly multicultural organization are clearly needed to succeed.

## Informal Support Systems and Networks

Sometimes assigning people to mentors may create too artificial a situation to succeed consistently. Instead, informal coaching and tutoring may provide more genuine support for individuals. Effective informal support networks are also helpful. Leaders and managers can encourage their formation and make sure that those who do not belong to them are not threatened by their effectiveness. (See Perspectives . . . Encounters with Bias in the Workplace.)

## Requiring Fairness and Prohibiting Discrimination

Fairness and valuing of diversity can become an integral part of the formal level of operations in an organization. Affirmative action committees to monitor the fairness of policies and their implementation; formation of advisory groups representing various minority groups within the organization; active recruitment, selection, and promotion of women and minorities; and monitoring of their progress are all formal ways to achieve more organizational equity.

> *When employers stop identifying workers by their ethnicity and instead see them as productive colleagues, businesses will be that much closer to achieving true workplace diversity.*
> —Arthur, 1998, p. 42

**Equal employment opportunity laws** at both the federal and state levels prohibit discrimination in hiring and paying employees. The Equal Pay Act of 1963, for example, prohibits paying women less than men for doing the same work. Other laws prohibit discrimination on the basis of age, disability, pregnancy, religion, and nation of origin (Arthur, 1998):

- *Age.* Despite assumptions to the contrary, older works have fewer on-the-job accidents, less work-related stress, and fewer avoidable absences than younger workers. Unless a job

## PERSPECTIVES . . .

### Encounters with Bias in the Workplace

A group of 10 highly successful senior managers of color were invited to participate in a *Harvard Business Review* roundtable discussion. Each participant shared his or her own personal experience with bias and how he or she overcame it successfully.

A few examples of their experiences of bias:

- "I remember when I was a child, a teacher telling me, 'Oh, Santiago, you can't be Mexican, you're too smart!' "
- "I sat there while an executive asked two associates who worked for me to go out and play golf at his country club . . . I remember thinking . . . 'He never asked if I could play!' "
- "What I have encountered many times is surprise-surprise that a person of color in authority like myself is the analytical, academic, or intellectual equal of my white peers."

How did they succeed? Here is a sampling of what they said about succeeding:

- "I always knew I had to believe in myself, because I couldn't assume that anybody else was going to believe in me."
- "Frequently, white supervisors are reluctant to give negative feedback . . . because they are afraid it will end up in a lawsuit or be misinterpreted as racism. But I signaled that it was okay—I would hear what they had to say, and I would act on it."
- "You can't underestimate the power of professional networks, because when they are positively focused, you no longer feel alone or isolated . . . and that can be tremendously helpful both personally and professionally."
- "People of color have a buddy-mentoring program for recent hires . . . they have a chance on a regular basis to talk about their careers with people like them who have been there and know the ropes."

*Source:* Thomas, D.A. & Wetlauer, S. (1997). A question of color: A debate on race in the U.S. workplace. *Harvard Business Review,* 118–132.

requires a high level of physical strength, they also perform as well and adapt to changing work demands. Until illness or advanced old age (the 80s or 90s) take effect, that saying, "You can't teach an old dog new tricks," simply does not apply to older workers.

- *Disability.* Most accommodations for people with disabilities (such as ADD, telephone devices for the deaf) are of minimal cost to employers. With minimal accommodation, most disabled have low absence rates and perform well on the job. One of the major barriers is the discomfort of other people with another's disability, which manifests itself in a number of ways from reluctance to hire to patronizing or overprotective behavior to exclusion from social activities.
- *Minorities.* Lower expectations, inadequate feedback that is overly harsh or patronizingly mild, and limits on opportunities for advancement continue to be problems for members of minority groups. Although overt bias has decreased, the more subtle forms continue to operate in many settings. Focusing on the ability of the individual, not on the individual as a member of a particular minority group, is the key to fairness in hiring, managing, and promotion.

What does the leader need to bring to this effort? Respect for differences in attitudes, values, and behavior is essential (Spicer et al., 1994) and includes a commitment to fairness; an antisexism, antiracism, antiethnocentrism, and antiageism attitude; in-depth understanding of diversity; openness to change; a vision of a genuinely multicultural organization; and the ability to model the behavior expected of others (Mai-Dalton, 1993).

## ● SUMMARY

Reflecting the society as a whole, the nursing profession witnessed discrimination against men, blacks, and other groups earlier in the twentieth century. Today, even though much progress has

## C A S E   S T U D Y

### Managing a "Tricultural" Unit

It was an oversimplification, Reuben admitted, but he often thought of his acute geriatric unit (AGU) as "tricultural": the nurses were primarily Hispanic, the patients (many of them over 90) were primarily of Russian Jewish extraction, and most of the ancillary staff had been born in the Caribbean islands, particularly Haiti. Ancillary staff often adapted a "parental" approach to the patients, scolding them when they "complained too much." Many of the patients preferred to speak Yiddish or Russian, languages completely incomprehensible to the Hispanic nurses or Haitian patient care assistants. Some days Reuben despaired of them ever understanding each other.

### Questions for Critical Reflection and Analysis

1. Why is the problem faced by Reuben a concern for a nurse manager?
2. If you were the nurse manager of the unit described, how would you determine the extent and seriousness of the cross-cultural "understanding" problem in the acute geriatric unit?
3. How would you approach resolving the cross-cultural understanding problem on the AGU? What strategies would you use?
4. What kind of response would you look for in the nurses, ancillary staff, and patients on the AGU? How would you know, in other words, that your plan for resolution of the problem was successful?
5. How would you ensure that the changes you brought about are neither superficial nor short-lived?

been made, diversity within the profession lags behind that of the population as a whole.

Recognizing and accommodating differences across groups enriches the entire organization. Indicators that tolerance of diversity has not occurred include lower pay, less mobility, and higher turnover among minority employees. A sociogram may be used to identify patterns of free mixing versus clustering by identified groups within an organization.

A person's culture includes all of the learned patterns of beliefs, values, and behaviors common to a group or society. Variations in beliefs about the nature of people, time orientation, and relationships to nature and to other people are found across cultures. Additional variations of particular interest to leaders and managers include relationship to people in authority, use of interpersonal space, eye contact, emotional expressiveness, language, modes of thinking, use of evidence, and preferred leadership and management styles.

Nurse leaders and first-line managers need to develop some insight into their own cultures and the cultures of the people with whom they work. Knowledge of self and others comes first, followed by learning to see the individual as well as the group, interpreting behavior more accurately, and distinguishing that which needs to be changed from that which can be accommodated.

Common errors in leading and managing diverse work groups include unequal performance standards, expecting assimilation, and looking for easy solutions. Helpful actions include raising cultural awareness, increasing contact across the clusters (groups) that can form in a work environment, encouraging the development of mentoring relationships and networks, and instituting policies and procedures that support fairness and prohibit discrimination.

## REFERENCES

Albert, R.D. (1992). Polycultural perspectives on organizational communication. *Management Communication Quarterly, 6*(1), 74–84.

Andrews, M.M. (1998). Transcultural perspectives in nursing administration. *Journal of Nursing Administration, 28*(11), 30–38.

Arnst, C. (1999, June 14). Will the 21st century be a woman's world? *Business Week,* 24.

Arrarte, A.M. & Barciela, S. (1993, February 22). Study discovers vast differences within racial and ethnic groups. *Miami Herald.*

Arthur, D. (1998). *Recruiting, interviewing, selecting and orienting new employees.* New York: AMACOM.

Axtell, R.E. (1991). *Gestures: The do's and taboos of body language around the world.* New York: John Wiley & Sons.

Blank, R. & Slipp, S. (1994). *Voices of diversity: Real people talk about problems and solutions in a workplace where everyone is not alike.* New York: AMACOM.

Burtt, K. (1998). Male nurses still face bias. *American Journal of Nursing, 98*(9), 64–65.

Carnegie, M.E. (1995). *The path we tread: Blacks in nursing worldwide, 1854–1994.* New York: National League for Nursing Press.

Fisher, H. (1999). *The natural talents of women and how they are changing the world.* New York: Random House.

Hall, E.T. & Whyte, W.F. (1976). Intercultural communication: A guide to men of action. In P.J. Brink (Ed.). *Transcultural nursing: A book of readings.* Englewood Cliffs, NJ: Prentice-Hall.

Kavanagh, K.H. & Kennedy, P.H. (1992). *Promoting cultural diversity.* Newbury Park, CA: Sage.

Kenton, S.B. & Valentine, D.C. (1997). *Crosstalk: Communicating in a multicultural workplace.* Upper Saddle River, NJ: Prentice-Hall.

Kluckhohn, F.R. (1976). Dominant and variant value orientations. In P.J. Brink (Ed.). *Transcultural nursing: A book of readings.* Englewood Cliffs, NJ: Prentice-Hall.

Kolb, D.A., Oslund, J.S. & Rubin, I.M. (1995). Organizational behavior: An experiential approach. Englewood Cliffs, NJ: Prentice-Hall.

Krebs, V. (1992). Measuring how your organization really works. *Healthcare Forum Journal, 35*(1), 34–39.

Leininger, M. (1986). *Transcultural nursing: Concepts, theories and practices.* New York: John Wiley & Sons.

Lynch, F.R. (1992, October 26). Multiculturalism comes to the workplace. *Wall Street Journal.*

Mai-Dalton, R.R. (1993). Managing cultural diversity on the individual, group and organizational levels. In M.M. Chemers & R. Ayman (Eds.). *Leadership theory and research: Perspectives and directions.* San Diego: Academic Press.

Malone, B.L. (1998). Diversity, divisiveness and divinity. *The American Nurse, 30*(1), 5, 27.

Moch, M.K. & Bartunek, J.M. (1990). *Creating alternative realities at work: The quality of work life experience at FoodCom.* New York: Harvard Business.

Negandhi, A.R. (1985). Management in the Third World. In P. Joynt and M. Warner (Eds.). *Managing in different cultures*. Oslo: Universitetsforlaget AS.

Pavlovich-Davis, S., Forman, H. & Smek, P.P. (1998, March 9). Nurse-physician relationship: Can it be saved? *Nursing Spectrum, 6, 7,* 16.

Preston, J.E. (1991). Foreword. In R.R. Thomas (Ed.). *Beyond race and gender*. New York: AMACOM.

Scarborough, J.C. (1998). *The origins of cultural differences and their impact on management*. Westport, CT: Quorum Books.

Shellenbarger, S. (1993, September 3). Work-force study finds loyalty is weak, divisions of race and gender are deep. *Wall Street Journal*.

Spicer, J.G. et al. (1994). Supporting ethnic and cultural diversity in nursing staff. *Nursing Management, 25*(1), 38–40.

Stewart, M. (1998, January/February) Mental disorders and culture-bound syndromes. *American Nurse,* 24–25.

Sue, D.W. (1981). *Counseling the culturally different: Theory and practice*. New York: John Wiley & Sons.

Thomas, D.A. & Wetlauer, S. (1997). A question of color: A debate on race in the U.S. workplace. *Harvard Business Review*, 118–132.

Triandis, H.C. (1993). The contingency model in cross-cultural perspective. In M.M. Chemers & R. Ayman (Eds.). *Leadership theory and research: Perspectives and directions*. San Diego: Academic Press.

Trossman, S. (1998). Diversity: A continuing challenge. *The American Nurse*.

Ward, L.B. (1992, December 27). In culturally diverse work place, language may alienate. *Miami Herald*.

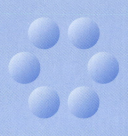

CHAPTER **8**

# Time Management

## LEARNING OBJECTIVES

*After completing this chapter, the reader will be able to:*

• Characterize his or her perception of time.
• Set short- and long-term personal and career goals.
• Analyze activities at work using a time log.

• Organize and streamline work to make more effective use of available time.
• Set limits on the demands made on his or her time.

**How Do You Perceive Time?**

1. Do you think of time more as a galloping horse, or a vast, motionless ocean?

2. Which of these words best describes time to you: sharp, active, empty, soothing, tense, cold, deep, clear, young, or sad?

3. Is your watch fast or slow? (You can check it with the radio.)

4. Ask a friend to help you do this test. Go into a quiet room without any work, reading material, radio, food, or other distractions. Have your friend call you in somewhere between 10 and 20 minutes. Try to guess how long you were in that room.

*Test Results Interpreted*

1. A person who has a circular concept of time would compare it to a vast, still ocean. A galloping horse would be characteristic of a linear conception of time, emphasizing speed and motion forward.

2. A fast-tempo, achievement-oriented person would describe time as clear, young, sharp, active, or tense rather than empty, soothing, sad, cold, or deep.

3&4. These same fast-tempo people are likely to have fast watches and to overestimate the amount of time that they sat in a quiet room (Webber, 1972; 1980).

Time urgency seems to be characteristic of our society today. Even if you have not yet been employed in a healthcare setting, you likely have experienced a hectic pace or overload of work, school, family, and personal responsibilities. Feeling rushed or lacking sufficient time to do your work well can lead to an increase in errors, omission of important tasks, and generalized feelings of stress and ineffectiveness (see Figure 8–1). For these reasons, we will look at ways to manage time in the workplace.

> *As a nation, we have a surfeit of "stuff" but an alarming dearth of time for ourselves and each other. Take our morning coffee: It now comes in 25— or is it 50?—flavors, but we haven't a minute to spare for a leisurely sip.*
>
> —Rublin, 1998

## ● THE TYRANNY OF TIME

In our society, calendars, clocks, computers, watches, newspapers, television, and radio all remind us of our position in time—how much of it we have used and how much we have left. How often do you look at your watch in a day? Do you divide your day into blocks of time? Do you

have separate activities planned for each hour or even for every few minutes? Or do you see the minutes, hours, and days as part of the whole of your life? Our perception of time is important because it affects our use of time and our response to time (see Test Yourself).

## Differing Time Perceptions

Most Western societies conceptualize time as linear, moving forward like an arrow. Other cultures perceive time as circular, measured in seasons and important events instead of in hours, minutes, and seconds. They see time as continuous and repetitive: if you have missed an opportunity, it will come around to you again someday. Western thinking on the other hand, emphasizes that once a particular time has passed, it will never be repeated again. If you were sick, for example, and missed a New Year's Eve celebration, you can never recapture that opportunity. You can celebrate another New Year, but it will be a different one. If you are a highly achievement-oriented person, with a Western perspective on time, you are more likely to have already set some career goals for yourself and to have a mental schedule of deadlines for reaching these goals ("become assistant administrator in 8 years").

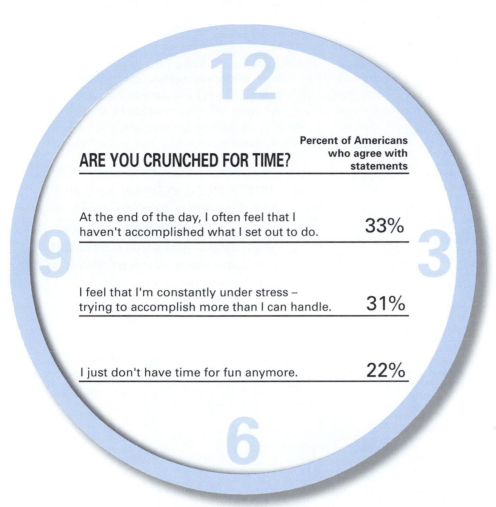

**ARE YOU CRUNCHED FOR TIME?**

**Percent of Americans who agree with statements**

At the end of the day, I often feel that I haven't accomplished what I set out to do.    **33%**

I feel that I'm constantly under stress – trying to accomplish more than I can handle.    **31%**

I just don't have time for fun anymore.    **22%**

**Figure 8–1**    Proportion of Americans who feel pressured by time.
*Source:* Adapted from *Miami Herald* (1992, October 25). With permission from Hilton Time Values Survey, 1991.

In some European countries, people like to brag that the trains are so punctual you can set your watch by them. Computers complete operations in a fraction of a second, and we can measure speed to the nanosecond. Time clocks that record the minute we enter and leave work are commonplace, and few excuses for being late are really considered acceptable. Time sheets and schedules are a part of most healthcare professionals' lives. We are expected to follow precisely set schedules and meet deadlines for virtually everything we do, from distributing medications to getting reports done on time. In community settings, nurses are asked to account for their time from entering the office to leaving in the evening, specify-

ing travel time, clinic time, home visits, meetings, recordkeeping, and so on. Many agencies produce vast quantities of computer-generated data that can be analyzed in terms of the amount of time spent on various activities. It is no wonder some of us feel obsessed with time.

Individual personality, culture, and environment all interact to influence our perceptions of time (Matejka & Dunsing, 1988). In Western cultures, we expect to get to the point quickly and reach a conclusion as soon as possible during a business meeting. In Eastern cultures, taking enough time to listen to everyone and keep the dialogue going is usually considered more important (McGee-Cooper, 1994).

Each of us also has a different internal tempo (Chapple, 1970). Some of us have fast tempos, others have slow ones. We can change our tempos, to some extent, in response to a variety of contexts (Davis, 1982). A fast-paced environment, for example, will influence most of us to work at a faster pace despite the difficulty or discomfort experienced if our internal tempo is much slower.

## Hurry Sickness

Excessive time urgency has been related to increased job stress and associated risks (Lee, Ashford & Jamieson, 1993). **Hurry sickness** is the term Larry Dossey (1994) uses for the deleterious effects of time pressure. McGee-Cooper (1994) defined hurry sickness as "habitual, un-necessary or compulsive rushing that leads to the speeding up of our natural body functions, ultimately damaging our health" (p. 13). The pressure to do more with less in health care can contribute to hurry sickness. Box 8–1 lists some of the signs of hurry sickness that you might want to watch out for in yourself and in your colleagues.

*We grow up believing that time is a "thing" that is external and objective, that flows from birth to death, and that we sooner or later will run out. This is one of the most pernicious and damaging ideas we ever develop. It can, in fact, be fatal.*

—*L. Dossey in McGee-Cooper, 1994, p. X*

---

## Box 8–1  Signs of Hurry Sickness

- **Rushing Whether or Not It Matters**
  *Example*:  Leaving a movie theater before the credits run at the end
  Wanting to be the first one off when the bus stops
- **Getting Angry When Someone Wastes Our Time**
  *Example*:  Losing your temper when someone cuts in front of you in line
  Becoming angry when you have to wait for a sales clerk to help you
- **Skipping Meals, Breaks**
  *Example*:  Working through break time on a regular basis
  Eating standing up or while talking on the telephone
- **Overscheduling Our Lives**
  *Example*:  Filling every free moment with organized activities, events
  Scheduling after-school classes and sports for your children every day of the week and on the weekend
- **Becoming Impatient If Someone Talks or Moves Too Slowly**
  *Example*:  Frequently urging people to "get to the point"
  Losing your temper when caught in a traffic jam
- **Addiction to Speed**
  *Example*:  Talking too fast or about several things at once
  Driving too fast
  Eating too fast
- **Failing to Savor the Moment**
  *Example*:  Being unaware of the first crocuses coming up in spring
  Not caring what you have for dinner
  Inattention to the people around you

*Source:* McGee-Cooper, A. (1994). *Time Management for unmanageable people.* New York: Bantam Books.

While many healthcare professionals are linear, fast-tempo, achievement-oriented people, simply working at a fast pace is not necessarily equivalent to accomplishing a great deal. Much energy can be dissipated in rushing about, stirring things up, but actually accomplishing little. The rest of this chapter considers ways in which you can use your time and energy to the best effect. We will begin by looking at how nurses spend their time.

## How Nurses Spend Their Time

Nurses are the largest single group of healthcare professionals. Sheer numbers alone warrant attention to the efficiency and effectiveness of their time management. The effect of rotating shifts, for example, has long been a concern in nursing. Nurses who rotate shifts are twice as likely to report medication errors than those who do not rotate. Night shift and rotating shift nurses also report getting less sleep, a poorer quality of sleep, greater use of sleep medication, and a problem with "nodding off" at work or while driving home after work (AJN, 1993).

A number of studies have looked at how nurses use their time, especially nurses in acute-care settings. One study by E.J. Murphy, Ltd., found that nurses engage in 93 different activities in a day compared with pharmacists, who are involved in an average of only 26 different activities in a typical workday, as illustrated by Figure 8–2 (AJN, 1992). Another study by Arthur Andersen and Co. found that only 35 percent of nurses' time was spent in direct patient care (including care planning, assessment, teaching, and technical activities). Documentation accounts for another 20 percent of their time. The remainder is spent on transporting patients, transaction processing, administrative responsibilities, and "hotel services"

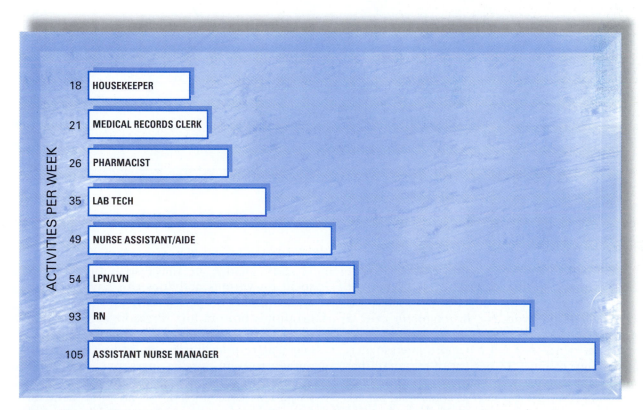

**Figure 8–2**   Average number of activities per week performed by nurses compared with other hospital employees.
*Source:* RNs do 93 different jobs, says hospital study. *American Journal of Nursing, 92*(12), 9. Used with permission.

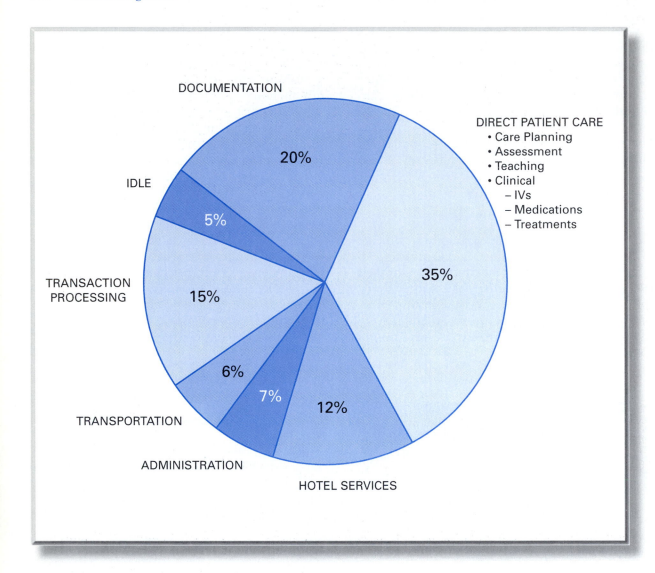

**Figure 8–3**   Nurse time allocation in direct patient care activities.
*Source:*  Brider, P. (1992). The move to patient-focused care. *American Journal of Nursing 92*(9), 29. Used with permission.

as indicated in Figure 8–3 (Brider, 1992). These categories change from study to study, but the amount of time spent on direct care is usually less than half of the workday. In long-term care, a larger proportion of nurses' time is spent in direct care (see Figure 8–4 ). Even more interesting is the amount of time (28 percent of the total) that nurses spend doing two or more things at once (Cardona et al., 1997), such as combining patient education with bathing or feeding. They also continued to do productive work such as directing ancillary staff or completing documentation during their meals and breaks.

Any change in the distribution of time spent on various activities can have a considerable impact on patient care and on the organization's bottom line. Prescott and associates (1991) offered an example: if more unit management responsibilities could be shifted from nurses to non-nursing personnel, about 48 minutes per nurse per shift could be redirected to patient care. In a large hospital with 600 full-time nurses, the result would be an additional 307 hours of direct patient care a day. A different way of describing the impact is even more impressive: the change would contribute

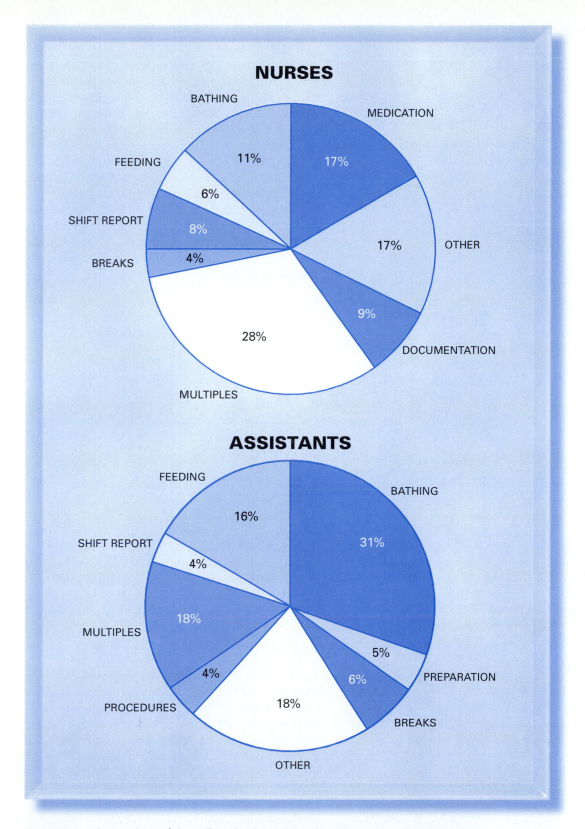

**Figure 8–4** Comparison of time allocation by registered nurses and nursing assistants. *Source:* Cardona, P. et al. (1997). Nursing staff time allocation in long-term care: A work sampling study. *Journal of Nursing Administration, 27*(2), 28–36. Used with permission.

the equivalent of 48 additional full-time nurses to direct patient care.

> *. . . being busy doing nothing much of value may indirectly contribute to patient suffering and could therefore be of ethical concern.*
> —Cave, 1998, p. 25

## ● ORGANIZING WORK ACTIVITIES

Now let's turn our attention to some specific ways to use time more effectively. Although some people are naturally more organized than others, a conscious effort can help any one of us avoid time-wasting disorganization. Kerzner (1998) created a list of more than 100 "time robbers." The following is a sampling of those he identified:

- Work done so poorly that it has to be done over again
- Misplaced report, records
- Failure to delegate
- Too many people involved in making a minor decision
- Unreliable employees, contractors
- Constant interruptions
- Too much record keeping, documentation, and other paperwork

Whether it is just eliminating extra steps or avoiding serious delays in finishing your work, organizing your work can reduce the amount of time spent doing things that are neither productive nor satisfying.

### Lists

One of the most useful organizers is a list of things to do. You can prepare this list either at the end of every day for the next day or first thing in the morning *before* you do anything else. Do not include the routine tasks because they will make the list too long and you will do them without an extra reminder. If you are a nurse manager, for example, it is not necessary to list the routine tasks of the day, such as mak-

ing assignments, giving reports, doing rounds, and so forth. Instead, put the unique tasks of the day on the list: preparation for a care-planning conference, telephone calls to families, discussion of a new project with the director of nursing, a stop at the library to research an unfamiliar diagnosis, or preparation of an employee evaluation. These tasks are the postponable ones that may not be done or will be done poorly in a last-minute rush if you do not allot the time to do them. Additionally, you may want to arrange them by priority, starting with those that must be done that day. To prioritize, you can consider the following points:

- What is the relative importance of each of these tasks?
- How much time will each task require?
- When must each task be completed?
- How much time and energy do I have to devote to these tasks? (Moshovitz, 1993)

If you find yourself postponing an item for several days, decide whether it should be given priority the next day or dropped from the list as an unnecessary task.

The list itself should be in a form most convenient for you: on your desk calendar if you spend most of your day in an office, or in your pocket or on a clipboard if you spend most of your day on a patient-care unit or in clients' homes. Checking the list several times a day for reminders will quickly become a good habit. It is also satisfying to be able to cross things off your list when they are done! Your daily list may become your most important time manager.

### Tickler Files

Tickler files are a kind of long-term list. The basic principle of a tickler file is that you create a system to remind yourself of approaching deadlines and due dates. For example, at the beginning of a school semester, you usually find out when exams will be given and assignments are due. Many students find it helpful to enter all of these dates on a semester-long calendar so that they can see in a glance what is due week by week, and look ahead to see what is coming, especially where several assignments or tests come at the same time. This long-range view allows you to see when you will have to begin preparation further in advance than usual or when it might be a good idea to request a change in the due dates to meet these multiple deadlines. Unlike the daily list, the tickler file may contain some regular assignments (such as budget report or the monthly summaries for long-term care patients) that you must prepare in advance.

Another useful technique is the daily reminder file, which is a set of file folders numbered 1 through 31 for each day of the month (some find weekly files just as useful). Simply drop a memo into your file to remind yourself of upcoming tasks. The trick is to make sure that you use these tickler files and look at them at the appropriate time.

Using a tickler file, you can anticipate coming deadlines and remind yourself when to begin preparation for a particular task. For example, the annual unit budget may be due on the first of July. Because you know that it takes about six weeks to finish the budget, you would write a note for your tickler file to begin work in the middle of May, allowing yourself enough time to get it done.

## Schedules and Blocks of Time

Without a schedule, you are much more likely to drift through a day or rush from one activity to another in a disorganized fashion. Assignment sheets, work sheets, flow sheets, and care plans are all designed to help you plan and schedule patient care time effectively. The care plan is the general design for the care of each individual patient or family. Assignment sheets indicate the patients or clients for whom each staff member is responsible. Work sheets are then created to organize the daily care that must be given to the assigned patients or clients. Flow sheets are lists of items that must be recorded for each patient.

Effective work sheets and flow sheets schedule and organize the day. They provide reminders of the various tasks and when they have to be done. The danger in them, however, is that the more they divide the day into discrete segments, the more they may fragment the work and impede a holistic approach. If the work sheet becomes the focus of attention, the perspective of the whole may be lost.

Some activities must be done at a certain time. They will structure your day or week to a great extent, and their timing may be out of your control. However, every job also contains tasks that can be done whenever you want to do them, as long as they are done on time. During available unstructured time you can schedule activities to suit yourself and your staff.

Several points merit consideration when scheduling discretionary time at work. First of all, certain tasks have earlier deadlines than others. Second, priorities in patient care, personal priorities, and your employer's priorities must be taken into account when deciding what to do first and how much time to spend on a task. Third, some activities are best done all at once. For these activities, you need to set aside **blocks** of time during which you can concentrate on the task. It is difficult, for example, to write a report or an evaluation by doing it 5 or 10 minutes at a time. By the time you reorient yourself to the task, the 5 or 10 minutes is over and nothing is accomplished. Doing such tasks all at one time or in several substantial blocks of time is a much more efficient use of your time. Finally, consider your own energy levels when scheduling your activities. A task that requires intense concentration should not be done at 4 P.M. if that is a time when your energy wanes. As much as possible, you should work *with* your energy levels, not against them.

Some people go to work early just to have a block of uninterrupted time to do a complicated task. Others take work home with them for the same reason. The drawback, however, is that you are extending your working hours at the expense of rest and leisure time. You may also be wasting time during your scheduled work hours, time in which you could have accomplished these tasks if you had rescheduled other activities, reduced interruptions, and avoided putting off difficult or unpleasant work.

## Time Lines

Although time lines are primarily a technique used in planning, they are also useful in time management. Time lines are usually project oriented, illustrating activities and the deadlines necessary to complete a project. If your work is primarily project oriented, a set of these time lines (one for each project) would be a helpful organizer. Project planning is discussed in Chapter 16.

## Filing Systems

Filing systems are particularly important to people with a great deal of paperwork, especially those at the coordinator or manager level. However, every professional maintains papers such as licenses, certificates, continuing education activities, current information for their specialty area, and so forth. Keeping these papers organized in easily retrievable files rather than in disorganized stacks saves much time when you have to find a particular piece of paper or information. Do not let unsorted papers accumulate. Instead, put them into files (manila folders, for example) right away so that you can find them easily when you need them again.

## ● SETTING LIMITS

In order to set limits, you must first know what your goals and priorities are. It can take quite a lot of determination to set limits and stick to them.

## Saying "No"

Saying "no" to nonpriority demands on your time is an important but difficult part of setting limits. Assertiveness and determination are necessary in maintaining limits.

Is it possible to say "no" to your boss? It may not seem so at first, but actually many requests from your manager or supervisor are negotiable. You may, for example, be asked to represent your division on a hospital public relations committee. The invitation is flattering and, if you have ambitions toward entering management in this organization, then this opportunity will probably help you move toward your goal. On the other hand, if your ambitions are focused on becoming an advanced nurse practitioner, membership on the committee would not further your goals, and you can, politely and regretfully, thank your supervisor and decline the invitation.

Can you refuse a burdensome patient assignment? Not directly but you can confront your su-

pervisor regarding the problem, particularly if you have been given more work than others on your team. You can also confront the issue of understaffing by filing an unsafe staffing complaint.

Some psychological needs can interfere with effective limit setting. For some people, ambition keeps them from saying "no" to any opportunities, no matter how overloaded they are. We call these people **workaholics,** but we may fail to see the symptoms in ourselves. Others have a great fear of displeasing people, especially their supervisors. They are afraid to question an assignment, negotiate a more reasonable workload, or accept a new task only when relieved of an old one. Still others have such a great need to be rescuers that they continually give of themselves, not only to clients but to their coworkers and supervisors, without replenishing themselves.

People who accept too much work hurt not only themselves but others as well. Out of sheer sensory overload or fatigue, their work will be inefficient and error prone, an unacceptable situation in a healthcare setting. Working extra hours on a regular basis can have a number of deleterious physical and emotional effects on the overworked individual, from headaches and frequent colds to injury and exhaustion (Trossman, 1998). It is the responsibility of the team leader or nurse manager to avoid overloading staff members despite the temptation to do so.

## Eliminating Unnecessary Work

Some work has become so deeply embedded into our routines that it *appears* to be required although it really is unnecessary. Some nursing routines fall into this category. Vital signs, baths, linen changes, dressing changes, irrigations, and similar basic tasks are more often done according to schedule rather than according to need, which may be much more or much less often than the routine.

Many meetings also fall into this category. If you are the leader of the group, then it is fairly easy to cancel unnecessary meetings, but if you are a member of the group, it may require a combination of diplomacy and persuasiveness to eliminate time wasters. Remember that some gatherings meet other needs—they provide a time to vent feelings, work on relationships, or get away from the pressures of the job for a short time. These needs are important, so it is a good idea to analyze the value of a meeting before dismissing it as worthless.

Much paperwork is duplicative; some is unnecessary altogether. You may find, for example, that some assessments or nursing interventions are charted in two or three different places on the patient record. Most of the time these duplications can be eliminated. Charting by exception is another way to eliminate unnecessary work. Each setting will have its own rituals, duplications, and well-established but unnecessary routines. It requires a critical eye to spot these activities and a persistent questioning of their purpose to eliminate them—another reason to be a critical thinker.

Social talk in the hallways, nurses' lounge, cafeterias, and by office coffee pots takes up a lot of time during the day. Some of this seemingly useless talk has a purpose (Duck, 1994). If you recall that most leadership theories emphasize both the relationship and task aspects of work, you will recognize that some of this talk meets important human needs. However, you must use your judgment about how much is good for working relationships and at what point it begins to reduce productivity. In times of crisis or heightened tensions, more attention to relationships will be needed; at other times, you can lead others back to the task by saying, "Let's get back to work."

You may also have created additional work for yourself without realizing it. Do you rewrite assignment sheets every day when they could be duplicated and have changes written in? Do you write long answers to memos when a brief note could be written right on the memo that was sent to you? Do you do work that you could delegate to other people? Do you drive to a client's home or walk down the hall to a patient's room when you could use the telephone or intercom system? Are you ritualistic in your care, doing procedures as you originally learned them, or do you modify them according to the principles behind them to eliminate unnecessary steps? Is your staff still collecting vital signs at predetermined intervals instead of making informed judgments regarding individual patients' needs for monitoring? Are they giving medications to rehabilitation patient's who should be learning how to do it for them-

selves before they go home? These examples are just a few of the kinds of work that take much time but may be unnecessary (Huey, 1986).

## Keeping Goals Reasonable

Do you plan to do more work than it is reasonable to expect of one person? Many people's time management problems stem from their failure to keep their goals reasonable. Only the rare superhuman individual can accept every challenge and excel in every endeavor. The rest of us need to limit our goals to those that are likely to be attainable and then to be satisfied with what we are able to do.

## Delegating

As you move up the organizational ladder, it will become more and more necessary for you to delegate work to other people. At the staff-nurse level, clerical tasks, cleaning, transport, and simple patient care tasks such as distributing meal trays should be delegated to patient care assistants. Complex tasks, those requiring specialized knowledge, should not be delegated. Consider the following important points when delegating work to others in order to save time:

1. *Delegate work but do not dump it.* Delegation is assigning work with the assurance that the individual has the necessary training, supervision, and authority to get it done; dumping is just getting rid of work in any way possible. It quickly becomes obvious if you attempt to get rid of unpleasant or boring tasks and keep the interesting work for yourself. (Making assignments is discussed in Chapter 11).

2. *Select the appropriate level of delegation.* The amount of supervision and control you maintain should be appropriate to the task and to the skill of the staff member. Delegation can range from telling the staff member exactly what needs to be done and how to do it and then following the person's work closely (level 1) to allowing some freedom to decide how to do it (level 2) to telling the staff members what has to be done and letting them decide how to best get it done (level 3) (Haynes, 1991). For example:

*If you delegate the task of ambulating an orthopedic patient to a patient care assistant (PCA), you will have to give explicit directions and observe how well they are carried out if the PCA is inexperienced (level 1). If the PCA is more experienced, you have only to remind the PCA of particularly important points such as limitations on weight bearing or prevention of falls (level 2). With a PCA who has received extra training, however, you may just delegate the task and confirm that the PCA is familiar with the patient's needs (level 3).*

3. *Maintain control and responsibility.* When you have delegated work, you are still ultimately responsible for the outcome. It is important to clearly communicate your expectations about the quality of care expected and ensure that performance standards are met.

A good many people try to do all the work themselves with the result that they are severely overloaded. Why do they do it? Occasionally the perfectionist demands of their supervisors make it difficult to delegate (Haynes, 1991). The reluctance to delegate may also be due to a person's own perfectionism, insecurity, desire for power or control, lack of leadership ability, or enjoyment of the task that could be delegated.

A frequent protest is that it takes too much time to give directions to other people. "It's easier to do it myself," is a common excuse. Sometimes it is true. A study by Booz-Allen found that 14 cents of every dollar a hospital spends on salaries goes for coordinating and scheduling care. Another 29 cents is spent on documenting care. Only 16 cents of the dollar goes to direct care (Brider, 1992). The patient-focused model for organizing nursing care (described in Chapter 12) has been developed in part to reduce the enormous amount of time presently spent on scheduling and coordination.

## ● STREAMLINING WORK ACTIVITIES

Many tasks can be neither eliminated nor delegated, but they can be done more efficiently. Many axioms in time management reflect the principle of streamlining work. "Work smarter, not harder," is a favorite. "Never handle a piece of paper more than once," reflects the need to avoid procrastination." "A stitch in time saves nine," reflects the degree to which preventive action saves time in the long run. "Time is money," reflects the organization's growing interest in streamlining work.

How can you streamline your work? A few general suggestions follow but the first one, a time log, can assist you in developing others unique to your particular situation. If you keep the log accurately a few surprises about how you really spend your time are almost guaranteed.

### Keeping a Time Log

Our perception of time is elastic. People do not accurately estimate the time they spend on any particular task, so we cannot rely on our memories for accurate information about how we have been spending our time (Adelman, 1997). (See Perspectives . . . Are We Really Overworked?) Once you see how large amounts of your time are spent, you may be able to eliminate or reduce the time spent on nonproductive activities (Drucker, 1967; Robichaud, 1986).

Figure 8–5 illustrates a general format for a time log in which you enter your activities every half hour. This format means that you will have to pay careful attention to what you are doing so that you can record it accurately every half hour. Do not postpone the recording—your memory of time is too elastic. A three-day sample may be enough for you to see a pattern emerging. Repeat the process in six months, both because work situations change and to see whether you have made any long-lasting changes in your use of time. If you work in a fast-paced environment, you should note what you are doing every 15 minutes instead of every half hour.

### Reducing Interruptions

Everyone experiences interruptions. Some are welcome, others are necessary, but too many interfere with your work. Interruptions should be kept to minimum. Closing the door to your office or to a patient room may reduce interruptions. You may also have to ask visitors to wait a few minutes before you can answer their questions; if you do, it is important to remain sensi-

## PERSPECTIVES . . .

### Are We Really Overworked?

Every 10 years, researchers from the Americans' Use of Time Project ask respondents to report how they spend their time by keeping time diaries. Their controversial conclusion: "Americans routinely overstate work and understate leisure time" (p. 1L). Although people generally say they have about 18 hours a week free, the diaries indicated it was closer to 40 hours a week. Women have less free time than men.

How can the researchers' conclusions differ so much from what the majority believe? A major factor seems to be how much time people believe they spend watching television. The researchers compared the diaries with Nielsen ratings that indicate Americans average 27 hours per week in front of the television.

They concluded that free time spent in front of the television was underreported by respondents. Another factor is that people exaggerate more than they used to. For example, people may say they worked from 8 to 6 but actually worked only 8 of those 10 hours. When asked about work, people rated it as both a high and a low of their day. One respondent compared work to golf: "You have a lot of bad times and frustrations, but you keep coming back for that one good hole . . . that makes you forget all your bad shots" (p. 6L).

The solution? Allocate your free time more carefully. Pay attention to the amount of time you spend watching television. Learn to savor the moment, the little pleasures like a beautiful sunset or biting into a fresh tomato. "There is, in fact, time for life."

*Source:* Adelman, K. (1997, August 31). Overworked? *Miami Herald*, 1L, 6L. Reprinted from *Washingtonian Magazine*.

**DAILY TIME LOG**

| ACTIVITIES | COMMENTS |
| --- | --- |
| 6:30 | |
| 7:00 | |
| 7:30 | |
| 8:00 | |
| 8:30 | |
| 9:00 | |
| 9:30 | |
| 10:00 | |
| 10:30 | |
| 11:00 | |
| 11:30 | |
| 12:00 | |
| 12:30 | |
| 1:00 | |
| 1:30 | |
| 2:00 | |
| 2:30 | |
| 3:00 | |
| 3:30 | |
| 4:00 | |
| 4:30 | |
| 5:00 | |

**Figure 8–5**  Time log.

tive to their needs and return to them as soon as possible. You can also ask the unit secretary to hold nonemergency telephone messages for you or answer your beeper calls temporarily so that you can have uninterrupted time to complete your caregiving. Referring nonemergency calls to another staff member during the blocks of time you set aside to get your work done is also helpful. (Remember, however, you will be asked to extend the same courtesy to your colleague another time.) Unavoidable interruptions from other people may be kept short by thanking the person for the information and saying you must get back to what you were doing. You may find that charting takes less time while you are still with the patient or immediately after seeing a patient—the information is fresh in your mind and you do not have to rely on notes or recall. Try to follow a task to completion before beginning another whenever possible.

## Dealing with Recurrent Crises

Recurrent crises are actually regular interruptions. Whether the interruption comes daily, weekly, or annually, if it is recurrent it is likely to be preventable or at least manageable with some planning. If you can predict a crisis you should be able to prepare for it and reduce its impact. A predictable crisis may be a staff shortage on holidays, an annual budget frenzy, or patient complaints of indigestion whenever a particular lunch menu is served. In each case, the problem can be avoided or ameliorated by preventive action.

## Categorizing Activities

Clustering similar activities together helps to eliminate the feeling of bouncing from one unrelated task to another. It also makes your managerial work and your caregiving more holistic. For example, try to complete your assessment of one newly admitted patient before turning to the next admission whenever possible. This continuity will not only save time but will probably result in more thorough assessments and in leaving the patient feeling that you really listened and cared.

## Finding the Fastest Way

A critical analysis of your group's work may reveal many ways to increase efficiency. Perhaps you can computerize some operations or limit the number of people who must handle an item such as a laboratory specimen or supply requisition. Counting narcotics, checking for missing medications, and keeping track of medication keys are time-consuming chores that can all be eliminated by an automated system. Such a system can reduce nursing time for medication distribution and increase time available for nurse-patient interaction (Meyer, 1992). Robots can be used to pick up and deliver medications or lab specimens once they are correctly programmed (Miller, 1997). The solution does not always have to be complex or expensive. Using preprinted NPO (nothing by mouth) stickers on patient records and at the bedside can save time by reducing the number of tests canceled because patients had been served their meals too soon.

Ask your team how their time is being wasted. Together you can analyze your tasks and experiment with various methods to find the most efficient one.

## Automating Repetitive Tasks

Automating repetitive tasks is similar to finding the fastest method, but it focuses on tasks that are repeated again and again. These tasks are not necessarily simple. Automatic blood pressure monitors, for example, not only record readings but store them in memory. A series of classes for families with infants requiring apnea monitors may contain enough standard material so that this content can be filmed, videotaped, or printed and repeated automatically each time it is needed. The nurse would then discuss the content, family concerns, and individual adaptations with each family. In this way, the nurse's time could be reduced by half without reducing the effectiveness of the teaching.

Even case management could be done more efficiently than it presently is. Computerized patient records can be accessed by community-based nurses automatically, saving time by eliminating the transfer of information to a discharge summary sheet that is then delivered to the home health agency. If patients have access to computer networks, they can communicate with their nursing care manager daily after discharge, complete follow-up interviews by computer, get answers to their questions via the computer, and receive reminders or alarm signals through their computers (Simpson, 1993).

## ● ENHANCING PRODUCTIVITY THROUGH LEADERSHIP

Effective time management requires analysis of the characteristics of the work and individual work habits of your team members, followed by intervention where a nonproductive use of time is found. To be successful, some of the strategies discussed in this chapter require a great deal of leadership on your part: first, in initiating the analysis; second, in involving team members and gaining their cooperation; and third, in guiding the work to its conclusion and successful implementation.

Sometimes the major blocks to effective use of time come from higher up in the organizational hierarchy rather than from your level or below. Your supervisor may not delegate effectively or may not allow you sufficient authority to implement more efficient work methods. This situation requires confrontation on your part and negotiation of a solution with the supervisor.

Another component of effective leadership is self-awareness. Keeping this aspect in mind, look for any personal blocks to effective time management, such as fear of failure, fear of success, or personal crises that drain your energy and interfere with your effectiveness. You may have unconsciously developed time-consuming rituals or work habits that unnecessarily fill your workday. An analysis of each task or project to find the shortest route to its completion is usually worth the effort. Nurses in general have had a tendency to equate looking busy, even harried, with being important (del Bueno, 1992). Recognition of this tendency in yourself or in your staff may be the first step in increasing the effectiveness of your time management.

*"Busyness" has become a status symbol. You make yourself important by claiming to be too busy to do something.*
—Adelman, 1997, p. 6L

Your leadership can make the work flow more smoothly for all around you, enhancing productivity through elimination of common time-wasting frustrations and frictions that divert energy and reduce satisfaction when leadership is absent.

A set of questions posed by Drucker (1967) is worth keeping in mind as you try to manage your time more effectively:

- What would happen if this task were not done at all?
- Which tasks could be done by someone else?
- What do you do that wastes your time and other people's time?

## ● SUMMARY

Different cultures view time in different ways. Time can be a tyrant if we do not learn how to manage it effectively. Time studies indicate that nurses typically are involved in many different activities in a day, sometimes in several at the same time.

Time management is accomplished through identifying and concentrating on the most important goals and making them your priorities for time allotment. Keeping a time log for several days can help you see how your time is spent. Time management is accomplished by organizing your work through lists, tickler files, time lines, and scheduling; by setting limits on the number of requests and assignments you accept and the number of interruptions that occur by delegating work appropriately to others; and by streamlining your work. Effective leadership can also lead to increased productivity.

# C A S E   S T U D Y

## Time for a Change?

"Do we have to change every sheet on every bed every day?" This question came from an exasperated, overworked patient care assistant (PCA) at the weekly unit meeting.

"Of course," replied the nurse manager.

"Why?" asked the PCA.

"Patients need clean sheets. They perspire, vomit, bleed, lose urine, have bowel movements, spill food, and so forth, that's why we change their sheets," explained the nurse manager.

"They don't all get their sheets soiled," a staff nurse added. "I'd say about half really need clean sheets every day on this unit. In fact, we often change sheets when something happens in the afternoon or evening, so why change them again in the morning if nothing else happens?"

"Infection control may object," the nurse manager said.

"Let's find out if there's a problem with infection control," suggested the staff nurse. "If

not, perhaps we could change sheets PRN on a trial basis, see how it works."

Note: Inspired by Westfall, N.L. & Burrow, C.M. (1997).

## Questions for Critical Reflection and Analysis

1. What is the primary barrier to effective time management in this example? Explain your reasoning.
2. What patient care concerns may have priority over saving time in this example? Are any of these concerns threatened by the proposed time-saving measures?
3. If you were given responsibility for evaluating the suggested time saver, how would you do it?
4. What other ordinary daily routines on inpatient units could be modified to save time without reducing the quality of patient care?

# REFERENCES

Adelman, K. (1997, August 31). Overworked? *Miami Herald*, 1L, 6L. Reprinted from *Washingtonian Magazine*.

*American Journal of Nursing* (AJN). (1993). Sleeping on the job. 93(2), 10.

*American Journal of Nursing* (AJN). (1992). RNs do 93 different jobs, says hospital study. 92(12), 9.

Brider, P. (1992). The move to patient-focused care. *American Journal of Nursing*, 92(9), 27–33.

Cardona, P., Tappen, R.M., Terrill, M., Acosta, M. & Eusebe, M.I. (1997). Nursing staff time allocation in long-term care: A work sampling study. *Journal of Nursing Administration*, 27(2), 28–36.

Cave, P. (1998). Busy doing . . . nothing much. *Nursing Standard*, 13(3), 25–27.

Chapple, E.D. (1970). *Culture and biological man: Explorations in behavioral anthropology*. New York: Holt, Rinehart & Winston. Reprinted as *The biological foundations of individuality and culture*. Huntington, NY: Robert Krieger, 1979.

Davis, M. (1982). *Interaction rhythms: Periodicity in communicative behavior*. New York: Human Sciences Press.

del Bueno, D.J. (1992). Delegation and the dilemmas of the democratic ideal. *Journal of Nursing Administration*, 23(3), 20–25.

Dossey, L. (1994). Foreword. In A. McGee-Cooper (Ed.). *Time management for unmanageable people*. New York: Bantam Books.

Drucker, P.F. (1967). *The effective executive*. New York: Harper & Row.

Duck, S. (1994). Steady as (s)he goes: Relational maintenance as a shared meaning system. In D.J. Canary & L. Stafford (Eds.). *Communication and relational maintenance*. San Diego: Academic Press.

Haynes, M.E. (1991). *Practical time management*. Los Altos: Crisp Publications.

Huey, F.L. (1986). Working smart. *American Journal of Nursing*, 86, 679–684.

Kerzner, H. (1998). *Project management: A systems approach to planning, scheduling, and controlling*. New York: Van Nostrand Reinhold.

Lee, C., Ashford, S.J. & Jamieson, L.F. (1993). The effects of type A behavior dimensions and optimism on coping strategy, health and performance. *Journal of Organizational Behavior, 14*(2), 143– 158.

Matejka, J.K. & Dunsing, R.J. (1988). Time management: Changing some traditions. *Management World, 17*(2), 6–7.

McGee-Cooper, A. (1994). *Time management for unmanageable people.* New York: Bantam Books.

Meyer, C. (1992). Equipment nurses like. *American Journal of Nursing, 92*(8), 32–36.

Miller, R. (1997, March). Using service robots to deliver medications. *Nursing Management, 28*(3), 49.

Moshovitz, R. (1993). *How to organize your work and your life.* New York: Doubleday.

Prescott, P.A., Phillips, C.Y., Ryan, J.W. & Thompson, K.O. (1991). Changing how nurses spend their time. *Image, 23*(1), 23–28.

Proportion of Americans who feel pressured by time. (1992, October 25). *Miami Herald.*

Robichaud, A.M. (1986). Time documentation of clinical nurse specialist activities. *Journal of Nursing Administration, 16*(1), 31–36.

Rublin, L.R. (1998, March 9). Too, too much! *Barron's,* 33.

Simpson, R.L. (1993). Case-managed care in tomorrow's information network. *Nursing Management, 24*(7), 14–16.

Trossman, S. (1998). Fighting the clock: Nurses take on mandatory overtime. *The American Nurse, 30*(3), 1, 12.

Webber, R.A. (1972). *Time and management.* New York: Moffat Publishing. Reprinted in 1982.

Webber, R.A. (1980). *Time is money: The key to managerial success.* New York: Free Press.

Westfall, N.L. & Burrow, C.M. (1997, November). Are daily bed linen changes necessary? *Nursing Management, 28*(11), 90–92.

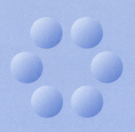

# CHAPTER 9

# Critically Reflective Thinking and Problem Solving

## LEARNING OBJECTIVES

*After completing this chapter, the reader will be able to:*

• Distinguish between clear and muddy thinking.
• Discuss common barriers to clear thinking.
• Define critically reflective thinking.
• Use critically reflective thinking in analyzing questions related to nursing leadership and management.

• Define problem solving and compare it with nursing process.
• Use problem solving to resolve difficult leadership and management situations.

Decisions . . . choices . . . problems . . . we face these every day. Leaders are constantly faced with the need to make decisions. What is wrong here? What is right? How should we resolve this disagreement? Which alternative is best? Does this new policy make sense? Nurse leaders and managers deal with complex human beings and work within highly complex systems; neither are completely predictable. The uniqueness of each person and each situation demands a newly formulated approach, not a preprogrammed one that may not fit.

Thought should precede action in leadership. Varying amounts of reflection and critical analysis of situations are needed before deciding the most appropriate action to take. Sometimes problem solving is also required. In this chapter, we will consider critically reflective thinking and problem solving as they relate to health care, leadership, and management.

## ● CRITICALLY REFLECTIVE THINKING

### Barriers to Clear Thinking

#### Assumptions

Clear thinking is essential to good practice, but muddy thinking is all too common in the workplace. Consider the following:

*When nursing case management was implemented, the case managers continued to use the SOAP (Subjective, Objective, Assessment Plan) format they had always used to com-*

*plete patient records. Eventually, they realized this format did not facilitate communicating what had occurred between case manager, patients, families, and others. Once they recognized the poor fit, a simple question, "What are the functions of a case manager?" led them to create a new format called ACID:*

| | |
|---|---|
| *Assessment:* | *information about the person's living arrangements, impairments, etc.* |
| *Collaboration:* | *with colleagues to meet placement, other needs* |
| *Interventions:* | *arrange transport, teach patient and family self-care skills, etc.* |
| *Discharge Plan:* | *future-oriented description of care that will be given after leaving the facility (Frakes, 1998)* |

Do you see the difference between the originally muddy thinking and the clearer thinking that followed? The muddy thinking was in the **assumption** that the old way of charting would still be suitable in the new role. The clear thinking was in the recognition that this assumption was mistaken and in the creation of the new format for recording patient care data (see Box 9–1).

> ### *Although we all can think, we can't all think clearly.*
> —*Ruchlis, 1990*

What else contributes to muddy thinking? Common contributors are mindsets, circular thinking, overgeneralizations and stereotypes, jumping to conclusions, misuse of statistics, mistaking

relationships for cause and effect, and allowing emotion to rule.

### Mindsets

At one time, healthcare "experts" declared that all ulcers were caused by stress, that infectious disease had been conquered, and that AIDS was limited to the gay population. How can apparently intelligent, well-educated people make such mistakes? One reason is that we all develop habitual ways of thinking and seeing the world around us. These ways of thinking become so much a part of us that we are no longer conscious of them or of their effect on our opinions and decisions.

The problems caused by such mindsets are related to the fact that we are not consciously aware of the extent to which they restrict our thinking. It would be as if we all wore permanent rose-colored contact lenses and saw the world in various shades of pinks and reds, losing sight of the blues, greens, and yellows. Anyone who talked about seeing blue would be considered mistaken and would be corrected. Why would someone see blue when everyone else saw pink? The person seeing blue is using a different set of lenses.

> ### *Individuals do not react to the world per se but to the world as they see it.*
> —*Schwarz, 1995, p. 345*

### Circular Reasoning

Like a dog chasing its tail, conclusions are often mere rephrasings of the original question or premise. Here is an example:

| | |
|---|---|
| *Staff Member:* | *Is it safe to do this procedure without gloves?* |
| *Nurse Manager:* | *Sure, just go ahead and get it done.* |
| *Staff Member:* | *Are you sure it's safe?* |
| *Nurse Manager:* | *Sure, I said it was safe, didn't I?* |

In fact, the nurse manager has said that the procedure was safe to perform ungloved because she'd already said it was safe. No evidence was offered to back up her statement.

---

**Box 9–1    Want to Avoid Muddy Thinking?**

- Stay alert for hidden assumptions
- Think before acting
- Keep an open mind
- Recognize the effect of your emotions
- Separate fact from opinion
- Weigh the evidence
- Look for errors in reasoning

## Overgeneralizations and Stereotypes

Assumptions made about individual people based on common characteristics of a group to which they belong are particularly dangerous in health care. It can lead to such errors as overlooking signs of a heart attack because the patient is a young woman or assuming that an unmarried staff member has fewer family responsibilities and can be asked to work extra overtime.

## Jumping to Conclusions

This type of muddy thinking occurs when little evidence, usually unverified, is used to draw a conclusion. For example:

> The coordinator of the emergency department observed that one of the most experienced nurses on the day shift seemed nervous lately. She noticed that the nurse's hands trembled as she inserted lines, even as she gave injections. The coordinator concluded that this nurse could no longer cope with the demands of emergency care and suggested she transfer to a less pressured environment. He was surprised to find out that she had some difficulty adjusting to her new thyroid medication and that the trembling was a temporary symptom, which was soon brought under control again. He nearly lost his best nurse by jumping to conclusions.

## Misuse of Statistics

While the old axiom that numbers don't lie may have some truth in it, the manner in which numbers are presented can be deceptive. Consider the following news item:

> NIMBY (Not in my Back Yard): Almost 80 percent of employers polled said they believed that workers can return to productivity given treatment for drug or alcohol abuse. But nearly 30 percent said they would fire an employee found abusing substances at work (Karr, 1998, p. 1).

Think about what this item is really reporting. Does it sound like an indictment of employers who say they believe in treatment for drug and alcohol abuse but fire anyone with that problem? Compare the percentages reported carefully: It amounts to barely a 10 percent discrepancy. Is that difference so bad? Does it demonstrate as serious an inconsistency as the "NIMBY" title suggests?

## Mistaking Relationship for Cause and Effect

A common misinterpretation of statistical evidence can result in this type of mistake. The statistics can be derived from research studies or they can be institutional data. The following is an example of misinterpretation of institutional data:

> Soon after new nurse managers were assigned to the three surgical units, the number of staff resignations jumped 200 percent on these units. "I think we've made a mistake in our selection of new nurse managers," the nursing director remarked. "It looks that way but let's investigate further before we change our selection process," responded the chief nurse executive.

Further investigation, primarily interviews of the people resigning, revealed the real cause of the sudden increase. Fearing the new selection process would bring in nurse managers who were too "tough" on their staff, many nurses had applied for positions in other institutions. By the time they realized that the new managers were fair and reasonable in their treatment of the staff, these nurses were already committed to new positions. The selection process, not the individual managers, had precipitated the resignation increase. In this example, the chief nurse executive was a critically reflective thinker; the nursing director was not.

## Allowing Emotion to Rule

Denying that emotion ever affects one's opinions is an example of the "ostrichism" to which Levy (1997) refers (see Perspectives . . . Pollution of the Mind). Recognizing that an appeal to emotions has been made and that you could be influenced by it is a more realistic approach. The following is an example:

> Denial of emotional appeal:
>
> I chose Martin's proposed project because of its superior rationale. It is well thought out and addresses a great

*need. This project will certainly be of greater benefit to the community.*

Recognition of emotional appeal:

*The two proposed projects are equally well developed. Both projects would be worthwhile but we have money to support only one. My heart goes out to these young homeless parents who are trying to raise children under the worst imaginable conditions. Martin's proposal will become our community service project for the year.*

## Defining Critically Reflective Thinking

The primary purpose of this section is to assist you in (1) developing an open mind and spirit of inquiry, and (2) encouraging others to do the same. People with closed minds miss many opportunities for positive growth and effective action by rejecting new ideas. It is equally ineffective to readily accept misguided notions because you did not critically analyze them first.

Why do people develop ineffective thinking habits? Ruggiero (1998) suggests that it begins when parents say "Don't ask so many questions!" and teachers reward correct answers more than creative ideas. Other factors that may limit critically reflective thinking include resistance to change, difficulty admitting you were mistaken, discomfort with uncertainty, pressures for conformity, and self-deception (Ruggiero, 1998). A critically reflective thinker tries to avoid these barriers to clear thinking.

Critically reflective thinking is both an attitude and a process. It is a willingness to give fair consideration to any idea, but to accept an idea only after you have reflected carefully on it and evaluated it in terms of the evidence to support it and its congruence with your value system. A hallmark of effective leaders and managers is the ability to make decisions reflectively without being influenced by current opinion or one's own dislikes or prejudices (Hinterhuber & Popp, 1992).

Ennis (1962) defined **critical thinking** as reflective, reasoned thinking "focusing on deciding what to believe or do" (in Miller & Mal-

## PERSPECTIVES . . .

### Pollution of the Mind

The president of the American Public Health Association listed some important barriers to clear thinking in the health professions:

**Complacency:** Allowing threats to the public's health that we could prevent: work-related injuries, poisonings, nosocomial infections, inadequate care, hunger and starvation

**Fragmentation:** Not seeing the whole person or the whole community

**"Ostrichism":** Refusing to confront serious problems—such as gun or auto-related injuries—hoping they will just go away

**Lack of Responsibility for Others:** Tolerating a decline in compassion for others; letting the safety net of public assistance diminish

**Uncritical Acceptance of Technology:** Believing that more technology is usually the best solution; believing everything one reads on the Internet

**Racism:** Permitting discrimination of any kind or pretending it no longer exists

**Isolationism:** Ignoring problems beyond our national borders such as air pollution or the export of unapproved drugs

**Professional Arrogance:** Thinking that only healthcare professionals can decide what is best for other people

*Source:* Adapted from Levy, B.S. (1997, September). Eliminating pollution of the mind. *The Nation's Health, XXVII*, (8), 2.

colm, 1990, p. 67). Mezirow (1990) used the term **critical reflection** instead of **critical thinking** to emphasize the importance of identifying and evaluating the assumptions underlying decisions. Another useful definition comes from Scriven and Fisher:

> *. . . skilled, active interpretation and evaluation of observations, communications, information, and argumentation as a guide to thought and action (in Fonteyn, 1998, p. 13).*

## Examples of Muddy Thinking from Health Care

It wasn't that long ago that nurses starched their caps, removed flowers from patient rooms at night, or kept women in bed for a week after childbirth. Hearing of these practices, today's nursing students shake their heads and think, "How silly they were! What were they thinking?" Of course, not every tradition or ritualized practice is misguided (Silberger, 1998), but all are worthy of critical reflection and analysis to decide whether they should be continued. A recent example:

> *Judah Folkman's original idea that tumors need blood to grow occurred to him in 1960 when he was only 27 years old.*
>
> *The idea has been tested and refined a great deal since then. Malignant tumor cells have been found to secrete a substance that induces the growth of capillaries and increases metastasis under certain circumstances. Early reaction to Folkman's idea was hostility and ridicule. Colleagues laughed or walked out when he presented his ideas at scientific meetings. Others would say to him, "You really don't believe that, do you?" (p. 56).*
>
> *Members of his research team have since discovered an inhibitory antiangiogenesis substance that may eventually be used to stop tumor growth and may even shrink existing tumors. His work is now described as an exciting breakthrough in the fight against cancer (Begley & Kolb, 1998).*

How could his colleagues have been so blind? Part of the reason is that biology has recently been focused on genes so their **paradigm** (their mental model for thinking about causes of cancer) differed from Folkman's. They thought he was headed in the wrong direction. They were not able to see the promise of his discoveries because they were looking at it through the lens of gene therapy, not through Folkman's lens of growth inhibition.

The effect of group norms may have been operating here as well. Folkman's colleagues were deeply committed to gene therapy and unwittingly had closed their minds to a promising alternative, which is not an unusual occurrence. People often remain loyal to a cherished paradigm (lens) even when evidence indicates it is not working out

well. This paradigm may continue until its holders are confronted with overwhelming evidence to the contrary and/or a general shift in the paradigm occurs within the group or society (Janis, 1997). Much of what we do in clinical practice demands reflection and critical analysis. Without it, we will continue our muddy thinking, making mistakes like those of Folkman's colleagues.

> **Many of our own practices will appear to our descendants as ludicrous and superstitious; and our descendants will be right.**
> —Dalrymple, 1998, p. W10

Perspectives . . . It Wasn't All That Long Ago That We . . . , has some other interesting examples of past healthcare practices that today make no sense.

## PERSPECTIVES . . .

### It Wasn't All That Long Ago That We . . .

- Treated pneumonia with oxygen bubbled through brandy.
- Used tobacco smoke for intractable asthma.
- Recommended fish boiled in milk for ulcers.
- Gave croton oil (a powerful laxative) to psychotic patients to sedate them.
- Removed ovaries to cure epilepsy.
- Removed the large intestine to clear the body of toxins.

*Source:* Dalrymple, T. (1998, April 3). This will hurt you more than it hurts me. [Review of book]. *The Wall Street Journal*, W10.

## An Example from Leadership

Failing to recognize the lenses through which we view the world can have unintended consequences in leadership as well, some of them negative, even harmful. The beloved "let's arrange our chairs in a circle" is an example suggested by Brookfield (1995).

> *In school and at work, group leaders often ask people to form a circle "so we can be informal" or "so everyone can see everyone else." The*

assumption is that sitting in a circle makes everyone equal because no one is at the head of the table or the front of the classroom. Sitting in a circle also makes it possible for each member of the group to see everyone else in the group. It is assumed that this is beneficial and agreeable to everyone. Is it?

Brookfield (1995) says that the circle can be a congenial, liberating experience for the self-confident, talkative group member. However, for the new or shy group member it may be torture, a painful, humiliating situation. A circle denies these individuals an opportunity to hide temporarily, to check out others before coming forward, to test group members and develop a level of trust in them before speaking out. It can have the unintended effect of putting too much pressure on people to participate or to disclose personal information before they are comfortable doing so (Brookfield, 1995).

The example also illustrates the different ways each of us experiences the world.

## Critical Analysis: A Guide

A guide to doing critical analysis follows (Ennis, 1962; Dressel & Mayhew (n.d.); Tripp, in Brookfield, 1995). To thoroughly understand what it entails, you may find it helpful to analyze a particular incident or issue that disturbed you in some way. Some examples of issues worthy of critical reflection and analysis: demand versus scheduled infant feeding, allowing children to sleep with their parents, gun control, violence on television, legalization of marijuana, assisted suicide, managed care.

1. *Issue: Describe the issue or incident, its meaning, and its significance.* Write down your description or share it with interested listeners so you can return to it later.
2. *Assumptions: Identify the assumptions and dominant paradigm* (lens) underlying the incident or issue.
3. *Alternative Paradigm: Suggest or find an alternative* lens (paradigm) through which to view the incident or issue. Creative thinkers consider multiple perspectives, look for similarities and differences, and seek alternative solutions and new ideas even when the currently

accepted ones are generally satisfactory (Lipman, 1985; Ulrich & Glendon, 1999). Looking for new relationships between different pieces of information or between different experiences can bring more meaning to what you observe and lead to the discovery of new meanings.

Searching for alternative paradigms can also help to eliminate the feeling that you have learned fragments of unrelated information and can lead to completely new connections. Many scientific discoveries, such as the relationship between an antihypertensive medication and the prevention of baldness, were made this way. The following is an example from women's health:

Profet, a woman biologist, wondered why females shed blood and tissue every month. Was hormonal fluctuation really an adequate explanation? Why would blood loss be an adaptive response? Was there another reason for it?

Adopting this critical new viewpoint, Profet continued to study the question. Through further research and reflection on the existing literature, she came up with a new explanation: menstruation cleans harmful pathogens from the uterus that had been carried in by sperm. This radical new view could transform the field of women's health (Downs, 1993).

Not every new connection is as important, but each adds creativity and the excitement of discovery to your practice.

4. *Evidence: Evaluate the strength of the evidence to support the viewpoints* outlined in #2 and #3. The evidence can be fact or opinion, accurate or inaccurate. Inconsistencies, contradictions, stereotypes, biases, and appeals to emotion are clear warning signals. A common bias in arguments is to promote the beneficial aspects and leave out potentially negative effects. Evidence should be evaluated in terms of its accuracy, consistency, linkages, and relationships to other ideas, cause and effect, relationships, and bracketing of prior judgments.
5. *Evaluate: Decide which viewpoint you support and justify your choice.* Include reference to your own value system in supporting your choice.

Let critical reflection and analysis become a habit of thinking. It will open up new perspectives and new possibilities that would never have occurred to you if you have a closed mind. Some risk, however, comes with being a critically reflective thinker. These risks are described in the next section.

## The Risk in Being a Critical Thinker

The insights derived from critical thinking are not *always* welcome. Brookfield (1993) warns of potential personal and professional risks in being a critical thinker. His warning is based on interviews of staff nurses, educators, and administrators. The interviewees described their surprise when colleagues not only did not thank them for their insights but reacted with indifference, discomfort, and sometimes open hostility. Some of the critical thinkers were even labeled as troublemakers.

One of the nurses interviewed said it was a serious mistake to believe that when people said they wanted constructive criticism, they really meant it. Another described colleagues as trying to end the conversation and escape, rather than appreciate the insight into a problem they were struggling to solve. Why would people react this way? People who have not been critical thinkers may find it threatening to examine their practice, especially the ambiguities that are still a part of our clinical decision making and management practices.

How can these insights be shared, then, without precipitating such a reaction? Brookfield (1993) suggests being open and affirmative rather than aggressively confrontational. He also suggests sharing your insights by telling a story about yourself, sharing how you arrived at your new ideas, and then letting your listeners decide how useful the insight would be for them.

## ● PROBLEM SOLVING

A problem exists when *the way to reach a goal is unknown or initial attempts to reach it have failed* (Dominowski & Dallob, 1995, p. 33). LeStorti and colleagues define a problem as "the difference or gap between the current state and a goal state" (1999, p. 62). The **initial state**, when a problem is first recognized, is the starting point of the problem-solving process; the **end point** or goal is resolution of the problem. In between are all the possible solution paths one can take to reach the goal, which is called the **problem space** (Halpern, 1997). Problems large and small arise constantly in the workplace. In some cases there is only one path, but in most situations there are many possible paths, some long and complex, others short but difficult. The selection of the best path is an important decision in problem solving. Some problems are easy to solve; the solution comes readily to mind and the goal is quickly attained. Others, the ones we are most concerned with in this section, require a *new* solution, one that does not come readily to mind, a solution not used before.

Problem solving is a strategy for organizing and sequencing your **thinking** as you work toward finding a solution. The **knowledge** or content comes from prior experience and education. Problem solving puts this knowledge to use in novel ways; it does not provide the answer but guides you in finding the answer.

## Steps in the Process

Problem solving is a deliberate, thoughtful way to deal with a situation that is creating some kind of difficulty that has no ready-made solution. It begins with an effort to sort out the complexities of the situation and then brings some structure to the search for a solution.

The well-known nursing process is based upon problem solving. Nursing process is the use of problem solving in relation to a patient, client, or group of clients. It is compared to problem solving in Table 9–1.

"Let's problem-solve" is often a useful response from the leader when a person or group is upset or confused. By the time the solutions are listed, you will feel at least partially in control of the situation and able to respond more constructively and calmly. You can help a client problem-solve, you can lead a group through the process, and you can problem-solve for yourself.

The steps in the problem-solving process are probably familiar to you.

| Table 9–1 | Comparison of the Problem-Solving and Nursing Processes | | | | |
|---|---|---|---|---|---|
| | Step I | Step II | Step III | Step IV | Step V |
| **Problem Solving** | Collect data | Define the problem | Generate possible solutions and select the best ones | Take action | Evaluate the results |
| **Nursing Process** | Assessment | Diagnosis | Plan | Implementation | Evaluation |

*Step 1. Collect data.*    As objectively as possible, list the information you have about the problem as it presently exists. Sometimes you will find that more data is needed before problem solving can proceed. Focus on relevant information; discard whatever is irrelevant.

*Step 2. Define the problem.*    Prepare a statement summarizing the situation as specifically and objectively as possible. Do not include possible solutions to the problem.

*Step 3. Generate a list of possible solutions and select the best one(s).*    First, list every possible solution you can think of. Allow any solution, however silly or improbable, to be listed so that a creative, novel way to solve the problem is not missed. When the possibilities are exhausted, evaluate each suggestion, selecting the strategy or combination of strategies most likely to work.

*Step 4. Take action.*    Now you are ready to take action. Implement the strategy devised in #3 but be ready to modify it if it is not effective.

*Step 5. Evaluate the results.*    Has the problem been resolved? If not, what went wrong? Is it necessary to go back and repeat the process? What did you learn for the next time this problem arises? Could it be prevented?

Don't skip this last step. Reflecting on the process and outcomes will leave you better prepared to deal with the next problem.

In addition to these simple steps, some additional information may enhance your problem-solving skills.

## Enhancing Problem Solving

### Ineffective Habits

Pesut (1998) reminds us that most problem solving looks back rather than forward. People have a tendency to choose a solution that worked in the past, continually reverting back to previously successful strategies rather than generating new strategies. It is also easy to become *fixated* on an ineffective solution, trying it again and again instead of abandoning it and moving on to try a new solution (Dominowski & Dallob, 1995).

Shouldn't every possible solution come up the first time? Typically, people end their search for a solution as soon as they have enough (or what seems like enough) information to generate what appears to be a workable solution. If the situation is extremely serious or the solution of great consequence, people are likely to search longer for a solution (Schwarz, 1995).

People also may tend to oversimplify a situation (Prescott, Dennis & Jacox, 1987). The desire for ease and simplicity is quite strong: people will ignore complications and try to make new facts fit old hunches in order to avoid having to redefine the problem. You should be alert for this pattern when problem solving.

### Individual Differences

Research also suggests that people generally use one fundamental, perhaps even innate, approach that does not change easily, even when they are taught a different method. One extensive study found that people generate hypotheses early in the problem-solving process despite recommendations not to do so. In other words, they do not wait until all the facts are in before coming up with solutions.

## How Hard Is It to Be Objective?

How hard is it to be objective? Much harder than you think, in some instances. Hammond, Keeney, and Raiffa (1998) describe a number of traps people fall into when making decisions.

The following are just a few:

*Recallability Trap:* It is much easier to remember an event with a high emotional valence than it is to recall an ordinary event. Their example: when read a list with an equal number of famous men and women, those who heard a list on which the men were more famous said the list had more men on it while those who heard a list that included women who were more famous said the list had more women on it. One problem with a violent patient or malfunctioning computer will stand out in our memories far more than hundreds of gentle patients or hundreds of hours on humming computers. Don't let one incident affect your judgment too much.

*The Wrong Heuristic:* Each of us uses these "mental shortcuts" to process complex information. The example from Hammond and colleagues is a heuristic for judging distance. Other things being equal, we assume that clearer objects are closer than those that appear fuzzy. Hazy weather can throw off our judgment—a serious problem for airline pilots who have to be trained to use other measurers of distance. Watch out for these shortcuts. While valuable most of the time, they can lead us to ignore important pieces of information.

*Status Quo:* The familiar is almost always more comfortable than the unknown. Furthermore, Hammond and colleagues point out that sins of commission (doing something) are almost always more severely punished than sins of omission (doing nothing) when something goes wrong.

*Sunk Cost:* This trap is closely related to the status quo trap. A sunk cost is an investment that cannot be recovered. It's often hard to admit one's mistakes or to give up on a project once you've begun it. For example, if you fire an employee, you are in effect admitting that you made a poor choice and/or failed to rehabilitate this employee. Unless the employee is actively causing trouble, it's easier (although unadvisable) to allow the person to stay.

*Source:* Hammond, J.S., Keeney, R.L. & Raiffa, H. (1998, September/October). The hidden traps in decision making. *Harvard Business Review*, 47–58.

These researchers also found that individuals are best at particular types of problems in particular situations (Elstein et al., 1978). One person may be particularly adept at solving problems with recalcitrant equipment while another is particularly good at working out creative staffing patterns when a temporary shortage occurs. One's profession also seems to affect how that person solves a problem (Holzemer, 1986). Not surprisingly, nurses usually focus on different aspects of a situation than a physician would.

People also vary in the amount of knowledge and experience that they have to apply to a particular problem. Knowledge and experience have considerable impact on the effectiveness of their problem solving. For some additional information on traps people fall into when solving problems, see Perspectives . . . How Hard Is It to Be Objective?

## ● SUMMARY

Clear thinking, keeping an open mind, and critically analyzing ideas and situations before acting are essential elements of effective leadership and management. Barriers to clear thinking include acting on assumptions, failing to recognize mindsets, circular reasoning, overgeneralization and stereotypes, jumping to conclusions, misinterpretation of statistics, mistaking relationships for causes, and allowing emotions to override reason.

Critically reflective thinking is defined as giving due consideration to any idea but accepting an idea only after weighing the evidence and congruence with one's values. Critical analysis begins with a clear description of the issue involved and

## C A S E   S T U D Y

### What's Wrong with This Policy?

An influential state senator was appalled by the quality of care his father-in-law received at a new subacute care facility in his state. As a result, he began asking questions of every nurse and physician he encountered in his travels through his district. Again and again he heard that many of the problems related to a lack of continuity of care. "How can we improve the continuity of care?" he finally asked his niece who had just finished nursing school. "More thorough assessment and better communication of patient information across shifts, across disciplines, and across institutions," she replied. His niece also showed him the interdisciplinary assessment form she'd used in school as an example of a way to improve communication.

With little change, this interdisciplinary assessment form (IAF) was adopted by the state legislature during the next session. All subacute units, whether freestanding or part of larger institutions, were required to use it for every person admitted. Unfortunately, this complex form used language understood only by those who were familiar with the terminology of the framework used. Administrators of most subacute facilities were perplexed by it but obligated to implement the IAF form. Some brought in consultants to teach the staff how to use the forms, but the majority hired part-time nurses to complete the forms. Familiarly called "IAF nurses," most of these nurses did thorough assessments and filled out the forms correctly. However, the administrators noted that the information on the forms was not being used by the rest of the staff. In effect, they said, the form was just an added expense for their institutions.

### Questions for Critical Reflection and Analysis

1. Use critically reflective thinking to analyze the problem that led to adoption of a state requirement to use the IAF form.
2. Identify the assumptions underlying adoption of the IAF form.
3. Using the steps of the problem-solving process, search for more effective solutions to the original problem described in the case study.
4. Identify the assumptions underlying the new proposed solutions and critically analyze them. Weigh the strength of the evidence to support them, compare them with your own values, and then decide what alternative you would support if you were an influential state senator.

identification of the assumptions underlying the issue and the paradigm through which it is usually seen. Then follows a search for alternative lenses and an evaluation of the different viewpoints and a decision on which viewpoint you support. Critical thinking is not without risk because it challenges the status quo, which can make some people uncomfortable.

Problem solving is a strategy for organizing and sequencing efforts to find a solution. It is a guide to finding solutions rather than a source of answers to one's problems. The process proceeds from the initial state—recognition of the problem—to a search for the best path through the problem space to the end goal, which is the solution to the problem. The nursing process is a specific example of the more general problem-solving process. Truncating the search for solutions, becoming fixated on an ineffective solution, and trying old solutions for new problems are common errors. Individuals differ in their preferred approaches and in the knowledge they bring to solving problems.

### REFERENCES

Begley, S. & Kolb, C. (1998, May 18). One man's quest to cure cancer. *Newsweek*, 55–61.

Brookfield, S. (1993). On imposters, cultural suicide, and other dangers: How nurses learn critical thinking. *The Journal of Continuing Education in Nursing, 24*(5), 197–205.

Brookfield, S.D. (1995). *Becoming a critically reflective teacher.* San Francisco: Jossey-Bass.

Dalrymple, T. (1998, April 3). This will hurt you more than it hurts me. [Review of book]. *The Wall Street Journal,* W10.

Dominowski, R.L. & Dallob, P. (1995). Insight and problem solving. In R.J. Sternberg & J.E. Davidson (Eds.). *The nature of insight.* Cambridge, MA: The MIT Press, 33–62.

Downs, F.S. (1993). Alternative Answers. *Nursing Research, 42*(6), 323.

Dressel, P. & Mayhew, L.B. (n.d.). *Critical thinking in social science.* Mimeo.

Elstein, A.S., Shulman, L.S., Sprafka, S.A. & Allal, L. (1978). *Medical problem solving: An analysis of clinical reasoning.* Cambridge, MA: Harvard University Press.

Ennis, B.H. (1962). A concept of critical thinking. *Harvard Education Review, 32,* 81.

Fonteyn, M.E. (1998). *Thinking strategies for nursing practice.* Philadelphia: Lippincott.

Frakes, K.L. (1998, March 23). SOAP is out, ACID is in. *The Nursing Spectrum,* 5.

Halpern, D.F. (1997). *Critical thinking across the curriculum.* Mahwah, NJ: Lawrence Erlbaum Associates.

Hammond, J.S., Keeney, R.L. & Raiffa, H. (1998, September/October). The hidden traps in decision making. *Harvard Business Review,* 47–58.

Hinterhuber, H.H. & Popp, W. (1992). Are you a strategist or just a manager? *Harvard Business Review, 70*(1), 105–113.

Holzemer, W.L. (1986). The structure of problem solving in simulations. *Nursing Research, 35,* 231–235.

Janis, I.L. (1997). Groupthink. In R.P. Vecchio (Ed.). *Leadership: Understanding the dynamics of power and influence in organizations.* Notre Dame, IN: University of Notre Dame Press, 163–176.

Karr, A.R. (1998, February 10). Work week: A special news report about life on the job—and trends taking shape there. *The Wall Street Journal,* 1.

LeStorti, A.J., Cullen, P.A., Hanzlek, E.M., Michiels, J.M., Piano, L.A., Ryan, P.L. & Hohnson, W. (1999). Creative thinking in nursing education: Preparing for tomorrow's challenges. *Nursing Outlook, 47*(12), 62–66.

Levy, B.S. (1997, September). Eliminating pollution of the mind. *The Nation's Health, XXVII,* (8), 2.

Lipman, M. (1985). Thinking skills fostered by philosophy for children. In J.W. Segal, S.F. Chipman & R. Glaser (Eds.). *Thinking and learning skills.* Hillsdale, NJ: Lawrence Erlbaum, 83–108.

Mezirow, J. (1990). *Fostering critical reflection in adulthood: A guide to transformative and emancipating learning.* San Francisco: Jossey-Bass.

Miller, M.A. & Malcolm, N.S. (1990). Critical thinking in the nursing curriculum. *Nursing and Health Care, 11*(2), 67–73.

Pesut, D.J. (1998, May 29). Future-think. Paper presented at conference of the Florida Organization of Nurse Executives and South Florida Organization of Nurse Executives. Fort Lauderdale, FL.

Prescott, P.A., Dennis, K.A. & Jacox, A.K. (1987). Clinical decision making of staff nurses. *Image, 19*(2), 56–62.

Ruchlis, H. (1990). *Clear thinking: A practical introduction.* Buffalo, NY: Prometheus Books.

Ruggiero, V.R. (1998). *The art of thinking.* New York: Addison-Wesley.

Schwarz, N. (1995). Social cognition: Information accessibility and use in social judgment. In E.E. Smith and D.N. Osherson (Eds.). *Thinking: An invitation to cognitive science.* Cambridge, MA: The MIT Press, 267–296.

Silberger, M.R. (1998). Tracing our rituals in nursing. *Nursing Leadership Forum, 3*(1), 8–12.

Tripp, D. (1993). Critical incidents in teaching: Developing professional judgment. New York: Routledge, 345–376.

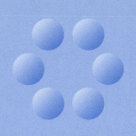

CHAPTER **10**

# Leading Change

## LEARNING OBJECTIVES

*After completing this chapter, the reader will be able to:*

- Identify the characteristics of a particular planned change.
- Apply the rational approach to change appropriately and effectively.
- Apply the participative approach to change appropriately and effectively.

- Apply the reframing approach to change appropriately and effectively.
- Evaluate the relative strengths and weaknesses of the three approaches to planning and implementing change.

## TEST YOURSELF

### How stressed are you?

*Holmes and Rahe developed this scale to rate the amount of stress caused by life changes:*

*major and minor, pleasant and unpleasant. To obtain your score, circle the ones that apply to you and then add up the total.*

| Events | Stress Value |
|---|---|
| Death of a spouse | 100 |
| Divorce | 73 |
| Marital separation | 65 |
| Jail term | 63 |
| Death of a close family member | 63 |
| Personal injury, sickness | 53 |
| Marriage | 50 |
| Fired from job | 47 |
| Reconcile marriage | 45 |
| Retire | 45 |
| Illness in family | 44 |
| Pregnancy | 40 |
| Sex difficulties | 39 |
| Gain new family member | 39 |
| Change in business | 39 |
| Change in financial state | 38 |
| Death of close friend | 37 |
| Change line of work | 36 |
| Change in number of family fights | 35 |
| Mortgage over $100,000 | 31 |
| Mortgage or loan foreclosed | 30 |
| Grown child leaves home | 29 |

| Events | Stress Value |
|---|---|
| Change in job duties | 29 |
| In-law troubles | 29 |
| Outstanding achievement | 28 |
| Wife begins or stops work | 26 |
| Begin or end school | 26 |
| Change living conditions | 25 |
| Revise personal habits | 24 |
| Trouble with boss | 23 |
| Change work hours or conditions | 20 |
| Move to new home | 20 |
| Change schools | 20 |
| Change recreation | 19 |
| Change church activities | 19 |
| Change social activities | 18 |
| Mortgage or loan under $100,000 | 17 |
| Sleeping habits change | 16 |
| Change in number of family get-togethers | 15 |
| Eating habits change | 15 |
| Vacation | 13 |
| Christmas | 12 |
| Minor violation of the law | 11 |

Scoring: *Follow-up studies show that people who accumulate more than 200 points in a year are high risks for physical or psychological stress-related illnesses.*

*How many of these changes have you experienced in the past year?*

*Source:* Holmes, T.H. & Rahe, R. (1967). The social readjustment rating scale. *Journal of Psychosomatic Research,* 2(4), 213. Used with permission.

The rapidity and enormity of the changes occurring in health care appear to have increased our concern about change: planning change, responding to change, initiating and leading change. The changes in the healthcare system make it more important than ever to anticipate change and prepare for it, despite the increased unpredictability. To some, change is an exciting opportunity, to others it is a threat of chaos.

To engage yourself actively in learning about change, you can think about your own experience with change or about a particular change you would like to initiate. Some examples of changes you could think about as you read this chapter include the following:

- Installing a new medication distribution system
- Introducing telehealth in a rural county
- Eliminating duplication in the patient record system
- Hiring APNs (advanced practice nurses) for the first time in your agency
- Closing inpatient units or discontinuing selected services

## ● DYNAMICS OF CHANGE

Change is a natural and continuous process according to open systems theory. Growth and development, for example, are a type of change that affects every human being throughout the life span. The reader may be aware of change occurring frequently and rapidly in his or her own life. Not every change in a system is obvious, however. Change may be as subtle as an imperceptible shift in a system's function or as obvious as a large-scale alteration in the pattern and organization of the system.

### Positive or Negative?

Change per se is neither inherently good or bad. Some changes have a positive effect on a system, others have a negative effect. Change can be as welcome as a holiday from work or as unwelcome as a speeding ticket.

### *Innovate or fall behind.*
—*Leonard & Straus, 1997, p. 111*

Positive change is growth producing and as necessary as order and regularity are in the function of a human system. If you find it difficult to accept this idea, consider extreme sensory deprivation as a situation in which a system is experiencing too little change.

Of course, not every change in a system is a positive one. In fact, resistance to change can sometimes be a healthy response. The following is an example:

*A midwestern community strongly resisted attempts to locate a new chemical waste treatment plant on the edge of town. Residents picketed, protested, and wrote letters to their representatives in order to block the potentially hazardous waste from coming into their community. They saw this change as a threat to the health of their friends and families.*

In this case, the change was considered a threat to the integrity of the system and resistance was a positive response in terms of the health and safety of the community.

### Potential for Change

The potential for change is inherent in every open system. People often make remarks such as, "nothing ever changes around here" or "people here refuse to change," which seem to indicate that these systems have not changed or will not change. What they really mean is that no rapid, large-scale changes have taken place or that members of the system have not shown much resistance to change. Whether the impetus comes primarily from within the system or from the environment, some kind of change is inevitable in open systems.

Change in one part of a system will affect the whole system. Furthermore, change that affects the entire system will also affect its relationship with the environment. Even the person who attempts to guide and influence a change in a system will in some way be affected by the change process.

### Characteristics of Change

Clearly, not all changes are alike, and we cannot lump all changes together in our analysis of change (Strebel, 1992). Change can vary in terms of type, intensity, pattern, and pace. The characteristics of change are a major factor in selecting a strategy for action.

#### *Type*

**Planned change** is a deliberate application of leadership skills to guide and influence the direction of change (Bennis et al., 1976). The opposite is spontaneous or **unplanned change**, which may evolve gradually or occur in an abrupt and dramatic manner (Samuelson, 1998).

The source of change may be within the organization or one of its subsystems or it may be external to the organization (Panel, 1994). For example, external economic forces may cause the bankruptcy and closing of a hospital, or they may stimulate innovations such as an array of attractive new services that bring in new patients and make the hospital thrive.

It is important to recognize that leaders and managers cannot control or even manage all these forces (Wilson, 1992). It is possible, however, to continuously monitor the environment in which your organization or team operates and to respond to signs of impending change in that environment. Maintaining the status quo in the face of sweeping changes may not be possible. For example:

> A voluntary, not-for-profit home health agency had always been proud of its ability to serve the community. "We have never turned anyone away for lack of money," the director declared proudly. Unfortunately, the charitable groups on which they depended for support were overwhelmed by the number of requests for support and reluctantly reduced their contributions to the agency, hoping that the government would make up the difference. The agency found, however, that many of the clients did not qualify under the government's increasingly stringent eligibility criteria.
>
> The home health agency's director refused to change the policy of serving everyone, saying it was "the cornerstone on which the agency was founded." A year later, the agency's board of trustees fired this director because the agency was deeply in debt and in danger of closing. The new director's first action was to put limits on the amount of free service the agency provided.

## Intensity

Change can be so subtle that it is almost imperceptible, or it can be so radical that it shakes the entire organization, sometimes destroying it. The level of intensity ranges from virtually nil to a major transformation (Koerner & Bunkers, 1992; McWhinney, 1992; Wilson, 1992). The degree of intensity can be described as one of the following four levels:

**Level 0: Status Quo.** No apparent change occurs.

For example, everyone one feels as if the structure and function of the organization and its subsystems have remained the same.

**Level 1: Expansion or Contraction.** The structure and purpose of the organization remain relatively stable but some operations change.

For example, a clinic may expand its hours to include evenings and Saturdays, or a rehabilitation center may see an increase in spinal cord injuries from gunshot wounds.

**Level 2: Transition.** Changes occur within the existing framework of the organization.

For example, a women's center may add cancer screening and management of menopause to its array of services to attract older women.

**Level 3: Transformation.** At this level, the structure and function change.

For example, a free-standing adult day center may be converted into an inpatient drug treatment center.

It is easy to imagine how much more stressful a Level 3 change is to the staff and administration of an organization than is a Level 1 change. In the Level 3 example, the staff and the administration would be faced either with needing an entirely new set of skills to function well or with being replaced by people who had these skills. Senge (1999) notes that the majority of large-scale efforts to transform organizations, which would be Level 3 changes, end in failure. They lose energy, momentum, and relevance (Purser & Cabana, 1998). A typical cycle is for the change effort to begin growing vigorously but soon whither and eventually die because the change process has not been nurtured and the limiting factors (resistance) have not been reduced or eliminated (Senge, 1999).

## Pattern

Change may be continuous, sporadic, occasional, or rare in its occurrence. Predictable changes allow time for preparation; sudden or unpredictable changes are more difficult to respond to effectively. Sudden change may be the most difficult to manage, especially if it is intense as well. Curiously, change may bring about increased homogeneity as well as increased diversity. For example, the trend to multihospital systems has led to greater uniformity across institutions.

## Pace

Not only the type but also the rate at which change occurs within a given time will affect the system's response. Holmes and Rahe's Stress Scale (1967) illustrates the cumulative effect of too many changes occurring in a short period of time (see Test Yourself at the beginning of the chapter). Some of the changes such as "outstanding achievement" have positive value, yet too many of these changes occurring together can be stressful.

Any change occurring at too rapid a rate may elicit resistance. The following is an example:

> A new director of rehabilitative services was hired for the outpatient services of a large healthcare center. In six months, the director had thoroughly organized and modernized the entire department. The director purchased new equipment, moved the department into attractive new quarters, expanded the services offered, raised salaries, improved therapists' roles and status within the center, and hired several new employees.
>
> The result? Although the changes were needed and desired, the tension level in the department rose rapidly. Several people resigned and the rest of the employees in the department organized themselves into a bargaining unit and sought union representation for the first time. The administrator of the complex summarized the reasons for the department employees' response this way: "We tried to make too many changes too fast. They couldn't take it."

## Resistance to Change

A system can respond in several different ways to an attempt to change it. If it is neutral toward the change and does not see it as a threat, a small push can move the system in a new direction. A small force can also lead to great changes in an unstable system. For example, little added force can make an angry mob turn violent and dangerous. On the other hand, if a system is stable and considers the change a threat to its existence, it may take a strong force to change it (Mathwig, n.d.). You can see that the way in which a change is perceived can be crucial to its successful implementation.

> *Stress is a normal response to change, but response to stressors is unique to each person.*
> —*Johnston, 1998, p. 13*

Systems do not always actively resist change. A mature, healthy individual, for example, seeks opportunities for further growth: perhaps a new career, learning a new sport, or meeting a person for the first time. Even the most bureaucratic organization can and does change voluntarily over time.

A system's response to change is influenced by many factors. People react to change as whole persons. Their past experiences, culture, values, roles, coping abilities, and present needs all have some influence on their responses. The same is true of groups, organizations, or communities as they respond to change. Some of the models for change take these factors into consideration more than do others.

An apparently positive value of a proposed change is not the only factor that influences the amount of resistance that will be encountered. Healthcare providers frequently fail to recognize this fact when proposing a change in lifestyle. The following is an example:

> Consider how difficult it is for some people to quit smoking despite overwhelming evidence of the positive benefits of doing so. The health benefits, encouragement of others, and the fact that other friends have quit reinforce the motivation to change, but habit, psychological craving, pleasurable handling, stimulation, tension reduction, and the physical effects of nicotine reinforce smoking behavior and create resistance to change. Advertising and the smoking habits of friends and colleagues further reinforce the habit.

The outcome of the attempt to change smoking behavior depends on which set of forces is finally more influential, those for change or those resisting change.

## ● MANAGING CHANGE

The complexity of the forces that exist within a system and in its environment makes it difficult to predict the results of a change unless you have made a thorough analysis of the change itself, that particular system, and its relationship to the environment. Although you cannot stop change or determine its course with any certainty, you can influence the course of change.

Surprisingly, with all of the interest and concern about change in the leadership and management literature, no "science of change" has emerged (McWhinney, 1992). With the exception of the rational model, which has a substantial research base (Rogers, 1995), many of the recommendations are still based more on experience than on research (Wilson, 1992). Three models are discussed: the rational mode, participative mode, and reframing mode.

### Rational Mode

The rational approach is built on the assumption that people and organizations are capable of acting in a reasonable, objective manner. It is analytic in the sense that much attention is paid to the design of the change to be implemented (McWhinney, 1992). It is not so analytic, however, in its approach to implementation.

According to this model, the target system—the group, organization, or other system in which the leader-manager proposes to bring about change—goes through five phases in adopting a new idea:

1. *Knowledge:* The target system learns of the existence of the new idea.
2. *Persuasion:* The target system develops either a favorable or unfavorable impression of the new idea.
3. *Decision:* The target system decides either to implement or to reject the idea.
4. *Implementation:* The idea is put to use.

5. *Continuance:* The change in behavior is either discontinued or becomes an adopted change (Rogers, 1995).

This approach is particularly concerned with assessment of the characteristics of the proposed change and how these characteristics influence the rate of adoption or rejection by the target system. The original research that led to the development of this mode came from such diverse sources as the study of the introduction of a new hybrid corn to farmers, the adoption of educational innovations such as adding the kindergarten year or adopting modern math, and the rate of adoption of a new drug by physicians.

### Assumptions

Developers of the rational approach originally assumed a passive or neutral attitude on the part of the system to be changed and, therefore, did not emphasize the use of strategies to overcome resistance to change. They assumed that people's behavior is usually reasonable and logical and that their behavior would be guided by rational self-interest once it was revealed to them. In other words, once you have informed people about a better or easier way to do something, they will adopt it.

Ignorance and superstition are considered the main stumbling blocks in the way of change. Once people become better informed, they should adopt the new change willingly. Passing on new information is typically done through the media or other educational channels. This approach (informing the people) appeals to the American belief in the ability of science and technology to solve a wide range of problems, from curing disease to improving the quality of life.

### Diffusion of Innovation

Rogers's **diffusion of innovation** (Rogers, 1995; Rogers & Shoemaker, 1971) is the best known of the rational models of change. Three phases make up the diffusion of an innovation:

1. Invention of the change
2. Diffusion (communication) of the information regarding the change
3. Consequences (adoption or rejection) of the change

**RESEARCH EXAMPLE 10–1** *Changing Nurses' Pain Management Practices*

Dufault and colleagues noted that, while information on effective pain management is readily available, it is not consistently used in practice. In response, they conducted a small research study to test use of the diffusion of innovation model to change nurses' behavior.

Altogether, 27 oncology nurses participated in the study. Fifteen nurses assigned to the experimental group participated in a series of collaborative research utilization activities within the diffusion of innovation framework. The activities included identifying a practice concern (pain management), reviewing the related research on the subject, designing an innovation based on this work (in this case, adapting an existing pain assessment instrument for their use), testing it, and then deciding whether to continue to use it.

Two thirds of the nurses in the experimental group reported changes in their practice at the end of the experiment. None in the control group did. A review of selected charts supported their self-reports.

The researchers concluded that their findings supported use of the diffusion of innovation model in transferring information from research studies on pain management into practice.

*Source:* Dufault, M.A., Bielecki, C., Collins, E. & Willey, C. (1995). Changing nurses' pain assessment practice: A collaborative research utilization approach. *Journal of Advanced Nursing, 21,* 634–645.

**Invention**   During this first phase, the leader or manager's attention is directed to thorough development of the proposed change. You might develop a new method, for example, to distribute medications more efficiently. Or you could find a new solution to a common clinical problem such as postoperative hypothermia through research on the subject. Another approach would be to collect all the information people would need to guide implementation of a particular change (see Research Example 10–1). The focus is on the change itself rather than on the target system.

The rational approach is frequently used in health education. An example from a community health program is used to illustrate its application:

*A community health center nurse noticed that many clients with hypertension were not following their prescribed reduced sodium diet. Most did avoid using the salt shaker but ate liberal quantities of fast food, deli meats, cheeses, and other hidden sources of sodium.*

*The nurse consulted references for the latest information about reduced sodium diets and spoke with the dietitian, who offered to assist the nurse in gathering educational materials. Together they developed an outline of the basic information needed to follow the diet correctly. They also collected and evaluated booklets from a number of sources to find the best materials to give to clients with hypertension.*

**Diffusion**   The next step is to diffuse or communicate the idea or information developed in the first phase. Rogers (1995) describes diffusion as a special type of communication in which the messages are concerned with a new idea. Diffusion involves selecting a way to communicate the change and estimating the characteristics of the change and their effect on the ease of diffusion. The primary goal is to ensure adequate dissemination of the information, reaching everyone in the target system. It should be presented in such a way that the people can understand it well enough to use it.

**Using Mass Media**   The mass media are effective channels of communication for increasing people's knowledge and awareness. You are probably familiar with these examples:

- Air pollution alerts
- Immunization campaigns
- Food and Drug Administration actions
- Health messages during Heart Month
- Antismoking posters, pamphlets, buttons, and bumper stickers
- Radio and television talk shows on various health concerns from infertility to cancer
- Newspaper articles and health columns

- Warning messages about sexually transmitted disease
- Long-term care insurance information

Although these methods are rapid and efficient in terms of reaching large numbers of people, personal face-to-face communication is usually more persuasive. This type of communication includes individual and small group methods. Rogers (1995) points out that adoption is "a very social process" (p. 18) in which people are persuaded as much by the experience of their friends and family as by the results of scientific studies.

The next step was to consider the different ways in which information about reduced sodium diets could be communicated to the people who need it (target system):

*The health center nurse and dietitian considered several options for disseminating the information they had put together. They could make copies of their outline for distribution, have the information printed in a colorful pamphlet, present it in a classroom format, or prepare a videotape to show to their clients. To be sure that everyone understood the information, they could review the material with each person individually or they could organize a class. They decided to try the classroom approach.*

*If the nurse and dietitian had decided to enlarge their target system to include the whole community, they could consider using mass media methods of communication. They could organize a campaign to inform the community they served by using radio spot announcements, newspaper columns and interviews, poster and pamphlet distribution, and so on.*

**Estimating Diffusibility**    The degree of difficulty in diffusing a new idea or information varies considerably. Every idea has certain characteristics that make it easier or harder to diffuse successfully. These characteristics include:

- *Relative advantage:* To what extent is it better?
- *Compatibility:* Is it consistent with the target system's usual behavior, values, beliefs?
- *Complexity:* How difficult is it to understand and use this new idea?
- *Trialability:* Can the idea be tested on a limited basis first?
- *Observability:* Can the benefits be easily seen?

Is the proposed idea or method in some way better than what it replaces? It is important that the change be perceived as having some advantage over the present method or information being used. There are many ways in which the innovation may be better: more efficient, more satisfying, easier, more attractive visually, faster, cheaper, or safer, to name just a few possibilities.

For example, what is the relative advantage of the reduced sodium diet?

*The diet itself has the advantage of improving health and reducing health risk (of stroke and heart attack, for example) if followed as part of a long-term treatment plan. This advantage can be noted in the printed material and in other communications.*

*The information put together by the nurse and dietitian also has some advantages. It is more complete, more accurate, and easier to understand than the old diet instructions that the health center had been handing out with little or no explanation in the past.*

To what extent is the innovation consistent with existing values and behavior patterns? Target systems that are generally open to communications from outside and have positive attitudes toward learning and change are usually more receptive to innovations. Some knowledge of the target system's culture, norms, values, and needs is necessary in order to evaluate the degree to which the innovation will be compatible. The system's past experiences with other changes may also affect its response. Compatibility, then, is a measure of the "fit" or congruence between the proposed change and the target system.

> **Obviously more than just a beneficial innovation is necessary for its diffusion and adoption to occur.**
> —Rogers, 1995, p. 8

For example, is the proposed class on sodium-restricted diets compatible with the health center clients' values and behavior patterns?

*This characteristic is a little more difficult to evaluate than was the first one. If the center's clients have been making some attempts to reduce their sodium intake, then the proposed change will be compatible with current behav-*

ior. If the clients have not been trying to follow the diet, then the proposed change lacks compatibility in this regard, which may be a problem area.

Compatibility will also be increased if the center's clients are accustomed to seeking information about their health problems and to using health information as a guide to behavior. It would also be helpful if they feel comfortable in a classroom setting.

Is this innovation difficult to use? If the target system perceives the proposed method or new idea as being hard to understand or difficult to use, they will be less accepting of the change. A simple change is easier to communicate and also easier to implement.

For example, how complex is a reduced sodium diet?

One factor that increases the complexity of the reduced sodium diet is that table salt is not the only dietary source of sodium. Another related factor that increases the complexity is that foods may contain a lot of sodium and yet not taste salty at all. A reduced sodium diet is also difficult to follow when eating outside the home.

If the diet could be reduced to a single, simple phrase such as, "Don't eat salt," it would be more easily communicated, but this command oversimplifies the information. Despite this drawback, if the information is communicated in a clear, concise manner, it should not be too difficult for most people to learn.

People are often more willing to try something new if they can do it on a trial basis first. They are more likely to be reluctant to implement a change if it requires a full-time commitment from the start.

For example, does a sodium-restricted diet have "trialability"?

This diet could be implemented gradually, although it is not going to be effective until it is followed on a full-time basis. Trial implementation is possible.

Observable results encourage people to continue their efforts to implement a change. Seeing positive results reinforces the innovative behavior. The old saying, "Nothing succeeds like suc-

cess," is another way of saying that the observability of results encourages the change activity.

How observable are the results of implementing a sodium-restricted diet?

Many people are not aware of their symptoms when they have elevated blood pressure, so they will also not be able to observe for themselves that the diet has helped lower the blood pressure.

However, a lower blood pressure reading at the next visit to the health center could provide observable results. Another good substitute for observable results would be praise and encouragement from the center's staff when a client follows the diet. Keeping a food diary is another way to produce observability of adherence to the diet, but the work involved reduces its effectiveness for all but highly motivated people.

**Consequences**   The result of the effort to diffuse an innovation throughout a target system is either adoption of the change or its ultimate rejection. A particular change is more likely to be adopted if it has the five characteristics described previously.

The adoption process usually has three stages: trial, installation, and institutionalization. Each successive stage indicates an increasing degree of acceptance of the change as follows:

- *Trial:* The change is first tried out on an experimental basis by the target system. The attitude of the target system at this stage is generally one of "OK, we'll try it once and see how it works."
- *Installation:* If the trial is successful, the change becomes accepted enough to make it part of the regular routine and the attitude becomes one of "From now, we'll do it this way."
- *Institutionalization:* The third phase begins when the once-new idea has become so deeply enmeshed a part of the system's behavior pattern that the attitude toward it can be described as "We always do it this way."

The health center's clients may go through these three stages of adoption in the following manner:

When the clients first attend the class and try to follow the reduced sodium diet correctly, the change is in the **trial phase.**

*If the clients accept the diet sufficiently to make it a part of their everyday routine, the change has become **installed.***

*If they follow the diet so well that they do not even need to think much about it anymore, it has become **institutionalized** and the change has been successfully implemented.*

## Discussion

When is the rational approach a good choice? The rational mode works well when widespread readiness for change characterizes the target system. For example, when the polio vaccine was developed years ago, most people were eager to obtain it because they had been worried about outbreaks of the disease and had great faith in the ability of medical research to develop an effective vaccine. Many technologies—all kinds of mechanical inventions and new ideas—have been quickly adopted using this model. Consider the success of the Internet!

However, the rational approach's assumption that people act logically ignores the fact that, as holistic beings, they also react emotionally to attempts to change them. Any change that violates a norm, threatens a cherished tradition, or even disturbs a comfortable routine is not going to be accepted as readily as one that does not. Entire groups can react on the basis of a shared group feeling or norm that has developed.

We return to the reduced sodium diet example once more to analyze the circumstances under which the rational mode will be effective.

*If the class consists of a highly motivated group of clients who are concerned about following their diets correctly, then the rational mode will probably be effective. However, food has emotional and social significance and is a part of many religious and cultural traditions. A restricted diet frequently conflicts with these meanings. Also, as was mentioned before, people often experience few symptoms when they have high blood pressure and, therefore, may not be motivated to even try following a restricted diet. It is also difficult to see or feel immediate benefits from following a restricted diet and some people are easily discouraged by this invisibility of change. The*

change project described ignores these potential sources of resistance.

The rational approach works best when the planned change is easy to understand, easy to implement, and provokes little resistance from the target system. It assumes readiness to change and a tendency to respond rationally; it virtually ignores social, cultural, and emotional responses to proposed changes. It is most useful when the situation is conducive to change. In the presence of more resistance to change, however, you will find that the next approach, which pays more attention to the twin problems of developing readiness to change and reducing resistance, will be a more appropriate choice.

> *The fundamental flaw in most innovators' strategies is that they focus on their innovation, on what they are trying to do—rather than on understanding how the larger culture, structures and norms will react to their efforts.*
>
> —Kleiner et al., 1999, p. 26)

## Participative Mode

The participative or normative approach to change seeks ways to increase acceptance of the change and to increase people's motivation to change. It recognizes that often more than one choice is available as to the type of change to implement. In that approach, the people who will be affected by the change are encouraged to engage in dialogue about the alternative (McWhinney, 1992). Resistance is considered natural (Harvey, 1990) and significant effort is made to identify its sources and eliminate them.

This approach focuses on the target system, or "changee," particularly the influence of people's needs, feelings, attitudes, and values on their response to change, the actions of the leader or manager as the change maker, and the characteristics of the change itself.

### Assumptions

Some resistance is anticipated, but it is expected that this resistance can be overcome without force. Both the leader-manager and the target system are expected to be active rather than passive participants in the change process.

The ability of the target system to resist, modify, or accept the proposed change is central to this approach, so stronger tactics are used. Rationality is not ignored but treated as one of many factors influencing behavior.

### Lewin's Phases of Change

The **force field model** originated with Lewin's (1951) work and was further developed by Schein and Bennis (1975) and many others since then. This model divides the change process into three phases: unfreezing, changing, and refreezing. The importance of analyzing the forces for and against change is a distinguishing feature of this model.

Driving and Restraining Forces    Lewin (1951) recommended beginning the change process by analyzing the **driving and restraining forces** within the system involved. This approach is quite different from beginning with the development of a new or better idea.

The forces that push the system toward change are the driving forces. Those forces that pull the system away from change are the restraining forces (Figure 10–1). When the restraining forces are the same or stronger than the driving forces, the leader or manager needs to use participative change strategies to reduce the restraining forces and increase the driving forces in order to implement the change.

To assess these opposing forces accurately, a thorough acquaintance with the target system, the environment, the characteristics of the change, and the potential responses to change is needed. The leader or manager may have to spend some time becoming more familiar with one or all of these elements before an accurate appraisal of the situation can be made. When this analysis is done,

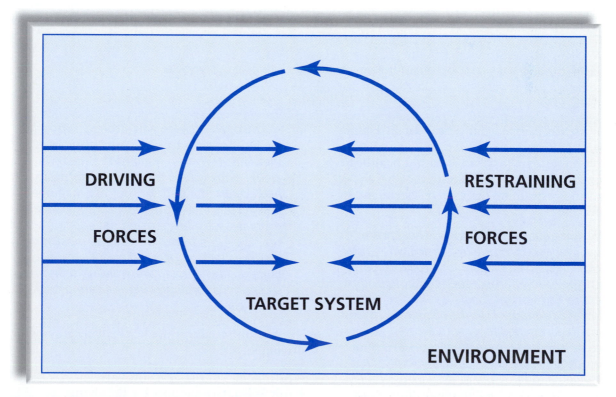

**Figure 10–1**  Opposing change forces in a system.
*Source:*  Adapted from Lewin, K. (1951). *Field theory in social science: Selected theoretical papers.* New York: Harper & Row.

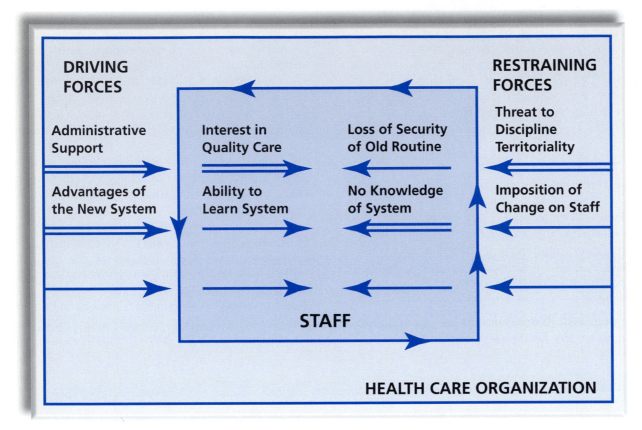

**Figure 10–2** Diagram of opposing change forces in computerized patient record example.

the forces are mapped out as shown in Figures 10–1 and 10–2.

A common type of change within healthcare organizations is used to illustrate the analysis of driving and restraining forces in a system and its environment.

*The nurse educator of a primary healthcare clinic was asked to take responsibility for installation and implementation of a radically different type of software for their computerized patient record system. The new software had several advantages over the old: it required less writing, eliminated repetition, allowed quicker access to stored information, combined notations from all disciplines into one format that provided a total picture of the client's progress and could be modified for use by the various services offered by the clinic and to share data with other agencies.*

*The new software was strongly supported by the administrators and executive board of the clinic. However, none of the staff who would actually be using the new software had ever used it before. They also had not expressed any interest in replacing the old software and were busy seeing patients the entire day. Aside from these issues, most staff members were concerned about providing high-quality care and were willing to listen to suggestions for improving the care provided at the clinic.*

The nurse educator identified the following **driving forces:**

- Advantages of the new software
- Administrative support for the change
- Staff concern about quality care
- Staff ability to learn the new software

On the other hand, the nurse educator also found the following **restraining forces:**

- Lack of staff participation in the selection of the software
- Little or no staff knowledge of the new software
- Potential threats to the staff's feelings of security when giving up their old routine
- Potential threats to territoriality of various disciplines because of equal access to the information in the new system

The opposing forces are diagrammed in Figure 10–2. The diagram shows you which factors will help and which factors will hinder your efforts to bring about change. In some situations you might also want to note which of the forces are especially strong by adding extra lines to the arrows, as was done in Figure 10–2.

Unfreezing    Target systems usually need a push to get them moving toward change. Technically, open systems are never really "frozen" but they can be amazingly resistant to change and so appear to be frozen to the individual trying to introduce change. Particular patterns of behavior can be so entrenched that it takes a great deal of energy to change them. You may have to deliberately stir things up to unfreeze the situation. Three kinds of tactics can be used to unfreeze the target system:

1. Create disconfirmation
2. Induce guilt and anxiety
3. Provide psychological safety

Introducing disconfirmation is actually confrontation with conflicting evidence. This confrontation makes the target system feel uncomfortable or dissatisfied with its present condition so that it will want to change. The disconfirming evidence may be any information, example, or experience that challenges the status quo.

People often resist disconfirmation. They may try to ignore the evidence or to rationalize that the evidence is ambiguous or atypical. Or they may blame the problem on someone else. These responses are often aimed at protecting security, esteem, or some other need.

Inducing guilt and anxiety will overcome resistance to disconfirmation through demonstrating that a goal or value that is important to the target system is not being met or upheld. This type of situation upsets the balance between the driving and restraining forces and raises the tension level within the target system.

Providing psychological safety is the third tactic. Making a change requires some risk on the part of the target system, so the leader or manager needs to provide sufficient security to minimize the risk. Is this point in conflict with the second tactic? It may be. Usually the guilt or anxiety induced is specific to the planned change, while the feeling of security is related to creating a general climate of trust and acceptance. Many changes are resisted primarily because they present some kind of threat to the target system. When the threat is reduced or removed, people usually feel comfortable enough to attempt the change. These tactics can be used separately or together to unfreeze the target system.

Much time and energy may be needed to unfreeze the target system enough to get it moving toward change. As a general rule, the most energy is needed to reduce or eliminate the strongest restraining forces and to strengthen the weaker driving forces. For a large-scale change, it may take weeks or even months to achieve unfreezing.

To unfreeze the staff, the nurse educator took the following actions:

| | |
|---|---|
| Disconfirmation | Meet with every staff member in a series of small group discussions of the inadequacies of the current software. |
| Inducing Guilt and Anxiety | Demonstrate ways in which the old software interfered with quality care. |
| | Indicate that the staff is not doing the best job possible in using the old software. |
| | Tell staff members how strongly administrators and board members support the new software. (This message implies that they |

Providing
Psychological
Safety

would be unhappy if
the new software
were not accepted).
Assure staff members
that they will have
ample time and op-
portunity to learn the
new software.
Indicate that staff will be
involved in deciding
how to implement the
change.
Point out similarities
between the old and
new software; that the
new software will not
change the routine
too much or be too
difficult to learn.
Express confidence in
staff's ability to mas-
ter the new software.
Ensure the continued
identity of each disci-
pline: use examples for
each one; show how
others will be better
able to see and appre-
ciate each discipline's
contribution with the
new software.

Each of the driving and restraining forces are dealt with in at least one of the three tactics.

Many situations have more or stronger restraining forces than this example does and may require more emphasis on the disconfirmation and guilt-inducing tactics than discussed here.

Changing    In the implementation phase of the change process, the target system is unfrozen and moving toward change and the leader can begin putting the planned change into effect.

The unfreezing process leaves people feeling off-balance. A natural response to such change efforts is a state of high energy called **hyper-energy** (Gillen, 1986). This energy needs to be directed into productive actions. If it is not, it can provoke serious resistance to the proposed change.

The leader or manager plays an active role in this phase. The following is a list of the activities in which he or she will be engaged during the changing phase:

1. Introduce any new information that is needed to implement the change.
2. Encourage the new behavior so that it becomes part of the system's regular patterns of behavior. Provide for practice and experimentation with the change behavior if possible. Allow people to make mistakes without negative consequences and provide opportunities for success (Manion, 1993; Schaffer & Thomson, 1992).
3. Continue to provide a supportive climate to minimize defensive behavior and resistance to the change.
4. Provide opportunities to ventilate the anxiety, anger, or hostility aroused by the change process.
5. Provide feedback on progress and reiteration of the goal to reinforce the change process and to keep people from getting sidetracked.
6. Present yourself as a trustworthy person to keep communication open.
7. Act as an energizer to keep interest high and to keep the change process moving forward.
8. Overcome any resistance that arises by using the unfreezing tactics again.

You can see that keeping everyone informed is an essential element of the participative mode. Open, honest, direct communication, including acknowledging the feelings associated with the effects of the change are key to the success of this approach (Wells et al., 1998). Demonstrating sensitivity can be a great deal of work for the leader or manager but failing to so greatly increases the likelihood of failure (Bolton et al., 1992). Most of the actions already listed are basic leadership skills derived from the components of effective leadership.

During the change phase, the nurse educator took the following actions:

Introduce new
information

Teach the staff how
to use the new
software.

Encourage the new
behavior

Begin with practice
using examples
from real
situations.
Then have the staff
begin using the

| | |
|---|---|
| | new software according to the plan they devised for implementation. |
| Continue the supportive climate | Allow adequate time for learning and practice before implementation. |
| | Point out how the staff is supporting its standards for care. |
| Provide opportunities for ventilation | Ask staff how they feel about the new software; listen and respond to what they say about it. |
| Provide feedback and clarification of goals | Check computerized patient records to evaluate progress. Ask staff how well the new software is working. Remind staff personally and through memos about the use of the software and why it is being implemented. |
| Present yourself as trustworthy | Make sure that all staff were included in the implementation planning as promised. |
| | Follow through on other promises as well. |
| | Keep communications open and honest. |
| Act as an energizer | Take every opportunity to promote the new software at meetings, men- |

| | |
|---|---|
| | tion it in newsletters, and so forth. Demonstrate interest in staff progress. |
| Overcome resistance | Repeat, increase, and if necessary, expand the tactics described in the unfreezing phase. |

**Refreezing**   The purpose of the refreezing phase is to stabilize and integrate the change so that it becomes a part of the regular functioning of the target system. It is similar to the institutionalization phase of the rational approach.

At the beginning of this phase, the situation is still fluid. Because the target system is still in the process of changing and could still take a course different from the planned change, guidance is needed to ensure that the new pattern of behavior persists. However, the leader role does become a less active one than it was in the preceding phases.

To facilitate the integration of the planned change, the leader-manager continues to act as energizer and guide but increasingly delegates responsibility for the change behavior to other people in the target system.

By the time this phase is reached, other interested and capable people should be ready to accept responsibility for continuing the new behavior. The leader or manager gradually reduces participation as other people become increasingly involved.

In some cases, the leader or manager relinquishes all responsibility for continued supervision at the end of this phase; in others, this supervision becomes part of his or her regular functions.

We return to the example once more to see how the refreezing phase is accomplished. Having succeeded in installing and beginning use of the new software, the nurse educator took the following actions to ensure its continued use:

| | |
|---|---|
| Continue acting as energizer | Continue to show interest in staff progress and response to the new software. |
| | Praise staff for genuine progress. |

| Continue guiding new behavior | Continue to check computerized patient records to see how well the new software is working and to intervene if problems arise. Help staff correct mistakes and provide needed information. |
| Delegate increased responsibility to others | Designate certain staff members as resources for staff to turn to for help. Turn over responsibility for checking implementation to supervisors. |

The nurse educator continued to show interest in the usefulness of the new software but otherwise turned over all other responsibility for the system to staff members and their supervisors by the end of this phase.

## Discussion

The participative approach to change is holistic, responsive, democratic, flexible, and adaptable. A number of variations of the model have been developed, often using entirely different terminology (see Perspectives . . . Another Change Model).

The participative approach is applicable to a wider range of situations than the reframing mode, which is discussed next. In Research Example 10–2, you can see that the researcher came up with recommendations that parallel the strategies of the participative approach. Although effective in a wide range of situations, it does not always work. Because it is basically a persuasive, problem-solving method, participative change works well in situations of low to moderate amounts of resistance to change. However, individuals and groups are sometimes not easily persuaded, and certain situations are problematic and not amenable to logical solution. In some of these cases, the reframing mode may be effective.

## PERSPECTIVES . . .

### Another Change Model

Any complete change theory has four parts: a procedure for diagnosing the problem, a process for devising a solution or innovation, strategies for implementing the solution, and a way to evaluate the outcome, according to Tiffany and Lutjens (1998) who have written about the use of change theories in nursing. Bhola's CLER model has all four of these.

Developed within an open systems framework, the CLER model employs participative decision making. The acronym CLER stands for:

**C**onfiguration of change

**L**inkages between the leader and target system and within the target system

**E**nvironment within which the change takes place

**R**esources including cognitive (understanding), power and influence, economic (money), personnel, infrastructure and time

The interrelated components of a planned change are:

**P**lanner or initiator of the change

**O**bjective or goal of the change

**A**dapters or target system (Bhola, 1995)

Sound familiar? Which of the models for change presented in this chapter does the CLER model most closely resemble?

---

*Sources:* Bhola, H.S. (1995). The CLER model: Thinking through change. *Nursing Management, 25*(5), 59–63.

Tiffany, C.R. & Lutjens, L.R.J. (1998). *Planned change theories for nursing: Review, analysis and implications.* Thousand Oaks, CA: Sage.

Sometimes, resistance to change is due to conflicting beliefs, norms, or values. The controversy over abortion is an example of conflicting values in which each side uses moral or ethical arguments to support its position. The participa-

## RESEARCH EXAMPLE 10–2  *Successful Planned Changes*

What factors facilitate planned change? What factors increase resistance? Schermerhorn (1981) asked middle managers from hospitals of different types in New England to rate the effect of a number of different factors on a typical planned change. Most of these changes were common events such as altering admission procedures, asking laboratory employees to begin wearing laboratory coats, or trying to change the attitudes of uncooperative employees. A total of 70 successful and unsuccessful attempts to implement change were analyzed.

The factors rated by the managers as having increased success included the presence of a felt need, providing information about the change, using coercion and personal attraction to induce change, frequent communication, direct assistance, and top-management support. It was interesting that they believed success in implementing change decreased when alternative actions were available. The managers found that coercion was effective but the use of special incentives (rewards) was not effective, which seemed to surprise the researcher.

The managers thought that conflict decreased when a problem existed, which created a felt need to change. Resistance was increased when alternatives to the change were available. On the basis of these results, the researcher suggested the following guidelines for implementing change:

- Build the change around a felt need.
- Use effective communication skills when presenting information and alternatives.
- Maintain good interpersonal relations with staff to capitalize on the influence of your personal attraction.
- Encourage free exchange of ideas to develop a sense of participation.
- Provide assistance and avoid overloading the group to facilitate the change process.
- Use coercion to help unfreeze a situation.

*Source:* Schermerhorn, J.R. (1981). Guidelines for change in health care organizations. *Health Care Management Review,* 6(3), 9.

tive mode will not work when people cannot eventually reach some kind of consensus.

In other situations, the resistance to change is strong because members of the target system feel that the change will be detrimental to their position or well-being. For example, many individuals and groups value their prestige, power, influence, or economic strength. A change that threatens any one of these aspects will be strongly resisted. In these situations, one must also deal with issues of power and conflict, discussed in a later chapter.

## Reframing Mode

The originators of the **reframing** or **paradoxical** mode of change have a background in psychotherapy that is apparent in their model (Watzlawick, Weakland & Fisch, 1974). This approach is

particularly concerned with the way in which problems arise and why some persist while others are resolved. It grew out of the observation of a paradox: that logical, reasonable approaches to change often fail whereas illogical, backward-seeming approaches sometimes succeed. The reframing approach destroys the logic of the opponent's argument, thereby eliminating a conflict rather than resolving it (McWhinney, 1992).

Underlying the reframing approach is the idea of two different types of change: first-order and second-order changes. First-order changes are those that seem logical; second-order changes appear to be illogical.

### First-Order Change

First-order changes are less intense, less profound types of changes in which the nature of the relationships between the people and systems involved remain virtually the same. The following example illustrates a first-order type of change:

> *The professionals on an interdisciplinary child abuse evaluation team have had difficulty relating to one another as peers. For example, instead of developing a pattern of communication between equals, the group has a superior-to-subordinate communication pattern.*
>
> *Two members of the team tried to change this pattern of communication. At a team meeting, they raised the issue of collegiality and equality among team members (a first-order attempt to bring about change). All team members agreed that they were colleagues and that no one was superior or subordinate to any of the others. Despite this enthusiastic endorsement of collegiality, whenever a member of the team approached another team member as an equal, the other member retreated either into a subordinate or superior position, so the overall pattern of interpersonal relationships remained the same. No permanent change in communication pattern occurred.*

The first-order change did not alter old behavior patterns and may actually have contributed to making them more entrenched than ever. Here, a paradox is operating: some attempts to bring about change can actually make the problem worse. When a well-entrenched behavior pattern needs to be changed (as in the example of the child abuse team), first-order change is often not adequate to change it. Let us return to the child abuse team example to see how other attempts at first-order change reinforced old behavior patterns:

> *The child abuse team has become divided into two groups: the lower-status professionals (teacher, nurse, social worker) and the higher-status professionals (psychiatrist, physician). This division is reinforced by the entrenched superior-subordinate communication pattern.*
>
> *The lower-status members also tried to improve their position on the team by writing excellent reports on each child evaluated by the team and by asserting themselves at team conferences. But the more they asserted themselves, the more the higher-status professionals used a superior tone of voice and ignored their input in making decisions, even to the point of dictating the team's recommendations.*
>
> *This team is caught in a status struggle. As a result, the valuable input of several team members is lost, impairing the function of the team.*

Another common paradox that operates on the individual level is the demand to "be spontaneous." It is a demand to engage in some kind of natural behavior that can only occur spontaneously. In fact, the harder you try to perform the required behavior, the harder it is to do so. For example, urging depressed patients to "Cheer up!" is asking them to do the impossible. Paradoxically, it can make them feel even worse because they are unable to please you by cheering up. Another interesting example is insomnia. Falling asleep is a natural behavior, but for many insomniacs the harder they try to fall asleep, the wider awake they feel. The more conscious efforts they make to get to sleep on time, such as counting sheep or going to bed earlier, the less likely they are to succeed.

Because of these paradoxes, when first-order changes fail to break up old behavior patterns, second-order change is needed.

## Second-Order Change

Shifting from first-order to second-order change requires **reframing**, that is, taking a new perspective on the problem or situation you are trying to change. Watzlawick and associates used a familiar puzzle to illustrate this shift from first-order change (Figure 10–3). If you have not seen the puzzle before, try doing it before proceeding.

The solution to the puzzle requires going outside the square. While the directions do not **prohibit** your doing so, most people cannot figure out the puzzle because the edge of the square represents a boundary line that keeps them from seeing the solution. It is an example of a first-order attempt to change. A second-order change, requiring that you go outside the logical boundaries of the square, is needed to solve this puzzle. Once you see the second-order solution, it becomes clear why you could not solve it with a first-order change.

the original problem are reviewed. They may at first appear to resemble the familiar problem-solving process, but they are *not* the same. Instead, they address the elimination of the paradoxes that keep you from solving the problem. This model can also be used when simple problem solving has failed to produce a lasting solution. The steps are as follows:

1. Define the problem in concrete terms.
2. List the solutions attempted so far.
3. Clearly define a realistic change.
4. Select and implement a second-order change strategy.

**Step 1: Define the Problem in Concrete Terms**  The purpose of this step is to help you concentrate on the specific, solvable aspect of the problem or situation and avoid trying to solve unsolvable problems. Some problems really are inevitable and cannot be changed, although you can change the way in which you cope with them. You cannot, for example, remove the threat of a hurricane or tornado but you can either prepare for them or move out of their path. A storm itself is not amenable to change, but your response to the storm is amenable to change. Many social problems are amenable to change only over the long term and are not sufficiently concrete to resolve directly and gain immediate relief. Let us return to the child abuse team example to illustrate reframing:

> Here is a list of three possible ways to define the problem from the point of view of the nurse, teacher, and social worker:
>
> * Our professional status is too low.
> * Our value to the team is not recognized.
> * Our input is ignored.

The first definition of the problem is too global to be amenable to immediate solution. It is a long-term problem that goes beyond the team and requires a change in societal attitudes. The second definition of the problem is more specific but still too general. The third one is the most concrete. It avoids analyzing the reasons behind the problem and specifically defines the present dilemma and immediate concern of the lower-status members of the team.

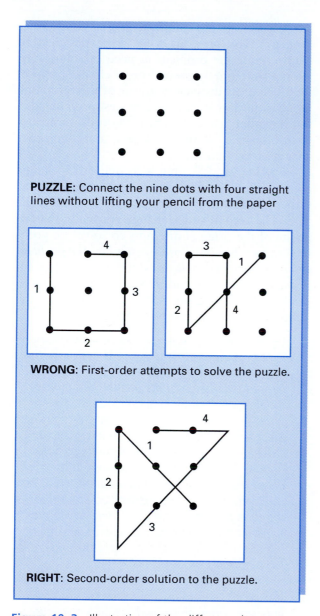

**PUZZLE:** Connect the nine dots with four straight lines without lifting your pencil from the paper

**WRONG:** First-order attempts to solve the puzzle.

**RIGHT:** Second-order solution to the puzzle.

**Figure 10–3**  Illustration of the difference between first- and second-order changes.
*Source:* Watzlawick, P., Weakland. J. & Fisch, R. (1974). *Change: Principles of problem formation and problem resolution.* New York: W.W. Norton & Co. Used with permission.

## *Reframing*

Second-order change requires a rethinking of a problem from a new perspective. Before considering more second-order solutions to problems, the steps suggested by Watzlawick for reframing

**Step 2: List the Solutions Attempted So Far**   Once you have defined the problem in concrete terms, you are ready to look for solutions to the problem. In most cases, the previously attempted solutions were first-order changes that failed to bring about any lasting change in behavior and may even have made the problem worse. The purpose of this step is to help you avoid repeating previous unsuccessful attempts to change the situation. For example:

*In the child abuse team, the lower-status professionals made several attempts to change their position on the team. They repeatedly tried to do the following:*

- *Relate to other team members as equals.*
- *Prove their expertise by writing high-quality evaluations.*
- *Demonstrate their worth by working harder and being more thorough than the rest of the team.*

None of these solutions worked. In fact, they made the situation worse because they had tried so hard and been so frustrated by the results of their efforts.

**Step 3: Clearly Define a Realistic Change**   In this step, you define the goal of the planned change. As in the first step, the emphasis is on the specific and concrete. To be avoided are goals that are too global or too vague, or attempts to solve the unsolvable aspects of the problem that are not amenable to change (the inevitable storms, for example).

*At the outset, the nurse, social worker, and teacher on the child abuse team wanted to achieve the following outcomes:*

- *Raise our status.*
- *Gain respect and recognition from the rest of the team.*
- *Increase use of our input in making recommendations.*

The first goal is global; it defines an attempt to change a social phenomenon and is a long-term goal. The second is more specific but still general in comparison with the third goal. The third goal, increased use of their input, is more specific and more amenable to change than the first two. It is the most realistic of the three goals listed.

**Step 4: Select and Implement a Second-Order Strategy**   The previous steps were designed to help reframe the problem in need of solution to allow a shift into the second-order change perspective. The most distinctive aspect of the reframing mode is this last step, the strategies recommended to bring about change. When first-order strategies have been tried without success, a second-order change is recommended.

The key to designing a second-order change comes from the list of unsuccessful solutions rather than from the problem, as is usually the case. The second-order change is usually the **opposite** of the original attempts to solve the problem. In fact, it *more closely resembles the problem than the original solutions!* Often, the second-order change is a solution that brings a smile to the face of the person who is to carry out the strategy. Here is an example of this:

*D.L. had developed a fear that he would faint in hot, crowded stores. He could not shake this fear no matter how hard he tried to reason with himself that he was quite healthy and unlikely to faint (a first-order change strategy).*

*Finally, a second-order change strategy was prescribed for D.L. He was told to go into a crowded department store at the busy noon hour and lie down flat on the floor in the middle of the main aisle as if he had fainted. When D.L. went to the store, he walked around looking for a place to pretend to faint, smiling to himself at the thought of deliberately stretching out on the floor, blocking traffic, and creating a hubbub.*

*D.L. did not actually carry out the prescription; he had no need to do it because the unshakeable fear had been converted into a private joke he was tempted to play on the department store (Watzlawick, Weakland & Fisch, 1974).*

You can see how closely the solution resembled the problem. It was almost the opposite of the original first-order change in which D.L. tried so hard to avoid feeling faint. The same strategy can be applied to the fear of speaking in public. Instead of trying to cover up your fear, which makes people more nervous because they are sure their fear is showing, try telling the audience how scared you are of speaking to them. By announcing your fear, you not only eliminate its worst consequence but also win the support of the group to whom you are speaking.

The "be spontaneous" paradox can be dealt with in the same way. Insomnia was mentioned as an example of the paradox. Insomniac patients who can't make themselves go to sleep are told to go to bed but to be sure to keep their eyes open. With their efforts turned away from trying to fall asleep, they are able to fall asleep naturally. Their original solutions (counting sheep, going to bed earlier, trying harder to get to sleep) had become part of the problem and were dealt with by reframing the problem: by trying to stay awake, the insomniac patients were able to fall asleep spontaneously.

Every situation or problem calls for its own unique second-order strategy. We return once more to the child abuse evaluation team example to see what kind of second-order change strategy could be devised for this problem:

*The nurse, teacher, and social worker had found that their attempts to prove their worth on the team only provoked more resistance and resulted in less recognition for their work rather than more. Using a second-order change approach, they redefined their goal to be "increased use of our input in making recommendations."*

*To implement a second-order change, the nurse, teacher, and social worker decided to use a second-order change strategy, one that was almost the complete opposite of their earlier unsuccessful first-order change efforts. Instead of working so hard to prove their ability, they started asking the psychiatrist and physician to do their work for them. They stopped trying to be recognized at the team conferences and began omitting important parts of their evaluations, asking the psychiatrist or physician to fill these parts in for them. Each one politely but insistently asked for time to meet with the psychiatrist and physician several times a week and telephoned them several times a day as well "just to check with you on this point."*

*Within two weeks, the psychiatrist and physician were telling the nurse, teacher, and social worker that they were quite capable of doing their own work. They also began to encourage them to contribute to the team con-ferences, saying, "You can't expect the two of us to do all the work!"*

Reframing is particularly suited to those situations in which logical solutions have failed. In fact, it was designed to deal with just this type of situation in which first-order change has not solved the problem.

Reframing does have some drawbacks. First, the person who carries out the second-order change strategy must be highly motivated to carry out a seemingly absurd strategy. Even though people often do feel a desperate need to change a situation and are willing to do almost anything to resolve their problems, the model does not provide a way to increase this motivation when it is lacking.

A second drawback is the risk that the strategy will backfire. People faced with a persistent problem may see the risk as negligible in comparison with the problem but the risk does exist.

Third, although reframing can be applied to larger systems, it does not address communicating the paradoxical message to large numbers of people. In this sense, the model is not complete in itself but can be used in conjunction with other change strategies.

Finally, reframing requires imagination, the kind of creativity needed to be humorous, and a willingness to alter one's perspective (to step out of the box). In a sense, it is the same kind of creativity Greene (1973) referred to when she talked about taking a stranger's point of view. In spite of these drawbacks, the creative leader or manager may find reframing an effective approach for dealing with the persistent and seemingly unresolvable dilemmas that prevented the solution to the problem.

## ● SUMMARY

Change is a natural part of life. Planned change is the deliberate application of knowledge and skills by the leader in order to bring about change. Change is inherent in open systems. It may be mild or extreme, positive or negative, welcome or resisted by the system. Many factors influence a system's response to change, including the perceived value of the change, the rate of change, and

# CASE STUDY

### You Can't Do That Here

Danny studied nursing at a small midwestern college. After graduation, Danny moved to the West Coast and accepted a staff nurse position at a large metropolitan hospital. Staff at this facility were busy but prided themselves on the high quality of nursing care they provided.

Finding new ways to improve patient care was a frequent subject of discussion at staff meetings. "Why don't we start a volunteer corps?" Danny suggested. "Volunteers! What would they do?" a staff nurse asked. "They could run errands, pass trays, help patients with their meals," Danny began to answer. "Our patients are too sick. We couldn't allow volunteers on this unit," interrupted another staff nurse. "Where I come from, they even have volunteers assigned to the critical care units," Danny explained. "Well, you're not in Kansas anymore, Dorothy!" a sarcastic tech replied. Everyone laughed, even Danny. "We couldn't get anyone to volunteer here, anyway," added another nurse.

Danny let the subject drop for the time being but kept thinking about the value of volunteers and all of the ways they could be helpful on his unit. "Somehow," he thought to himself, "I've got to convince them that a volunteer corps is a good idea."

### Questions for Critical Reflection and Analysis

1. Why did the other staff members criticize Danny's suggestion?
2. Create a scenario in which Danny uses one of the change models described in this chapter to bring about the establishment of a volunteer corps.
3. Critique the usefulness of the change model you chose.
4. Would the scenario you created succeed in real life? Why or why not?

the needs, experiences, culture, values, and coping abilities of the system within a given environment.

The rational mode assumes that people will respond in a logical fashion to change. It works best when faced with little resistance to change. This model has three phases: invention, diffusion, and consequences. A change is more easily diffused or communicated if it has an advantage over the old way, is compatible, is not too complex, can be tried out on a limited basis, and provides observable results. In the last phase, the change may be either accepted or rejected. If it is accepted, it will usually pass through three stages: trial, installation, and institutionalization.

Participative change focuses on people's needs, feelings, values, and potential resistance to change. The force field model, derived primarily from Lewin's work, begins with an analysis of the driving forces for and restraining forces against change. The leader or manager then proceeds to work through the unfreezing, changing,

and refreezing phases of change. This approach works best when the resistance to change is low to moderate and when some consensus on the planned change can be reached.

The reframing mode divides change strategies into two types: first-order and second-order changes. The logical solution to a problem of the first-order type often fails to break up old patterns of behavior and paradoxically may even make the problem worse. The second-order change strategy is usually the opposite of the logical first-order change. By reframing the problem, the second-order change can resolve the paradox that prevented resolution of the problem.

## REFERENCES

Bennis, W.G. et al. (1976). *The planning of change*, 3rd ed. New York: Holt, Rinehart & Winston.
Bhola, H.S. (1995). The CLER model: Thinking through change. *Nursing Management, 25*(5), 59–63.

Bolton, L.B., Aydin, C., Popolow, G. & Ramseyer, J. (1992). Ten steps for managing organization change. *Journal of Nursing Administration, 12*(6), 14–20.

Dufault, M.A., Bielecki, C., Collins, E. & Willey, C. (1995). Changing nurses' pain assessment practice: A collaborative research utilization approach. *Journal of Advanced Nursing, 21,* 634–645.

Gillen, D.J. (1986). Harnessing the energy from change anxiety. *Supervisory Management, 31*(3), 40–45.

Greene, M. (1973). *Teacher as stranger.* Belmont, CA: Wadsworth.

Harvey, T.R. (1990). *Checklist for change: A pragmatic approach to creating and controlling change.* Boston: Allyn & Bacon.

Holmes, T.H. & Rahe, R. (1967). The social readjustment rating scale. *Journal of Psychosomatic Research, 2*(4), 213.

Johnston, B.C. (1998). Managing change in health care redesign: A model to assist staff in promoting healthy change. *Nursing Economics, 16*(1), 12–17.

Kleiner, A., Roberts, C., Ross, R., Roth, G., Senge, P. & Smith, B. (1999). The challenges of profound change. In P. Senge (Ed.). *The dance of change.* New York: Doubleday, 21–34.

Koerner, J.G. & Bunkers, S.S. (1992). Transformational leadership: The power of symbol. *Nursing Administration Quarterly, 17*(1), 1–9.

Leonard, D. & Straus, S. (1997, July/August). Putting your company's whole brain to work. *Harvard Business Review,* 111–121.

Lewin, K. (1951). *Field theory in social science: Selected theoretical papers.* New York: Harper & Row.

Manion, J. (1993). Chaos or transformational? Managing innovation. *Journal of Nursing Administration, 23*(5), 41–48.

Mathwig, G. (n.d.). *The nurse as a change agent* (mimeographed). New York: New York University.

McWhinney, W. (1992). *Paths of change: Strategic choices for organizations and society.* Newbury Park, CA: Sage.

Panel. (1994). The role of the CFO in CQI. *Healthcare Financial Management, 48*(4), 60–72.

Purser, R.E. & Cabana, S. (1998). *The self-managing organization.* New York: The Free Press.

Rogers, E.M. (1995). *Diffusion of innovations,* 4th ed. New York: The Free Press.

Rogers, E.M. & Shoemaker, F.F. (1971). *Communication of innovation,* 2d ed. New York: Free Press.

Samuelson, R.J. (1998, January 12). The way the world works. *Newsweek,* 52.

Schaffer, R.H. & Thomson, H.A. (1992). Successful change programs begin with results. *Harvard Business Review, 70*(1), 80–89.

Schein, E.H. & Bennis, W. (1975). *Personal and organizational change through group methods.* New York: John Wiley & Sons.

Schermerhorn, J.R. (1981). Guidelines for change in health care organizations. *Health Care Management Review, 6*(3), 9.

Senge, P. (1999). The life cycle of typical change initiatives. In P. Senge (Ed.). *The dance of change.* New York: Doubleday, 5–10.

Strebel, P. (1992). *Breakpoints: How managers exploit radical business change.* Boston: Harvard Business School Review.

Tiffany, C.R. & Lutjens, L.R.J. (1998). *Planned change theories for nursing: Review, analysis and implications.* Thousand Oaks, CA: Sage.

Watzlawick, P., Weakland, J. & Fisch, R. (1974). *Change: Principles of problem formation and problem resolution.* New York: W.W. Norton & Co.

Wells, N., Barnard, T., Mason, L., Ames, A. & Minnen, T. (1998). Work transitions. *Journal of Nursing Administration, 28*(2), 50–56.

Wilson, D.C. (1992). *A strategy of change: Concepts and controversies.* London: Routledge.

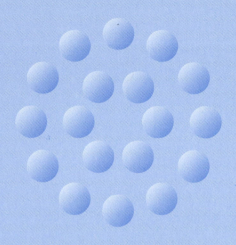

UNIT **III**

# Nursing Management

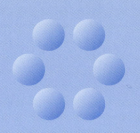

# Components of Effective Management

## LEARNING OBJECTIVES

*After completing this chapter, the reader will be able to:*

- Name the components of effective management.

- Discuss the importance of each component of effective management.

- Evaluate his or her own effectiveness in terms of the components of effective management.

- Evaluate managers in terms of the components of effective management.

## TEST YOURSELF

**Which of the following roles does an effective first-line nurse manager play?** Place a check mark alongside all that you think apply and then check your answers.

____ 1. Coordinator

____ 2. Boss

____ 3. Integrator

____ 4. Negotiator

____ 5. Administrator

____ 6. Monitor

____ 7. Salesperson

____ 8. Teacher

____ 9. Dictator

____ 10. Placator

____ 11. Diplomat

____ 12. Coach

____ 13. Motivator

____ 14. Bureaucrat

____ 15. Tyrant

____ 16. Spokesperson

____ 17. Sergeant

____ 18. Organizer

____ 19. Mother

____ 20. Politician

*Source:* Inspired by Hill, J. (1992). *Becoming a manager.* Boston: Harvard Business School Press.

*Answers*

1. Yes 2. Yes 3. Yes 4. Yes 5. No 6. Yes 7. Yes, sometimes 8. Yes, sometimes 9. No 10. No 11. Yes 12. Yes 13. Yes 14. No 15. No 16. Yes 17. No 18. Yes 19. No 20. Yes, sometimes

---

**W**hat makes a person an effective manager? Leadership is a prerequisite for effective management and the first of the seven components of effective management. The other components of effective management are: planning, direction, monitoring, recognition, development, and representation (Figure 11–1). Together they summarize the fundamental concepts of management. Each of the seven components is discussed in this chapter.

> *. . . like an outstanding conductor who facilitates that stunning performance, the nurse manager is the pivotal element in the delivery of high-quality patient care.*
>
> —Frank, Eckrich & Rohr, 1997, p. 14

## ● EFFECTIVE MANAGEMENT

A manager works through others. For example, a nurse manager may not actually dispense medications, monitor central lines, or give immunizations, but the manager is responsible for ensuring not only that this care is given but that it is done well. This task is not simple; it requires considerable knowledge and skill to be an effective manager. In this chapter, we will look at the areas in which managers must be well prepared in order to be effective. The effective manager

1. assumes **leadership** of the group.
2. actively engages in **planning** the current and future work of the group.

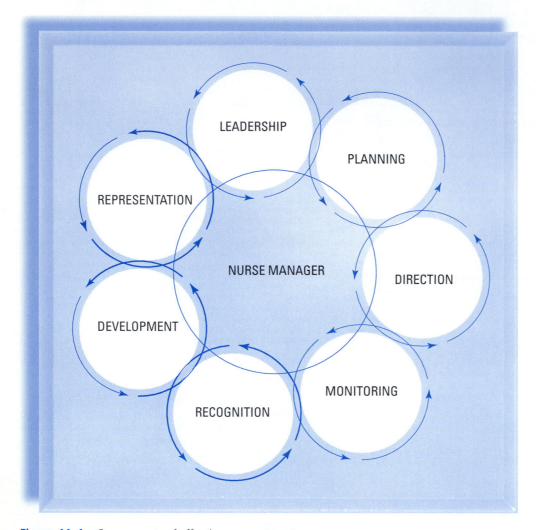

**Figure 11–1**  Components of effective management.

3. provides **direction** to staff members regarding the way the work is to be done.
4. **monitors** the work done by staff members to maintain quality and productivity.
5. **recognizes** and **rewards** quality and productivity.
6. fosters the **development** of every staff member.
7. **represents** both administration and staff members as needed in discussions and negotiations with others.

The contrast between an effective and ineffective manager is illustrated by this set of comments often heard in work situations.

Manager (frustrated): "It would be easier to do the work myself!"

Subordinates (complaining): "We do all the work. All our manager does is sit at a desk all day!"

Ineffective managers frustrate both themselves and their staff members. These managers feel as though they are doing all of the work and getting little cooperation from staff members. The staff members, on the other hand, feel as though they are not only doing all of the work themselves but that their managers are making it harder for them to get it done. Effective managers, in contrast, make it easier for staff to complete their work.

## Defining Management

In 1916, Henri Fayol (Wren, 1972) wrote that the functions of a manager are to plan, organize, command, coordinate, and control. Although often modified, Fayol's original list of functions appears regularly as the outline of management functions and the organizer for many management textbooks. In fact, many managers who learned this list in school will tell you that that is exactly what they do: plan, organize, direct, and control (Wren, 1972). Yet this list is in danger of becoming irrelevant if not obsolete in today's organizations (Purser & Cabana, 1998).

Mintzberg (1975; 1997) says that although managers *say* that they plan, organize, direct, and control, what they actually *do* is quite different. Managers fill four different types of roles according to Mintzberg: interpersonal, informational, decisional, and entrepreneurial. The **interpersonal role** includes ceremonial duties such as attendance at an awards dinner, leadership, and the role of liaison. The **informational role** includes scanning the environment for any useful information and seeking ways to improve work methods. The **decisional role** includes deciding how to allocate resources such as space or the amount of money available for giving raises, negotiating and resolving conflicts, and handling disturbances. Finally, the manager is also an **entrepreneur,** always alert to new ideas and new opportunities to expand and improve the effectiveness and profitability of the unit or the whole organization. The seven components of effective management are derived from the ideas of both Fayol and Mintzberg.

> **If you ask managers what they do, they will most likely tell you that they plan, organize, coordinate, and control. Then watch what they do. Don't be surprised if you can't relate what you see to these words.**
>
> —Mintzberg, 1997, p. 35

From the outside, the nurse manager's job looks easier than the staff nurse's job. To staff members, the nurse manager appears to sit in the office writing reports, goes to a lot of meetings, and occasionally makes rounds, asking questions about the work being done. The manager does not have to shift attention from medications to monitors, respond to call lights, watch critical patients, get charting done, or stabilize new admissions. From the nurse manager's viewpoint, however, the situation is quite different.

Imagine that you have become the nurse manager of a pediatric critical care unit. As a first-line manager, you are responsible for all of the care given by your staff (see Research Example 11–1). It is impossible for you to do all of this work yourself, even if you wanted to. Therefore, you are not only responsible for your own work but also for the work of many other people, and you must answer to many more people (more physicians, more parents, etc.) for the quality of the work than you did as a staff nurse. Although you do have some authority over staff members, you are also dependent on them to get the work done.

What will the manager of the future do? As we move further into the Information Age, much discussion centers around the effect of current management functions. Porter-O'Grady (1997) predicts a dramatic change from planning, organizing, and leading the work of others to a new manager who will become a "process leader" who coordinates, facilitates, and integrates:

> *Once taught, staff can self-manage the data system and their relationship with other providers, using the information infrastructure to facilitate both relationship and work. Furthermore, the staff can measure the fit between what they do and the resources available, the outcomes of their work, and the value of their activities in relationship to the organization's mission and purpose (Porter-O'Grady, 1997, p. 287).*

Moss (1999) goes one step further, suggesting that managers of the future will focus on managing knowledge, which is quite different from managing employees or processes:

> *. . . the next generation of knowledge worker is going to be very different from the worker of*

## RESEARCH EXAMPLE 11–1    *Tasks of First-Line Nurse Managers*

What do first-line nurse managers do? Beaman (1986) developed a questionnaire based on a list of tasks done by nurse managers in acute-care settings in Los Angeles. The list included tasks in each of the traditional functional areas of management: planning, staffing, controlling, directing, and organizing. Altogether, 109 questionnaires were mailed and 73 (67 percent) were returned.

When the responses were analyzed, Beaman found that 31 tasks had been selected by more than 50 percent of the people responding. The tasks included the following (some are combined):

- Assist inservice to prepare orientation schedule.
- Discuss the program of orientation with the new staff member.
- Decide when orientation is complete.
- Write counseling reports and discuss them with staff members.
- Discuss the need for termination.
- Terminate after approval has been obtained.
- Submit time schedule for three shifts.
- Assign patients, teams for day shift.

- Make recommendations about budget to nursing administration.
- Calculate nursing hours used and justify them.
- Call in extra help when needed.
- Prepare reports about budget variances.
- Make daily patient rounds.
- Attend and participate in first-line nursing management meetings.
- Conduct meetings with own staff for problem solving and learning.
- Set goals for individual unit.
- Participate in setting goals for the nursing department.
- Discuss unit problems with physicians regularly.
- Participate in all levels of quality assurance, including designing studies, collecting data, and preparing reports.

The reader may want to compare these activities to the components of effective leadership and management discussed in this book.

*Source:* Beaman, A.L. (1986). What do first-line nursing managers do? *Journal of Nursing Administration, 16,* 6–9.

*today—their requirements will be different, what they find of value will be different. . . . Knowledge workers will place a high value on their own creativity and demand more participation in the decision process (Moss, 1999, p. 61).*

An example from nursing practice is the clinical pathway, which Moss calls a "richly detailed repository of knowledge gleaned from experience," (1999, p. 58). Sharing such knowledge on line across institutions and geographical boundaries is different from labeling it "proprietary" and limiting access to it, which is common today.

Instead of spending much of his or her time closely supervising others' work, the manager of the future will primarily be responsible for helping others get their work done. In other words, the emphasis will shift from traditional management functions to highly supportive and facilitative leadership functions.

## ● LEADERSHIP

Because managers work through other people, their leadership skills are the *sine qua non* of management: without leadership skills, one cannot be an effective manager. Some people believe it is possible to be a generic manager, one who can effectively plan the work, direct, monitor, and evaluate any group of people no matter what kind of work they do. Others argue it is difficult to provide good direction if you do not know how to do the work yourself. True or not, this notion of a generic manager emphasizes the importance of the manager's leadership skills.

Without leadership skills, a manager may develop appropriate plans for the group, post a fair working schedule, and reward people equitably but still have difficulty getting people to work well together because the manager ignored the relationship aspects of the situation. Personality conflicts, communication problems, and immature groups are common problems that do not go away if they are ignored. In fact, they usually get worse. As you will recall from Chapter 3, being an effective leader means developing self-awareness, acquiring adequate knowledge, using critical thinking, practicing good communication, recognizing and reconciling differences in goals, and using personal energy wisely in taking action—**prerequisites** to being an effective manager. In short, it is possible to be a **manager** without being a leader, but it is not possible to be a **good manager** without being a leader.

## ● PLANNING

Planning is the component of effective management that is hardest to do and easiest to ignore. Because it deals primarily with the future, planning can be postponed unless deadlines are set or you make it an explicit objective. In fact, if you do not specifically set aside time or are not specifically required by your administration to do it, you probably will not do much planning despite its importance, because other more immediate demands fill your day.

Planning is the essential link between good intentions and action (Kraegel, 1983). Without it, good ideas rarely become realities. Good planning requires a broad knowledge of the organization's operations and goals, detailed knowledge of your own department or unit, technical knowledge, and intuition, together with a keen awareness of changes and current trends affecting your area of health care. Good planning is useless without an adequate implementation plan that includes the commitment of higher-level management, adequate resources, and a set of well-conceived strategies for putting the plan into action (Christensen, 1997).

The popular image of a manager who has time to sit quietly in the office thinking and planning has no basis in reality according to Mintzberg (1975), who found that a manager's pace is unrelenting and that managers are bombarded with telephone calls, interruptions, problems, and crises all day long. The manager's response to these immediate demands is called "putting out the brush fires." Fighting fires can take up all of the manager's time if the manager does not get control of these situations. As a result, planning is often in managers' heads and produces only tentative ideas of what they would like to see done next, either immediately or in the future. Despite these obstacles, planning is an important component of effective management.

> *Managers are paid to . . . make tough decisions intelligently in environments of shifting uncertainty.*
> —Shapiro, 1997, p. 142

Several types of planning need to be done. First, it is important to engage in careful personal time management. Second, it is important to plan the work done by your group. Third, it is important to plan the future direction of your unit or department.

### Time Management

An effective manager not only manages his or her own time well but also helps staff members analyze their own habits and workloads in order to do the same. As a manager, there are some time demands you simply will not be able to control, although you can manage them. Examples are a mandatory meeting, an outbreak of flu among staff, or a patient's cardiac arrest. If the meeting really is mandatory, then you can think about how you can get the most out of the meeting. For time demands that constitute a serious problem or crisis, you need to have worked out a contingency plan in advance. For example, should you request temporary personnel to replace your ill staff members or ask other staff members to work overtime? Should you fill in yourself? Each of these alternatives has its advantages and disadvantages. Is your arrest team well prepared? Is the crash cart well stocked and readily accessible? Knowing these answers ahead of time will prepare you to respond quickly and efficiently during a crisis.

### Planning Current Work

Work done haphazardly is usually work done inefficiently. The workload is simply too great in most healthcare settings to tolerate inefficiencies. In planning the most efficient way to do current work, you need to consider several factors: priorities, allocation of scarce resources, timing and sequence, deadlines, organizational goals, skill mix of staff, and characteristics of the work.

- *Priorities.* The work must be organized and completed according to priorities, beginning with the most important and urgent tasks. Some work must be done before the day is over, no matter what else happens. Other work can be postponed. When necessary work is postponed, however, it is important that it is not forgotten. Physical care, for example, is usually given priority over emotional care in acute-care settings. Yet the emotional needs of many patients may actually be the most acute need, and the effects of its postponement will soon become apparent.
- *Allocation of Scarce Resources.* The allocation of scarce resources is one of the greatest challenges faced by the nurse manager. For example, getting the "right amount of labor resources to the right place at the right time and in the least costly manner" (Cavouras & McKinley, 1997, p. 34) is not only a budget concern but also a personnel and quality of care concern for the nurse manager. Achieving both quality and efficiency is not a simple matter in the management of patient care. It may require careful analysis of the work that needs to be accomplished and a consequent restructuring of the way in which that work is done. At some point, the resources may become too scarce to provide quality care. If care is jeopardized, the manager becomes responsible for making these needs clear to administration and obtaining the resources needed to preserve quality.
- *Timing and Sequence.* Some tasks must be done before others are begun. For example, consents must be signed before preoperative medication takes effect and shift reports must be given before patient care begins.
- *Deadlines.* Deadlines are imposed times by which a task must be done. The time may be specified within a physician order, by another department, or by upper-level management.
- *Organizational Goals.* Priority goals of the organization, such as a renewed emphasis on

risk reduction or on good patient-provider relations, should also be considered.
- *Skill Mix of Staff.* The preparation and experience of staff members are also important. Some assignments simply cannot be given to unlicensed staff according to legal and professional standards of practice. Individual ability and experience must also be considered.
- *Characteristics of the Work.* Some nursing tasks require technical skill and precise timing, such as the administration of intravenous medications. Others require a high level of knowledge and judgment but have flexible timing, such as parent education. The timing of the first needs to be exact; the timing of the second needs to be flexible. The selection of the appropriate staff member to carry out these two different tasks should consider the abilities, preferences, and availability of individual staff members.

The preceding list may contain a large number of factors to keep in mind, but each is important. The first-line manager considers each one in planning the daily and weekly work of the unit or department.

## Planning for the Future

The effective manager plans for the future rather than waiting to see what the future will bring. Change is rapid in health care. Some nursing units or teams have been reduced or eliminated altogether (Wells et al., 1998). Some services such as healthy baby visits have become obsolete while others, such as intensive care units, have multiplied rapidly. The manager must be aware of these general trends as well as more specific local ones that could affect the work, even the existence, of the unit. For example:

*The nurse manager of the obstetrics unit watched the census statistics carefully and realized that the number of births at the hospital was declining slowly but steadily. Several neighborhood hospitals had been talking about closing their maternity units. It was clear that the population of the community was aging and could not support all of the existing services; some obstetric units would soon close.*

*The nurse manager knew the staff was highly skilled and provided excellent care. But the community did not recognize any difference between their services and those at other hospitals. The nurse manager decided to embark on a campaign to keep the unit open. The first step was to enlist the support of the nursing staff and the obstetricians who agreed to keep sending their patients to the unit. The nurse manager met with administration and with the nursing staff to plan ways to make their unit particularly attractive to expectant parents so that they would request this particular hospital. With the staff, a plan was formulated to add birthing rooms, grandparent classes, and sibling visitation. Prenatal classes were videotaped so that working women could watch them at home or on their own time at the hospital and then meet for just one or two question-and-answer sessions. The new services were so well received that the local newspaper ran a story about them titled, "Local Hospital Caters to Needs of Expectant Mothers."*

Some plans may involve highly complex organizationwide change, whereas others are formulated on a far smaller scale, involving such things as a new piece of equipment, a new staffing pattern, or an improved technique. Whether on a small or grand scale, planning for the future is an important part of the effective manager's functions.

## ● DIRECTION

The effective manager provides direction to staff members. The amount of direction needed varies with the knowledge, experience, and initiative of individual staff members and the group as a whole. Everyone needs some direction, no matter how small. People need to know (1) what is expected of them, and (2) how to do it. The knowledgeable staff member will know how to do the assigned task or how to obtain the needed information, but still needs information about how the work has been divided among members of the team. The less experienced, less knowledgeable staff member will need assistance with the how-to-do-it part of the assignment. This assistance does not necessarily have to come from the nurse manager; it may be delegated to other experienced staff members.

## Work Assignments

Assigning work is one of the most fundamental of all managerial responsibilities. Only the most passive manager might fail to make work assignments. Assigning work effectively, however, requires consideration of a number of factors, the most important being the capabilities of staff members and distribution of the workload. Failing to take these factors into account is dangerous to patients and demoralizing to staff. Other factors to consider include efficiency, continuity, staff preferences, and learning opportunities for staff members.

Another important principle in making work assignments is to assign to strength, not away from weakness. The difference is subtle but important. Assigning to strength means selecting the person who can do a job well. Assigning away from weakness means that you focus on avoiding staff limitations when delegating. For example:

*You know that Nurse X has had a great deal of difficulty being supportive to families of terminally ill patients and yet can handle a crisis situation with calm assurance and skill. If you assigned from weakness, you would avoid assigning Nurse X to any terminal patients because their families were frequently present and required much support. In doing so, you are likely to give Nurse X a subtle message that Nurse X cannot be trusted with the care of grieving families, or even with the terminally ill. A more positive approach is to give Nurse X an assignment that requires dealing with patients in crisis, an area where Nurse X excels.*

Staff members are sensitive to these subtleties. Assigning to strength will contribute to positive esteem and higher morale among staff members, whereas doing the opposite reduces esteem and morale.

Although it is a fundamental managerial responsibility, delegating work is rarely a simple task. A number of conflicting demands may confront you when trying to make a fair assignment, including staff shortages, special requests from various staff members, and unpleasant or undesirable work that must be done. Some managers have difficulty delegating work at all. They try to do too much of the work themselves and wind up exhausted and frustrated, unable to fulfill their managerial responsibilities while trying to do other people's work. More information on these and other dilemmas in making work assignments can be found in Chapter 12.

## Job Descriptions

A job description is a formal document describing the work expected of an individual. Although a patient care assistant's job description is quite different from a nurse executive's, both should have job descriptions for several reasons.

A job description defines what is expected of a person in a particular position and, consequently, what that person can expect of other people in their positions. This information is helpful when considering a new job or when disagreement arises about a person's responsibilities.

A job description also clarifies expectations when they are vague. People in newly created positions may find it worthwhile to take the time to write their own job descriptions and obtain administrative approval for them. It is usually not necessary to create descriptions in staff positions. You will find that some organizations have already developed clear job descriptions for all positions.

## Staffing and Scheduling

Much time and effort have been put into devising workable staffing and scheduling patterns for nurses, particularly for nurses in acute-care settings. The variety of approaches (12-hour shifts, weekend staff, 4-day weeks, permanent pools, and job sharing are a few examples) demonstrates just how complex and difficult it has been to find a method that is cost effective, ensures quality, and is satisfactory to staff.

Rapid turnover, retrenchment (reduction in the total number of budgeted staff positions), large numbers of unlicensed staff, use of temporary personnel, and the increased sophistication of nursing interventions all make staffing and scheduling a matter of achieving a delicate balance among pa-

tient, staff, and organizational needs. The needs and wishes of individual staff members, for example, have to be weighed against the needs of the unit as a whole. As a team leader or nurse manager, you will wish at times that you had the wisdom of King Solomon.

Even when decisions are centralized and computerized, requests for changes have to be considered. You will have to distinguish, for example, between a true emergency and a desire to get an additional weekend day off. Be careful about making exceptions for an individual employee. It can create a troublesome precedent for future requests (Hill, 1992). Your evenhandedness in approving and denying requests will impact on the smooth operation of your unit.

One approach to reducing the number of conflicts arising from staffing and scheduling is to use participative management. The participative manager may allow staff members as a group to plan their own schedules or may invite staff comments and suggestions and incorporate them in the scheduling or staffing routine. Whichever way you choose (your choice may be restricted by administrative policies), you will probably find that staff members have some creative ideas and that when their ideas are implemented, they will be far more committed to them and cooperative in keeping the unit adequately staffed than they would be under imposed routines. Given the opportunity, staff members can assume a great deal of responsibility for self-policing.

## Technical Direction

Giving technical direction is a somewhat tricky business. Some nurse managers give far too much, and end up interfering with the functioning of their units by constantly "suggesting" better ways to do things. In the extreme case, this interference can immobilize the unit staff. Staff members feel as if they should not take a single step without the manager's approval. In truth, most activities can be done correctly in more than one way, and the manager who steps in too often may be correcting individual style more than substantive mistakes.

The opposite, of course, is the nurse manager who gives no technical direction at all, often in the belief that people should take initiative to learn on their own. Although encouraging initiative is important, it can be carried to extremes and staff members can be deprived of the information needed to perform well.

Much information circulates within any organization, some of it critical to the operation of the unit. The nurse manager can help the staff deal with it by summarizing and sharing it with staff. The means by which information and direction are shared is also important. For example, an effective manager avoids taking over or saying "Let me show you how to do it" (Lashbrook, 1986). Although well meant, it is often irritating to professional staff because of its implied message, "I can do this better than you can." The goal in giving direction and technical assistance is to inform without criticism, whether implied or direct.

The work climate influences the way people seek information. In some work settings, admitting a need for information is equal to admitting inadequacy. The result is that learning needs are concealed and people seek information indirectly and surreptitiously. In contrast, an open, trusting climate encourages people to freely and spontaneously seek and share information. Information seeking and learning are rewarded in this type of environment, as they should be.

## ● MONITORING

Once you have given directions to staff members, can you sit back and wait for results? Of course not. The effective manager monitors the unit's operation and progress continuously.

The first-line nurse manager has responsibility to several constituencies, each with its own concerns. The three major ones are the staff, the patients or clients, and the administration of the organization (Figure 11–2). In addition, the first-line nurse manager must also consider the needs and interests of other departments or units, medical staff, patients' families and significant others, the community, the nursing profession, and so forth.

The staff's major concerns are to serve the clients well and to be treated well themselves. The patients' or clients' major concern is with the quality of the care given by the staff. The administration's major concern is with the effectiveness of the staff, the resulting satisfaction of the clients, and the success of the organization as a whole. Some of these interests are primarily served by the monitoring function of the nurse manager; others are primarily served by the representation function, the seventh component of effective management.

The nurse manager is concerned with the functioning of individual staff members and of the unit as a whole. A number of different aspects of the individual staff members' and the unit's functioning should be monitored. Some that might need regular scanning by the nurse manager are found in the following list.

### Individual Staff Members

The following is a list of items to consider in monitoring the work of individual staff members:

- Excellence in provision of patient care
- Excellence in recording patient care and its outcomes
- Adherence to standards of ethical behavior
- Adherence to professional standards
- Conformity to legal standards of practice
- Ability to work with other staff members
- Absenteeism
- On-time arrival and departure
- Leadership
- Pursuit of professional growth

The type of unit, type of care given, ability and experience of the staff, and related factors will help determine how often each of the items needs to be monitored. Some, such as absenteeism, require daily scanning. Others, such as adherence to professional standards, require weekly or monthly scanning unless a problem has arisen that alerts you to the need for more frequent monitoring.

### The Unit as a Whole

The following is a list of some items to consider in monitoring the unit as a whole:

- Patient census
- Patient length of stay
- Number of clinic visits, home visits

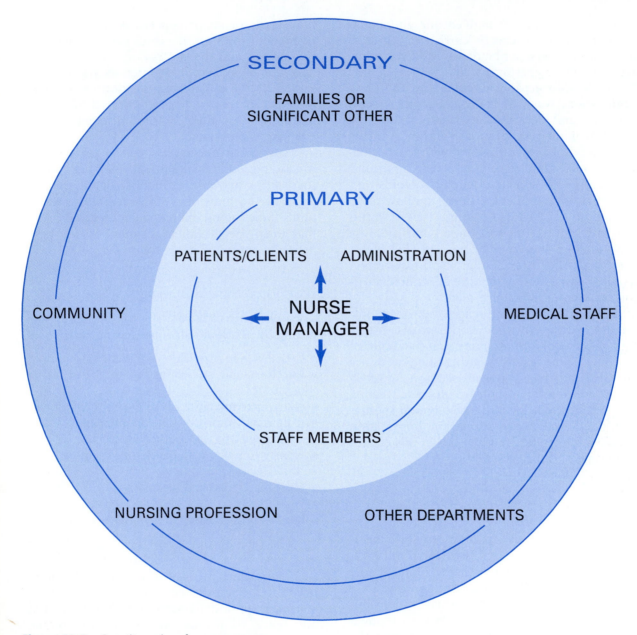

**Figure 11–2**   Constituencies of nurse manager.

- Incidence of nosocomial infections
- Incidence of other adverse events such as falls, decubiti, medication errors, and so forth
- Unplanned readmissions
- Injuries to staff
- Relationships with other departments
- Comparison with other units
- Cost overruns
- Staffing requirements

- Compliance with regulatory requirements
- Compliance with professional standards (such as the National League for Nursing or the Joint Commission on Accreditation of Health Care Organizations)

Most organizations have formal procedures in place to assist the first-line manager in monitoring these multiple aspects of unit function. (see

Perspectives . . . Measurement: The Subjective Aspect.

---

# PERSPECTIVES . . .

## Measurement: The Subjective Aspect

A troublesome myth in management thinking today is the myth of the **objectivity of measurement,** according to Henry Mintzberg (1996) who says we have embraced this myth "with almost religious fervor" (p. 79). But many important outcomes are not as easily measured as this myth implies. Even when they are, the interpretation of the results still has an element of subjectivity in it. To illustrate, Mintzberg cites an example from England's National Health Service, paraphrased here:

> *Ten people received liver transplants; two of the 10 died, eight survived. One of the eight survivors had a recurrence of an earlier cancer and also died. Another needed a second transplant when the new liver failed. Three of the remaining six were actually able to return to work. What was the success rate?*
>
> *The surgeon claimed an 8 out of 10 success rate. An immunologist rated it as a 7 in 10 success rate. Thinking about the cost of liver transplants, the hospital administrator concluded the rate was 6 in 10. Considering patient quality of life post surgery, the nurses rated the success of the transplants as 3 in 10.*

Who was right? Is there one right answer? Mintzberg says no, no one has a "magic envelope with the one right answer in it" (p. 79).

---

*Source:* Mintzberg, H. (1996, May/June). Managing government; governing management. *Harvard Business Review,* 75–83.

---

## Monitoring Methods

Collecting the information needed to monitor the activities and outcomes on your unit can be done a number of ways. Direct observation is one of the most important, which can be done through management rounds, often called "management by walking around" (Pagonis, 1992; Hansten &

Washburn, 1997). A manager who is often seen and heard makes his or her presence felt. Unit staff know that their manager is interested in them and that the quality of their work is being noted. As you make your rounds, you can identify potential problems, make on-the-spot suggestions and corrections as needed (providing informal feedback is discussed in detail in Chapter 13), develop staff through coaching and role modeling, build trust with staff, physicians and patients, and reinforce your vision and the mission of the organization (Hansten & Washburn, 1997).

Nurse managers are usually expected to collect staff and patient data for their units or departments. Absenteeism rates, nurse-patient ratios, skill mix (the proportion of RNs, LPNs, and unlicensed staff), and medication errors are common types of staff data monitored by nurse managers. Falls, decubiti, and nosocomial infection rates are common types of patient data collected and monitored by nurse managers.

You can also ask individual staff members to tell you how they are progressing. This type of interaction is particularly useful when a staff member has experienced some difficulty that you are trying to resolve together or when implementing a new or particularly complex task. Checking and rechecking may be necessary with a low-output or poor-output staff member (McVey & Moore, 1993). This level of supervision can take a considerable amount of the nurse manager's time.

More formal methods of monitoring include peer review procedures and chart audits, which may be used to monitor adherence to standards of care. Formal employee performance appraisals are held at regular intervals to inform employees about whether they are performing at expected levels. Pay raises and promotions are based on these formal evaluations.

Finally, numerous reports obtained from other departments as well as those generated by the nurse manager regarding the incidence of accidents or infections, budget overruns, or other occurrences need to be tracked regularly. Comparisons with statistics for other units and with previous years for your unit usually indicate areas where improvement is occurring or, conversely, where a problem is developing. If the purpose of monitoring can be summarized in one sentence, it is to identify trends and problems

**RESEARCH EXAMPLE 11–2**    *Providing Recognition to Staff Nurses*

What types of rewards are most important to staff nurses? Cronin and Becherer (1999) distributed questionnaires on this subject to 987 staff nurses and nurse managers in three institutions in the Midwest. The surveys were attached to their paychecks and collected in an envelope left in each unit. Altogether, 342 usable responses were received, a 35 percent response rate.

The highest ranked category derived from items on the list provided to respondents was salary. The second highest was provision of private verbal feedback, which ranked higher than public

acknowledgment. Opportunities for growth and development had the lowest ranking.

The authors conclude that pay commensurate with performance is the key to any reward system and suggest that, given budgetary limitations, the available funds should be used strategically. They also point out that nonmonetary rewards such as feedback are not only low cost but easy to provide and can be highly motivating.

*Source:* Cronin, S.N. & Becherer, D. (1999). Recognition of staff nurse job performance and achievements. *Journal of Nursing Administration, 29*(1), 26–31.

early, when they are still small, in order to prevent them from becoming big problems.

## RECOGNITION AND REWARDS

The effective manager uses recognition and rewards to encourage desired behaviors (including innovation and creativity) and to retain good employees (Beckhard, 1997). It would seem obvious that people who do the best work should receive the most rewards and that employers would reward the behavior that is most desired; often, however, subjectivity in reward systems and some paradoxical reasoning (often, lack of reasoning) govern the ways rewards are given. Before considering how rewards are determined, however, let us look first at what kinds of rewards are available to the first-line nurse manager.

### Types of Rewards

The effective manager uses as broad a range of rewards as possible. The most positive and powerful ones include raises and promotions, but many others also serve to reward desired behavior. Simple positive feedback is an underestimated means to reward desired behavior. "The weight of managers' feedback," says Huntsman, "has credibility beyond a manager's wildest dreams" (1987, p. 52).

The nurse manager can build peer recognition by announcing achievements at staff meetings and using the organizational newsletter to recognize achievements. It is also possible to reward staff members by giving them challenging assignments and seeking interesting opportunities for them either within the unit or somewhere else within the organization. See Research Example 11–2 for some information on which of these rewards mean the most to staff nurses.

A creative manager can find many ways to reward deserving staff members. McNeese-Smith (1993) offers a good example:

> A patient care unit manager used part of her bonus to take the staff out for lunch to celebrate. The manager explained why: "It was the staff who really did it" (p. 39). Staff were so eager to work on this manager's unit that it had a waiting list.

This manager remembered that effectiveness cannot be achieved alone but is dependent in large part on the staff.

Negative rewards are also available to the nurse manager. Termination of employment is the most extreme example. Other examples include negative feedback, a necessary component of the manager's repertoire; formal and informal warnings and reprimands; and the omission of challenging assignments or other special recognition for those who have not earned it.

## Determining Rewards

To the nonmanager, a manager's ability to give or deny rewards makes the manager seem quite powerful. In reality, however, a manager faces a number of restrictions in giving these rewards. Both the policies and preferences of upper management (the first-line manager's bosses) are some of the most common and sometimes severe restrictions. In some organizations, first-line managers evaluate staff members but the recommendations for raises and promotions come from individuals higher up the management chain who may or may not agree with the first-line manager's recommendations. Almost every organization restricts the number of promotions and the amount of salary increases that can be given.

Upper-level management, however, is not the only source of restrictions. First-line managers must also carefully consider the effect of how rewards are given. If staff members see rewards being given in a fair and objective manner, those rewards can be an effective motivator; but if rewards seem to be subjective, staff can become destructively competitive, apathetic, or confused about what is really expected of them.

A common saying, "the squeaky wheel gets the grease," if true, means that the staff member who demands attention or complains loudly gets more attention than the quieter staff members. Other staff members will notice, and the inequitable treatment will likely become a source of resentment and reduced motivation. The complainer is being rewarded for complaining while the noncomplaining, more cooperative staff members receive no reward. This situation is an example of what one writer calls the "folly of rewarding A while hoping for B" (Kerr, 1986, p. 417). The manner in which rewards are given is probably as important as the size and frequency of the reward.

## ● DEVELOPMENT

### Two Schools of Thought

Staff development is not found in the traditional plan, organize, command, coordinate, and control lists of manager's functions.

Of the two schools of thought about staff development, the first views staff members as a valuable resource of the organization who should be developed to their fullest extent. Staff development is considered a wise investment in the future growth and development of the organization. The opposing point of view is that as little as possible should be spent on staff development. If a particular skill is needed, go out and look for someone who already has that expertise. Staff members are kept as long as they are useful; when they are no longer useful, they are discarded.

> *People are the intellectual assets that make things happen and the cost of mismanaging them can be disastrous.*
> —Rosen, 1997, p. 304

The first approach to staff development clearly resembles Theory Z (described in Chapter 2) (Ouchi, 1981). Employees are expected and encouraged to work cooperatively and to remain with the organization a long time. When an employee's skills become obsolete, the employee is retrained, not discarded. The result is a loyal staff with a much higher level of commitment to the organization. Employees feel valued and they function accordingly. This management practice is not just altruism: high employee turnover is costly and high employee satisfaction can increase productivity (Shellenbarger, 1998).

The second approach encourages competition and fosters a climate of insecurity. Under the second, "use-and-discard" approach, staff members often feel threatened and are far more concerned about their own future than about the future of the organization.

### Encouraging Staff Development

The effective manager takes responsibility for development of individual staff members and for the group as a whole as well as his or her own development. Training meets specific, immediate learning needs while staff development is a long-term strategy. The numerous ways staff development can be supported will vary somewhat according to what your organization is willing to support financially.

Capable staff members should be encouraged to continue their education, particularly if the organization can assist them in paying their tuition. All staff members should be encouraged to attend continuing education programs even if not required for license renewal in your state. The educational gain, not license renewal, should be the major motivator for attendance at continuing education programs. Staff members should be given time off for continuing education rather than being asked to use their days off or vacation time to pursue continued learning.

Some nurse managers, unfortunately, develop the habit of attending all of these programs themselves. Being sent to these programs is usually perceived by staff as a sign of positive regard from the manager. Anyone who attends a continuing education program should be encouraged to share the new knowledge with the rest of the staff in formal and/or informal ways.

Much learning can take place within the unit or team itself as well. The nurse manager can encourage staff members to "stretch" themselves (Tichy, 1997), to grow beyond their present capabilities. Staff members can learn from each other and from other members of the interdisciplinary team. The informal sharing of expertise can occur at the bedside, in hallways, and in meetings and conferences.

Team meetings can be designed to be learning experiences. Different staff members, for example, may be assigned to prepare agendas on a rotating basis to share the work and the leadership experience. Some groups of nurses have formed lunchtime or after-work discussion groups to network and share information.

A frequent complaint about staff development programs is that what is taught is often not put into practice after the person has returned to work. Typically, the staff member or manager returns from the workshop full of enthusiasm for new ideas, only to find them so difficult to implement that the enthusiasm quickly dies and the idea is soon forgotten. Sharing workshop experiences with other staff members can help prevent this loss of enthusiasm, but the nurse manager should also actively assist the staff member in applying potentially useful new ideas to the work setting.

## ● REPRESENTATION

Like staff development, representation is another component of effective management not found on the traditional organize, plan, control, and direct list of managers' functions. And yet, as Mintzberg (1975) points out, a manager can spend a great deal of time representing his or her group of staff members. In fact, how their manager represents them is a matter of vital interest to most employees. It can also be a source of conflict for nurse managers who find themselves caught in the middle between staff and upper management (Boston & Forman, 1994). We will first consider the many different ways in which a manager represents staff members and administration and then look briefly at the ways in which conflict can arise in fulfilling this function.

### Representing Staff Members

The first-line manager typically represents staff in discussions with other departments and with upper-level management. The nurse manager should be an articulate spokesperson for staff (Frank, Eckrich & Rohr, 1997) speaking on behalf of their needs, requests, and rights. The following are examples of how a nurse manager fulfills the role of spokesperson in some ordinary situations:

*For security reasons, the administrator of a large city hospital was considering the enforcement of limited visiting hours. Keeping visiting hours confined to 5 hours in the late afternoon and early evening would make it possible to control the flow of people in and out of the hospital. When this policy was announced, the nurse manager of the pediatric unit said that the nursing staff would find this restriction on parents nontherapeutic and therefore strongly inadvisable. The nurse manager of the oncology unit agreed. The idea was reconsidered in light of their comments and then dropped.*

*The physical therapy department decided to open at 7:00 A.M. so that their staff could finish and go home early. The rehabilitation unit's nursing coordinator, however, pointed out that this practice would mean the night shift staff on the nursing units would have to begin morning care, which it did not have enough personnel to do. The physical therapy department had to give up their plan to begin at 7:00 A.M.*

*A small county public health unit had expanded its services to include primary care. This change meant an extension of the working day to include some evenings and Saturday work for the existing staff. The public health nursing supervisor successfully negotiated overtime payments for the public health nurses who would be working more than their regular 40 hours per week and made the overtime voluntary instead of mandatory.*

In the three examples just given, the nurse managers acted primarily as **advocates** for their staff members and patients. The second nurse manager also acted as a **coordinator** ensuring adequate communication and smooth operations between different departments within the organization. Coordination may involve outside agencies as well.

> **The primary role of the leader-manager is to influence others' performance by helping to shape an organization in which people can realize and express their capabilities and, in so doing, contribute more fully.**
>
> —Napolitano & Henderson, 1998, p. xxv

A third important role is to act as **promoter** for the unit, convincing others of the value and quality of the work done by the unit and seeking opportunities to expand or to improve the function of the unit. This last role is a new but important one for most nurses, one that is in keeping with the competitive spirit of the times. Patient education is an area that provides a good example of the promoter role:

*The coordinator of patient education was shocked to see that the proposed budget for the patient education department had been cut in half for the next year. Two diabetes educators and one childbirth educator would lose their jobs if this budget was implemented. The coordinator demanded an explanation and was told that the hospital would no longer support departments that did not contribute to the organization's profits. At the very least, the patient education department would have to support itself, that is, bring in enough money to cover the cost of operating the department.*

*This new requirement demanded a radical change in thinking for the patient educators. They had thought of themselves as professionals who provided a needed service but had not considered the cost of the individual patient teach-*

*ing that was their primary activity. After a series of brainstorming sessions, the group as a whole decided that they would do more group teaching, design more self-learning materials, and use the closed-circuit television system more effectively. They developed a series of programs for the community for which a reasonable fee would be charged. They could also market their services to corporations who would pay for their health promotion programs. The coordinator began planning and publicizing these programs. In addition, the patient educators made an increased effort to be responsive to as many units and departments in the hospital as possible to gain their support for the continued operation of their department.*

## Representing Administration

Everyone who works has at least one boss, and many people have more than one boss. The first-line manager, for example, usually reports to second-line managers, such as supervisors, assistant directors, or directors of nursing. As a first-line manager, you would be expected to contribute to the achievement of the organization's goals and to carry out whatever functions and tasks have been delegated to you by upper management. You would also be expected to support the organization's policies and procedures. When policies or procedures are poorly designed or implemented, however, the effective manager has a responsibility to challenge them and work on changing them.

> **New managers tend to focus on managing their immediate subordinates, not realizing they must also manage the perceptions of bosses and managers in other departments.**
>
> —Lancaster, 1998

Managers are often expected to represent administration when a new policy is put into practice. New policies can range from employee sign-in procedures to a change in the way that families are informed when a patient dies. The nurse manager is expected to inform staff members of the change, explain the policy, and then ensure that it is implemented.

First-line managers are also expected to represent administration in communicating such personnel decisions as granting raises and promoting and firing people. When the decisions have been made in a fair and reasonable manner and the manager's recommendations have been given serious consideration, this responsibility causes little conflict. However, when the manager does not agree with the decision, he or she can feel caught between responsibility to administration and to the staff. Evaluating the relative cost and benefit of nursing care on individual units is an additional responsibility that may lead to conflict between staff and administration (Mark, 1994). Choosing sides and supporting one against the other is not the best approach because it may lead to long-term alienation from the other side. Autocratic administrators sometimes try to force managers into this position. A better way to handle the situation is through negotiation of differences with either or both sides.

## ● MANAGEMENT EFFECTIVENESS CHECKLIST

Like the Leadership Effectiveness Checklist, the Management Effectiveness Checklist (Figure 11–3) is meant to provide a method for reviewing your actual or potential management effectiveness in a deliberate and thoughtful way. It is not a quiz that produces high, medium, and low scores, but a review of the major characteristics and behaviors of the effective manager. If you are not in a managerial position at present you can evaluate your readiness for one using the checklist and save it as a self-evaluation tool for the future should you attain a managerial position.

## ● SUMMARY

Management is often defined as planning, directing, coordinating, and controlling, but in reality it includes much more. Effective management consists of seven components: leadership, planning, providing direction, monitoring operations, distributing rewards fairly, developing staff, and representing both staff members and administration.

The effective first-line manager sets aside time for planning. The time of both manager and staff should be put to the best use possible, which can only be done with planning and organization. Planning of current work requires consideration of a number of factors, including priorities, allocation of scarce resources, timing and sequencing of work, deadlines, organizational goals, the skills of the staff, and the characteristics of the work. The future of the unit should be well thought out in terms of current trends, both general and specific.

Staff members need to know what is expected of them and how to carry out their assigned work. The effective manager sees to it that staff are well informed about the operation of the unit and that staffing and scheduling plans are both fair and adequate to meet the demand.

The work of individual staff members, the quality of the care given by the unit as a whole, and a number of other factors are monitored on a regular basis by the effective manager. Both formal and informal methods can be used, including direct observation, peer review, formal performance appraisals, a variety of specific reports, and so forth.

Rewards can be either positive or negative. The first-line manager actually experiences a number of restrictions in carrying out this managerial responsibility, particularly from upper management. The effective manager also carefully considers staff response to reward distribution, attempting as much as possible to reward desired, not undesirable, behavior.

Both the manager and staff members should continue to grow and develop as professionals. The effective manager not only provides a number of opportunities for this growth and development but also provides challenges to capable staff members and ensures that the environment of the unit is conducive to implementation of new ideas.

Finally, the effective manager actively represents his or her staff, acting as an advocate, coordinator, and promoter in dealings with other departments, upper management, and other agencies. When conflicts arise between the needs, requests, and rights of staff members and the desires of administration, the effective manager attempts to negotiate a fair and equitable agreement between these two important constituencies.

|  | Very Much | Somewhat | Not At All |
|---|:---:|:---:|:---:|

**A. Leadership**

1. Have you reviewed the leadership checklist? Are you...

| | | | |
|---|:---:|:---:|:---:|
| developing self-awareness? | ☐ | ☐ | ☐ |
| acquiring adequate knowledge? | ☐ | ☐ | ☐ |
| using critical thinking? | ☐ | ☐ | ☐ |
| practicing good communication? | ☐ | ☐ | ☐ |
| recognizing and reconciling differences in goals? | ☐ | ☐ | ☐ |
| using your energy wisely? | ☐ | ☐ | ☐ |
| 2. Do you give your attention to both the human (relationship) and business (task) aspects of your responsibilities? | ☐ | ☐ | ☐ |

**B. Planning**

| | | | |
|---|:---:|:---:|:---:|
| 1. Do you set aside time for planning? | ☐ | ☐ | ☐ |

2. Do you manage your time by...

| | | | |
|---|:---:|:---:|:---:|
| preparing for emergencies and crises? | ☐ | ☐ | ☐ |
| making the best use of your time? | ☐ | ☐ | ☐ |
| helping staff members manage their time well? | ☐ | ☐ | ☐ |

3. Do you plan current work and consider...

| | | | |
|---|:---:|:---:|:---:|
| priorities? | ☐ | ☐ | ☐ |
| timing and sequence? | ☐ | ☐ | ☐ |
| deadlines? | ☐ | ☐ | ☐ |
| organizational goals? | ☐ | ☐ | ☐ |
| skill mix of the staff? | ☐ | ☐ | ☐ |
| characteristics of the work? | | | |
| 4. Do you plan for the future of your department? | ☐ | ☐ | ☐ |

**C. Direction**

1. Do you communicate clearly to staff...

| | | | |
|---|:---:|:---:|:---:|
| what is expected of them? | ☐ | ☐ | ☐ |
| how to do the work? | ☐ | ☐ | ☐ |
| 2. Do you provide direction in a nonthreatening manner? | ☐ | ☐ | ☐ |
| 3. Do you ensure that everyone has a job description? | ☐ | ☐ | ☐ |

4. Do you prepare schedules that are...

| | | | |
|---|:---:|:---:|:---:|
| fair and adequate to meet the needs of the unit? | ☐ | ☐ | ☐ |
| developed in consideration of staff suggestions? | ☐ | ☐ | ☐ |

**Figure 11–3** Are you managing effectively?

(continued)

|  | Very Much | Somewhat | Not At All |
|---|:---:|:---:|:---:|

**D. Monitoring**
1. Do you monitor...

| | | | |
|---|:---:|:---:|:---:|
| the care given by your staff? | ☐ | ☐ | ☐ |
| individual staff members' performance? | ☐ | ☐ | ☐ |
| the budget? | ☐ | ☐ | ☐ |
| operation of the unit as a whole? | ☐ | ☐ | ☐ |
| 2. Do you use a variety of both formal and informal monitoring methods? | ☐ | ☐ | ☐ |

**E. Rewards**

| | | | |
|---|:---:|:---:|:---:|
| 1. Do you use a variety of both positive and negative rewards? | ☐ | ☐ | ☐ |
| 2. Do you use rewards to reinforce only the behaviors that are desired and not other, less desirable behavior? | ☐ | ☐ | ☐ |

**F. Development**
1. Do you encourage staff development by...

| | | | |
|---|:---:|:---:|:---:|
| rewarding it? | ☐ | ☐ | ☐ |
| making opportunities available? | ☐ | ☐ | ☐ |
| supporting implementation of what is learned? | ☐ | ☐ | ☐ |
| 2. Have you furthered your own professional growth and development? | ☐ | ☐ | ☐ |

**G. Representation**
1. In representing staff members and the unit as a whole, do you function as...

| | | | |
|---|:---:|:---:|:---:|
| an advocate? | ☐ | ☐ | ☐ |
| a coordinator? | ☐ | ☐ | ☐ |
| a promoter? | ☐ | ☐ | ☐ |
| 2. Do you support administration's actions and represent them fairly to your staff? | ☐ | ☐ | ☐ |
| 3. Do you enforce administration policy? | ☐ | ☐ | ☐ |
| 4. When an administration's action or policy is ineffective in some way, do you work to change it? | ☐ | ☐ | ☐ |
| 5. When differences between your staff and the administration occur, do you negotiate an acceptable settlement? | ☐ | ☐ | ☐ |

**Figure 11–3** *(continued)*

# C A S E   S T U D Y

## The Nurse Manager's Constituents: Who Are They?

As Miguel Santera entered the elevator that would take him to his appointment with the medical center chief executive officer (CEO) and the vice-president (VP) for nursing, he thought about his first three months as director of critical care services. Miguel had been a "crackerjack" critical care nurse and respected nurse manager of the open heart unit before his promotion. The VP for nursing had expressed satisfaction with his work so he was not especially nervous about the meeting, but he was curious about the purpose of it. He had only met the CEO a few times and wondered why she was going to be present.

The CEO and VP for nursing were both cordial but wasted little time on social amenities. "Miguel," said the CEO "you know we have been through several waves of downsizing and restructuring here. Through it all, the critical care units, while not entirely unaffected, have been pretty well protected from staffing reductions. In fact, we have the highest level of master's prepared advanced practice nurses in your area."

"We should," Miguel responded, "because we have the sickest patients."

"Well, the ED and ORs have very sick people, too," the CEO responded.

"What Erica is trying to tell you," interrupted the VP for nursing, "is that we are asking you to carefully review your personnel budget and personnel needs with the goal of reducing your overall personnel budget by 15 per-cent by the end of the year. You don't have to do it alone. All of us are available to help you make the decisions and work out the details. You are very popular with your staff. We know you can handle their reactions to this necessary move." The CEO nodded in agreement. They both smiled at Miguel, and stood to indicate the meeting was over.

Miguel was stunned. He had been spending some of his time preparing a request to bring in more intensivists and APNs, not to reduce staff. Both the physicians and nursing staff knew of his plan and enthusiastically supported it. What would they think of this new development? How should he handle it? For the first time since he accepted the director position, he wondered if it was right for him.

## Questions for Critical Reflection and Analysis

1. How many of Miguel's constituencies will be affected by the planned budget cuts? In what way would each be affected?
2. Analyze the dilemma Miguel faces in responding to the administration's request. Take each of the seven components of effective management and discuss the issues related to each of these functions.
3. If you were Miguel, how would you handle this situation? Predict the likelihood of success of your proposed response.
4. Evaluate the CEO and VP for nursing's management approach in this scenario in terms of each component of effective management. What could they have done differently?

# REFERENCES

Beaman, AL. (1986). What do first-line nursing managers do? *Journal of Nursing Administration, 16,* 6–9.

Beckhard, R. (1997). The healthy organization: A profile. In F. Hesselbein, M. Goldsmith & R. Beckhard (Eds.). *The organization of the future.* San Francisco: Jossey-Bass, 325–328.

Boston, C. & Forman, H. (1994). A time to listen: Staff and manager views on education, practice, and management. *Journal of Nursing Administration, 24*(2), 16–18.

Cavouras, C.A. & McKinley, J. (1997). Variable budgeting for staffing. *Nursing Management, 28*(5), 34, 36, 39.

Christensen, C.M. (1997, November/December). Making strategy: Learning by doing. *Harvard Business Review,* 141–156.

Cronin, S.N. & Becherer, D. (1999). Recognition of staff nurse job performance and achievements. *Journal of Nursing Administration, 29*(1), 26–31.

Frank, B., Eckrich, H. & Rohr, J. (1997). Quality nursing care: Leadership makes the difference. *Journal of Nursing Administration, 27*(5), 13–14.

Hansten, R. & Washburn, M. (1997 ). Managerial rounds: Getting in touch. *Nursing Management, 28* (6), 72.

Hill, J. (1992). *Becoming a manager.* Boston: Harvard Business School Press.

Huntsman, A.J. (1987). A model for employee development. *Nursing Management, 18*(2), 51–54.

Kerr, S. (1986). On the folly of rewarding A while hoping for B. In J.N. Williamson (Ed.). *The leader-manager.* New York: John Wiley & Sons.

Kraegel, J.M. (1983). *Planning strategies for nurse managers.* Rockville, MD: Aspen Systems.

Lancaster, H. (1998, February 10). New managers get little help tackling big, complex jobs. *Wall Street Journal,* B1.

Lashbrook, S.B. (1986). Management as a performance system. In J.N. Williamson (Ed.). *The leader-manager.* New York: John Wiley & Sons.

Mark, B.A. (1994). The emerging role of the nurse manager. *Journal of Nursing Administration, 24*(1), 48–55.

McNeese-Smith, D. (1993). Leadership behavior and employee effectiveness. *Nursing Management, 24*(5), 38–39.

McVey, C. & Moore, L.E. (1993). Managing mediocrity. *Nursing Management, 24*(6), 68I–68N.

Mintzberg, H. (1975, 1997). The manager's job: Folklore and fact. *Harvard Business Review, 53,* 49–61.

Mintzberg, H. (1996, May/June). Managing government; governing management. *Harvard Business Review,* 75–83.

Moss, M.T. (1999). Management forecast: Optimizing the use of organizational and individual knowledge. *Journal of Nursing Administration, 29*(1), 57–62.

Napolitano, C.S. & Henderson, L.J. (1998). *The leadership odyssey.* San Francisco: Jossey-Bass.

Ouchi, W.G. (1981). *Theory Z: How American business can meet the Japanese challenge.* Reading, MA: Addison-Wesley.

Pagonis, W.G. (1992). The work of the leader. *Harvard Business Review, 70*(6), 119–126.

Porter-O'Grady, T.P. (1997). Process leadership and the death of management. *Nursing Economics, 15*(6), 286–293.

Purser, R.E. & Cabana, S. (1998). *The self-managing organization.* New York: The Free Press.

Rosen, R.H. (1997). Learning to lead. In F. Hesselbein, M. Goldsmith, & R. Beckhard (Eds.). *The organization of the future.* San Francisco: Jossey-Bass, 325–328.

Shapiro, E. (1997, March/April). Managing in the age of gurus. *Harvard Business Review,* 142–146.

Shellenbarger, S. (1998, July 22). Companies are finding it really pays to be nice to employees. *Wall Street Journal.*

Tichy, N.M. (1997). The leadership engine: How winning companies build leaders at every level. New York: HarperCollins.

Wells, N., Barnard, T., Mason, L., Ames, A. & Minnen, T. (1998). Work transitions. *Journal of Nursing Administration, 28*(2), 50–56.

Wren, D.A. (1972). *The evolution of management thought.* New York: Ronald Press.

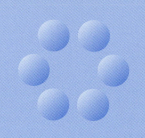

CHAPTER *12*

# Directing and Organizing Patient Care

## LEARNING OBJECTIVE

*After completing this chapter, the reader will be able to:*

- Compare and contrast the most commonly used models for organizing nursing care staff.
- Explain the purpose of critical pathways.
- Discuss the impact of staffing decisions on patient outcomes.
- List factors affecting staffing decisions.
- Analyze advantages and disadvantages of various scheduling options.

- Describe scope of responsibility and appropriate assignment for unlicensed assistive personnel.
- Apply the five rights of delegation in the practice setting.
- Discuss the advantages and disadvantages of cross-training and floating.

## TEST YOURSELF

1. Which of the following models for delivering patient care demands the most coordination of direct caregivers?
   A. Team nursing
   B. Patient-focused care
   C. Case method
   D. Primary care nursing

2. The key feature of patient-focused care is:
   A. All-professional staff that provides the highest level of care possible
   B. A holistic orientation that includes alternative and complimentary treatment
   C. Highly specialized care delivered by an interdisciplinary team
   D. Bringing services to the patient instead of the patient to the service

3. Which statement is correct regarding appropriate staffing?
   A. It is based only on patient census.
   B. All registered nurse staffing is the only way to provide safe care.
   C. The nurse manager has an ethical and financial responsibility when making staffing decisions.
   D. The budget is the most important part of staffing.

4. Which statement is correct regarding effective scheduling?
   A. Staff nurses should not have input into the process.
   B. Self-scheduling enhances staff satisfaction.

   C. All nurses should be scheduled according to flex-time requests.
   D. Temporary personnel should not be used in the hospital setting.

5. When delegating to unlicensed assistive personnel, it is important to:
   A. Allow the unlicensed assistive personnel autonomy in practice.
   B. Communicate with unlicensed assistive personnel once per shift.
   C. Have the unlicensed assistive personnel participate in patient teaching.
   D. Remember that the registered nurse remains responsible and accountable for the outcome.

6. The registered nurse needs to be aware of the following when delegating tasks:
   A. State Nurse Practice Act
   B. Unlicensed Assistive Personnel Code of Ethics
   C. Nurse managers' preference
   D. Chief nurse executive's role in the decision

7. When delegating tasks to a licensed practical nurse, the registered nurse needs to consider:
   A. The preference of the licensed practical nurse.
   B. That failure to delegate effectively increases patient safety.
   C. The State Nurse Practice Act.
   D. The role of the licensed practice nurse in the area of independent clinical judgement.

8. Which statement is correct regarding cross-training?
   A. It is always a benefit for the nursing staff and patient.
   B. It can be cost effective and increases marketability for the registered nurse.
   C. It is readily accepted by registered nurses.
   D. It increases the level of specialization for the registered nurse.

9. Which statement best describes floating practices?
   A. Registered nurses are assumed to be specialists.

B. Registered nurses are qualified to practice in any area because they passed the licensure examinations.
C. Registered nurses have the responsibility to evaluate their own competencies when asked to float.
D. Registered nurses are protected from licensure violations if the hospital has a policy on floating.

*Answers*

1. A  2. D  3. C  4. B  5. D  6. A  7. C  8. B  9. C

**S**taffing and scheduling decisions represent one of the major challenges for nurse managers in the current healthcare environment. The combination of demand for greater cost efficiencies and decreased reimbursement for care has put healthcare facilities and home health agencies under extreme pressure to find ways to reduce expenses. Because labor represents approximately 54 percent of an average hospital's costs and the nursing staff accounts for 70 percent of these labor costs (Williams & Torrens, 1998), many hospital administrators reduce the number of registered nurses employed within their organizations to save money (Ketter, 1994). Some cut too far too quickly without considering the impact of doing so.

Cost concerns have prompted a widespread substitution of unlicensed assistive personnel or licensed practical nurses for registered nurses, particularly in areas with a high saturation of managed care (Shindul-Rothschild, Berry & Long-Middleton, 1996). This phenomenon is known as **deskilling.** When the Balanced Budget Act of 1997 reduced reimbursement to home health agencies, they too responded with staff reductions and deskilling (Harris, 1998). Many also consolidated or closed their doors (Haydel, 1998), unable to survive on greatly restricted funding.

The related **speed-up** phenomenon affects nurses in all healthcare facilities and may have an equal or greater impact on the quality of care and patient outcomes. The term **speed-up** refers to administrative efforts to increase productivity by expecting fewer workers to provide more care (Shindul-Rothschild, Berry & Long-Middleton, 1996). In home health, nurses have also been faced with increased productivity quotas as well as cutbacks and layoffs (Reed, 1999). All these systemwide forces and events further challenge the nurse manager.

In order to provide cost-effective care while maintaining quality and sustaining staff morale, the nurse manager needs to become proficient in deploying and scheduling staff. The information in this chapter on nursing care delivery systems, patient census, patient acuity, DRGs, classification systems, scheduling options, unlicensed assistive personnel, cross-training, and delegation strategies will serve as an introduction to the many issues and decisions involved in staffing, scheduling, and delegating patient care.

## ● NURSING CARE DELIVERY SYSTEMS

How can we best utilize professional nurses across various practice settings? Professional nursing staff and support staff are assigned to patient care according to their educational preparation, specialization, level of autonomy, and patient acuity. The six basic models for organizing the delivery of nursing care are case, functional, team, primary nursing, nursing care management, and patient-focused care (Table 12–1) (Bower, 1992; Brider,

| Table 12–1 | Comparison of Common Models for Delivering Patient Care | | |
| --- | --- | --- | --- |
| Model | Nurses Are Called | Description | Where the Model Is Used |
| Case or Total Patient Care | Nurse | Each nurse is assigned to the total care of one or more patients. | Home care<br>Private Duty<br>Specialty Intensive Care Units<br>Student Assignments |
| Functional | Medical Nurse<br>Treatment Nurse<br>Lactation Consultant<br>Diabetes Educator | Nurses are assigned to specific tasks rather than to specific patients. | Hospitals<br>Nursing Homes<br>Nurse Consultants<br>Operating Rooms |
| Team | Team Leader<br>Team Member | Nursing staff members are divided into small groups responsible for the total care of a given number of patients. | Hospitals<br>Nursing Homes<br>Home Care |
| Primary | Primary Nurse<br>Associate Nurse | Nurses are designated as the primary nurse responsible for a patient's care, or as the associate nurse who assists in the implementation of the nursing care plan. | Hospitals<br>Specialty Intensive Care Units<br>Specialty Services, such as<br>Dialysis and Hospice<br>Home Care |
| Case Management | Care Manager<br>Case Manager | Nurses provide coordination of services as well as direct care for patients. | Hospitals<br>Health Departments<br>Home Care |
| Patient-Focused Care | Care Pair | Nurses are paired with other caregivers. Both may be cross-trained to provide as many nursing and non-nursing services as possible. | Hospitals<br>Home Health Agencies<br>Transport Teams |

1992; Brown, 1980; Rowland & Rowland, 1980). While the "pure" versions of each model are described here, each can be—and often is—modified to meet the goals of a particular organization, its staff, and its patients. Innumerable combinations and variations on these models are found in clinical settings (see Perspectives . . . Which Model Is It?).

## Case Method

The case method involves the assignment of one nurse to the total care of one or more patients or clients. The assigned nurse is responsible for providing all the nursing care that is needed.

The work of the private duty nurse is one example. Community health agencies often use this method to assign cases to individual nurses, and intensive care units often use a modified version of this method for delivering nursing care. It is also used extensively for student assignments.

### Advantages

Although it is the oldest of the six models, many still consider the case method to be the ideal way to deliver nursing care. Its primary advantage is that the care given is comprehensive, continuous, and usually holistic. The likelihood of the care being fragmented, discontinuous, or full of serious gaps is greatly reduced. It is simple and direct in comparison with the others, does not require the complex assignment planning that some others do, and has clear lines of responsibility.

### Disadvantages

With so many advantages, why is the case method not used universally? It is less efficient than some of the other methods because it uses highly skilled, higher-paid professionals to do work that can be done by less skilled, lower-paid people including unlicensed assistive personnel (UAPs). In most instances, the case method cannot be used to assign patients or clients to these ancillary staff members. In addition, with the number of specialties that have developed in the healthcare field, it is difficult for an individual professional to be knowledgeable in all areas and to provide the most expert care for a patient or client who has a wide variety of needs.

Some disadvantages relate specifically to inpatient and intensive home care. Continuous around-the-clock care cannot be done by one employee. Inpatient units are organized in such a way that interaction with many different departments is necessary for obtaining such services and supplies as drugs, linens, meals, laboratory tests, and various therapies. Having a large number of different nurses independently interacting with each of these departments can overload their systems. In such complex organized settings, more coordination than the case method offers is needed.

## Functional Method

The functional method of delivering nursing care is based on a division of labor similar to an assembly line. Individual caregivers are assigned to do specific tasks rather than being assigned to certain patients or clients.

Assignments are based on the criterion of efficiency: tasks are given to the lowest-skilled, lowest-paid worker who is available and able to do the work. The usual result on inpatient units is that one nurse is assigned to be in charge of the unit; another administers all medications; a practical nurse takes blood pressures; and a nursing assistant bathes patients, passes out meal trays, and so forth.

In a home health agency, implementation of the functional method would mean that a nurse would visit a client to counsel, teach, or carry out complex care techniques while a home health aide would visit to assist with bathing and personal care. Nursing care in the home is rarely divided into as many discrete pieces because of the inefficiency of making multiple visits.

### Advantages

The major advantage of the functional method is its efficiency. This method makes it possible to use more unskilled or lesser-skilled people to get the work done. Also, when caregivers are given the same tasks on a regular basis, each person becomes quite adept at them and can finish them quickly.

It is easy to give clearly defined assignments and to check later to ensure that the assignments were completed with the functional method. Once the tasks are defined and the assignments are made, little overlap or confusion arises over who is expected to do a particular job. This clarity minimizes the time required for coordination of staff members. It is interesting to note that even when team or primary nursing is the usual mode for delivering care, organizations frequently fall back on the functional method to deliver care if a serious shortage of staff occurs.

### Disadvantages

The functional method may not be as efficient as it is generally thought to be. From the point of view of getting the work done (efficiency), the need for coordination may be kept to a minimum; but the need for it is increased from the point of view of the recipient of this care (effectiveness). Consider, for example, how inefficient it is to have three different staff members enter a room, one to give a medication, the second to take a blood pressure reading, and a third to check a dressing.

An even more serious drawback of this method of care is the extreme fragmentation of care that results. The functional approach is mechanistic, impersonal, and emphasizes the more technical aspects of nursing care. Decisions regarding the difficulty of a task and to whom it should be assigned are usually based on its technical rather than interpersonal aspects (Adams, Bond & Hale, 1998). Both staff and patients are likely to be dissatisfied with the way care is given.

For the staff, the work becomes repetitious and boring. Doing the same disconnected tasks prevents them from experiencing the satisfaction of seeing anything done completely from beginning to end. For example, if a patient has a quick and uneventful recovery from surgery, no one staff member can take pride in having assured the patient's comfort and prevented postoperative complications. The patient, too, is confused and sometimes irritated by the large number of people going in and out of the patient's room or home, each one doing only one or two things and refusing to do others because it is someone else's job.

Potentially more serious for the patient is the fact that communication between staff members may be minimal, so that no one is aware of everything that is happening to an individual patient. Although the nurse in charge is theoretically responsible for all care given, responsibility is so diffused among various caregivers that a serious gap in care can occur without anyone realizing it. Holistic care is virtually impossible under the functional model.

## Team Nursing

Team nursing is the delivery of nursing care by a designated group of staff members including both professional nurses and nonprofessional (ancillary) staff. Several elements are considered necessary:

1. The team leader is delegated authority to make assignments for team members and guide the work of the team. The leader of the team should be a registered professional nurse, not a practical nurse.
2. The leader is expected to use a democratic or participative style in interactions with team members.
3. The team is responsible for the total care given to an assigned group of patients or clients.
4. Communication among team members is essential to its success, and includes written patient care assignments, nursing care plans, reports to and from the team leader, team conferences in which patient care problems and team concerns are discussed, and frequent informal feedback among team members (Kramer, 1971; Lambertsen, 1953).

Team nursing was created at the end of World War II to make the best use of the limited nursing staff available and alleviate the problems created by the functional method. As more workers with minimal on-the-job training were hired in the healthcare field, it became necessary to reorganize the delivery of care. It was also hoped that the use of team nursing would increase both staff and patient satisfaction and improve the quality of care.

In hospitals and nursing homes, the nurse manager selects the team leaders and designates the scope of the team's responsibility. The nurse manager is also responsible for overall management of the nursing unit, meeting the more formal education needs of staff, and formal evaluation. In community settings, the supervisor usually fulfills these roles.

The team leader has a pivotal role in team nursing and is expected to closely supervise ancillary staff and to provide informal training for them as needed. The leader is also expected to be thoroughly acquainted with the needs of every patient or client assigned to the team, even if not directly involved in their care.

### Advantages

Although patient care is still divided among several people, it is far less fragmented than in the functional method because of the increased communication and extensive coordination efforts of the team leader. The team nursing approach allows comprehensive, holistic nursing care when the team functions at its best.

Although team nursing was not designed to make up for inadequate staffing, it does make it possible to deliver quality care using a relatively large proportion of less costly ancillary personnel (Sherman, 1990). In comparison with the functional method, it is far more satisfying to both patients and staff when it is done well. The abilities of each staff member are more likely to be recognized and fully used. The increased amount of cooperation and communication among team members can raise morale, improve the functioning of the staff as a whole, and give team members a greater sense of having contributed to the outcomes of the care given. Most nurses working on teams find that they know both their patients and fellow staff members better than when using the functional method.

### Disadvantages

One of the greatest disadvantages of team nursing is that it is often poorly done, resulting in fragmented care and lack of accountability (Pontin, 1999). Team nursing is far more than simply dividing staff into equal parts and then assigning an equal number of patients to each group. Yet this method is often called team nursing even though it may be much like the functional method in everything but name.

Team nursing requires a great deal of cooperation and communication from all staff members. It demands even more of the team leader, who spends much time coordinating and supervising team members and who must be highly skilled both as a leader and as a practitioner. Not every nurse practicing today is prepared to assume these roles. Some efficiency is lost due to these demands for increased interaction among staff members. The large number of people attending the same patient under the functional method is not substantially reduced in team nursing.

Although the team leader is a professional nurse, a large proportion of the staff is not, and much of the care is given by persons other than nurses. In contrast, both the case method and primary nursing emphasize care given by professional nurses.

## Primary Nursing

Primary nursing incorporates the case method's concept of assigning full responsibility for a patient or client into a modality designed for inpatient care but adaptable to ambulatory care. Under primary nursing, every patient has a designated primary nurse who is responsible for planning the care and ensuring that the plan is implemented around the clock, seven days a week. The name and responsibilities of this primary nurse should be known to the patient (Steven, 1999). When the primary nurse is not at work, the implementation of the care plan is delegated directly to an associate nurse. The primary nurse is still responsible and in some institutions may be called on if a serious problem arises (Marram, Barrett & Bevis, 1979). Primary nurses are accountable for the **outcomes** of the nursing care given, not just for the fact that care is given (Zander, 1985).

When primary nursing is implemented, the inpatient unit is usually divided into districts or small modular units with a primary nurse assigned to each district. The nurse manager assigns the direct care of the patients to the primary care nurses. Nursing assistants provide personal care for patients, assist the primary nurse with patients with complex care needs, keep water pitchers filled, answer call lights, and convey messages to the primary nurse about patients' needs.

The primary nurse does all initial assessments and then develops care plans for assigned patients. The primary nurse may have other staff members to call on for assistance. She or he organizes the work and assigns parts of it to other staff members. Primary nurses may help one another with development of care plans. They provide complex treatments, coordinate the nursing care plan with other disciplines (including the physician's care plan), administer medications, prepare patients for discharge, provide needed education, and evaluate the efficacy of the interventions.

### Advantages

Primary nursing has many of the advantages of the case method. Nurses have more autonomy than in the functional or team approaches and are challenged to work to their full capacity. They spend less time in coordinating and supervising activities and more time in direct care activities. The primary nurse is also more accountable because responsibility is focused rather than diffused.

After becoming accustomed to this mode, primary nurses generally believe that they are more effective working under this system. In fact, many studies have shown that both cost and turnover are reduced, though evidence of the impact of primary nursing on the quality of care is inconclusive (Fairbanks, 1981; Melchior et al., 1999). Nurses also gain more satisfaction from being involved in the entire care of a patient and from being able to give more holistic care.

Patients also seem to appreciate the more personalized and holistic care that is given in primary nursing. They are especially pleased to be able to say, "This is my nurse." People from other disciplines also appreciate the fact that they can consult with one particular, identifiable nurse who knows all about the patient.

### Disadvantages

As with team nursing, most of the disadvantages of primary nursing come from problems with implementation. Although proponents of primary care nursing argue that it is no more costly than other ways to deliver care, its detractors point out that it requires a much higher proportion of professional nurses to ancillary personnel. It has also been noted that, even with primary nursing, a hospitalized individual is cared for by at least six nurses (three nurses to cover the three 8-hour shifts in a day and another three associates to substitute for them on their days off). The result is that the promise of continuity of care often goes unfilled (Gray & Smedley, 1998).

Primary nursing demands increased independence, accountability, and the ability to make thorough assessments and plan nursing care accordingly. Unfortunately, not every nurse feels prepared for this responsibility, especially those who are accustomed to the functional method's routines. Some are threatened by these additional demands; others find that they need additional education before assuming the primary

nurse role. Ancillary workers often feel a sense of loss when their direct care activities are reduced or eliminated under primary nursing.

One of the major differences between primary nursing and team nursing is the conceptualization of the way care is given, especially by whom. Team nursing was developed in order to include ancillary personnel in caregiving roles appropriately and emphasizes the supervising, teaching, and coordinating functions of the nurse. Primary nursing, on the other hand, focuses on the nurse as the caregiver and does not clearly define the roles of ancillary personnel. In fact, much disagreement surrounds the issue of licensed practical nurses (LPNs) assuming the primary nurse role. Many variations of primary nursing have arisen from attempts to make appropriate use of ancillary personnel.

## Nursing Care Management

Some confusion exists over the terms **case management, managed care,** and **nursing care management.** Managed care is an approach to providing a range of services in such a way that use of services and resulting costs are carefully controlled. Health maintenance organizations (HMOs) and preferred provider organizations (PPOs) are examples of managed care systems, as are the newer primary care systems developed by individual corporations to reduce the cost of healthcare benefits for their employees. It is a healthcare system-level approach with a population-wide perspective, not a method for organizing nursing care. Case management, on the other hand, has an individual client perspective.

Case management has its roots in community health nursing and social work. Its focus is coordination of services for the individual and his or her family. The process includes engaging the client, setting goals, accessing services, coordinating these services, and finally, disengaging (Ballew & Mink, 1986). Some models include direct hands-on care as well as coordination, others do not. Traditional community-based case management has been adapted to outpatient and acute-care settings. One adaptation is nursing care management.

Nursing care management in inpatient settings is a combination of primary nursing (Zander, 1990) and case management. In nursing care management, the primary care nurse assumes responsibility for both the clinical and economic outcomes of a patient's stay. In other words, nurses provide both direct care and case management services to assigned patients and their families. Some versions of this model separate case management and staff nurse roles (Biller, 1992); others do not.

A key feature of nursing care management is that care is organized around the patient, not around the geographic unit on which the patient has been placed or the particular medical team serving that patient. Another important feature is improved continuity and coordination of nursing care across traditional discipline lines.

The concept of nursing care management can be extended by crossing departmental as well as disciplinary boundaries. For example, Stillwaggon (1989) described a maternity service in which nurses are assigned to patients rather than to a unit within the service. Using this nontraditional approach, a nurse can admit a woman to the obstetric service of the hospital, care for her during labor, move with her to the delivery room, and then provide postpartum care. Imagine the difference when the patient has the same nurse through all of these different stages. These innovative modes may be extended even further to cross institutional boundaries (Lamb & Rapacz, 1991; Tappen et al., 1997). With this kind of continuity, that same nurse can follow the new mother and baby after discharge to assure a successful transition.

## Critical Pathways

Patient progress toward recovery and discharge is carefully monitored through the use of mechanisms such as critical pathways (Robinson, Robinson & Lewis, 1992). For example, a patient admitted with diabetic ketoacidosis may be expected to achieve control of blood glucose levels by the second day, learn self-care techniques by the third day, and be ready for discharge by the fifth day (Leebov & Ersoz, 1991). As with critical paths in project planning (see Chapter 16), the critical pathway identifies the intermediate goals that must be achieved within a certain length of time in order to continue progress to-

ward the ultimate goal of recovery and discharge within the time allotted by the diagnostic-related group (DRG) or other reimbursement system. When they are used, critical pathways become blueprints for providing and monitoring care. When a specified goal along the way is not met, a variance has occurred (Hill, 1992). A negative variance, or failure to meet a goal, may be due to a system problem (inability to promptly schedule diagnostic tests or treatments), or due to a patient problem. Monitoring the causes of variances assists in tracking the quality of care, particularly the timeliness and adequacy of the care and the resultant outcomes.

Standard critical pathway documents may be purchased or they may be developed by multidisciplinary teams within an institution. Those developed by multidisciplinary teams within institutions are more likely to succeed because a consensus has to be achieved during their development (Birdsall & Sperry, 1997), thus staff have a "buy-in" to the process.

## Advantages

The holistic orientation of nursing care management yields an enormous amount of satisfaction for both the nurse and the patient (Turkel, Tappen & Hall, 1999). Not only can the nurse follow patient progress from admission to discharge and even beyond, but the nurse can also influence the overall course of treatment far more than in the other models. The patient can identify with a particular nurse as in primary care and has someone to turn to who understands all facets of his or her care. Better coordination and better access to needed services are additional advantages.

## Disadvantages

As with many innovations, a number of healthcare organizations are prepared to give lip service to nursing care management but not to fully support its implementation. Commitment may falter when a physician complains about being called for consultation by a nurse rather than a fellow physician (Daly, Phelps & Rudy, 1991), or when the chief financial officer complains that its implementation may require the investment of scarce dollars. With administrative support, cooperation

| CP: Non-healing Lesion—Diabetic. ELOS: 3 Days—Variations from Designated Pathway Should Be Documented in Progress Notes | | | | |
|---|---|---|---|---|
| **ND and Categories of Care** | **Adm Day 6/28** | **Day 1 6/29** | **Day 2 6/30** | **Day 3 7/1** |
| Impaired skin/ tissue integrity | Actions: Goals: | Actions: Goals: Verbalize understanding of condition Display blood glucose WNL (ongoing) | Actions: Goals: Be free of signs of dehydration Wound free of purulent drainage Verbalize understanding of treatment need Perform self-care tasks No. 1 & 3 correctly Explain reasons for actions | Action: Goals: Wound edges show signs of healing process Perform self-care tasks: No. 2 correctly Explain reason for actions Plan in place to meet discharge needs |
| Referrals | | Dietician & Determine need for: Home care Physical therapy Visiting nurse | | |
| Diagnostic studies | Wound culture/sensitivity Gram stain Random blood glucose Fingerstick BG hs | CBC, electrolytes Glycosylated Hb Serum lipid profile → Fingerstick BG qid Chest X ray (if indicated) ECG (if indicated) | ↑ | Fingerstick BG bid if stable |
| Additional assessments | VS qid I&O/level of hydration qd Character of wound tid Level of knowledge and priorities of learning needs Observe for signs of antibiotic hypersensitivity reaction | ↑ ↑ ↑ | → VS Qshift ↑ ↑ ↑ | ↑ → D/C ↑ |
| Medications | Antibiotic: *Diclocacillin 500 mg PO q6h* Antidiabetic: *Humulin N insulin 10cc SC hs* Other NS soaks tid | Anticipated discharge needs Antibiotic: same Antidiabetic: *Humulin N insulin 10u SC q AM/hs DiaBeta 10 mg PO bid Glucophage 500 mg PO qd* Other same | Antibiotic: same Antidiabetic: same Other same | Antibiotic: same Antidiabetic: same Other same |

**Figure 12–1** Sample critical pathway.

**CP: Non-healing Lesion—Diabetic. ELOS: 3 Days—Variations from Designated Pathway Should Be Documented in Progress Notes** *(continued)*

| ND and Categories of Care | Adm Day 6/28 | Day 1 6/29 | Day 2 6/30 | Day 3 7/1 |
|---|---|---|---|---|
| Patient education | Provide *Understanding Your Diabetes* | Film *Living with Diabetes* Demonstrate and practice self-care activities: 1. Fingerstick BG 2. Insulin admin 3. Wound care 4. Routine foot care | Group sessions: *Diabetic management* | Practice self-care activities *2-insulin admin* Review discharge instructions |
| Additional nursing actions | Up ad lib Dressing change tid | → → | → → | → → |
| Pain | Goals: State pain relieved or minimized with 1 hr of analgesic administration (ongoing) Verbalize understanding of when to report pain and rating scale used Verbalize understanding of S/C measures No. 1–2 | Goals: Verbalize understanding of S/C measures No. 3 Explain reason for actions | Goals: Able to participate in usual level: *ambulate full weight bearing* | Goals: State pain-free/controlled with medication Verbalize understanding of correct medication use |
| | Actions: Explain reason for actions | Actions: → → → | Actions: → → → | Actions: → → → |
| Additional assessments | Characteristics of pain Level of participation in activities Individual analgesic needs | | | |
| Medications Allergies: 0 | Analgesic: Darvocet-N 100 mg PO q4d PRN | Analgesic: same | Analgesic: same | Analgesic: same |
| Patient education | Orient to unit/room Guidelines for self-report of pain and rating scale 0–10 Safety/comfort measures 1 elevation of feet 2 proper footwear | Safety/comfort measures *3 prevention of injury* | | Review discharge medication instructions: dosage, route, frequency, side effects |
| Additional nursing actions | Bed cradle as indicated | | | |

**Figure 12–1** Sample critical pathway. *(continued)*

from other disciplines, and some patience, however, these models have proved to be highly successful both in terms of staff and patient satisfaction and in cost effectiveness. If too much emphasis is placed on cost control, however, much of the improvement in quality of care could be lost.

Nursing staff may initially feel some of the same discomforts that were mentioned under primary care. Those who are more comfortable with the indirect kind of influence that they have in more traditional models may be uncomfortable with the autonomy and direct decision-making responsibility inherent in nursing care management models. In addition, when the same nurse cares for a patient across multiple phases of care, that nurse needs to be more knowledgeable and more flexible than a nurse assigned to a particular unit and a particular shift. Nursing care management makes greater demands on the individual nurse but offers the opportunity for greater professional rewards as well.

## Patient-Focused Care

As its name implies, patient-focused care brings as many services as possible to the patient rather than bringing the patient to these services. Most direct care is provided by a **care pair,** usually a nurse and technician, who share responsibility for a given group of patients. Members of the care pair are cross-trained to provide basic respiratory therapy, physical therapy, phlebotomy, and electrocardiography (ECG) as well as the usual bedside nursing care. The care pairs are expected to do as many things for the patient as possible: the same person who admits a patient one day may be giving him a bath the next morning. This mix of responsibilities is unheard of on a traditional unit (Brider, 1992; Townsend, 1993). Each caregiver provides a wider range of services than they would on a traditional unit. Teamwork and sharing of responsibility are encouraged but delegation is discouraged.

Strictly speaking, patient-focused care is not a model for organizing nursing care because it involves non-nursing staff as well. Patient-focused care developed in response to the proliferation of specialized healthcare personnel and an almost desperate drive to rein in the costs of operating acute-care patient units. It is designed to streamline what has become the complex organization of a patient care unit.

Most hospitals need to embark on a thorough redesign in order to implement patient-focused care. Patients who need similar services are clustered together for greater efficiency. Satellite pharmacies, mini-laboratories, and radiology rooms are located on or near the patient care unit. Patient care supplies and medications are located in or near the patient's room. A bedside computer terminal is used to complete documentation formerly done at the central nurses' station.

### Advantages

The patient-focused model offers a refreshing simplification of the patient care team and reduction of the bureaucratic tangle of services found in acute-care facilities. The parade of new faces into a patient's room is greatly reduced. The patient can ask virtually anyone for help and receive it from that same person. Far less time is spent on coordination of services and patient transport. Costs are reduced by the more efficient use of each employee and reduced need for such staff as unit clerks, ECG technicians, and so forth. Many care pair staff express increased satisfaction with their caregiving under this system. Considerable excitement is also generated by the innovative nature of the extensive departure from the traditional care models.

### Disadvantages

Start-up costs for patient-focused care are considerable, both in terms of staff retraining and in redesign of the physical facility. Staff response to these wide-reaching changes needs to be dealt with proactively to keep resistance to a minimum. The model can be implemented gradually, which may reduce tensions and spread the cost over a greater period of time.

Some serious concerns include the blurring of distinctions between nurses, respiratory therapists, physical therapists, and other healthcare professionals with this model. Not only is the requirement for licensure to carry out specific procedures a problem, but the expertise of each of these separate professions may be lost in the on-the-job cross-training and cross-assignment of patient care responsibilities. The result may be an unwelcome homogenization of staff and decline in quality of care to the lowest common denominator within the team. Patient-focused care could be a trade-off of quality for efficiency.

## Discussion

No single nursing care model works in all settings, or even necessarily across a single, multi-service setting. The organization's mission, philosophy, structure, resources, patient and community needs, and staff availability and expertise must all be considered when choosing a model of care. In every setting, the nurse manager must evaluate the appropriateness of the nursing care delivery model to ensure safe, effective nursing care (Cherry, 1999).

Marrelli (1997) suggests that the following questions be asked when evaluating nursing care delivery models:

- Are patients and families satisfied with their care?
- Are patient outcomes being achieved in a timely, cost-effective manner?
- Are physicians and other health team members satisfied with the care?

## ● STAFFING

Despite the wide variety of healthcare personnel in organizations today, nurses remain the core staff of any healthcare facility. Not only do they minister to patients around the clock, they also constitute the facility's early warning system, alerting physicians when a problem arises and intervening rapidly to prevent injury and often death for many of their patients. Without registered nurses, healthcare facilities as they are today could not exist. Yet many questions remain about optimal staffing numbers and the effectiveness of various scheduling methods.

The problem nurse managers face is how best to adjust nurse staffing to meet patient care and nursing staff needs while simultaneously staying within the budget. Although some nursing staff adjustments may be justified as inpatient days fall,

excessive or inappropriate cuts may adversely affect both patient care quality and staff morale. The issue of staffing and scheduling is even more complex when nurse managers are responsible for providing sufficient numbers of qualified nursing personnel to ensure adequate, safe nursing care for all patients 24 hours a day, seven days a week, every week of the year.

The Joint Commission on Accreditation of Healthcare Organizations' Standard HR.2 states, "The hospital provides an adequate number of staff members whose qualifications are consistent with job descriptions" (Kobs, 1997). Other than the model of nursing care used to organize staff, the major factors that should be considered in making staffing decisions are patient census, patient acuity, skill mix, allowing for "nonproductive" time, and the adequacy of the budget. Use of this information allows the nurse manager to best meet staffing needs.

## Patient Census

The number of patients to be cared for is obviously a major factor affecting staffing decisions. All other factors being equal, a unit of 40 patients requires more staffing than a unit of 25. The census of any unit can fluctuate within a given shift and from one day to the next. For example, on a busy telemetry unit, as many as eight or nine patients can be admitted and discharged within an eight-hour shift.

Additional patients may be admitted on **observation status,** staying anywhere from a few hours to two days before discharge to home. Nurse managers need to be aware of the number of observation patients on their individual units and to understand how the hospital's information system captures the number of observation patients when allocating budgetary resources to the individual unit. The nurse manager is expected to avoid both understaffing and overstaffing as the unit census fluctuates. If nursing staff are sent home early because of a decreased census, a sudden influx of admissions can create a severe shortage as the shift progresses.

*Twelve-hour day shift staff in the obstetrical department are often frustrated when they learn that the census has dropped and staff members are being sent home early without being paid for the remainder of the shift. They know they could receive multiple deliveries or an emergency C-section as soon as "excess" staff members leave, and the unit could become severely understaffed.*

Adjusting for staffing levels by census assumes that the nurse manager can forecast census accurately. If census fluctuates in an unpredictable manner, efforts to match staff levels with patient care needs will be thwarted.

Percentage of occupancy is one way of assessing staffing needs based on unit census. This figure is calculated by dividing the number of beds on a unit into the number of beds actually occupied. For example, if a medical-surgical unit has 45 beds and 40 of those beds are occupied, the occupancy rate is 88.8 percent. Knowing the average occupancy rate allows for more accurate predictions about the number of staff needed.

## Patient Acuity and Complexity of Care

Census numbers alone are not sufficient to determine staffing needs and in fact can leave a unit severely understaffed. Twenty acutely ill patients can have far more nursing needs than 40 less acutely ill patients.

One of the questions that must be answered before staff can be appropriately assigned to care for a particular group of patients is "Exactly what kind of care do they need?" In other words, how many patients need frequent monitoring or suctioning? How many patients have Swan-Ganz lines? How many need assistance with basic tasks like bathing, toileting, feeding themselves, and getting in and out of bed? How many have special skin care needs, are confused and disoriented, need to be taught how to care for themselves because of a condition they have not had before (for example, diabetes, hypertension, or a colostomy)? Answering these questions in an organized way produces an **acuity index,** which enables the nursing unit manager to determine quickly how many staff members are needed, and then how many should be registered nurses (RNs), licensed practical nurses (LPNs), or aides.

The patient can then be assigned to an acuity or complexity category to estimate how many hours of nursing care will be needed during a particular shift. When that information is collected for every patient on the unit, the total number of hours of care required will provide an indication of the number and type of nursing staff needed on the unit for that shift. However, if the scoring system used becomes too detailed or must be done too often, it can demand too much of the nurse manager's time and divert attention from other responsibilities, or not be used correctly.

## Diagnostic-Related Groups (DRGs)

In contrast to the acuity and complexity approach, the Medicare DRG (prospective payment) system tells the hospital the amount of money that will be reimbursed for a particular diagnosis. DRGs are based on the medical diagnosis of the patient. Examples of DRG categories include **DRG 209 (SURG) Major Joint Procedures–Lower Extremity,** which includes hip replacement; **DRG 210 (SURG) Hip and femur procedures,** which includes repair of hip fracture; and **DRG 127 (MED) Heart Failure** (*Federal Register,* 1998). These categories are consistent across settings and hospitals.

The amount of money a facility is reimbursed for a particular DRG has to cover the cost of all supplies, equipment, tests, procedures, and staff needed to care for the patient during the entire hospital stay. For example, a hospital is reimbursed $8,400 for a hip replacement but the average cost for a prosthesis is around $5,100. That means only $3,300 is left to cover the costs of nursing care, physical therapy, medications, X-ray procedures, and lab tests for the next seven days. Another example: the reimbursement for repair of a hip fracture is $7,900 for an average length of stay of 5.9 days, and the reimbursement for a medical diagnosis of congestive heart failure is $4,468 for an average length of stay of 4.2 days. Although the nursing care needs of these patients are similar, you will notice a wide variation in reimbursement.

It is evident that DRGs do not take into account the patient's actual self-care deficits or nursing need. They do not consider, for example, what kinds of disabilities the patients come in with, what psychological factors might interfere with their learning to care for themselves, or other problems that are not indicated by their DRG allocation but impact on the number and kinds of nursing needs. Examples of differences between patients not identified by DRG classification include the following:

- Feeds self with little or no assistance *versus* requires total assistance
- Emotionally stable *versus* subject to panic attacks
- Ambulatory *versus* bed bound
- Receiving oral medication *versus* intravenous medication
- Requires partial *versus* complete isolation
- Requires a simple dressing change *versus* complex wound care
- Alert and oriented *versus* confused and disoriented
- Needs vital signs measured every four hours *versus* every 15 minutes

## Patient Classification Systems

Clearly, different patients with the same medical diagnosis require different amounts of nursing care. To account for these differences, patient classification systems were developed. Patient classification is defined as "the categorization or grouping of patients according to an assessment of their nursing care requirements over a specified period of time" (Hilliard & Marrelli, 1997). In other words, patients are classified based on the projected number of nursing hours required to provide care.

Many patient classification instruments are being used today. Most fall into two categories: the prototype evaluation and the factor evaluation methods. The **prototype** evaluation method determines nursing resource requirements by assigning patients to predetermined categories based on a description of patient care needs. For example, one patient could be described as ambulatory and able to perform all activities of daily living independently. At the opposite end is the patient who requires almost constant monitoring and total assistance with all activities of daily living and so on.

The prototype method is simple and is probably the most commonly used system in the United States (Halloran & Vermeersch, 1987; Swansburg & Swansburg, 1999). Variability between raters can be a problem, with some raters being overly optimistic about a patient's level of need and others "padding" the ratings to make the unit's workload seem higher than it actually is.

The **factor evaluation** method identifies pertinent patient care attributes and assigns predetermined weights or relative value units (RVUs) to them. These weights are then summed to classify the patient into one of several homogeneous groups.

*Typically, the RVU has an arbitrarily set value of 6 or 10 minutes. This means that a patient who needs 60 RVUs would need 360 minutes of nursing care in a 24-hour period, depending on the given value of the RVU.*

A wide variety of patient classification systems are in use in hospitals across the country. Some have been developed specifically for a particular institution. Internally developed systems with four categories of classification, such as self-care, minimal care, moderate care, and extensive care are the most frequent type used (Nagaprasanna, 1988) (see Table 12–2). Others such as GRASP, Medicus, and Patient Intensity for Nursing Index (PINI) are commercially available, computer-generated programs that can be purchased from vendors. However, these systems are expensive, and fail to capture the complexity of nurses's work (O'Brien-Pallas, Cockerill & Leatt, 1992). Because other variables, such as experience and competency of the staff and the presence and quality of ancillary services within the hospital also impact on nursing care hours, it is often difficult to transfer a patient classification system from one hospital to another.

Regardless of the system in use, it is the responsibility of the nurse manager to become familiar with the system. The nurse manager must also recognize factors affecting a unit's staffing needs that are not reflected in a patient classification system. In addition to those already mentioned, such factors would include years of experience of unit staff, educational preparation of registered nurse staff, competency level of nursing staff, number of new graduates assigned to

**Table 12–2** Example of a Patient Classification System Using Four Categories of Classification

| Area of Nursing Care | Level 1 Self-Care | Level 2 Minimal Care | Level 3 Moderate Care | Level 4 Extensive Care |
|---|---|---|---|---|
| Eating | Feeds self | Needs some help in opening containers, cutting food, or requires encouragement to eat | Cannot feed self but is able to swallow without difficulty | Cannot feed self Requires constant observation during meals because of swallowing difficulties |
| Ambulation | Walks by self without assistive device | Walks by self with use of assistive device such as cane or walker | Requires assistance of 1 staff member to ambulate | Requires assistance of 2 staff members to ambulate |
| Bathing | Bathes self Able to shower | Bathes self with minimal assistance of staff Needs help in gathering supplies, setting up | Requires bed bath with moderate assistance Able to wash hands, face | Requires bed bath with maximum assistance Completely dependent |
| Medication Administration | Receives medications only once a shift Medications received require no pre or post evaluation | Receives medication more than once a shift Medications received require pre or post evaluation such as cardiac medications or anti-coagulation therapy | Receives medications at least every 4 hours or on IV therapy Medications received require pre or post evaluation such as cardiac medications or anticoagulation therapy | Receives medications via a central line, such as hyperalimentation Receives IV medications that require frequent observation and titration such as an insulin drip |

the unit, and the number of agency nurses and nursing students on the unit.

A valid and reliable patient acuity classification instrument is an ideal tool for determining the cost of nursing care. Regardless of which classification method is employed, each acuity level represents a group of patients who require, within a given range, similar nursing resources. Using these classifications is a step toward "costing out" nursing services. Nursing has fallen behind in the movement toward being a revenue-reproducing rather than revenue-absorbing department, compared with other disciplines that can charge directly for their services (e.g., speech therapy, physical therapy). Use of these systems can move us closer to this goal.

## Staff or Skill Mix

Once the number of patients and the patients' acuity levels are known, a third factor is the mix of staff members assigned to care for the patients. How many RNs, LPNs, and aides have been assigned to provide direct patient care on

that unit? Who can safely provide for the particular needs each patient has? Who would provide the optimal level of care for each patient?

As was mentioned earlier, in some institutions, nonprofessional staff were eliminated and replaced with a lesser number of professionally prepared staff. The idea behind this was that RNs can provide more complex care than either LPNs or aides and so can be assigned to meet all of the patients' needs. In other institutions, the prevailing wisdom has been that professional staff are expensive and their skills can be used more efficiently if the nonprofessional tasks are done by ancillary personnel. In this case, fewer RNs are available to care for patients and relatively more LPNs and aides are used. Both approaches have disadvantages. In the case of the all-professional staff, nurses may be spending considerable time doing relatively routine tasks that could be done for less cost by nonprofessional staff. The nurses are also left with less time for the tasks that require the skills and judgment of a nurse. In the opposite situation with fewer RNs and more paraprofessionals, enough professional staff may not be available for the tasks that require a nurse's skill. Either way, the nursing needs of the patient may not be adequately addressed. As staff and skill mix change in the wake of restructuring, nurse managers need to assess the impact of these changes on their individual units.

> ### We must ask a lot more questions. All RN-staffing is no longer in the cards.
> —Davis, 1996, p. 67

The use of an acuity index may help in determining the proper staff mix. The unit with a high acuity or complexity index may be able to make the most efficient use of a high proportion of RN staff because those patients have a high number of complex care needs (a critical care unit, for example). Some ancillary staff on the unit can assist with routine tasks, such as making beds or answering call lights. On the other hand, if the acuity index indicates that patients have a high proportion of chronic care needs requiring considerable help with the basic activities of daily living (bathing, dressing, toileting, and so forth), then the unit may operate more efficiently with relatively more paraprofessional staff, with fewer RNs needed to plan and manage care, carry out higher-level assessment and complex interventions, and develop appropriate discharge plans (for example, a long-term care facility).

Finding the right staff mix can determine the quality of care the patients receive and how quickly they get better. It can also help the nurse manager stay within the unit budget. Several research studies have documented the positive impact of relatively high registered nurse to nonprofessional staffing on patient outcomes (Kovner & Gergen, 1998; Lichtig, Knauf & Milholland, 1999). See Research Example 12–1, Does a Higher Proportion of Registered Nurse Staffing Produce Better Patient Outcomes? However, nurse managers continue to be challenged by demands for both efficiency and effectiveness in staffing and scheduling on their individual units.

## Productive Versus Nonproductive Time

In planning for staffing, the nurse manager also needs to identify the number of full-time equivalents (FTEs) needed to run the unit. A full-time equivalent is an employee who works full-time, 40 hours per week, or 2,080 hours per year. This figure would include productive as well as nonproductive time. Productive time is the time actually worked by the employee. Nonproductive time or benefit time includes paid time off such as funeral leave, vacation, sick, holiday, or education time. Although the organization pays an FTE for 2,080 hours of work, that employee does not actually work those hours. This concept is an important one for nurse managers to consider when calculating the unit's staffing needs, and is further discussed in Chapter 14, which covers budgeting.

Consideration must also be given to demands on staff time that are not directly related to patient care. Staff development programs and performance appraisals, for example, are necessary for ensuring quality of care, but they take time away from the direct care of patients.

Time is also spent on a number of other tasks and functions that are not direct patient care, including charting, counting narcotics, giving reports, waiting for elevators, getting supplies, and traveling for home visits. This "nonproductive" time can also be affected by an institution's organization of support services, such as who transports patients, picks up medications from the pharmacy, or serves meal trays. Even the placement of laundry chutes, medication/supply carts, and layout of the nursing stations affects nonproductive time.

Some types of nonproductive time can be predicted and planned for, whereas others cannot. For example, if a 20-bed unit can be adequately staffed by eight people (four nurses, two LPNs, and two aides), more than eight staff are actually needed to cover for days off, sick days, and so forth. Someone else has to be assigned to the patients whenever a staff member has a day off, calls in sick, or attends a staff development program.

Some organizations attempt to make up for their inefficiency by paying staff for eight hours of work but actually requiring more time each shift. For example, the home health nurse may be expected to complete paperwork on his or her own time or a charge nurse may be required to come in a half hour early to inventory narcotics and receive reports. Such solutions ease the agency's budget strictures but force nurses to involuntarily donate

**RESEARCH EXAMPLE 12–1    *Does a Higher Proportion of Registered Nurse Staffing Produce Better Patient Outcomes?***

What impact does the level of registered nurse staffing have on patient outcomes? To answer this question the American Nurses' Association commissioned a large-scale study to examine the effect of registered nurse staffing levels on patient outcomes. In this study, data were collected from 502 hospitals in three states (Network Inc., 1996). Higher nursing hours and higher levels of professional staff were found to be significantly related to reduced length of stay, suggesting that the increased cost of more skilled staff may be offset by savings related to length of stay. Patient outcomes (pressure ulcers, pneumonia, postoperative infections, and urinary tract infections) were also related to registered nurse skill mix. The researchers found that a higher proportion of registered nurse staffing resulted in better patient outcomes (Lichtig, Knauf & Milholland, 1999).

Another large-scale study examined the relationship between nurse staffing and adverse events experienced by patients during their hospitalization (Kovner & Gergen, 1998). In this study, the sample included data from 589 acute care hospitals in 10 states. A large and significant relationship was found between the number of registered nurses and number of postoperative complications that occurred. A higher number of registered nurses resulted in patients having fewer urinary tract infections and less pneumonia, respiratory compromise, or thrombosis after surgery. Findings from this study indicate a clear relationship between nurse staffing levels and avoidable adverse events (Kovner & Gergen, 1998).

What do these results mean? Clearly, patients in hospitals with higher registered nurse staffing ratios are less likely to experience preventable complications. While replacing registered nurses with unlicensed assistive personnel may reduce the cost of staffing a unit, in the long term the costs may be higher because patients who develop preventable complications have to stay longer and require more expensive treatment. This type of information is needed to secure the future of professional nursing practice.

*Sources:* Kovner, C. & Gergen, P.J. (1998). Nurse staffing levels and adverse events following surgery in U.S. Hospitals. *Image, 30*(4), 315–321.

Lichtig, L.K., Knauf, R.A. & Milholland, D.K. (1999). Some impacts of nursing on acute care hospital outcomes. *Journal of Nursing Administration, 29*(2), 25–33.

Network, Inc. (1996, December). *Implementation of a nursing report card for acute care settings.* Final report presented at meeting of American Nurses Association.

---

their time to cover an inadequate staffing budget. In a unionized agency, this requirement often constitutes a violation of the labor contract.

## Adequacy of the Budget

Nurse managers have the dual responsibility to provide sufficient numbers of staff to care for patients and to be mindful of the costs with respect to the unit's budget. In order to best accomplish these goals, the nurse manager needs to be involved in planning the unit budget.

The staffing budget is often determined by financial administrators and based on prior year census and productivity. Allocations in the budget for overtime, temporary staff, changes in salary scales, and unexpected increases in census or patient referrals allow greater flexibility to adjust staffing to need. Failure to allow for such contingencies in the budget may make it impossible to respond adequately to the fluctuations in patient need, leaving patients inadequately cared for and the nurse manager and the staff frustrated and worn out.

It is usually possible to stay within a staffing budget and meet the care needs of the patient. However, it requires that the nurse manager be involved in the budget process to assure that the budget is adequate to begin with and to focus on patient acuity and census fluctuation on a daily basis. The dual responsibility of nurse managers, then, is first, to the nursing staff and patients to increase staffing when patient acuity and census are high, and, second, to the organization to decrease staffing when patient acuity and census are low.

## Unlicensed Assistive Personnel

Unlicensed assistive personnel (UAP) are bedside healthcare workers who are not licensed; they include nursing aides or assistants and technicians of various kinds (Barter, McLaughlin & Thomas, 1994). In an effort to control labor costs, administrators have increased the number of UAPs assigned to a unit and decreased the percent of registered nurses (RNs) and licensed practical nurses (LPNs) (Marks, Dennis, Borozny & Ferrone, 1999). According to a survey conducted by the American Hospital Association, 97 percent of surveyed hospitals currently employed UAPs (Siehoff, 1998). It is usually the nurse manager who is ultimately responsible for the assignment of clinical responsibilities on a designated unit. To best accomplish this task, the nurse manager must understand the educational preparation, the scope of responsibility, and the appropriate assignment for UAPs.

### Educational Preparation

The preparation of UAPs varies considerably (Ventura, 1999). Certification standards vary between the states, and hiring and training standards are often determined by individual institutions. For example, at Duke University Medical Center, UAPs complete eight weeks of instruction at a community college, are state certified, and then receive additional training at the hospital (Zimmerman, 1996a). Conversely, other hospitals require no formal classroom education for UAPs and provide only one to three weeks of on the job training. The UAPs' prior experience typically includes such jobs as storeroom clerk, housekeeper, dietary aide, security, or unit clerk, many of which do not prepare them for direct patient care.

This "upskilling" of auxiliary staff has worked well for specified tasks such as assisting with bathing or transporting patients (Porter-O'Grady, 1998). However, UAPs lack the multifocal skill sets and educational preparation needed to make complex clinical decisions. For example, nurses report that some UAPs don't have the educational preparation to recognize abnormal vital signs when they take them.

> They do not have the background to understand that while 96/50 may be normal for a 100-pound young woman, it should be reported if it is found in a 240-pound middle-aged man with chest pain. One time an unlicensed worker was continuing to attempt obtaining a patient's pulse and blood pressure, oblivious to the fact that the monitor had changed to asystole and the patient was unconscious (Zimmerman, 1996a, p. 2).

### Scope of Responsibility

Nurse managers need to understand that the role of UAPs is to **complement** the care provided by the registered nurse rather than to **substitute** for the registered nurse. Guidelines for the role of UAPs vary between hospitals, and at times these guidelines expand into professional level responsibilities. For example, at some hospitals UAPs perform the following tasks: sterile procedures, suctioning, inserting catheters, complex wound care, and starting intravenous lines. Given this inconsistency in guidelines it is often difficult for nurse managers to determine an appropriate assignment for UAPs. Nurse managers also need to consider the time spent by RNs instructing, evaluating, and following up on the care provided by UAPs.

### Appropriate Assignment

Clearly, appropriately assigning UAPs requires the establishment of practice guidelines for this role within the individual organization. Prior to establishing these guidelines it is important for nurse educators and nurse managers to be familiar with state imposed practice parameters. Currently, 25 states have bills that regulate what UAPs can and cannot do (Sheehan, 1998). Once the specifics of the state regulations are known, the nurse educators can assist the nurse managers and the nursing staff in developing organization-specific guidelines for UAPs.

It is important that the tasks assigned to UAPs do not require professional judgment or interpretation. The nursing division of the University of Iowa Hospital identified the following as examples of tasks appropriate for UAPs: ambulate and transport patients, answer call lights, make beds, position and feed patients, obtain urine and sputum specimens, take routine vital signs, administer enemas and perform baths/oral care, environmental tasks, and simple dressing changes (Gould et al., 1996).

A second component of appropriate assignment is orientation of UAPs to ensure technical competencies and understanding of job responsibilities. Competency-based training ensures that UAPs meet a certain standard of performance within a given time frame (Williams, Donaldson & Watts, 1998). Skills checklists can be used by the registered nurse to validate the competence of UAPs. The UAP must demonstrate the skill or procedure correctly in order to be checked off by the registered nurse preceptor or nurse educator.

The role, responsibilities, and limitations on UAPs must be clearly explained to them during the orientation process. Failure to do so results in lack of understanding by some UAPs and failure to adhere to the role by others. One complaint related to this issue is that some UAPs set their own priorities after the registered nurse has determined the proper nursing interventions (Zimmerman, 1996a). A Chicago emergency room nurse shared the following experience:

> During our heat crisis, I had three ambulance patients arrive at the same time. I assigned complete vital signs to the unlicensed worker for one of the newly arrived possible heat stroke patients. He only did the blood pressure, which he assumed was most important. He then proceeded to transport another patient for a routine X-ray, something he had judged as more important. The new patient had a 105.8 degrees F rectal temperature (Zimmerman, 1996a, p. 2).

In order for registered nurses to work effectively with UAPs they must first understand their respective roles and responsibilities. Secondly, many registered nurses may require further education to develop supervisory and delegation skills.

## Cross-Training

In order to ensure appropriate staffing levels during times of fluctuating census or increased patient acuity, many hospitals have instituted the concept of cross-training to create a more flexible nursing workforce. The difference between cross-training and indiscriminate floating is that cross-training involves formal orientation to two or more "like" units, such as intensive care and the emergency room or postpartum and antepartum units (Trossman, 1999) or, in the patient-focused model of care, to competencies of those in a related discipline such as preparing staff nurses to do ECGs or provide respiratory therapy (Ventura, 1999). Under the former approach, when staffing shortages occur, nurses are then floated only to those units for which they have been cross-trained. The aim of this type of cross-training is to broaden the competencies of nurses already employed by the hospitals, not to train employees across disciplines.

### Pros and Cons

Cross-training can increase nursing staff flexibility, and allow for efficient, cost-effective use of staff. In one hospital where medical-surgical nurses were cross-trained to intensive care, employee morale increased and staffing costs decreased (Snyder & Nethersole-Chong, 1999). By combining like units, nursing staff can maintain clinical competencies in their area of specialization. Another benefit of cross-training is the elimination of indiscriminate floating where a nurse is sent to any type of unit without any orientation. Cross-training is valuable for registered nurses because it gives them an opportunity to broaden their skills and enhance future marketability.

> *The valuable nurse in the next millennium is the one who can do more—who has the knowledge base to function as a specialist but also as a generalist working in multiple areas.*
> —Shumaker, cited in Trossman, 1999, p. 1

Nurses are often critical of cross-training because they fear hospitals will fail to provide the required training and education needed. This fear was the reason registered nurses at a Michigan hospital rejected any management proposal that would require cross-training (Trossman, 1999). Another criticism is that cross-training will dilute highly specialized nursing care by creating nurses who know something about everything and not enough about any one area of specialization.

> *Hospital administrators forget that nursing practice is a continually evolving process. In labor and delivery there are changes that impact my practice every week. If you are cross-trained to several units, you can't keep up your own specialty skills. You end up being an expert at the little things, and don't know anything in depth.*
>
> —Armstrong, cited in Trossman, 1999, p. 2

### Floating

The practice of floating staff from one unit to another has raised many issues and concerns for both staff nurses and managers. Floating is a staffing strategy whereby nurses are assigned wherever they are needed, regardless of their training or unit orientation. It is based on the assumption that nurses are generalists. However, most nurses don't see themselves as generalists. In one study, 73 percent of the nurses surveyed stated they disliked, resented, or even hated floating (Orstein, 1992). A randomized survey of 135 nurses identified the following concerns about floating: inadequate orientation, concern about omissions and mistakes, lack of resources, unrealistic assignments, and unfriendly receiving unit (Nicholls, 1996). Intensive care nurses have identified floating as a major source of job stress (Davidhizar, Dowd & Brownson, 1998).

Staff nurses often find themselves in a situation where they are required to agree to float or be in jeopardy of losing their job. To avoid being placed in a litigious situation or violating the Nurse Practice Act, a nurse can keep the guidelines developed by the Florida Nurses Association in mind when asked to float. These guidelines suggest clarification, assessment, and option identification (Ketter, 1994). **Clarification** involves understanding what is being expected of you and includes knowing the number, diagnoses, and acuity level of the patients for whom you will be responsible and the other resources available for providing their care. **Assessment** refers to evaluating your current knowledge and job competencies prior to accepting the assignment. **Option identifi-**

**cation** means accepting the assignment if you believe you can provide safe care, realizing that by doing so you are ethically and legally responsible for the nursing care of the assigned patients (Ketter, 1994). If you feel that you are unable to accept the assignment based on competency concerns, you need to discuss it with nursing administration to negotiate other options.

Many state nurses' associations have developed Assignment Despite Objection (ADO) forms for use in case of unsafe floating practices (Trossman, 1999). Staff nurses need to be aware of state guidelines and individual hospital policies regarding floating. While state associations have indicated that nurses have the right to accept or reject assignment, nurses can be disciplined by the hospital for "abandoning an assignment" (Ketter, 1994).

### Role of the Manager

The nurse manager needs to make sure that the nurses floated to his or her individual unit have the required skills and have received adequate orientation. Floating should take place only in an emergency situation. It should not be used as a quick fix solution by administration to avoid hiring the necessary number of nurses for individual units. Nurse managers can implement strategies to make floating to their unit less difficult for the nurse and safer for the patients. Examples of such strategies include matching the "float" nurse's assignment with the nurse's competencies, having a buddy system for all floats, providing "cheat sheets" with basic unit information, identifying available resources, and avoiding assignments where the float nurse is given the most difficult patients on the unit (Banks, Hardy & Meskimen, 1999).

## ● SCHEDULING

Once the appropriate number and skill mix of staff needed on a given unit are determined, then the best method for scheduling the nursing staff can be selected. Scheduling of nursing staff is an important issue to both nurse managers and nursing staff. A 1990 survey of nurse managers found that 11.1 percent of their time, concern, and worry was centered around the topic of scheduling (Barrett, 1991). Nursing staff are also concerned about the effect of scheduling on their personal lives and are particularly frustrated when they lack input into decisions about their work schedules. Nurse managers should periodically evaluate how satisfied nurses are with the current scheduling system.

Scheduling options include 8-, 10- or 12-hour shifts, flex-time, self-scheduling, and use of temporary staff including agency or float pool staff.

> **Be open to scheduling options.**
> **There is more than one way to create**
> **a schedule/staffing pattern that is**
> **cost-effective and meets the goal of**
> **providing quality patient care.**
> —White-Fletcher, 1995, p. 437

## Centralized Versus Decentralized

The two basic approaches to scheduling of staff within an organization are centralized and decentralized scheduling. When scheduling is centralized, one or more individuals in a central staffing office schedule staff on all the units or teams within the organization. Many organizations use clerical staff and computer programs to assist with staff scheduling. However, accountability for scheduling still rests with the nurse manager. The role of the nurse manager is to communicate special staffing needs and assist in obtaining additional staff for call-ins or changes in patient census or acuity. This type of staffing is fairer to all staff because policies tend to be employed more consistently and impartially. It also allows the nurse manager time to focus on other management responsibilities. However, centralized scheduling lacks responsiveness to individual staff needs and variations in unit census and acuity.

Decentralized scheduling is done either by the nurse manager or by the nursing staff when self-scheduling (explained later) is used. When scheduling is decentralized, the nurse manager is responsible for preparing monthly unit schedules, providing coverage for holiday, vacation, and sick time, and adding staff during periods of high patient census or acuity. An advantage of decentralized staffing is that the nurse manager

is aware of the special needs of the unit and the unit staff. Another is that staff members feel more in control of their work environment when they can make requests to their nurse manager.

A major disadvantage to decentralized scheduling is that it is time consuming for the nurse manager, especially if a variety of scheduling options are available to the staff. If not handled well, employees may perceive that some staff members receive better treatment than others or that the schedule becomes a way for the nurse manager to reward or punish staff.

## Traditional Versus Nontraditional

The traditional approach to scheduling involves nursing staff working eight-hour shifts, five days a week, with alternate weekend coverage. This method worked well when nurse managers staffed units based on average patient census. Typically, nurses were assigned to a single shift based on seniority or rotated shifts on a monthly basis (less senior staff were assigned to evenings and nights). Rotating shifts has been identified as a major contributor to job dissatisfaction and burnout (Davidhizar, Dowd & Brownson, 1998).

Nurse managers are beginning to recognize that more flexible scheduling is needed to deal with the current environment of fluctuating census and higher patient acuity. Nursing staff are now assigned in a more flexible manner in most organizations. Assignments may take the form of 4-day weeks of 10-hour shifts or 3-day weeks of 12-hour shifts. The following is an example:

> *You are the nurse manager of a 12-bed intensive care unit, and the unit currently uses eight-hour shifts. A 12-hour shift alternative has been requested by a number of the nursing staff. Their main reason for wanting this change was so that they could work overtime when the unit is short-staffed or patient acuity is high. A major concern to you is the desire to work overtime as a reason for switching to 12-hour shifts. Research studies have shown that 12-hours shifts improve patient care, increase nurse satisfaction as nurses have additional time off for their personal lives, and reduce the number of call-ins (Bowers-Hutto & Davis, 1989; Fagin, 1982; Todd, Reid & Robinson, 1991). Research findings are contradictory*

*in the area of 12-hour versus 8-hour shifts in the area of fatigue and clinical judgment. Several studies have found no differences between the two systems (Fields & Loveridge, 1988; Washburn, 1991). However, other studies have shown that working 12 hours can result in fatigue and errors in clinical judgment (Mills, Arnold & Wood, 1983; Ugrovics & Wright, 1990).*

*The solution? You can meet with the staff and discuss the various research findings on 8-hour and 12-hour shifts. You then explain to the staff that overtime would have to be limited to one shift per week if 12-hour shifts were implemented. This way a balance between work and personal time and avoidance of adverse effects on fatigue levels and clinical judgment could both be achieved.*

These longer shifts make it possible to have more staff on duty during the heavy-need hours of the day, early in the morning and at supper time. It also allows staff to work shorter weeks and have more consecutive days off, which some people have found helpful for restoring energy levels.

## Flex-Time

Flex-time is a system that allows nursing staff to select time schedules that best meet their personal needs, while still meeting work responsibilities. For example, an occupational health nurse may work from 10 A.M. to 6 P.M. instead of the traditional 8 A.M. to 4 P.M. shift. This schedule would allow the nurse to get the children ready for school in the morning while expanding availability of services for the evening shift. This creative scheduling option increases nurses' job satisfaction and allows the organization to meet the needs of a diverse workforce (Wulff, 1997).

Flex-time is easier to incorporate in some work settings than in others. It can be instituted without much difficulty in settings where the nurses work independently. For example, in some home healthcare agencies, nurses may adjust their hours to suit the needs of their patients, making it possible to provide a broader range of services. Flexible working hours may make it easier for nurses to provide early morning or evening teaching to new diabetic patients who are learning to give themselves insulin but also need to go to work.

The option of flex-time may pose organizational and management challenges for the institution or agency. More supervision and clerical support over longer hours may also be needed. In areas such as hospital settings where the nursing coverage is continuous and nurses work as part of a group, flex-time is more of a challenge to implement. In these areas flex-time is best accomplished by providing a number of prescheduled shift starting and quitting times that vary from the traditional start times of 7 A.M., 3 P.M., and 11 P.M. For example, a nurse may be assigned from 10 A.M. to 3 P.M. or 10 A.M. to 6 P.M. depending on the number of hours the nurse wishes to work. In both variations the nurse would be available to cover busy times on the unit and still match work and home life schedules. Another example may be a nurse choosing to work only four hours per day from 12 P.M. to 4 P.M. to cover peak time for admissions and discharges.

Another type of flex-time allows nurses to work nine months a year and have the summer off while retaining seniority and healthcare benefits. Summers-off programs tend to work well in hospitals that experience a predictable seasonal decline in census from May through September.

## Self-Scheduling

Self-scheduling has been introduced as an alternative to the traditional approach to staffing. With self-scheduling, the responsibility for staffing is delegated to the staff in the unit. Guidelines for self-scheduling are mutually agreed on by the staff of the unit. Staff members are permitted to negotiate and trade times within the guidelines. In the beginning, the nurse manager usually works with the group to make the schedule. However, the ultimate goal is for a staff nurse or scheduling committee to oversee the process. An example of a form for self-scheduling is shown in Figure 12–2.

Initial implementation of self-scheduling may be time consuming for the nurse manager, but the process becomes smoother as the staff gain experience with it. Eventually the amount of time spent on scheduling by nurse managers is significantly reduced. Research has shown an increase in job satisfaction, autonomy, and control, and a

| NAMES | Sunday | Monday | Tuesday | Wednesday | Thursday | Friday | Saturday |
|-------|--------|--------|---------|-----------|----------|--------|----------|
| **7A-3P** | | | | | | | |
| | | | | | | | |
| | | | | | | | |
| | | | | | | | |
| **7A-7P** | | | | | | | |
| | | | | | | | |
| | | | | | | | |
| **3P-11P** | | | | | | | |
| | | | | | | | |
| | | | | | | | |
| **7P-7A** | | | | | | | |
| | | | | | | | |
| | | | | | | | |
| **11P-7A** | | | | | | | |
| | | | | | | | |
| | | | | | | | |
| | | | | | | | |

Nursing Unit _____
Date _____

**Figure 12–2** Form for self-scheduling by nursing staff.
(*Source:* Sovie, M.D.: Hospital restructuring's impact on outcomes (HRIO). Paper presented at the Invitational Conference for Nurse Executives, Philadelphia, PA, June 9–11, 1999.)

decrease in turnover and absenteeism when self-scheduling is implemented (Abbott, 1995). In one hospital, self-scheduling led to a savings of $614,400 over a three-year period (Davidhizar, Dowd & Brownson, 1998). These savings resulted from a decrease in turnover rate and in the number of nurses calling in sick.

A disadvantage to self-scheduling is the extra time spent by the nursing staff on scheduling and negotiating changes in the schedules. The negotiation process can be difficult if some staff members refuse to participate. Another issue identified as problematic is how to deal with staff members who fail to follow the established guidelines.

## Specialization

Another way to increase the efficiency of staff assignments is to group patients with the same diagnosis or nursing care needs on the same unit. Whereas physicians have been quite specialized for some time, nurses have only begun to develop specialties such as critical care, gerontological nursing, trauma care, or neonatology. These nurses become experts in providing nursing care for patients with a particular set of problems or needs. When nurses are assigned to a specialty unit, they develop a high level of expertise in caring for patients with a particular problem. Neonatal intensive care, spinal cord injury units, acute geriatric units, and open-heart surgery teams are examples of this type of specialization.

Because staff members are taking care of patients with similar needs so consistently, they also become more efficient in identifying the common needs these patients are likely to have and in providing specific interventions to meet these needs. Many aspects of care become routine and can be accomplished in less time than it would take the nurse who is not so accustomed to caring for this particular patient population. It may even be possible to discharge patients in less time if teaching is begun sooner and the patient becomes independent in caring for himself or herself sooner. This system may be seen as a good way to provide cost-efficient, quality care.

Many hospitals are developing more specialty care units (such as alcohol-abuse treatment units and diabetic treatment centers) rather than try to offer care for every type of patient who might be admitted to the general hospital. By focusing on specialties, they also establish a reputation for providing better care for patients with special needs than the general hospital can.

Some debate, however, centers on the long-term benefits of specialization. The following is an example of a debate in a public health agency:

*The current method of assignment in this agency is generalist; that is, each nurse is responsible for all the nursing care given in the assigned geographic area. The nurse receives all the referrals and makes all initial visits for patients with a specific diagnosis who require nursing care in conjunction with a medical regimen. In addition, the nurse is responsible for all the health guidance and public health care that is required by individuals or groups in the assigned geographic area, including immunization and well-baby clinics, contact investigations for tuberculosis, and consultation on the best long-term care for elderly clients.*

*Recently this agency has been piloting a new method of assignment in two of its four field offices. In each office, a team of two nurses has been assigned to provide all public health and health guidance care for the entire geographic area served by the field office. The remaining staff have been given larger geographic areas than they had previously but are now responsible only for the care of patients with a diagnosis requiring supportive home care or rehabilitation and teaching.*

*In some respects, community health nurses have retained a generalist focus long after their institutional counterparts have specialized in the care of patients with particular needs. They have been expected to be experts in many technical procedures that were formerly the province of institutional settings only but now frequently occur in the home, as well as the principles and practice of preventive health care and public health procedures. The specialist assignment is seen as an opportunity for community health nurses to become more expert in one area of nursing in the community, with the expectation that the care given will be of higher quality, the satisfactions greater, and the frustrations less. But many nurses find great reward in the generalist role and worry that they will become bored by confining their practice to one arena.*

## Temporary Personnel

In some situations, such as a high level of staff vacancies or periods of unexpectedly high demand for services, additional staff may be hired or assigned temporarily to supplement existing staff. Temporary staff may also be obtained directly from the organization's temporary pool or obtained from a registry or temporary agency if the need is great enough. The use of temporary staff has been widespread. It allows a facility to respond efficiently to changing staffing needs resulting from census fluctuations, increased acuity, or staff vacancies.

Although the use of temporary staff offers cost advantages because the organization does not pay benefits to the staff or guarantee hours worked, it is not without disadvantages. Use of temporary staff poses a considerable threat to continuity of care. It is also thought that pool employees lack the commitment to the organization that is found with permanent employees. In response, many facilities have developed their own "in-house" nursing pools as opposed to using "agency" nurses from an outside source. An in-house pool affords the facility greater control over who will work (the selection process), as well as the ongoing education of these pool employees. The ability to fill staffing needs on a demand basis also depends on the availability of budgeted funds and of temporary staff in the community.

## Developing a System

Every healthcare organization needs to develop a responsive system for scheduling staff, preferably one based on a well-developed nursing-sensitive patient classification system. Although the number of beds on a unit may not change, the acuity and complexity levels will undoubtedly fluctuate from day to day and week to week.

The organization's mission and goals also affect staffing. A home care agency that does not provide emergency services and uses alternative support systems for their clients on evenings and weekends will not need to plan for as much staff flexibility but still must be prepared to handle a large influx of new referrals. For this type of situation, an on-call system may be adequate to meet infrequent needs for extra staff, but it is easily abused and often creates personal difficulties for staff members. Maintaining staff on call and paying overtime can become expensive and may push staff to physical and mental extremes of exertion and fatigue. The same can be said for making a habit of asking staff to work double shifts, an inexcusable action in anything but an emergency. A reordering of staff priorities can also be used to handle minor increases in demand but cannot be continued on an indefinite basis.

Any hospital staffing system must take into account the 24-hours-a-day, 7-days-a-week nature of the need for staff. Some institutions establish a policy of every third weekend off and mandatory rotation to ensure adequate staffing for the less popular working hours. These policies ignore the needs and preferences of the staff members. Others hire sufficient staff and develop their own pool of temporary staff to maintain the needed flexibility and, at the same time, to keep their staff satisfied.

Both the organization's management philosophy and budget have a great deal of influence on its staffing policies. You can see that scheduling of staff is a complex function that does not yield to easy or consistent formulas.

## ● DELEGATION

Once the right mix and necessary number of staff have been scheduled for an individual unit, it is the role of the charge nurse to delegate tasks and assignments. The issue of delegation of tasks and responsibilities either to other registered nurses or to licensed practical nurses and unlicensed assistive personnel can also be a challenge. Multiple concerns regarding delegation include patient safety, license protection, and accountability for the completion and outcome of the delegated tasks. According to the American Nurses Association (ANA, 1997a), delegation is defined as "the transfer of responsibility for the performance of an activity from one individual to another while retaining accountability for the outcome" (p. 3). Thus, even though the leader or manager delegates a task to another employee, he or she remains responsible and accountable for the outcomes.

## What You Can and Cannot Delegate

The nurse manager is responsible and accountable for decisions on whether to delegate certain patient care activities. Consider the following when delegating: patient safety, the patient's condition, complexity of task, complexity of assessment, level of problem solving and judgment required, predictability of outcome, and competency of the registered nurse, licensed practical nurses or UAPs (Zimmerman, 1996b; ANA, 1997a). In order to delegate safely, the nurse manager needs to know the legal scope of nursing as defined by the State Nurse Practice Act, as well as which activities can be performed only by a registered nurse, and which may be performed by either a registered nurse, licensed practical nurse, or unlicensed assistive personnel. The activity delegated needs to fall within the scope of practice for the person to whom it is delegated. In turn, that person needs to have the skills, knowledge, and judgment to carry out the activity.

It is beyond the scope of this chapter to define the various state laws and state nursing board's guidelines on what tasks can or cannot be delegated to a licensed practical nurse or unlicensed assistive personnel. However, in a broad sense a registered nurse can only delegate tasks that are within his or her scope of practice and within the job description and training of the person to whom it is delegated. The National Council of State Boards of Nursing has issued a position statement specifying that tasks that involve nursing judgment and assessment of the patient's response to care must not be delegated to nonprofessional staff (Sheehan, 1998). A similar position has been taken by the ANA. According to the ANA (1997a), "any nursing intervention that requires independent, specialized, nursing knowledge, skill or judgment cannot be delegated" (p. 2). Those interventions would include patient teaching and health counseling activities.

## How to Delegate

Once a decision is made to delegate a patient care activity to either another registered nurse, licensed practical nurse, or unlicensed assistive personnel, it is important to know how to delegate effectively. Effective and safe delegation allows all members of the team to work together toward a common goal, which in turn fosters employee commitment and job satisfaction. Failure to delegate effectively and safely can result in job dissatisfaction, lack of team cohesion, patient harm, legal ramifications, and disciplinary action.

The ANA (1997a) suggests using the Five Rights of Delegation as a framework for effective and safe delegation. The five **rights of delegation** (Hansten & Washburn, 1992) are:

- Right task
- Right person
- Right direction or communication
- Right supervision or feedback
- Right circumstances

The **right task** means that the agency, state Nurse Practice Act, or nursing board does not prohibit the task from being delegated. Even if a licensed practical nurse or an unlicensed assistive personnel is permitted to perform a task it is important to consider whether this particular licensed practical nurse or unlicensed assistive personnel is the **right person.** Consider the level of experience, education, and competency of the individual licensed practical nurse or unlicensed assistive personnel, and determine whether they are comfortable performing the task. The **right direction** involves giving a clear, concise description of the task, including your expectations. **Right supervision** means that either you or another registered nurse is available to monitor, evaluate, and intervene if needed. For example, don't assign a task to the unlicensed assistive personnel who requires supervision if you will then be away from the unit for an educational meeting. The **right circumstances** includes considering the overall situation of the nursing unit: Is the unit understaffed? Is patient acuity high? Is the skill-mix inappropriate?

This framework is intended as guidelines, not mandates for delegation. The nurse who has the responsibility for the patient must retain the final decision regarding delegation.

## Role of the Manager

The nurse manager needs to ensure that adequate educational programs are available for all staff who delegate tasks to others. According to the ANA (1997b), content for these programs needs to include appropriate utilization of licensed practical nurses and unlicensed assistive personnel, effective teaching and supervision, roles and relationships, cultural diversity, decision making, delegation and assignment definitions, and liability issues.

All members of the nursing staff need to understand each other's roles and responsibilities. The nurse manager needs to provide ongoing support and training to all members of the nursing staff as patient care continues to be restructured.

## ● SUMMARY

Case method, functional method, team nursing, primary nursing, nursing care management, and patient-focused care are common ways to organize nursing care. The case method involves total care for one or more patients by one nurse. It does not allow for 24-hour coverage or roles for ancillary personnel. The functional method is an assembly-line division of tasks often selected for its apparent efficiency, but often results in fragmented care. Team nursing focuses on the coordination and supervision of care given by the team, including ancillary staff. Primary nursing returns to the focus on the nurse as caregiver with associate nurses covering the other hours of the day. Both team and primary nursing are more difficult to implement than the functional or case methods. Nursing care management is designed to coordinate the many different services provided to a patient and to help the patient move through the system more easily. Patient-focused care decentralizes services, bringing them to the patient by the least number of caregivers possible. It focuses on the receiver of care rather than on the provider of care.

Many factors must be considered in planning the staffing for a nursing unit or healthcare organization: the acuity or complexity of patient care, the mix of ancillary and professional staff, and patient classification systems. Other factors include the number of patients on a unit (census), limitations imposed by the budget, and allowing for the effect of nonproductive time.

Patient classification systems include the prototype method, which simply categorizes patients according to their level of need, and the factor evaluation method, which calculates the amount of time needed to carry out specific procedures and expresses these amounts in standard units. This database is then used to create a staffing system to suit the individual organization. Staff nurses, clinical specialists, and nurse managers should be involved in the development of the classification schemes and staffing systems.

The use of unlicensed assistive personnel has increased in many healthcare facilities. It is important for nurse managers, nurse educators, and staff nurses to understand the educational preparation and scope of responsibility for unlicensed assistive personnel when making assignments.

Cross-training and floating are used in many healthcare facilities to respond efficiently to census fluctuation and changes in patient acuity levels. Both have advantages and disadvantages. It is important for staff nurses to be involved in the implementation of either approach and to know their role and responsibilities when accepting an assignment. The unit manager is responsible for ensuring that only qualified staff are floated to the unit. They also need to make sure that floating is not used to avoid hiring the needed number of staff.

Scheduling of staff may be either centralized or decentralized. Both methods have advantages and disadvantages. Flex-time, nontraditional shift times, and self-scheduling are different ways in which people's schedules can be made more flexible to meet the needs of both the staff and the institution. Temporary or pool staff can be used to supplement the staff during periods of vacations or peak census.

Delegation can occur between professional staff if only registered nurses are providing direct patient care. However, most often registered nurses delegate tasks to either licensed practical nurses or unlicensed assistive personnel. In either case, the five rights of delegation—right task, right person, right direction, right supervision, and right circumstances—can be used to guide the process.

# C A S E   S T U D Y

## Learning How to Delegate

"How are we going to make assignments now that we are changing from primary care to team nursing on the medical-surgical units?" This question came from a frustrated, overwhelmed group of nurse managers at the monthly nursing management meeting.

"Your registered nurses will need to learn how to delegate effectively," explained the vice-president of nursing.

"What do you mean by that?" asked a charge nurse.

"Do you remember the five rights of delegation?" replied the vice-president of nursing.

"Yes, they are right task, right person, right direction or communication, right feedback, and right circumstances," a nurse manager replied.

"I'm still not sure how to use this information when making assignments," said another nurse manager.

"Let me give you an example," the vice-president said. "You are the charge nurse on a 40-bed medical-surgical unit and have a census of 40 with six admissions scheduled to come in. Each team has one registered nurse, one licensed practical nurse, and two nursing assistants. You may consider the following when delegating tasks to the team members. The registered nurse can perform the initial assessment on the new admissions, review discharge planning, initiate patient teaching, evaluate care delivery and documentation, administer intravenous medications, and perform the complex procedures. The licensed practical nurse can perform routine vital signs, administer oral medications, perform simple treatments, and assist with personal care needs. Tasks for the nursing assistants include assist with personal care needs, transport patients, make beds, answer call lights, and assist patients at meal times."

"Let's try this out on our individual units. Then we can talk about it at next month's meeting," suggested a nurse manager.

## Questions for Critical Reflection and Analysis

1. How have the five rights of delegation been used in this example? What would you add to what the vice-president for nursing said to the nursing managers?
2. What other factors do you need to consider when making an assignment?
3. How would you handle the situation if someone on the team refused an assignment?
4. What would you do if the patient acuity level increased during the eight-hour shift?

# REFERENCES

Abbott, M. (1995). Measuring the effects of a self-scheduling committee. *Nursing Management, 26*(9), 64A–G.

Adams, A., Bond, S. & Hale, C.A. (1998). Nursing organizational practice and its relationship with other features of ward organization and job satisfaction. *Journal of Advanced Nursing, 27*(6), 1212–1222.

ANA (1997a). *Registered nurse utilization of unlicensed assistive personnel.* Washington, DC: American Nurses Association.

ANA (1997b). *Registered nurse education relating to the utilization of unlicensed assistive personnel.* Washington, DC: American Nurses Association.

Ballew, J.R. & Mink, G. (1986). *Case management in the human services.* Springfield, IL: Charles C. Thomas.

Banks, N., Hardy, B. & Meskimen, K. (1999). Take the plunge: Expanding the float pool to "closed" units. *Nursing Management, 30*(1), 51–55.

Barrett, S. (1991). *Executive summary of 1990 national nurse manager study by American organization of nurse executives.* Chicago, IL: American Hospital Association.

Barter, M., McLaughlin, F. & Thomas, S. (1994). Use of unlicensed assistive personnel by hospitals. *Nursing Economics, 12*(2), 82–87.

Biller, A.M. (1992). Implementing nursing case management. *Rehabilitation Nursing, 17*(3), 144–146.

Birdsall, C. & Sperry, S.P. (1997). *Clinical paths in medical-surgical practice*. St. Louis: Mosby.

Bower, K.A. (1992). *Case management by nurses*. Washington, DC: American Nurses Association.

Bowers-Hutto, C. & Davis, L. (1989). 12-hour shifts: Panacea or problem? *Nursing Management, 20,* 56B–H.

Brider, P. (1992). The move to patient-focused care. *American Journal of Nursing, 92*(9), 27–33.

Brown, B.J. (1980). *Nurse staffing: A practical guide*. Germantown, MD: Aspen.

Cherry, B. (1999). Nursing care delivery models. In B. Cherry & S.R. Jacob (Ed.). *Contemporary nursing: Issues, trends and management*. St. Louis, Mosby.

Daly, B.J., Phelps, C. & Rudy, E.B. (1991). A nurse-managed special care unit. *Journal of Nursing Administration, 21*(7/8), 31–38.

Davidhizar, R., Dowd, S. & Brownson, K. (1998). An equitable nursing assignment structure. *Nursing Management, 29* (4), 33–36.

Davis, C. (1996). IOM panel demands proof that cuts are hurting care. *American Journal of Nursing, 96* (3), 67–70.

Fagin, C. (1982). The economic value of nursing research. *American Journal of Nursing, 82* (12), 1844–1849.

Fairbanks, J.E. (1981). Primary nursing: More data. *Nursing Administration Quarterly, 5*(3), 51.

*Federal Register* (1998). *List of diagnosis related groups, 63* (89). Washington, DC: U.S. Government Printing Office.

Fields, W. & Loveridge, C. (1988). Critical thinking and fatigue: How do nurses on 8 and 12 hour shifts compare? *Nursing Economics, 6,* 189–191.

Gould, R., Thompson, R., Rakel, J., Hasselman, E. & Young, L. (1996). Redesigning the RN and NA role. *Nursing Management, 27* (2), 37–31.

Gray, R. & Smedley, N. (1998). Assessing primary nursing in mental health. *Nursing Standard, 12*(21), 35–38.

Halloran, E. & Vermeersch, P. (1987). Variability in nurse staffing research. *Journal of Nursing Administration, 17* (2), 26–34.

Hansten, R. & Washburn, M. (1992). How to plan what to delegate. *American Journal of Nursing, 92* (4), 71–72.

Harris, M.D. (1998). The impact of the Balanced Budget Act of 1997 on home healthcare agencies and nurses. *Home Healthcare Nurse, 16*(7), 435–437.

Haydel, J. (1998). Help for home health strategies. *Nursing Management, 29*(12), 30–32.

Hill, L. (1992). *Becoming a manager*. Boston: Harvard Business School Press.

Hilliard, L. & Marrelli, T. (1997). Day-to-day operations. In T. Marrelli (Ed.). *The nurse manager's survival guide*. St. Louis: Mosby, 105–137.

Ketter, J. (1994). The ethical and legal implications of restructuring: Floating without being properly trained. *American Nurse, 26* (7), 23.

Kobs, A. (1997). The adequacy of nurse staffing. *Nursing Management, 28* (11), 16–20.

Kovner, C. & Gergen, P.J. (1998). Nurse staffing levels and adverse events following surgery in U.S. hospitals. *Image, 30* (4), 315–321.

Kramer, M. (1971). Team nursing—A means or an end? *Nursing Outlook, 19*(10), 648–652.

Lamb, G.S. & Rapacz, K. (1991). *Nurse case management model: Curriculum and sample model*. Tucson: Carondelet St. Mary's Hospital and Health Center.

Lambertsen, E.C. (1953). *Nursing team: Organization and functioning*. New York: Teachers College Press.

Leebov, W. & Ersoz, C.J. (1991). *The health care manager's guide to continuous quality improvement*. Chicago: American Hospital Association.

Lichtig, L.K., Knauf, R.A. & Milholland, D.K. (1999). Some impacts of nursing on acute care hospital outcomes. *Journal of Nursing Administration, 29* (2), 25–33.

Marks, L., Dennis, R., Borozny, M. & Ferrone, K. (1999). The new team triad. *Nursing Management, 30* (2), 44–46.

Marram, G.D., Barrett, M.W. & Bevis, E.O. (1979). *Primary nursing: A model for individual care*. St. Louis: C.V. Mosby.

Marrelli, T.M. (1997). *The nurse manager's survival guide*, 2d ed. St. Louis: Mosby.

Melchior, M., Halfens, R.J.G., Aker-Saad, H.H., Philipsen, H., Van den Berg, A.A. & Gassman, P. (1999). The effects of primary nursing on work-related factors. *Journal of Advanced Nursing, 29*(1), 88–96.

Mills, M., Arnold, B. & Wood, C. (1983). Core 12: A controlled study of the impact of 12-hour scheduling. *Nursing Research, 32,* 356–361.

Nagaprasanna, B. (1988). Patient classification systems: Strategies for the 1990s. *Nursing Management, 19* (3), 105.

Network, Inc. (1996, December). *Implementation of a nursing report card for acute care settings*. Final report presented at meeting of American Nurses Association.

Nicholls, D. (1996). Nurse's attitudes about floating. *Nursing Management, 27* (1), 56–58.

O'Brien-Pallas, L., Cockerill, R. & Leatt, P. (1992). Different systems, different costs. *Journal of Nursing Administration, 22* (2).

Orstein, H. (1992). The floating dilemma. *Canadian Nurse, 88* (9), 20–22.

Pontin, D. (1999). Primary nursing: A mode of care or a philosophy of nursing? *Journal of Advanced Nursing, 29*(3), 584–591.

Porter-O'Grady, T. (1998). Health care's best value. *Nursing Management, 29* (11), 3.

Reed, L. (1999). Important changes in home health care. *Rehabilitation Nursing, 24*(1), 4–5.

Robinson, J.A., Robinson, K.J. & Lewis, D.J. (1992). Balancing quality of care and cost-effectiveness through case management. *ANNA Journal, 19*(2), 182–188.

Rowland, H.S. & Rowland, B.L. (1980). *Nursing administration handbook.* Germantown, MD: Aspen.

Sheehan, J. (1998). Directing UAPs safely. *RN, 61*(6), 53–55.

Sherman, R.O. (1990). Team nursing revisited. *Journal of Nursing Administration, 20*(11), 43–46.

Shindul-Rothschild, J., Berry, D. & Long-Middleton, E. (1996). Where have all the nurses gone? *American Journal of Nursing, 96* (11), 25–39.

Siehoff, A. (1998). Impact of unlicensed assistive personnel on patient satisfaction: An integrative review of the literature. *Journal of Nursing Care Quality, 13* (2), 1–10.

Snyder, J. & Nethersole-Chong, D. (1999). Is cross-training medical-surgical RNs to ICU the answer? *Nursing Management, 30* (1), 58–60.

Sovie, M.D. (1999, June 9–11). *Hospital restructuring's impact on outcomes (HRIO).* Paper presented at the Invitational Conference for Nurse Executives, Philadelphia, PA.

Steven, A. (1999). Named nursing: In whose best interest? *Journal of Advanced Nursing, 29*(2), 341–347.

Stillwaggon, C.A. (1989). The impact of nurse managed care on the cost of nurse practice and nurse satisfaction. *Journal of Nursing Administration, 19*(11), 21–27.

Swansburg, R.C. & Swansburg, R.J. (1999). *Introductory management and leadership for nurses,* 2d ed. Boston: Jones & Bartlett.

Tappen, R., Turkel, M., Hall, R., Stahura, P. & Morgan, F. (1997). Nurses in transition: A response to the changing health care system. In S. Moorhead & D.G. Huber, Nursing roles: Evolving or recycled, *Series on Nursing Administration, 9,* 117–127.

Todd, C., Reid, N. & Robinson, G. (1991). The impact of 12-hour nursing shifts. *Nursing Times, 87,* 47–50.

Townsend, M.B. (1993). Patient-focused care: Is it for your hospital? *Nursing Management, 24*(9), 74–80.

Trossman, S. (1999, January/February). Staffing smart: A difficult proposition. *The American Nurse, 31* (1), 1–2.

Turkel, M., Tappen, R. & Hall, R. (1999). Moments of excellence: The experience of nursing home nurses following their patients home after discharge. *Journal of Gerontological Nursing, 25*(1), 7–12.

Ugrovics, A. & Wright, J. (1990). 12-hour shifts: Does fatigue undermine ICU nursing judgment? *Nursing Management, 21,* 64A.

Ventura, M. (1999). Staffing issues. *RN, 62*(2), 26–31.

Washburn, M.S. (1991). Fatigue and critical thinking on eight and twelve hour shifts. *Nursing Management, 22* (9), 80A–F.

White-Fletcher, K. (1995). A manager's viewpoint. In P. Yoder-Wise (Ed.). *Leading and managing in nursing.* St. Louis: Mosby, 437.

Williams, M., Donaldson, C. & Watts, J. (1998). Educate ICU assistive personnel. *Nursing Management, 29* (12), 32B–H.

Williams, S. & Torrens, S. (1998). *Introduction to health services,* 5th ed. Albany, NY: Delmar.

Wulff, K. (1997). Flex-time and self-scheduling: Transitional leadership tools. In J. McCloskey & H.K. Grace (Eds.). *Current Issues in Nursing,* 5th ed. St. Louis: Mosby, 397–402.

Zander, K. (1985). Second generation primary nursing: A new generation. *Journal of Nursing Administration, 15*(3), 18–24.

Zander, K. (1990). Managed care and nursing case management. In G.G. Mayer, M.J. Madden & E. Lawrenz, (Eds.). *Patient care delivery models.* Rockville, MD: Aspen.

Zimmerman, P. (1996a). Use of unlicensed assistive personnel: Anecdotes and antidotes. *Journal of Emergency Nursing, 22* (1), 42–48.

Zimmerman, P. (1996b). Delegating to assistive personnel. *Journal of Emergency Nursing, 22* (3), 206–212.

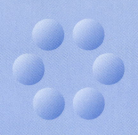

CHAPTER *13*

# Individual Evaluation Procedures

## LEARNING OBJECTIVES

*After completing this chapter, the reader will be able to:*

- Provide both positive and negative feedback in a constructive manner.
- Write objectives that are appropriate and include observable outcomes.
- Define management by objectives and list its advantages and disadvantages.

- Conduct a formal performance appraisal.
- Evaluate the objectivity and constructiveness of evaluation procedures.
- Participate in peer review procedures.

## TEST YOURSELF

**Which of the following evaluative comments from a team leader to a member of the team are appropriate (OK)? Which ones are not (NOT OK)?**

____ 1. The lab sent Mr. Bassano's stool specimen back as "quantity insufficient to test."

____ 2. You missed the last three team meetings.

____ 3. Tell me why you did that.

____ 4. Your handwriting is just awful.

____ 5. I can't read your handwriting.

____ 6. Stop! You're going to kill him.

____ 7. What the h _ _ _ do you think you're doing?

____ 8. You are 15 minutes late for your lunch break.

____ 9. Everyone is finished with their assignments except you.

____ 10. I like the way you work.

*Answers*

1. OK: Statement of fact. 2. OK: Statement of fact. 3. OK: Implies a problem but allows opportunity to explain. 4. NOT OK: too general. 5. OK: Specific problem communicated. 6. NOT OK: Too strong and no explanation of why the action was incorrect. 7. NOT OK: Angry, blaming. 8. OK: Statement of fact. 9. NOT OK: Implies blame without seeking explanation. 10. NOT OK: Too general, based on personal opinion, not a standard of care.

Everyone needs to know how well they are doing. From the chief executive officer to the lowest-paid clerk, people need to know where they stand and what impact they have on the organization. They need to know how valued they are, how others respond to them, how well they have solved a problem, whether they have been helpful to other people, and more generally, how effective their work has been.

You may recall that giving feedback was one of the actions listed in the components of effective leadership and that monitoring work was one of the components of effective management. These components are considered in detail in this chapter.

The term **informal evaluation** is used to distinguish it from formal procedures such as performance appraisals and/or peer reviews that are mandated by organizations or by accrediting agencies. Informal evaluation occurs during the give and take of other work activities. It is a continuous process, an action that should occur often, whenever it is needed rather than according to schedule. It is also an integral part of the activities of a well-functioning team and the responsibility of every member of the team, not just the team leader. The team leader or manager has the extra responsibility of ensuring that it does occur and that it is done appropriately.

**Formal evaluation** procedures may occur only once or twice a year. They usually have an explicit structure, including specific forms to fill out and timetables for carrying out the procedures. Alone, this structure is inadequate to provide the continuous guidance and recognition that people need at work, but with frequent informal feedback it meets these needs.

## ● INFORMAL INDIVIDUAL EVALUATION

### Purpose of Providing Evaluative Feedback

People function better when they receive constructive feedback about their performance. From a leadership perspective, feedback equals information, information that is valuable, often critical, to the individual (Napolitano & Henderson, 1998). Failing to give or receive feedback reduces the immediate risk of being exposed to criticism but increases the risk of later failure. Evaluative feedback serves many purposes. It clarifies performance expectations, reinforces constructive behavior, corrects negative behavior, provides recognition, increases self-awareness, and promotes growth and change (Mager & Pipe, 1970).

- *Clarify Performance Expectations.* No matter how clearly job descriptions are written (and sometimes they do not even exist), all the details of what a particular job entails are difficult to describe in writing. Informal feedback is an effective way to communicate these details. Feedback verifies for people either that they understand what is expected of them or that they need to clarify these expectations.
- *Reinforce Constructive Behavior.* Evaluative feedback can confirm that people are performing well. Providing positive feedback encourages constructive behavior, increases motivation, and promotes job satisfaction.
- *Correct Unsatisfactory Behavior.* Poor performance must be acknowledged and steps taken to correct it. Pointing out such performance is often mistakenly assumed to be the only purpose for evaluation.
- *Provide Recognition.* Recognition for work well done is a powerful and inexpensive reward for good performance (Cronin & Becherer, 1999). It meets those needs for esteem and recognition that all people have, whether they

make it apparent or not. The power of praise is frequently underestimated (Glaser, 1994).
- *Increase Self-Awareness.* Feedback helps people identify their strengths and weaknesses so that the efforts of the individual can be directed toward building on strengths and working on improving in areas of weakness.
- *Promote Growth and Change.* Frequent feedback challenges caregivers to continually do their very best. It also encourages people to use their resources when they face a problem or a difficult decision and to look for opportunities to upgrade their knowledge and skills.

### Guidelines for Providing Constructive Feedback

Evaluation involves making judgments and communicating these judgments to others. People make judgments all the time about all types of things yet are often uncomfortable sharing them in a work setting.

Sometimes these judgments are based on opinions, preferences, or inaccurate or partial information. Biased, hasty judgment offered as objective feedback has given evaluation a bad name (Messmer, 1998; Williams, 1998). Poorly communicated feedback has an equally negative effect. In fact, you will find that many of the people who are uncomfortable with evaluation have been the recipients of thoughtless, biased, or poorly communicated evaluations in the past.

When poorly done, evaluation can be destructive. It can reinforce ineffective work habits, reduce self-esteem, and destroy motivation. On the other hand, when it is done well, it can reinforce motivation, strengthen the team, and improve the quality of care given.

> *[Effective] Leaders make it clear that there is no failure, only mistakes that give us feedback and tell us what to do next.*
> —Warren Bennis, 1984, quoted in Fitton, 1997

Evaluative feedback is most effective when it is given immediately, frequently, and privately. To be constructive, it must be objective, specific, based on observed behavior, and skillfully communicated. The feedback message should include the reason why a behavior has been judged good or poor. If the message is negative it should be nonthreatening and include suggestions and support for change and improvement. Each of these criteria is discussed further.

### Provide Both Positive and Negative Feedback

Leaders and first-line managers often neglect to provide positive feedback. If questioned, people who do not give positive feedback usually respond, "If I don't say anything, that means everything is okay." Unfortunately, some people assume that everything is *not* okay when they receive no feedback. Many more will assume that no one is aware of how much effort has gone into their work unless it is acknowledged with positive feedback.

Most people want to do their work well. They also want to know that their efforts are recognized and appreciated; it is a real pleasure to be able to share the satisfaction of a job well done with someone else. Kron (1981) called positive feedback a "psychological paycheck" and pointed out that it is almost as important to people as their actual paycheck.

It is often claimed that nurses do not do enough to support each other as colleagues. Whether or not that statement is true, giving positive feedback is an important way to support your colleagues.

Negative or corrective feedback is just as necessary as positive feedback. Too often, negative feedback is critical rather than constructive. It is easier to just tell people that something has gone wrong or could have been done better than it is to make the feedback a learning experience by suggesting ways to make the needed changes or working together to develop a strategy for improvement.

Providing no negative feedback at all is the easiest but least effective solution to the problem of being too critical. Unsatisfactory work must be recognized and discussed with the people involved. The "gutless wonder" who silently tolerates poor work encourages it to continue and undermines the motivation of the whole team (Del Bueno, 1977).

### Give Immediate Feedback

The most helpful feedback, positive or negative, is given as soon as possible after the behavior has occurred for several reasons. Immediate feedback is more meaningful to the person receiving it. If it is delayed too long, the person may have forgotten the incident altogether or assumed that your silence indicated approval. Like other confrontation situations, problems that are ignored often get worse. In the meantime, a lot of frustration and anger can build up. When feedback is given as soon as possible, this buildup of negative feelings is prevented.

### Provide Frequent Feedback

Feedback should not only be immediate but also frequent. Frequent constructive feedback keeps motivation and awareness levels high and avoids the possibility that problems will grow larger and more serious before they are confronted.

Giving feedback becomes easier with practice. If giving and receiving feedback is a frequent and integral part of team functioning, it will be easier to do and less threatening to most people. It becomes an ordinary, everyday occurrence, one that happens regularly and is familiar to everyone on the team. Giving negative feedback privately rather than in front of others prevents embarrassment. It also avoids the possibility that those who overhear the discussion may misunderstand it and draw erroneous conclusions from it. It has been suggested that a manager should praise staff in public but correct them in private (Matejka, Ashworth & Dodd-McCue, 1986).

### Be Specific

It is easier to make broad, critical comments, such as "You're too slow," than it is to specifically describe the behavior that needs improvement, such as saying to an assistant "Waiting in Mr. D.'s room while he finishes his breakfast takes up too much of your time," and then adding a suggestion for change such as "You could get your bath supplies together while he finishes eating."

Specific information serves as a guide to improvement. Overly general comments leave a person wondering exactly what is wrong. It also leaves the person without any guidelines for improving his or her work.

Furthermore, if what you say is too vague or ambiguous, then it is open to interpretation. In other words, if you are not specific about what the problem is and what the solution could be, then you leave people free to interpret what you said in whatever way might occur to them—clearly not the purpose when providing evaluative feedback (Robbins & Finley, 1995).

## Be Objective

It can be difficult to be objective when giving feedback to others. Using critical reflection and analysis (Chapter 9), avoiding emotional arguments, and assuring that data are adequate can be helpful here. People should be evaluated on the basis of job expectations and not compared, favorably or unfavorably, with other staff members.

Another way to increase objectivity is to always give a reason why you have judged a behavior as good or poor. Reasons should be given for both positive and negative messages. For example, if you tell a coworker, "that was a good interview," you have told that person nothing except that the interview pleased you. However, when you add to the message, "because you asked many open-ended questions that encouraged the client to explore personal feelings," you have identified the specific behavior and reinforced it.

Finally, to the extent possible, use generally accepted standards for judgments to avoid basing evaluation on personal likes and dislikes. Objectivity can be increased by using standards that reflect the consensus of the team, the organization, the community, or the profession as a whole. Formal evaluation should always be based on an agreed-upon, written standard of what is acceptable behavior. Informal evaluation, however, is usually based on unwritten standards. If these standards are based on personal preferences, the evaluation will be highly subjective. Here are some examples:

*A team leader who thinks a female social worker has a professional appearance because she wears dark suits instead of bright dresses is using a personal standard.*

*A supervisor who asks an employee to stop wearing jewelry that could get caught in the equipment used is applying a generally accepted standard of safety.*

*The nursing home administrator who insists that staff include every resident in the weekly birthday party game is applying a personal standard. In comparison, the administrator who insists that staff members offer every resident the opportunity to participate in weekly activities is applying a professional standard.*

## Base on Observable Behavior

An evaluative statement should describe observed behavior, not personality traits or interpretations of behavior. The observation is much more likely to be factual and accurate than the interpretation is. It is also less likely to evoke a defensive response. Here is an example:

*Saying, "You were impatient with Mrs. G. today," is an interpretive comment. Saying, "You interrupted Mrs. G. before she finished explaining her problem," is based on observable behavior. It is not only specific but may be more accurate as the caregiver may have been trying to redirect the conversation to more immediate concerns, not feeling impatient.*

## Communicate Appropriately

An evaluative statement is a form of confrontation. Any message that contains a statement about the behavior of a staff member is confronting that staff member with information. All the guidelines given in Chapter 4 about the appropriate way to confront another person or group apply to giving evaluative feedback.

As with other confrontations, the leader who gives evaluative feedback needs to be prepared to engage in active listening and to receive feedback in return. Active listening is especially important because the person receiving the evaluation may respond with disagreement and high emotion. Here is an example of what may happen:

*Let's say that you point out to Mr. S. that his patients need to be monitored more frequently. Mr. S. responds emotionally that he is doing everything possible for the patients and does not have a free moment all day for one extra thing. In fact, Mr. S. tells you he never even takes a lunch break and goes home exhausted. Active listening and problem solving with this employee aimed at relieving his overloaded time schedule are a must in this situation.*

When you give negative feedback, allow time for ventilation of feelings and then for problem solving with the individual to find ways to improve a situation. This two-part approach is particularly important if the problem has been ignored long enough to become as serious as in the example given.

### Include Suggestions for Change

When you give feedback to an employee that indicates a change in behavior is needed, it is helpful to suggest alternative behaviors. Making suggestions is easier when the change is a simple one.

When complex change is needed (as in the previous example), you may find that the person is aware of the problem but does not know how to solve it. In such a case, oversimplified solutions are inappropriate but an offer to engage with the person in searching for a solution is appropriate. A demonstrated willingness to listen to the other person's side of the story and to assist in finding a solution also indicates that your purpose was to help rather that just to criticize the individual.

### Communicate in a Nonthreatening Manner

When the feedback is negative, the focus of the message should be on the specific behavior, not on the person as a whole, which devalues and threatens self-esteem. Threatening messages reduce motivation and inhibit learning by diverting people's energies into activities aimed at reducing the threat. Although a small degree of anxiety may increase learning, too much immobilizes people. The ultimate purpose for providing informal evaluation is, after all, to improve the function of the team and its individual members.

> **Advice is like castor oil—easy enough to give, but difficult to take.**
>
> —Anonymous, quoted in Fitton, 1997

Negative feedback may contain hints of dire consequences, probably in the mistaken belief that it will increase the person's motivation to change. The following are some common examples:

*"You're not going to last long if you keep doing that."*

*"People who want to do well here make sure their assignments are done on time."*

*"Don't argue with the doctors; they'll report you to the nursing office."*

When a person's behavior actually does threaten job security, a formal warning stating this fact and proposing needed change is appropriate.

You may have assumed that people in the ranks above you (manager, supervisor, director, and so forth) could not be threatened by feedback from you. It is not true. They are all human and as susceptible to feeling threatened as you are. You need to follow the same guidelines in giving feedback to people above you in the organization as you do with people below you in organizational hierarchy.

## Seeking Evaluative Feedback

Just as important as knowing how to give feedback is knowing when to look for it and how to take it. The purposes for seeking feedback are the same as those for giving it to others. The criteria for evaluating the feedback you receive are also the same.

### When Evaluative Feedback Is Needed

In a number of different situations you need to seek feedback. For example, you could find yourself in a work situation where you receive little feedback from any source other than your own evaluation of your work. Or you may be getting only positive and no negative comments, or vice versa.

Another time when you need to look for feedback is when you feel uncertain about how well you are doing or whether you have correctly interpreted the expectations of the job. The following are some examples of these situations:

*You have been told repeatedly that good patient care is the first consideration of your job but feel totally frustrated by never having enough staff to give good care.*

*You thought you were expected to do case finding and preventive care in your community, but receive the most feedback on the number of home visits made and the completeness of your records.*

An additional instance in which you should request feedback is when you feel that your needs for recognition and job satisfaction have not been met adequately.

Requests for feedback should be made in the form of "I" messages. If you have received only negative comments, ask, "In what ways have I done well?" If you receive only positive comments, you can ask, "In what areas do I need to improve?" Or, if you are seeking feedback from a patient, you could ask, "How can I be of more help to you?"

## Responding to Evaluative Feedback

At times, it is appropriate to critically analyze the feedback you are getting. If the feedback seems totally negative or you feel threatened by what you are being told, ask for further explanation. You may have misunderstood what the person meant to say.

It is hard to avoid responding defensively to negative feedback that is subjective or laced with threats and blame. But if you are the recipient of a poorly done evaluation, it may help both you and your supervisor if you try to guide the discussion into more constructive areas. You can ask for reasons why the evaluation was negative, what standard it is based on, what the person's expectations were, and what the person suggests as alternative behavior.

When the feedback is positive but nonspecific, you may also want to ask for some specifics so that you can find out what that person's expectations are. Do not hesitate to seek that psychological paycheck. Tell other people about your successes—most are happy to share your satisfaction in a successful outcome or positive development in a patient's care.

**We protest against unjust criticism, but we accept unearned praise.**

*—Anonymous, quoted in Fitton, 1997*

## ● FORMAL INDIVIDUAL EVALUATION

As a first-line manager you will be expected to do formal evaluations. In addition, whether or not you are a nurse manager, you may also be involved in setting up evaluation procedures. To be effective, you need to know the purposes of formal evaluation, how to develop and use standards, and how to write objectives. Even more important is the ability to be objective in your evaluation and to use communication skills effectively in sharing the information with the person who was evaluated. These aspects are so important that many organizations hold workshops on evaluation and schedule skill-training sessions for people who do performance appraisals (formal employee evaluations).

As an employee, you will also be the **subject** of evaluation procedures. When you are evaluated, you need to know what constitutes an objective evaluation and how to communicate effectively (see Box 13–1).

---

**Box 13–1   Performance Appraisal Failures**

**Typical Mistakes Made by Managers in the Conduct of Performance Appraisals**

- Using incomplete or inaccurate information
- Ambiguous performance measures
- Irrelevant criteria
- Overemphasis on neatness, punctuality, or courteousness for people at the professional level
- Subjectivity (influenced by personal preferences, personality, gender, race, ethnic group)
- Halo effect, either positive or negative
- Avoidance of sensitive or "touchy" subjects
- Failure to reward excellent performance
- Failure to correct poor performance

*Sources:* Based on Messmer, M. (1998). *The fast forward MBA in hiring: Finding and keeping the best people.* New York: John Wiley & Sons; Williams, R.S. (1998). *Performance management.* London: International Thomson Business Press.

## Purpose of Formal Evaluation

The purposes of informal evaluation described earlier (providing recognition, increasing self-awareness, and so forth) also apply to formal evaluation. Formal evaluation has additional purposes related to the function of the organization, to the regulatory and accrediting bodies that require such procedures, and to the professions represented by those who are involved in the procedures.

### Accountability

Evaluation is an important demonstration of both the employee's and the healthcare organization's sense of responsibility for the services provided. It is a demonstration to the public that efforts are being made to provide quality care.

Individual healthcare professionals are accountable for the care they give. Participation in evaluation procedures in which the caregiver is judged against an accepted standard is one way to achieve this accountability.

### Administrative Intervention

Evaluation that is taken seriously by upper-level management can be a stimulus for change. Regular evaluation of individual staff members identifies weaknesses before they become major obstacles to achieving desired objectives. If these evaluations are based on the goals and standards of the organization, they can answer a number of questions, including the following:

- Are expected objectives being achieved?
- Are patients' needs being met?
- Is care being given both efficiently and effectively?

Because the leadership of any organization can be crucial to its effectiveness, upper-level management people should also be evaluated.

### Rewards

Formal evaluations should serve as the basis on which employees are given raises and promotions to reward satisfactory or better performance. Evaluations are also the basis for termination of employment when consistently poor appraisals follow substantial efforts to remedy the problem.

### Identification of Educational Needs

The data resulting from formal evaluation procedures can be used to analyze the continuing education and developmental needs of the people who work in an organization and the success of any training programs or other initiatives undertaken to improve performance (Hannigan, 1998). For example, such an analysis could point out a specific need such as improving the leadership skills of members of interdisciplinary teams.

For an alternative view on the value of performance appraisals, see Perspectives . . . Abolish Performance Appraisals?

## Performance Appraisals

**Performance appraisals** are formal evaluations of employees by a superior, usually a manager or supervisor of some kind. The employee's behavior is compared with a set of objectives or standards describing how the employee is expected to perform. Employees need to know *what* has to be done, *how much* has to be done, and *when* it has to be done (Hansen, 1986). Actual performance is evaluated, not intentions.

Ideally, performance appraisal is an ongoing activity, not a once-a-year event. It should begin with the translation of organizational goals into clear expectations for each employee (Kolb, Osland & Rubin, 1995). Based on a written job description (see Box 13–2), the employee and manager discuss the expected standard of performance (see Table 13–1) or write a set of objectives (for examples, see Table 13–2) that they think the employee can reasonably accomplish within a given time. The objectives should be written at a level of performance that demonstrates that some learning, attainment or refinement of a skill, or advancement toward some long-range objective has taken place. The following are examples of objectives that could be set for a patient educator to accomplish in six months:

- Conduct a survey of patient use and response to the closed-circuit television programs.
- Include staff in development of a proposal for a neuropsychological rehabilitation program.

# PERSPECTIVES . . .

## Abolish Performance Appraisals?

The well-known quality management "guru" W. Edwards Deming suggested that performance appraisals have a "ruinous" effect on people. They cause "humiliation, crush out joy of learning, innovation, joy on the job" (quoted by Messmer, 1998, p. 199) he said in an interview. In addition, because much of what any employee can accomplish is determined by the system in which he or she is operating, any evaluation is really an appraisal of what has occurred between individual, organization, and the constraints under which they operate, it is argued. Hannigan (1998) described performance appraisal as subjective, difficult, full of problems, and unpopular with all involved (p. 233).

A harsh judgment of performance appraisal? Messmer says maybe not if you consider all the pitfalls of performance appraisal. Consider these drawbacks:

- Traditional performance appraisal of an employee by a manager has no relevance to self-directed teams of professionals and has an authoritarian air that is incompatible with modern ways to motivate people (Foust, 1999).
- If the appraisals are too positive, the employee may take it easy or be promoted and, therefore, lost to the department or unit. If they are too negative the employee may leave or be fired. Neither is a win-win situation.
- No matter how specific the criteria are, performance appraisals are always at least partially subjective.

It is difficult to obtain consistent ratings for the same level of performance across a number of different managers. Therefore, the employee working for a lenient manager will get a higher rating than an employee doing equally good work for a demanding manager.

Messmer is not alone in this opinion. Kolb and colleagues (1995) note that many total quality experts suggest focusing on providing continuous feedback and coaching of employees and stop doing performance appraisals (p. 488).

Do you think we should abandon performance appraisal? If we did, what do you think we should use instead?

*Sources:* Messmer, M. (1998). *The fast forward MBA in hiring: Finding and keeping the best people.* New York: John Wiley & Sons. Kolb, D.A., Osland, J.S. & Rubin, I.M. (1995). *Organizational behavior: An experiential approach.* Englewood Cliffs, NJ: Prentice Hall. Hannigan, T.A. (1998). *Managing tomorrow's high-performance unions.* Westport, CT: Quorum Books.

- Continue to conduct birthing classes for the community.
- Implement a cancer support group.

Six months later, at the previously agreed-upon time, the employee and supervisor sit down again and evaluate the employee's performance in terms of the previously set goals or standards. The evaluation should be based on both the employee's self-assessment and the supervisor's observation of specific behaviors. A copy of the performance appraisal and plan for the next year must be available to the employee so that he or she can refer back to them and check on progress toward the agreed-upon goals.

## Setting Objectives and Standards

### Using Objectives

The purpose of using objectives in formal evaluations is to set forth expectations by clearly specifying what direction the employee's work should take and what specific accomplishments (outcomes) are expected within a given time. The objectives serve first as a guide to the planning of the work and later as a guide to evaluating that work.

When objectives are used as a part of a formal system of management, they may be written not only for individual employees but also for larger work groups, including committees, departments, and the organization as a whole (Table 13–2 shows some examples). Congruence between these different levels of objectives is sometimes difficult to achieve.

### Essentials of Management by Objectives

The essentials of management by objectives (MBO) are quite simple: set meaningful goals written in the form of objectives, work on carry-

> **Box 13–2  Sample Job Descriptions**
>
> **Clinical Nurse I (CN I)**
>
> The clinical nurse I supports the philosophy of primary nursing by planning and coordinating nursing care for a group of patients within his/her district. It is the CN I's responsibility to direct auxiliary personnel for full implementation of the plan of care. The CN I supports the management of the unit and uses resource persons and/or materials when the need arises. He/She has satisfactorily mastered the basic skills required to work on the assigned unit. The CN I's scope of nursing practice is focused on his/her assigned group of patients and does not extend into the administrative aspects of the unit at large.
>
> **Clinical Nurse IV (CN IV)—Unit Clinician**
>
> The CN IV is an advanced clinical nurse who supports the practice of primary nursing on the unit, as well as hospitalwide. He/She is recognized within the specialty area, as well as throughout the hospital, as being proficient in the delivery of complicated nursing care. The CN IV has mastered the many facets of nursing care required at the CN II and CN III levels. This qualification is validated through the acquisition of national certification in the appropriate specialty area.
>
> The CN IV coordinates and directs emergency situations, seeks out learning opportunities for the unit staff, and serves as a resource for all aspects of nursing care delivery.
>
> The CN IV collaborates closely with physicians on the unit for the implementation of the plan of care. This collaboration may be facilitated through assessing special equipment needs, as well as planning multidisciplinary programs.
>
> The CN IV works closely with the nurse manager in planning unit goals and objectives and unit specific orientation programs, as well as assisting with staff performance evaluations.
>
> The CN IV acts as a liaison between his/her unit and the departments of nursing education and patient education.
>
> *Source:* Adapted from Baptist Hospital of Miami, FL, Professional Nursing Advancement Program. Used with permission.

ing out the objectives, then evaluate how well the objectives have been met. The procedure assumes that a thorough assessment of the needs of the work situation has already been done.

The first step in MBO is to create a set of objectives for a given time period. The objectives should begin with an action verb and describe an activity that can be observed and, if possible, measured. They should be specific, timebound, and state a measurable or observable end result in order to increase the objectivity of the evaluation.

The objectives should also be **meaningful** and **congruent** with the goals of the system. Meaning-

less objectives tend to describe the routine activities that accompany any job or specify no action at all, such as "have a positive attitude toward work." The objectives should be challenging but achievable (Conrad, 1990). Often the less quantifiable objectives such as "increasing team cohesion" are left out because they are difficult to write and even more difficult to measure (Kerr, 1997). Nevertheless, attempts should be made to include them and to specify evidence that indicates they have been achieved.

The **time** set for completing the objectives depends on the nature of the work being planned.

**Table 13–1** Sample Performance Standards

| Responsibility to Patient | CN I | CN II | CN III | CN IV |
|---|---|---|---|---|
| **1.** Plans care for duration of stay on clinical unit | a. Addresses family/social concerns in the assessment process, as evidenced by nursing care documentation<br>b. Records all admission documentation on assigned patients<br>c. Reviews history as it reflects information relevant to current hospitalization<br>d. Updates patient problem/outcome statements and/or designates as achieved<br>e. Documents patient teaching, transfer, and/or discharge preparation | a. through e.<br>f. Utilizes nursing history for care planning by auditing charts for integration of problem statements<br>g. Assesses supplies/equipment and has them readily available for patient use<br>h. Initiates discharge summary sheet prior to discharge | a. through h.<br>i. Identifies need for and/or initiates appropriate family/social referrals with documentation<br>j. Assesses and documents cultural differences, patient support systems, and expectation for hospitalization<br>k. Documents patient's response to teaching as identified in nursing care documentation | a. through k.<br>l. Collaborates with the Department of Patient Education in designing and revising patient teaching materials |
| **TO PEERS**<br>**1.** Avails himself or herself to coworkers at all times | a. Notifies peers when required to leave the clinical area<br>b. Assumes responsibility for I.V.s and orders of LPN on assigned patients<br>c. Responds promptly to all emergency situations that arise in the district | a. through c.<br>d. Takes initiative to offer assistance to other nurses and with assigned patients<br>e. Serves as preceptor to students/orientees | a. through e.<br>f. Acts as senior resource coordinator in absence of nurse manager | a. through f.<br>g. Coordinates/teaches two programs in conjunction with the Dept. of Nursing Education annually<br>h. Conducts staff conferences to evaluate clinical competencies of personnel with documentation |

Adapted from Professional Nursing Advancement Program, Baptist Hospital, Miami, Florida, with permission.

| **Table 13–2** | Examples of Individual, Group, and Organization-Level Objectives |
|---|---|
| **Level** | **Objective** |
| Individual Staff Nurse | Complete a course on infection control in the home. |
| Nursing Team | Review all cases for the past six months in which occurrence of infection is documented. |
| Nursing Supervisors | Update all policies and procedures related to infection control. |
| Home Health Agency (Organizational level) | Reduce incidence of readmissions due to infection in current agency caseload. |

The proportion of the workday dedicated to work on these objectives and other factors will affect the speed with which the work can be done. Common time frames used in most healthcare organizations are one month, three months, six months, and one year.

If your organization uses MBO, you may be given a set of objectives, asked to write your own objectives, or asked to write them with your immediate supervisor. Of course, being encouraged to set your own objectives is different from being handed a prepared set of objectives. The first approach increases motivation and encourages self-management; the second discourages self-management and often becomes primarily a means for control (Levinson & LaMonica, 1980).

Involvement of the employee in developing a plan for professional growth has a number of benefits:

- Increased control over one's own professional growth
- Increased job satisfaction
- Opportunities for dialogue between manager and employee
- Mutual agreement on goals and expectations (Barnes et al., 1999)

The following objectives would be appropriate for a discharge planning coordinator:

| One month: | Invite a speaker on in-home services to the next discharge planning meeting. |
| Three months: | Design a method for surveying existing in-home services in the community. |
| Six months: | Survey the existing in-home services in the community. |
| One year: | Prepare a directory of in-home services in the community. |

It is less common and yet probably more important for healthcare teams as a whole to develop a set of objectives because they can easily become immersed in their daily routines and lose sight of future goals or direction for improvement and change. The following list is one example:

1. Invite people from other agencies to agency staff education conferences.
2. Plan, organize, and initiate a support group for families of developmentally disabled children.
3. Design a new crash cart system to shorten response time.
4. Revise outpatient chemotherapy procedures to decrease waiting time.

A humorous performance appraisal form from Kerzner (1998) may be found in Figure 13–1.

## Using Job Descriptions and Standards

You can see by comparing Box 13–2 and Table 13–1 that the job description is a general statement, whereas the standards are specific behaviors that can be observed and recorded.

Writing useful job descriptions and measurable standards of performance is an arduous but rewarding task. It requires a clarification and explication of the work nurses actually do that goes beyond our usual generalizations about what nursing is and what nurses do. Under effective group leadership and with strong administrative support for this process, it can be a challenging and stimulating experience. Without support and

| PERFORMANCE FACTORS | EXCELLENT (1 out of 15) | VERY GOOD (3 out of 15) | GOOD (8 out of 15) | FAIR (2 out of 15) | UNSATISFACTORY (1 out of 15) |
|---|---|---|---|---|---|
| | Far Exceeds Job Requirements | Exceeds Job Requirements | Meets Job Requirements | Needs Some Improvement | Does Not Meet Minimum Standards |
| QUALITY | Leaps Tall Buildings with a Single Bound | Must Take Running Start to Leap over Tall Buildings | Can Only Leap over a Short Building or Medium One without Spires | Crashes into Building | Cannot Recognize Buildings |
| TIMELINESS | Faster Than a Speeding Bullet | Is as Fast as a Speeding Bullet | Not Quite as Fast as a Speeding Bullet | Would You Believe a Slow Bullet? | Wounds Self with the Bullet |
| INITIATIVE | Stronger Than a Locomotive | Stronger Than a Bull Elephant | Stronger Than a Bull | Shoots the Bull | Smells Like a Bull |
| ADAPTABILITY | Walks on Water Consistently | Walks on Water in Emergencies | Washes with Water | Drinks Water | Passes Water in Emergencies |
| COMMUNICATIONS | Talks with God | Talks with Angels | Talks to Self | Argues with Self | Loses the Argument with Self |

**Figure 13–1**  Guide to Performance Appraisal: How Do You Rate Your Own Performance? *Source:* Kerzner, H. (1998). *Project management: A systems approach to planning, scheduling, and controlling.* New York: VanNostrand Reinhold. Reprinted with permission.

leadership, however, it becomes frustrating when the group gets bogged down in details and disagreements or isn't given sufficient time to do this work.

Once the job descriptions and performance standards for each level have been developed and agreed upon, a procedure for their use must also be worked out. An evaluation form listing the performance standards can be completed by the nurse manager to determine pay raises and promotions.

In some organizations, the standards are considered the minimal qualifications for each level. In this case, additional activities and professional development are expected before promotion to the next level. The candidate for an advanced-level position may prepare a promotion portfolio for review (Schultz, 1993). The promotion portfolio may include a self-assessment, peer review, management performance appraisal, and evidence of professional growth. Evidence of professional growth, for example, may be documented by participation in the quality improvement program, evaluating a new product or procedure, serving as a translator or disaster volunteer, or making postdischarge visits to patients from the unit.

## Implementing the Plan

Once the objectives or standards have been determined, the next step is to carry out the work indicated. The objective or standard itself defines the expected outcome, but it does not tell you what action will be needed to get this result. For example, the healthcare team objective of including people from other agencies in client-oriented conferences tells you that these people should be invited, but it does not tell you exactly which people, how many people, or how to extend the invitation. In other words, the objective serves as a directional guide, telling you what to do but not how to do it.

Some of the examples given have included an indication of the time in which the objective is expected to be completed. Time lines (like the ones discussed in Chapter 16 on planning) are particularly helpful in working out the specific objectives leading to a long-term goal. When the objective is a complex one, it may also be necessary to break it down even further into separate steps or components in order to have an adequate guide for your work and for evaluating your progress as you go along.

The job expectations, objectives, and time estimates should be flexible guides, not unbending requirements. Circumstances change and external factors can interfere with fulfilling expectations within a projected amount of time. For example,

if you needed one more course to complete an advanced nurse practitioner program but the course was canceled at the last minute, you could not be expected to fulfill your objective in the originally estimated amount of time. You might, however, be expected to investigate the possibility of an alternative schedule for completing the program requirements on time.

## Evaluating Outcomes

It is important to set aside adequate time for the appraisal review and development of the plan for the next year. Both the employee and the supervisor bring data for use at this session. These data should include a self-evaluation by the employee and observations by the evaluator of the employee's activities and their outcomes. Data may also be obtained from peers and patients or clients. Some organizations use surveys for getting this information from patients.

The guidelines for providing informal evaluative feedback discussed earlier apply to the conduct of performance appraisals. Although not as frequent or immediate as informal feedback, formal evaluation should be just as objective, private, nonthreatening, skillfully communicated, and growth promoting. The results of a research study described in Research Example 13–1 illustrate just how difficult it is for a manager to be fair and objective in performance appraisals.

Evaluation of accomplishments is based on the degree to which an outcome was met. This outcome may or may not have been specifically described in the objective. For example:

*An objective set by the discharge planning coordinator was to increase the number of comprehensive discharge plans completed before the day of discharge for patients on the traumatic injury and spinal cord rehabilitation units. If only 25 percent of the comprehensive discharge plans were completed before the day of discharge in the past, then an outcome of 50 percent completed would indicate the objective had been met. However, if the objective had been to have all of the plans complete the day before discharge, then a 50 percent completion rate would not have met the objective.*

The degree to which the individual or work group has control over all of the factors that affect

### Research Example 13–1    *Subordinate Influence on Managers' Appraisals*

Can managers be influenced by subordinates' self-ratings? Much effort has gone into ensuring the fairness and objectivity of systematic performance appraisals but questions have been raised about factors that affect the evaluation. Blakely (1993) designed a study to test the degree to which the manager's rating could be influenced by the employee's own self-rating, particularly a low self-rating.

Ninety-six undergraduate business majors were given an "in-basket" task of prioritizing and responding to 17 memos and letters in a half hour. Each student was observed for 5 minutes by another student designated as his or her "supervisor." The students were paid for their participation and told that they would receive training in performance appraisal or managerial decision making as part of the study. They were also led to believe that it would be an ongoing "subordi-

nate-supervisor" relationship. After the "subordinates" completed the task and a self-evaluation, the researcher prepared bogus ratings either higher or lower than the original self-ratings done by the "subordinates" to show to the "supervisors." Altogether, 11 "supervisors" lowered their ratings after seeing the bogus self-ratings from the "subordinate."

Blakely concluded that subordinates' formal self-evaluations can influence supervisors to modify their original rating. Blakely suggested that managers may be influenced in order to avoid an uncomfortable confrontation; however, they need to be aware of this potential source of influence on their rating.

*Source:* Blakely, G.L. (1993). The effects of performance rating discrepancies on supervisors and subordinates. *Organizational Behavior and Human Decision Press, 54*(5), 57–80.

the fulfillment of the objective is a source of concern in the evaluation phase of MBO, especially when the objectives are used as a basis for formal evaluation of employees and affect decisions about raises, promotions, and so forth. For example:

> *A public health nursing director's goal of reducing waiting time in the immunization clinic to 15 minutes or less seemed reasonable until an unforeseen outbreak of measles occurred in the high schools. The resulting flood of high school students going to the health department for further immunization made it virtually impossible to meet this goal until the outbreak was brought under control.*

Concern about external factors that can influence the progress toward a stated objective has led to the development of more complex appraisal systems. For example, any major obstacles that stood in the way of completing the objectives within the given time can be listed separately to recognize the possibility of their occurrence. The types of support and resources that are needed from others in order to fulfill objectives are also listed separately at the time

that the objectives are set in order to increase the fairness of the expectation set out as evaluation criteria.

### Ensuring Fair, Uniform Procedures

Unfortunately, many organizations have employee evaluation procedures that are far from ideal. Their procedures may be inconsistent, subjective, and even unknown to the employee in some cases. The following is a list of standards for a fair and objective employee evaluation that you may want to use to judge your own or your employer's procedures:

1. Standards are clear, objective, and known in advance.
2. Criteria for pay raises and promotions are clearly spelled out and uniformly applied.
3. Conditions under which employment may be terminated are known.
4. Appraisals are part of the employee's permanent record and have space for employee comments as well as signature.
5. Employees may inspect their own personnel files.

6. Employees may request and be given a reasonable explanation of any rating and may appeal the rating if they do not agree with it.
7. Employees are given a reasonable amount of time to correct any serious deficiencies before other action is taken, unless the safety of self or others is immediately threatened.

In some organizations, collective bargaining agreements are used to enforce adherence to fair and objective performance appraisals. However, collective bargaining agreements often emphasize seniority (length of service) over merit in giving raises and promotions, a situation that does not promote growth and change.

## Peer Review

Peer review is the evaluation of an individual by his or her colleagues (peers). A peer is someone who has similar education, experience, and occupational status. The purpose of peer review is to provide the individual with feedback from those who are best acquainted with the requirements and demands of that particular position.

On an informal basis, professionals frequently observe and judge their colleagues' performance. But many feel uncomfortable about telling others what they think of their performance and so their evaluative feedback is often not shared with the individual unless a formal system is established. Reluctance to provide honest feedback is a critical problem in the implementation of a peer review system (Barnes et al., 1999).

Whenever staff members meet to audit records or otherwise evaluate the quality of care they have given, they are actually engaging in a kind of peer review. Formal individual peer review programs are less common but may be effective (See Perspectives . . . Peer Review of an Employee Dismissal).

### *Fundamentals of Peer Review*

Formal peer review begins with precisely defining the scope of professional practice and setting standards for quality care. Observations of performance are made by one or more peers, compared with previously set standards, and then shared with the person being reviewed. The reviewer is

## PERSPECTIVES . . .

### Peer Review of an Employee Dismissal

This is the story of Ruth Hatton who had been a waitress for Red Lobster restaurants for 19 years when the incident occurred. Ms. Hatton was fired because she had removed a comment card on which she was described as "uncooperative" from the comment box and the customer complained about the incident. Apparently the customer, who is black, sent back her prime rib because it was too fatty and undercooked. Ms. Hatton, who is white, had the meat cooked further but the customer was still displeased. The customer reported that she felt "violated" when the incident happened; Ms. Hatton said "it felt like a knife going through me" when she was fired.

Instead of suing, Ms. Hatton requested a peer review of her firing. The peer review panel included a general manager, server, hostess, and bartender. Ms. Hatton testified that she forgot about the card and threw it away by mistake. The peer review panel deliberated for an hour and half. They noted that the policy forbidding retrieval of the comment cards had not been enforced at that restaurant. They concluded that putting a reprimand in Ms. Hatton's file would have been sufficient but thought that the supervisor might have felt she had to do more. "Red Lobster is sensitive to race on a corporate level and [they] could have said, 'Whack her. You have someone who [upset] a guest,' " said the peer reviewer who was a general manager. "I think the whole thing snowballed." The panel did refuse to grant her back wages, however, because she had violated a company policy. Her supervisor reported "it didn't bother me a bit that she got her job back." Ms. Hatton concluded that the review process had worked. "The panel took my claim seriously," she said. The corporation reported that using peer review of employee dismissals had cut a million dollars (a 25 percent reduction) from their legal expenses for employee disputes.

*Source:* Jacob, M.A. (1998, January 20). Red lobster tale: Peers decide fired waitress' fate. *Wall Street Journal,* B1, B4.

expected to look for those items indicated by the standards and to avoid making judgments based on personal standards or feelings.

Observations may be shared only with the person being reviewed, with the person's supervisor, or with a review committee. The evaluation report may be written by the reviewer or it may come from the review committee. The use of a committee defeats the purpose of peer review, however, if the committee members are not truly peers of the individual being reviewed.

### Uses of Peer Review Data

There are a number of possible variations in the peer review process. Peer review systems can simply be informal feedback shared among colleagues or comprehensive systems that are fully integrated into the formal evaluation structure of a healthcare organization. When a peer review system is fully integrated, the evaluative feedback from one's peers may be joined with the performance appraisals done by the nurse manager, and used in combination to determine pay raises and promotions for individual staff nurses. This style of formal evaluation is far more collegial than the traditional hierarchical one in which each employee is only evaluated by the manager above him or her in the administrative hierarchy.

In some organizations, the evaluation from one's peers is used for counseling purposes only and is not taken into consideration in determining pay raises or promotions, an approach that provides useful feedback but weakens the impact of peer review on the individual or the system as a whole.

An alternative approach uses a professional practice committee. This committee, composed of colleagues selected by the nursing staff, reviews the evaluation forms and makes its recommendations to the chief nursing officer, who then makes the final decision regarding the appropriate rewards (raises, promotions, commendations) or punishment (demotion, transfer, termination of employment). It may surprise the reader who has not participated in such a peer review process that the recommendations of one's peers may be harsher than the recommendations made by management (Dison, 1986).

A comprehensive peer review system can be an effective mechanism for both evaluation and staff development. It demands a great deal of analysis of the nursing care delivered within the organization, objectivity and fairness in dealing with one's peers, and leadership on the part of both staff members and management. Done well, it can provide many opportunities for increased professionalism and learning and ensure appropriate rewards for high performance levels and professionalism on the job.

## Evaluating the Marginal Staff Member

Conducting the performance appraisals of highly motivated, competent staff members is usually a satisfying experience for the first-line manager. The appraisal meeting provides an opportunity to recognize and reward the individual for work well done and to plan for further growth and development. Generally, the meeting reaches an agreeable conclusion even if it begins with some tension on your part or that of the staff member being evaluated.

Evaluation of a staff member whose performance has not been satisfactory is an entirely different story. Few people find it easy to sit down and discuss a person's shortcomings with him or her directly. It is usually an uncomfortable but necessary experience for both the evaluator and employee under evaluation (see Perspectives . . . An Easy-Going Manager Turns Tough).

### Excuses for Inaction

It is quite easy to rationalize your failure to confront unsatisfactory performance. You may rationalize that the person's poor performance is just a temporary lapse, one that will soon disappear, or that it is due to a personal problem at home. Or you may tell yourself that the employee really is trying hard and any negative feedback may discourage him or her from trying any longer. Both of these excuses imply that negative feedback cannot be helpful, that you are doing the employee a favor by not acknowledging any problems.

Often, just the fact that this employee is a nice person can inhibit a manager. The employee

## An Easy-Going Manager Turns Tough

Alan Robbins runs a small factory that converts old milk and soda bottles into plastic "lumber." The factory is located in a rundown section of Akron, Ohio. He considered himself an "enlightened" employer, breaking out beer at the end of a shift and giving personal loans to employees but now says he was too lax. Now he is more businesslike, no more loans, no alcohol in the workplace. Why did he change his approach? The turning point occurred when two factory workers were fighting and one was spotted coming after the other with an iron bar in his hand.

After that incident, Robbins developed an employment manual and demerit system that not only lets workers know what is not tolerated but also is the basis for building a case for dismissal if necessary. Originally, he had been reluctant to put anything in writing but now realizes that it is a valuable defense if a lawsuit arises. He also hadn't wanted to spend money on preemployment drug tests, but an alarming injury rate convinced him of the necessity. He has also hired some disabled workers, some of whom have become his most dedicated workers.

Has this drastic change in policy solved all of Mr. Robbins' problems? Not at all. Most workers have adapted, some have become success stories, but difficult situations still arise—and they probably always will.

*Source:* Aeppel, T. (1998, January 14). Losing faith: Personnel decisions sap a factory owner of his early idealism. *Wall Street Journal.*

may be the person who always has a cheerful smile early in the morning, the one who never complains, or the one who can lighten up a serious staff meeting with a funny story. The problem with these excuses is that you are confusing personality with performance (Hansen, 1986).

Inaction is further encouraged when the unsatisfactory employee is thought to be leaving, transferring out of the department, or retiring. One may question the point of raising the issue when the employee is leaving soon. In the meantime, however, the employee is drawing a salary but not doing a fair share of the work.

### Importance of Intervention

The importance of intervening with the marginal performer should be clear. Like the failure to confront problems generally, failure to confront unsatisfactory performance is likely to result in the problem growing larger, not smaller. The longer unsatisfactory behavior is tolerated, the more difficult it is to change.

Remember the unsatisfactory performer is still being paid as if performance were satisfactory. This fact alone makes the employee a liability to the organization. Unless another staff member is doing the employee's work (which is obviously not fair to that other staff member), that person's work is not being done. Can your unit afford to allow this employee to continue performing poorly? Is it not affecting patient care? Or morale within the team?

Excessive tolerance of poor performance also affects your image as a nurse-manager. The nurse-manager who fails to confront problems affecting the group may be seen as laissez-faire, uncaring, ineffective, powerless, cowardly, or simply lazy. Some of these interpretations may be true. Failure to confront poor performance results in increased cost to the organization, an unfair work burden on other staff members, work bottlenecks within the team, lower quality of care to the clients being served, and the potential for reduced morale among the employees whose performance is satisfactory (Pulick, 1986).

### Factors Leading to Marginal Performance

The cause of poor performance is not necessarily found in the employee. An open systems perspective makes this point clear. Consider the elements of a management situation: the manager, the employee, the work to be done, and the environment in which they interact. The problem may have begun all the way back at the **selection and hiring** process. The employee may not have been carefully screened and interviewed, or the requirements for the position may not have been clear at the time. The employee may not have had enough prior experience, education, or both to be ready for the responsibilities of the position. The orientation and training provided may also have been inadequate.

Sometimes the manager's or organization's expectations are **vague or unrealistic.** Vagueness is especially problematic in a newly created position unless both the employee and manager make deliberate efforts to clarify expectations through initial discussion, written job descriptions, and frequent feedback. Nurse managers may assume that an experienced nurse needs little orientation to a new unit. Other times, the expectations for a single individual or person with limited preparation are far too high. For example, a new graduate should not be placed in charge of a unit on the evening or night shift, yet it is still done when staff shortages occur, which is the worst time! One nurse cannot provide good primary care for 10–15 patients on most acute-care units, yet this unrealistic standard is often used. The employee may also have had unrealistic expectations of self and may have tried to take on too many responsibilities too quickly.

A **lack of communication or miscommunication regarding priorities and expectations** may be another factor in poor performance. Managers often do not realize that their attention to such details as a clean utility area or tidy patient units can inadvertently communicate to employees that appearance rather than substance is a priority. Poor management can certainly be a factor in poor employee performance.

**Poor work habits** also contribute to poor performance. Time management skills may be undeveloped: procrastination and delay are a source of much poor performance. Other problems may include defensiveness, frequent absenteeism or lateness, frequent complaints (which may be legitimate), lack of confidence, or failure to take the initiative. Each of these factors requires investigation to determine how the problem can be resolved.

## Resolution of the Problem

The first step in correcting marginal performance is to observe and objectively document the problem. Documentation should be of the behavior itself, not your interpretation of the behavior. Remember also that your concern is with the employee's performance, not personality traits that you might find unattractive. Behavior that disrupts team or department function, however, is a legitimate management concern.

Once the problem behavior is carefully documented, it is time for a counseling session with the employee. Both positive and negative (corrective) feedback should be given to the employee, but the emphasis should be on the behavior that is cause for concern. The purpose of the session is to communicate the problem and to develop a plan for resolution of the problem. It is important that the employee's point of view be heard and that the employee be treated with respect and concern. During the session, your support in resolving the problem should be offered, but the employee must also be clearly informed of the consequences of continued poor performance (no raise, no promotion, a cut in pay, a demotion, or termination of employment). Before the session is ended, guidelines for reevaluation should be agreed on. Some of the actions to be taken before that time could be further orientation or education, reassignment of the employee, a change in either or both parties' expectations, a change in the work environment, or some combination of these alternatives. A transfer to another unit may be a solution, but too often it is used as an escape from confrontation, leaving the fundamental problem unresolved. The counseling session should, of course, be carefully and thoroughly documented.

Minor problems can usually be resolved through discussion between the first-line manager and the employee. However, any serious or long-standing difficulty should be discussed with your second-line manager or supervisor before you conduct a counseling session. For most first-line managers, especially new ones, it is a relief to have someone to turn to for guidance and support in handling these situations. Furthermore, upper-level management may have to make a decision regarding demotion or termination if the problem is sufficiently serious and cannot be resolved. For this reason alone, they must be involved in this process from the beginning.

Every employee should be given at least a second and perhaps third opportunity to improve. A clearly spelled-out improvement plan leaves no doubts about the areas in which the employee is weak or the improvements that are necessary to retain his or her position. The plan should include specific areas in which improvement is needed and the time frame in which it must be accomplished. Again, it is important to warn the marginal employee of the consequences of failing to improve (Smith, 1993). Several recounseling sessions may be necessary, and your support and guidance may be needed over a long period of time. However, if all efforts to resolve the problem and improve performance have failed, then demotion or termination of the employee, however difficult and painful it may be to all concerned, may be the only solution to the problem.

A number of alternatives may be used to handle this situation. One would be to first provide an oral reminder about standards employees are expected to live up to. If no change is made in performance, the employee is given a written reminder. The third step differs considerably from the traditional approach: the employee is given a day off with pay—called the "day of decision"—to think about the standards and whether he or she will accept and adhere to them (Rogers, Hutchins & Johnson, 1990). If the employee decides not to accept the standard or fails to meet them after accepting them, employment is terminated. This nontraditional approach is meant to shift the responsibility to change from the manager to the employee.

## Fear of Firing

An increase in wrongful dismissal suits has made managers more reluctant than ever to terminate an employee. Other factors include difficulty finding a qualified replacement, the effect on other employees, and the emotional toll on everyone involved. However, failure to terminate when indicated sends a message that incompetence and nonproductive behavior is tolerated. "Why should I work so hard when so-and-so gets away with doing practically nothing?" is not an unreasonable question for other employees to ask if a poor performer is retained indefinitely. Failure to terminate an incompetent employee not only places an unfair work burden on others but, in extreme cases, puts patients and clients at risk, a situation that should not be tolerated.

In some instances, these problems can be prevented through proactive management. To minimize the risk of a wrongful dismissal lawsuit, consider the following points (Forman, 1998).

- Do not fire a person immediately. Warnings with time to improve are usually warranted. When the behavior is so dangerous that the person should be removed from the scene immediately, a suspension pending investigation can be imposed.
- Document the actions of the marginal performer carefully and objectively. Never backdate any noted observation; always use the current date.
- If past documentation was inadequate, review past problems in the explanation of the current reprimand.
- Review the reasons for termination from all possible angles. Be certain it is not due to any characteristics related to age, disability, pregnancy, gender, religion, race, or national origin.
- Obtain a legal opinion and administrative guidance to be certain the procedure is done correctly. Do not do it on your own.

This situation is another in which proactive management prevents problems later. To avoid having to dismiss employees too often, consider the following points (Messmer, 1998):

- Select new employees carefully. Investigate their previous employment records thoroughly and match their skills and experience to the position available.
- Provide adequate orientations for new employees. While a "sink or swim" approach works for some people some of the time, too often it leaves new employees unprepared for the challenges they face.
- Review the history of resignations and terminations for your unit and the organization as a whole. Look for patterns that may indicate a problem unique to your group or setting.

These actions won't eliminate the need to terminate an employee occasionally but they can decrease the number of times it has to be done and can reduce the repercussions when it must be done.

## ● SUMMARY

Informal evaluation is a continuing process of seeking and providing feedback that should be an integral part of team function. The purposes of this type of evaluation are to provide recognition, increase self-awareness, clarify expectations, promote change and growth on the job, facilitate team function, and challenge staff members to improve their performances.

People need both positive and negative (corrective) feedback. Constructive feedback is immediate, frequent, private, objective, based on observable behavior, appropriately communicated, nonthreatening, and includes suggestions for change. Seeking feedback is as important as providing feedback and follows the same guidelines. Responding to feedback that is given is also important and may help to clarify both positive and negative feedback.

Formal evaluation procedures in organizations serve as a source of data, a demonstration of accountability, the basis for the reward system, and identification of educational needs for administrative intervention.

A performance appraisal begins with setting goals to be accomplished within a specified period of time. The degree to which these objectives were met is evaluated at the end of this time, reasons for success or failure are discussed, and new goals are set. The goals serve as a guide to planning the work, setting priorities, and evaluating effectiveness. Objectives may be used as the basis of a formal evaluation. Objectives should begin with an action verb and include observable outcomes. The objectives may be long or short term; individual, group, or organizational; and used in an autocratic or participative manner. When using objectives to evaluate outcomes, it is important to recognize the effects that organizational and external factors may have had on individual and group success in meeting the objectives. The resources and support needed to achieve the objectives may be added to make the evaluation fairer.

Peer review is another mechanism for formal evaluation and staff development. It is done by one's equals or peers, rather than by one's manager, and supports a collegial relationship between the evaluator and the employee under evaluation. It also should be based on clear, measurable written expectations and standards for a particular position. The results of peer review may be used for counseling purposes only or for determining appropriate rewards (pay raises, promotions, or commendations) or punishments (reassignment, demotion, termination of employment) within the organization.

This entire process becomes more difficult when the staff member to be evaluated has been a poor performer. In this case, counseling sessions may need to be scheduled more frequently, more support and guidance from the manager are needed, and the consequences of failing to meet the objectives must be clearly spelled out.

Firing an employee is difficult but sometimes necessary. Failure to do so can place an unnecessary burden on other employees and, in health care, sometimes put patients or clients at risk. Employees in danger of termination should usually be given adequate warning and opportunities to improve. Documentation of a fair process is essential. Prevention of the problem is preferable. Careful selection, thorough orientation, and constructive evaluation procedures can eliminate the necessity of employee terminations in many cases.

# C A S E   S T U D Y

## An Unfair Evaluation?

Carlene Thomas is an experienced nurse manager. While not lenient, most who worked for her said she was demanding but fair. Her expectations were high but she also worked hard for her staff, supporting them when an undeserved complaint was lodged by an upset family member or physician, providing opportunities to attend conferences, adjusting schedules so people could go back to school, and so forth.

Carlene reported to the director of Obstetrical and Gynecological Services. The director reviewed all of Carlene's performance appraisals before they were shared with the employees and rarely questioned her conclusions. This increased the director's surprise when confronted with an angry LPN from Carlene's unit.

"What's the problem?"

"That evaluation was completely unfair. I can't believe you signed it."

"How was it unfair?"

"Carlene put me on warning."

"Did she explain why?"

"She claims I didn't achieve the goals."

"Did you?"

"How should I know?"

"What do you mean? Didn't you review those goals with Carlene?"

"No. I never heard about any goals. This was the first time I'd ever heard about any goals."

"Are you certain of that?"

"I never heard about goals before. How am I supposed to work on goals I never saw? She can't put me on warning for that."

Wisely, the director ended the interview at this point and said she would speak with Carlene and get back to the employee as soon as possible.

Carlene and the director reviewed the employee's personnel record the next morning. Carlene had several concerns about this individual, particularly his higher than average medication error rate, a penchant for long coffee breaks, and many complaints from staff and patients about his impatience and slow response to call lights. Carlene showed the director the list of goals she had written and discussed with him at the last performance appraisal.

"Did he see these?"

"Of course, we talked about them quite a while and he said he would work hard to improve."

"He told me that he'd never seen these goals."

"That's just not true!" Carlene exclaimed.

"Did he sign them?"

They both looked at the personnel record. It was clear that the employee had signed the rating form. The list of goals was attached but not signed.

"He's going to file a grievance," the director predicted.

"He can't win, can he? We reviewed those goals together."

"It's your word against his. You have no written evidence and he is adamant. You really need to be more careful in the future."

The director ended the meeting with this comment.

## Questions for Critical Reflection and Analysis

1. Review Carlene's handling of this situation. What did she do well? What mistakes did she make?
2. Now take the employee's point of view. Why does he believe he was treated unfairly? In what ways could he have handled the situation more effectively?
3. Pretend you are the director in this situation. How would you proceed to resolve this dilemma?
4. Again as director, how would you prevent a similar problem in the future?
5. Review the purposes of formal performance appraisal and the disadvantages mentioned in Perspectives . . . Abolish Performance Appraisals. What are your thoughts on the value of performance appraisals?

# REFERENCES

Aeppel, T. (1998, January 14). Losing faith: Personnel decisions sap a factory owner of his early idealism. *Wall Street Journal.*

Barnes, B., Leis, S., Brammer, J.M., Gustin, T.J. & Lupo, T.C. (1999). A developmental evaluation process for nurses: Enhancing professional excellence. *Journal of Nursing Administration, 29*(4), 25–32.

Blakely, G.L. (1993). The effects of performance rating discrepancies on supervisors and subordinates. *Organizational Behavior and Human Decision Press, 54*(5), 57–80.

Conrad, C. (1990). *Strategic organizational communication: An integrated perspective.* Fort Worth: Holt, Rinehart & Winston.

Cronin, S.N. & Becherer, D. (1999). Recognition of staff nurse job performance and achievements. *Journal of Nursing Administration 29*(1), 26–31.

Del Bueno, D. (1977). Performance evaluation: When all is said and done, more is said than done. *Journal of Nursing Administration, 7*(10).

Dison, C. (1986). *Professional nursing advancement in the work place.* Paper presented at the Annual Nursing Research Conference, Sigma Theta Tau, Beta Tau Chapter, Miami, FL.

Fitton, R.A. (1997). *Leadership: Quotations from the world's greatest motivators.* Boulder, CO: Westview Press.

Forman, E. (1998, February 27). Improper firings can cost fortune, employers warned. *Sun-Sentinel,* Miami, FL

Foust, D. (1999, May 3). Man on the spot. *Business Week,* 150–151.

Glaser, S.R. (1994). Teamwork and communication. *Management Communication Quarterly, 7*(3), 282–296.

Hannigan, T.A. (1998). *Managing tomorrow's high-performance unions.* Westport, CT: Quorum Books.

Hansen, M.R. (1986). To-do lists for managers. *Supervisory Management, 31*(5), 37–39.

Jacob, M.A. (1998, January 20). Red lobster tale: Peers decide fired waitress' fate. *Wall Street Journal,* B1, B4.

Kerr, S. (1997). On the folly of rewarding A, while hoping for B. In R.P. Vecchio (Ed.). *Leadership: Understanding the dynamics of power and influence in organizations.* Notre Dame, IN: University of Notre Dame Press.

Kerzner, H. (1998). *Project management: A systems approach to planning, scheduling, and controlling.* New York: VanNostrand Reinhold.

Kolb, D.A., Osland, J.S. & Rubin, I.M. (1995). *Organizational behavior: An experiential approach.* Englewood Cliffs, NJ: Prentice Hall.

Kron, T. (1981). *The management of patient care: Putting leadership skills to work.* Philadelphia: W.B. Saunders.

Levinson, H. & LaMonica, E.L. (1980). Management by whose objectives? *Journal of Nursing Administration, 10*(2), 22.

Mager, R.F. & Pipe, P. (1970). *Analyzing performance problems.* Belmont, CA: Lear Sigler/Fearon.

Matejka, J.K., Ashworth, D.N. & Dodd-McCue, D. (1986). Discipline without guilt. *Supervisory Management, 31*(5), 34–36.

Messmer, M. (1998). *The fast forward MBA in hiring: Finding and keeping the best people.* New York: John Wiley & Sons.

Napolitano, C.S. & Henderson, L.J. (1998). *The leadership odyssey.* San Francisco: Jossey-Bass Inc.

Pulick, M.A. (1986). What to do with incompetent employees. *Supervisory Management, 31*(3), 10–16.

Robbins, H. & Finley, M. (1995). *Why teams don't work.* Princeton, NJ: Peterson's/Pacesetter Books.

Rogers, J.E., Hutchins, S.G. & Johnson, B.J. (1990). Nonpunitive discipline: A method of reducing absenteeism. *Journal of Nursing Administration, 20*(7/8), 41–43.

Schultz, A.W. (1993). Evaluation for clinical advancement system. *Journal of Nursing Administration, 23*(2), 13–19.

Smith, M.L. (1993). Defensible performance appraisals. *Journal of Management Engineering, 9*(1), 128–135.

Williams, R.S. (1998). *Performance management.* London: International Thomson Business Press.

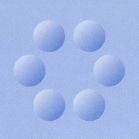

# Managing a Budget

## LEARNING OBJECTIVES

*After completing this chapter the reader will be able to:*

- Explain why financial management is important to the nurse manager.
- Identify the individuals within an organization who have responsibility for budget preparation, approval, and monitoring.

- Distinguish zero-based budgeting from incremental budgeting.
- Read and explain a simple budget variance report for a nursing unit.
- Understand the factors that influence productivity at the unit level.

## TEST YOURSELF

**Do you know the answers to these budget-related questions?**

1. The average daily census (ADC) on a unit is 33. The productivity standard (HPPD) is 3.8. How many FTEs do you need in a 24-hour period to staff this unit?

2. The census on a unit is 36. The number of people who worked yesterday in the 24-hour period was 10. What was unit productivity (HPPD)?

3. Your variance report indicates an increase in spending in medical-surgical supplies. What are some possible explanations?

*Answers*

1. ADC × 33 HPPD = 33 × 3.8 = 125.4, 8 hours = 15.6 FTEs in a 24-hour period 2. Ten persons worked eight hour shifts, 10 × 8 = 80 hours. 80 hours divided by the census 36 = 2.2 HPPD 3. Increased census, accounting error, increased patient acuity, increased cost of item, waste, etc.

---

**A**nyone who believes it is not necessary to be aware of the financial side of health care is like those proverbial ostrichs who stick their heads in the sand and hope that what they can't see won't hurt them. Budgeting decisions affect everyone who works in an organization. Furthermore, with decentralization of some administrative responsibilities, most first-line managers are expected to prepare and monitor their unit budgets. They also need to fully understand how to make the necessary changes to control costs or show where revenue is produced to justify retaining personnel and maintaining services. This complexity has come as a surprise to many new nurse managers who find themselves learning how to prepare a good working budget by trial and error.

Nurse managers today need to have a working knowledge of the budgetary process so they can anticipate changes and adapt to decisions made based on the financial status of the organization. Effective resource management is a necessity, not a luxury, in the current healthcare environment. In this chapter, we will consider the growing importance of financial management for the nurse manager, the different roles and responsibilities of people in the budgeting process, and the budgeting process itself.

## ● IMPORTANCE OF FINANCIAL MANAGEMENT

Why is the budget of a healthcare organization so important to the nurse manager? Just a few of the most important reasons are outlined in this section.

## Effect on People's Work

The financial management of the organization affects many aspects of work: the salaries paid, the benefits offered, the number of people available to do the work, and the quality and quantity of equipment and supplies available (see Box 14–1 for components of an operating budget). The following are some examples of important organizational decisions based primarily on budgetary factors:

*A rehabilitation hospital decided to use fewer physical therapists and more physical therapy techs to save money. This change decreased salary costs but led to increased workload for the remaining therapists who had to supervise the techs.*

*Directors of a home health agency elected to serve only private-pay and Medicare clients because Medicaid does not pay as much as it actually costs the agency to make visits. The agency also put strict limitations on time allowed per visit in order to increase efficiency and realize a profit.*

*A nursing home kept nursing staff levels to the minimum required by law in order to reduce costs and increase profits. As a consequence, this facility lost its superior rating from the state.*

Budgetary decisions such as these affect both the people working in the organization and those who are served by it. You can see that they also reflect the goals and values of the organization.

---

**Box 14–1   Components of the Operating Budget**

**Costs (Expenses)**

| | |
|---|---|
| **Payroll:** | salary, vacation, holidays, social security, tuition reimbursement, unemployment, other employee benefits |
| **Supplies:** | office supplies, treatment supplies, and so forth |
| **Overhead:** | building maintenance, water, electric |
| **Other:** | mortgage interest, loans, insurance, marketing efforts |

**Revenue (Income)**

| | |
|---|---|
| **Payment sources:** | private pay, Medicaid, Medicare, commercial insurance, managed care organizations |
| **Contributions:** | philanthropic, grants-in-aid, research and program grants |
| **Other:** | interest, rent, sale of equipment |

---

## Blaming the Budget

The budget itself is just a management tool. On paper, it is simply a compilation of information on money spent and received in the past and a projection of the same for the future. How future monies will be spent is also outlined in the budget and reflects decisions made by certain people within the organization. Once completed, the budget is used as a roadmap to assist in decision making and as a scorecard to monitor progress throughout the year. Because it reflects the extent of the resources available and how they will be distributed, the budget has a great deal of power associated with it (Dillon, 1979).

You might hear that "the budget won't allow us to hire more nurses" or that "the budget won't allow us to modernize the NICU this year." If you understand the rationale behind the decisions that entered into creating the budget then you will know whether these statements are true or whether the budget is being used as an excuse for diverting funds to other areas. Managers should be able to defend the validity of the decisions made in creating the budget, not hide behind it or use it as an excuse for unpopular decisions. If one blames the budget, power and authority are ascribed to the budget itself rather than to the people in the organization who created the budget and who enforce adherence to it.

## Planning

A budget is a plan for the management of monetary resources. To create this budget, one must predict how much money the organization will generate in the next fiscal year and how much it will need to spend in order to continue operation. (A fiscal year differs from a calendar year in that it may or may not begin in January. It may, for example, begin July 1 and end June 30 (Finkler, 1992). Healthcare organizations, like other enterprises, depend on adequate revenues for their continued survival and growth. Organizations that manage their resources efficiently and effectively thrive; those that do not cease to operate entirely.

> ***At the level of nursing operations, management's responsibility should be to help the care delivery organization reduce its cost to a competitive level while achieving acceptable quality of care.***
>
> *—Hankins et al., 1998*

Whether the financial goals of the organization are stated directly or implied by the allocation of funds for certain projects and the lack of funds for others, the budget is a statement in monetary terms of what the organization and its various departments expect to do in the next year. Any new service or activity that has money allocated for it in the budget is far more likely to be carried out than one that requires a special request for funds during the year, even for a relatively small amount of money. Simply knowing when budgets are being prepared, and by whom, and then getting your project included in the budget can be an important step in accomplishing your goal.

In some cases, it may be necessary to prepare a detailed **business plan** to obtain budgetary approval for a new project (Finkler & Kovner, 1993). This plan should include a description of the project, analysis of the market for the service, estimates of the costs and predicted income, description of how the project would be implemented, and alternatives to the proposed project. The business plan should provide sufficient information to allow a thorough evaluation of its potential for success. It should be persuasive but realistic in its projections.

The people who are involved in preparing a healthcare organization's budget must look ahead as well as looking at past costs and income. It is essential to consider trends such as economic inflation or recession, community needs, public demands, availability of qualified staff, anticipated healthcare reform measures, changes in healthcare methodologies, and competition from other organizations. Failure to consider any of these factors can result in poor budget decisions. With the rapid changes in the healthcare system, it is especially difficult to accurately plan for the financial survival of any healthcare organization. The more knowledgeable you are about your organization's financial plan, the more likely your budget will reflect organizational goals and support success.

## Roles, Responsibility, and Authority

Those individuals or groups in the organization who decide how resources will be allocated have a great deal of influence over the operation of the organization. These decisions greatly affect individual employees, the growth or stagnation of various departments, and the direction of the organization as a whole. The decision to use more per diem staff because of budgetary limitations, for example, or to eliminate staff positions because of a reduction in Medicaid reimbursements affects many people, staff and clients alike.

Two fundamental principles underlie resource allocation (Hannigan, 1998). The first is that resources are always scarce to some degree in relation to the wants and needs of those to whom they will be distributed. In other words, organizations almost never have enough money to do absolutely everything you would like to do in the best way possible. The second is that alternative ways to allocate resources can always be found. In other words, no one right way guides the design of a budget for your unit or for the entire organization but there are several potentially effective ways to do this.

Budgeting is not a mechanical process. Rather, it is one that requires thought about the consequences of the way in which resources are allocated. Because of the powerful impact of these budgetary decisions, the resource allocation that is done when a budget is prepared can be a complex and often politically intense process (Hannigan, 1998).

Nursing care is the major service offered by most healthcare institutions. The primary reason for patients entering into a hospital facility is for 24-hour nursing care. If you think about it, almost all other services (physical therapy, occupational therapy, physicians' visits, X rays, and even much surgery) can be done on an outpatient basis. Historically, patient care units have been budgeted in a way that nursing service is viewed as an expense. Nursing care does not generate revenue that is identified as an income source to the unit. Consequently, the nursing salary budget is frequently a target when cost containment is a priority (Hendricks & Baume, 1997).

A comparison with the billing done by other departments illustrates this difference. Every treatment given to a patient by speech therapists can be recorded and billed separately. The result is that these departments can easily show that they generate income for the hospital, even a profit, that offsets the cost of running these departments. It has been more difficult for nursing to do this. Although nursing service does not generate revenue directly, it has a significant impact on patient satisfaction and patient outcomes. Also a direct relationship can be demonstrated between budget decisions and the quality of care provided (Stone, 1998).

Thus, budgetary decisions related to nursing can have a profound effect on organizational success. Nursing service's power base in an organization does not come from its ability to generate revenue, but from the ability to impact patient satisfaction and the outcomes of care. A shrewd nursing leader can quantify nursing service's impact in many domains within the organizations, demonstrating the value of good nursing care.

For some time, the general trend has been toward larger and larger multihospital, multiagency corporations. In these large systems, a facility may be only one of many owned by a corporation. Many activities that were formerly done by each agency are done at the centralized corporate level to increase efficiency and take advantage of potential economics of scale, eliminate duplication, and attract lower bids for large quantities of various materials and supplies. For example, a large corporation can bargain for lower prices on supplies bought in large quantities. Other activities that affect nursing, such as the development of policies and procedures or the planning of education programs, may also be done at the corporate level rather than in your individual facility. These corporate procedures can limit the nurse manager's flexibility in making budgetary decisions. For example, if you want to keep some education funds in your individual unit's budget, you need to do your homework and justify why this would be more cost-effective than using corporationwide resources for staff education.

The reader should not assume that other services are immune to the impact of centralization. For example, several national laboratories are contracting with hospitals to do all their laboratory work, which has led to drastic shrinkage of the in-hospital laboratory. The national laboratories are able to perform the tests at a lower per unit rate because of the efficiency derived from doing a high volume of work on expensive machines and the reduction in the number of people in highly paid managerial positions. The projected budget savings has persuaded hospitals to contract with these corporations. The same approach is being used with other departments as it proves to be a successful way to contain costs.

## RESPONSIBILITY FOR FINANCIAL MANAGEMENT

Budgeting is a management responsibility. In some organizations, the budgeting process is highly centralized, involving only a small number of people at the higher levels of administration. In others, it may be widely decentralized, involving all managers within the organization, who in turn seek input from their staffs. Decentralization empowers the nurse manager to make more decisions about the unit budget, and increases ownership of the finished product. Whether centralized or decentralized, the final authority for the organizationwide budget rests with the governing board and chief executive officer (CEO). The CEO may actually prepare the final master budget in small agencies. We will focus here on the division of responsibility typically used in the participative approach (Bean & Laliberty, 1980).

### Chief Executive Officer (CEO)

Whatever the title—president, executive director, or other name—the CEO has general responsibility for the overall budget. The CEO sets the process in motion, determines the extent of involvement of others in the organization, assigns responsibilities, and sets deadlines.

The long-range goals of the organization must be determined before decisions can be made about allocation of financial resources. For example:

> *A hospital may have a long-range goal of expanding into long-term care services to broaden its income source, or it may have decided to concentrate on the specialized intensive care services that are not offered by other facilities in the community.*
>
> *A health department may have a long-range goal of expanding beyond its current function to offer comprehensive primary care or to add mental health care to its array of services.*

Forecasting future needs and demands in the healthcare market is an important part of the process for determining long-range goals. Internal factors also affect the budget goals: proposed changes in departmental activities, expansion or renovation of existing facilities, addition of new services and equipment, and so forth, affect the way the organization's money will be spent. Deliberate efforts may be made to increase revenue by expanding services or improving collection of money due and to reduce the cost of current operations (Finkler, Knickman & Hanson, 1994). All these factors must be taken into consideration by the CEO when giving direction regarding preparation of the budget.

## Governing Board

Although the members of the governing board or board of trustees are not usually involved in the actual preparation of the budget, they are responsible for working with the CEO in setting the long-range goals of the organization, in recommending changes in the budget, and in giving final approval to the organizational budget. In most organizations the CEO must report regularly (usually quarterly) to the governing board to ensure oversight of the fiscal goals and objectives.

## Chief Financial Officer (CFO)

This individual, often called the comptroller, provides the information on past budgets, past expenses, and revenues needed to begin the process of preparing a new budget (Kiser, 1988; Needles, Anderson & Caldwell, 1984). The CFO ensures that acceptable accounting practices are employed. In larger organizations, a set of budget guidelines is prepared by the chief financial officer to assist managers in completing their portions of the budget. These guidelines include explanations of the budget forms and reporting procedures; formulas for calculating the cost of employee benefits; cost and income figures for the past year; predictions of the rate of inflation and other cost increases (for anything from new equipment to the cost of electricity); and, of course, the deadlines for submitting budget requests.

Financial officers and their departments are also responsible for providing an analysis of the financial health of the organization and predicting its future financial status. They are responsible for the continuous management of the financial aspects of the organization, from paying employees and suppliers to collecting payments from patients or third-party payers.

They also are involved in producing reports (usually biweekly and monthly) that help departments monitor their total expenses as compared to what they planned to spend. These reports are called **variance reports** (see Tables 14–1 and 14–2). When specific costs run over or under what was projected for the month, or year to date (YTD), a variance occurs. A variance is simply a difference, either more or less, from what was planned (Porter-O'Grady, 1987). As a nurse manager, it is important to understand variances because you will most likely be required to explain any variances that exceed a certain dollar or percent amount.

> *[A sound cost accounting system] . . . not only reveals our mistakes—it shows us who's doing a good job!*
> —Bror R. Carlson in Eigen & Siegel, 1989, p. 2

As an example, let's say your organization has determined that all variances of 5 percent or greater must be explained in writing. Last month's variance reports show that $2,800 was spent on rental equipment for your unit and you had budgeted only $1,900 for last month, a 32 percent variance. It would be important to know why a variance occurred. Two factors that would increase rental equipment costs might be a high census (more patients than expected) or a high number of acute patients. Another factor might be that the business office inadvertently charged your unit for a rental item used by another unit. Whatever the cause, it is important to know why a variance occurred and to be able to explain why it was necessary.

## Managers

In the decentralized, participative approach to budgeting, every manager is responsible for preparing his or her section of the budget in detail. This budget should reflect the needs of the unit or department and be congruent with the goals of the organization. All of the departmental budgets prepared at this level are eventually combined into the master budget. To keep the subject of financial management relatively simple, we will concentrate primarily on describing

**Table 14-1** Monthly Budget Report

| Account Name/ Salary Expense: | Present Month | | | | Year to Date | | | |
|---|---|---|---|---|---|---|---|---|
| | Actual | Budgeted | Variance[a] | Percent Variance[b] | Actual | Budgeted | Variance[a] | Percent Variance[b] |
| RNs | $19,931.27 | 28,902.00 | 8,970.73 | 31.03 | 55,110.63 | 87,670.00 | 32,559.37 | 37.13 |
| LPNs | 1,481.72 | 0.00 | −1,481.72[c] | 100.00 | 3,861.36 | 0.00 | −3,861.36[c] | 100.00 |
| CNAs | 9,148.71 | 14,687.00 | 5,538.29 | 37.70 | 26,348.98 | 44,550.00 | 18,201.02 | 40.85 |
| Dietary expense | 525.82 | 943.00 | 417.18 | 44.23 | 1,763.10 | 2,829.00 | 2,065.90 | 37.67 |
| Office supplies/Equipment | 545.21 | 477.00 | −68.21[c] | −14.29 | 545.21 | 1,431.00 | 885.79 | 61.90 |

[a]Formula for variance: Budgeted amount − Actual amount = Variance.

[b]Formula for percent variance: Variance ÷ Budgeted amount = Percent variance.

[c]A negative number indicates over budget.

**Table 14–2** Monthly Budget Variance Summary

Month August

Department Rehabilitation
Prepared by AH

Variances for Month
10% and greater than
$200.00

| Cost Center/ Account Name | Month | | | Year to Date | | | Explanation/Action |
| | Actual | Budget | % | Actual | Budget | % | |
| | | | $ | | | $ | |
| | | | Variance | | | Variance | |
| 1010-3 LPN | $1,481.72 | 0.00 | 100 −1,481.7 | $3,861.36 | 0.00 | 100 −3,861.36 | Shift salary budgeted for RN to LPN category |
| Supplies/Equipment | 545.21 | 477.00 | 14.29 68.21 | 545.21 | 1,431.00 | 61.90 885.79 | Temporary variance—unit census high for this month, within budget for the year |

302

the components of a budget that would be prepared by a nurse manager.

> *Even though not all nurse managers are responsible for budget development, an understanding of underlying dynamics is necessary to have any input to the budget and control processes.*
>
> —Grohar-Murray & DiCroce, 1992

## ● TYPES OF BUDGETS

We will consider two different approaches to preparing the budget: incremental and zero-based budgeting. Incremental, or historical, budgeting is by far the most common.

### Incremental Budgeting

Incremental, or historical, budgeting is the traditional process in which budgets are prepared every year on the basis of what was spent the year before (Berman & Weeks, 1979). The two most basic components of the budget are **income** by its source (contributions, private payment, Medicare, Medicaid, and other third-party payers) and **expenses** (salaries, benefits, equipment, supplies, overhead, staff education, and so forth).

The budget process begins with the validation of certain assumptions, and includes an analysis of the income and expenses of the previous fiscal year. Special attention is given to departments and categories that were substantially over budget or under budget and the reasons for these deviations (variances) from the previous budget. The reasons for the deviations are taken into consideration in projecting the next year's income and expenses.

A variance indicates that historical expenses did not reflect what was predicted. It is necessary to analyze these variances to make sound management decisions. The analysis of variances may demonstrate that assumptions were inaccurate because of either internal or external factors. For example:

> A hospital orthopedics unit did a staffing budget based on the assumption that the average daily census (ADC) would remain at 22 patients. A new orthopedic surgeon came on board and the census went to 30, which increased the demand for nursing FTEs. The result was a variance in the anticipated expenses for nursing salaries. But there was also an increase in revenues, another variance.

You can see that a variance is not necessarily a negative. Budgeting projections are also based on plans to expand or limit services, add new staff, and so forth. Any of these actions require a change in the budget, usually an increase, which is the reason it is called an incremental budget. In incremental budgeting, the projected changes in costs and income are simply *added* to the previous year's budget.

After analysis of the organization's past budget and future plans, dollar figures are assigned to all departments and to all categories on both the income and expenditure sides of the budget. In some organizations, individual departments are given some flexibility in allocating funds to various categories. In other organizations, departments are restricted to using funds only as designated in the budget unless a modification is requested and approved.

### Zero-Based Budgeting

Zero-based budgeting is designed to require even more justification from each department for any funds budgeted for the next year. This approach is based on the idea that no expense should be assumed to be absolutely necessary.

The use of the **decision package** is the core of the zero-based budgeting process and the feature that particularly distinguishes it from the incremental process (Pyhrr, 1973). Decision packages consist of several basic elements: a listing of all current and proposed objectives or activities of a given team, nursing unit, or department; alternative ways of carrying out these activities and the different costs for each alternative; the advantages of continuing the activity; and the consequences of discontinuing the activity. The following is a sample from a decision package (without cost figures) for a staff development department:

| | |
|---|---|
| **Objective:** | Provide CPR (cardiopulmonary resuscitation) instruction for all employees. |

| Advantages: | Prepares all employees to respond immediately to an emergency situation |
| | Saves lives and reduces insurance premiums |
| | Additional benefit to employees |
| | Retain Joint Commission Accreditation |
| Disadvantages: | Time away from work for CPR class |
| | Cost of part-time CPR instructor |
| **Alternative 1:** | Require each employee to acquire CPR instruction from a community organization |
| Major Advantage: | No cost to organization |
| Major Disadvantage: | Employee resistance and resentment of control of off-duty hours |
| **Alternative 2:** | Do not require CPR |
| Major Advantage: | No cost, no employee resentment |
| Major Disadvantage: | Potential loss of client life, jeopardize accreditation, increased insurance rates, and potential lawsuits |

All of the listed activities, such as providing CPR instruction in the previous example, are ranked or arranged by priority, from the most essential activities required to maintain minimal operation of the nursing unit to those that are nonessential but desirable if sufficient money is available to support them. The packages are then compiled for the entire organization and further prioritizing is done on the basis of organization-wide goals and resources.

*Money is of no value; it cannot spend itself. All depends on the skill of the spender.*
—Ralph Waldo Emerson, 1803–1882, in Eigen & Siegel, 1989 p. 3

Zero-based budgeting requires more documentation and justification than does incremental budgeting. More attention is given to identifying activities and expenses that are assumed to be essential but are actually avoidable. It requires the nurse manager to review the way in which business has been conducted and to decide whether it is the most cost efficient, appropriate way to do business.

## ● THE BUDGET PROCESS

### Phase I. Planning

As was mentioned earlier, the planning phase is an important part of the overall financial management of a healthcare organization (Table 14–3). No facility operates in a vacuum: the current economic picture, growth of competition, regulatory changes, and other factors can have a great impact on the future costs and income of every organization. It is important that the nurse manager be aware of these trends and their effect on nursing within the organization. An understanding of the goals of the organization is also critical. Is future growth and expansion an important goal? Or are short-term profits considered more important? Are employees considered a valuable resource to be nurtured and developed or are they considered a short-term resource to be pushed to their limits for as long as they can endure it?

Priorities must be established, specific guidelines need to be developed, past performance analyzed, responsibilities assigned, a budget committee selected, and deadlines for completing the budget established. Once these tasks are done, a draft of the budget can be prepared.

As the nurse manager you know the needs of your unit. Talk to your staff before you are

**Table 14–3** The Budgeting Process

| Phase I. Planning | Phase II. Drafting | Phase III. Modification & Approval | Phase IV. Monitoring |
|---|---|---|---|
| 1. Set short- and long-term goals<br>2. Obtain input from staff<br>3. Prioritize objectives<br>4. Analyze past performance<br>5. Predict future costs and revenues<br>6. Review time lines for budget completion<br>7. Ascertain estimates, compare costs<br>8. Identify capital equipment needs | 1. Translate objectives into projected costs and revenues<br>2. Write justifications for all requested expenses<br>3. Present proposed budget<br>4. Submit capital requests | 1. Receive back preliminary budget from management review<br>2. Eliminate lowest-priority items if necessary<br>3. Approve final budget<br>4. Communicate final budget to all departments | 1. Review monthly summaries of departmental expenses and revenues<br>2. Compare actual expenses with budgeted expenses to determine variances<br>3. Investigate and provide justification for any variance within your budget guidelines<br>4. Readjust budget and/or improve performance as necessary<br>5. Continue to monitor on monthly basis |

handed the budget packet. During the course of the year document unit needs, such as equipment, education, and so on.

## Phase II. Drafting

Each manager develops goals and objectives for his or her department or unit. These objectives are then translated into probable cost and revenue figures. For the nurse manager, most of the calculations required to do this kind of translation involve predictions about the staff and supplies needed to do the work and the amount of patient service or patient days and associated income that will be generated. Basic concepts regarding the nursing budget include the following:

1. *Full-time equivalents (FTEs).* A full-time employee is one who is paid 40 hours per week over the calendar year. One full-time employee represents 2,080 hours of pay in a calendar year.

   An FTE of 1.0 refers to a payroll unit equal to a 40-hour week. This unit of time and pay does not represent a person specifically, but does represent the hours worked. For example, the full-time worker on a traditional unit works five eight-hour days per week. On a particular unit that 40-hour period may be covered by two different part-time individuals, one working 2 days (16 hours) and one working 3 days (24 hours). The total FTE is 1.0; each individual makes up a portion of that FTE. The person who works 16 hours a week is a .4 FTE, and the person who works 24 hours is a .6 FTE.

2. *Actual hours worked.* When preparing the budget, the difference between hours worked and hours paid is important. Most regular full-time employees are paid for more hours than they actually work. **Hours worked** is the actual hours spent working. **Hours paid** is the amount of time paid for, including vacation and sick time (Box 14–2).

   An FTE receives 2,080 hours of pay in a year. This figure represents 40 hours per week multiplied by 52 weeks per year. Any time that an individual is paid but is not working on the unit due to sick time, holidays, vacation, jury duty, or funeral leave is considered nonproductive time. Those hours must then be covered by another person if staffing levels are to be maintained. The net effect is that the manager must adjust the needed FTEs to cover all anticipated nonproductive hours. Those organizations that provide generous vacation benefits that increase with longevity (length of time employed) may find that units with stable workforces have increased numbers of nonproductive hours and therefore increased FTE needs.

3. *Productivity standard/Staffing requirement.* A factor that is needed to establish a staffing budget is referred to as the **productivity standard.** The standard is a number that is established by historical experience, validated by the time/work studies and authorized by management. It equals the number of hours of care each patient will receive in a 24-hour period. The name for this standard is **hours per patient day,** or HPPD. It is important to un-

derstand this number because it is useful in evaluating whether more or less care is being delivered than expected. HPPD is a direct reflection of the number of staff needed in relation to the number of patients on the unit (census). The average HPPD multiplied by the number of patients will yield your total hours of nursing care needed in a 24-hour period (see Box 14–3).

The example shown in Box 14–3 permits you to use 12.5, 8-hour people over a 24-hour period. Depending on how you distribute the workload of a unit, it may be typical for you to assign 5.5 staff on day shift, 4 on evenings, and 3 on nights. The distribution of the 12.5 persons over a 24-hour period is a management decision. Obviously, a .5, or half person does not exist. It simply means one person works 4 hours that day. To determine FTE needs for an annual budget, you must multiply the productivity standard (in our example, Box 14–3,

> ### Box 14–4   Hours into FTEs for One Year (Annually)
>
> $$\frac{\text{Total required hours} \times 365 \text{ days in a year}}{\text{Actual hours worked in a year}}$$
> $$= \text{FTEs needed}$$
>
> ### Example:
>
> $$\frac{100 \times 365 = 36,500 \text{ Nursing care hours}}{1,799 \text{ (productive hours per FTE)}}$$
>
> $$= 20.2 \text{ FTEs to staff the unit annually to provide the HPPD}$$
>
> Note: Total required hours was calculated on the basis of 4 hours per patient day × average daily patient census of 25 (see Table 14–4).

4 hours per patient day, PPD) by the average census (25) to get the total hours of care needed (4 × 25 = 100 hours PPD) per day. Then you multiply hours needed per day by 365 days per year (100 HPPD × 365 days/year = 36,000 hours/year). This number is divided by the productive hours an FTE at the respective facility actually works. In our example, that is 1,799 hours (Box 14–2). Box 14–4 shows this calculation. The result is that 20.2 FTEs are needed to provide the care and staffing coverage to the level of hours we have accepted as the standard on this unit (4 HPPD on this unit). Translating these hours into people (FTEs) is how you calculate your staffing requirements.

4. *Staffing budget.* We will continue the example to develop a simplified annual staffing budget for this unit. In the example given, it was esti-

mated that 20.2 FTEs would be needed to give direct care. In addition, a nurse manager, assistant nurse manager, and support services for the unit are needed (Table 14–4). Employee benefits, such as continuing education costs, membership in professional organizations, health insurance, and retirement benefits as well as social security and state and federal unemployment taxes are calculated by the facility at a rate of 30 percent of the annual salary (this percentage will vary from one institution to another). The grand total of $1,014,228 is the amount budgeted for the personnel who work on the rehabilitation unit. A separate summary sheet would be used for other expenses such as office supplies, medical supplies, equipment, and overhead (repairs, maintenance, electricity, and so forth).

### Table 14–4   Annual Staffing Budget Summary

#### Rehabilitation Unit

| Staff | A. FTEs | B. Annual Salary | C. Benefits 30%* | D. Total A (B + C). |
|---|---|---|---|---|
| Nurse manager | 1 | $46,500 | $13,950 | $60,450 |
| Assistant nurse manager | 1 | 41,000 | 12,300 | 53,350 |
| Unit clerk | 2 | 20,000 | 6,000 | 26,000 |
| FTEs:   RNs | 14 | 553,000 | 165,900 | 718,900 |
|        LPNs | 2 | 49,800 | 14,940 | 64,740 |
|        CNAs | 4.2 | 81,900 | 24,570 | 106,470 |
| Total | 23.2 | | | Total salary costs = $1,029,860 |

*Benefits including shift differentials.

| Table 14–5    Shift Differential Calculation* | | | | | | | |
|---|---|---|---|---|---|---|---|
| Staff | | Average Salary | | Differential | | | Total Yearly Cost of Differential |
| Days: | | | | | | | |
| 9 staff members | × | $23,944 | × | 0% | | = | 0 |
| Evenings: | | | | | | | |
| 7 staff members | × | $20,785 | × | 10% (0.10) | | = | $14,579 |
| Nights: | | | | | | | |
| 4.2 staff members | × | $20,000 | × | 20% (0.20) | | = | $16,800 |
| Total = 20.2 FTEs | | | | | | | |

*Number of staff × average salary × shift differential = total annual costs.

If you wanted to further determine what your differential costs were per shift, see Table 14–5.

5. *Expenses.* Expenses include such items as office supplies, medical supplies, equipment, and overhead (repairs, maintenance, rent, electricity, etc.). Some of these expenses vary with census and some are fixed expenses throughout the year. For example, as the census increases, the utilization of medical supplies will increase, while the rent does not change. To predict the dollars that should be budgeted for variable expenses one can use a simple formula. First, determine the annual total of the item in question from the previous year's history. For example, last year the unit spent $500 on trash bags. Next find the total patient days for that year. Let's say it was 9,125 (ADC = 25 × 365 days = 9,125 patient days/year). Divide the dollar amount of $500 by the total patient days of 9,125 to get a factor of (.06). Multiply that factor (.06) by the total number of patient days predicted for the new budget year, 9,625 (total assumed patient days) × .06 = $577.50. So, $577.50 is the amount to budget in the new year for trash bags.

6. *Capital expenses.* You also need to justify capital expenses for the unit (Porter-O'Grady, 1987). A capital expense usually involves a large sum of money or equipment with a lifetime of one year or more, such as a portable X-ray machine. Specific definitions of what belongs in the category of capital equipment will vary from organization to organization.

Managers usually have to provide administrators with a brief written explanation of the rationale behind such budget requests.

The completed budget usually includes a breakdown of monthly costs and revenues as well as the totals for the year. The completed budget, along with the written justification, is then submitted.

## Phase III. Modification and Approval

The budget requests for your unit will compete with requests from other nursing units and other departments in the institution when they are combined into the master budget. The total amount requested from all departments must be compared with the amount of revenue that could reasonably be expected to be earned in the next year. Budget requests often have to be reduced to achieve a balance between expected costs and expected revenues. Generally, the lowest-priority items are cut first, although when resources are limited even high-priority items must be eliminated. Skillful politicking can result in low-priority items being retained at the expense of higher-priority items.

Sometimes the budget committee simply will say, "Reduce all budgets by 5 percent." It is important to have a good working knowledge of your budget so that you can make the appropriate reductions with the least possible negative effect.

Next, the final budget is prepared, approved by the administrator and governing board, and then sent to each department to serve as the financial guide for the coming year.

## Phase IV. Monitoring

Financial management is far more than the annual rite of preparing the budget. The budget is a working document, a guide to the financial component of unit and department management, and a yardstick by which to evaluate the effectiveness of management.

Monthly summaries of expenses and income are usually distributed to every manager and should be carefully reviewed for two reasons. The first reason is to catch any possible errors made by the accounting department. For example, expenditures made by other departments may erroneously be charged to your unit. It is important to spot these errors and to be sure that they are corrected.

Second, the monthly summaries usually report both the budgeted amount and the amount actually spent for each category. Any differences between these two figures should be checked, especially those that are 5 percent or more over the budgeted amount (generally 10 percent under the budgeted amount in the case of revenues). Sometimes the variance appears because a large expenditure was made in one month (for example, the purchase of a new monitor) and will not appear again for the rest of the year. When averaged over the year, this expense should equal the budgeted amount. In other cases, however, you might note that expenses are over budget for items such as supplies or temporary personnel and that these need to either be brought under control or further justified to administration, depending on the situation. This regular surveillance should occur every month.

Another important aspect of monitoring that goes beyond the surveillance of the monthly summaries is an in-depth analysis of various financial aspects of your unit's operation. A number of factors are worthy of analysis. You could, for example, analyze the cost of using disposable versus reusable supplies or the difference between leasing and buying an expensive piece of equipment (computerized monitors, the unit ice machine, a copier, and so forth). Mention of the cost of various procedures and tests can be added to the usual clinical data presented on patient rounds if staff need to become more budget-conscious (West, 1994). The effectiveness of an all-RN staff compared with a mixture of aides, practical nurses, and RNs is a perennial issue that has financial implications. The savings realized by using nurse practitioners rather than physicians is another issue with budgetary implications that frequently comes up as does the cost of making home visits versus providing care during clinic visits. Attention to issues of accountability and efficiency can also help to improve care despite limitations in resources. In larger organizations, the budget or accounting office will assist first-line managers to do these analyses.

The results of the financial analyses can be used to support your arguments in favor of needed improvements, better management of nursing staff, and increased recognition of the contribution of nursing to the overall success of the organization. One example of how this analysis can lead to improved treatment of staff is the cost of staff turnover in the organization. Although many different reasons might explain why a staff member leaves an employer, one of the major ones is dissatisfaction with working conditions (salary, opportunities for advancement, and so forth). The cost of replacing just one nurse can be quite substantial. This cost includes advertising and recruiting activities, interviewing, processing the application, orientation (salaries of instructional staff, supplies, staff time, and so forth), and a temporary replacement until the position is filled. All together, it could cost an organization $4,000 or more per new nurse hired. In a large organization that hires 100 nurses in a year, turnover alone would cost the organization $400,000 a year. Suggestions for action to improve working conditions and reduce this expense should fall on receptive ears and lead to improvements in working conditions for the current staff. You can see that financial analyses of the operation of a unit are time-consuming but often provide persuasive data to support requests for changes in the budget or management of the unit.

Financial management as a whole is a complex but important subject. Professional nurses who assume responsibility for leadership need a basic understanding of the budget and its implications to enable an appropriate response in defense of an adequate budget.

## ● SUMMARY

The financial management of a healthcare organization affects the work of every professional in that organization. Finances need to be considered when doing any kind of planning. Organizational members who control the budget control an important source of power within the organization.

Responsibility for financial management begins with the governing board and administration of the organization. When participative management is used, it extends to every nurse manager and his or her staff.

The incremental type of budget is built on past budgets, whereas zero-based budgeting assesses objectives for the coming year and demands that every expenditure, no matter how basic, must be justified. No matter which budget strategy is used, cost analysis in regard to quality outcomes must be employed. The budgeting process begins with these objectives, which are then translated into projected costs and revenues, modified as needed, approved, and then monitored throughout the year for any variance from planned costs and revenues.

## REFERENCES

Bean, J.J. & Laliberty, R. (1980). *Decentralizing hospital management: A manual for supervisors.* Reading, MA: Addison-Wesley.

Berman, H.J. & Weeks, L.E. (1979). *The financial management of hospitals.* Ann Arbor, MI: Health Administration Press.

Dillon, R.D. (1979). *Zero base budgeting for health care institutions.* Rockville, MD: Aspen.

Eigen, L.D. & Siegel, J.P. (1989). *The manager's book of quotations.* New York: AMACOM.

---

## C A S E   S T U D Y

### Shifting Staff

You are the nurse manager of a 25-bed rehabilitation unit. You routinely staff the 7:00 A.M. to 3:00 P.M. shift with 5.5 people, 3:00 P.M. to 11:00 P.M. with 4 people, and 11:00 P.M. to 7:00 A.M. with 3 people. The night staff has been expressing great frustration, and the patients have complained of long delays in answering call lights at night. You cannot add another FTE staff member because your budget for personnel covers only 12.5 FTEs total per day. Given this limitation, if you put an additional person on the 11:00 P.M to 7:00 A.M. shift your choice is to take one off the day shift or evening shift.

### Questions for Critical Reflection and Analysis

1. If you add 1.0 FTE to the night shift staff, what tasks can be moved to the 11:00 P.M. to 7:00 A.M. shift to reduce the overload created by the reduction on either the 7:00 A.M. to 3:00 P.M. shift or the 3:00 P.M. to 11:00 P.M. shift?

2. How could you explain the loss of an FTE in a positive way to the shift that "loses" a staff member?

3. What tasks could potentially be eliminated altogether? How would you determine which tasks?

4. If no one permanently assigned to the 7:00 A.M. to 3:00 P.M. shift or 3:00 P.M. to 11:00 P.M. shift volunteers to change shifts, what are the implications? How would you handle it?

5. Other than shifting one person from day or evening shift to the night shift, what else could you do to resolve the night shift problem?

6. To whom in the organization would you go for guidance on how to respond to this problem?

Finkler, S.A. (1992). *Budgeting concepts for nurse managers.* Philadelphia: W.B. Saunders.

Finkler, S.A., Knickman, J.R. & Hanson, K.L. (1994). Improving the financial viability of primary care health centers. *Hospital and Health Services Administration, 39*(1), 117–131.

Finkler, S.A. & Kovner, C.T. (1993). *Financial management for nurse managers and executives.* Philadelphia: W.B. Saunders.

Grohar-Murray, M.E. & DiCroce, H.R. (1992). *Leadership and management in nursing.* CA: Appleton & Lange.

Hankins, R., Brady, T. & Saucier, B. (1998). Finance and accounting applications in nursing and clinical services, *Nursing Management, 4*(8), 18–21.

Hannigan, T.A. (1998). *Managing tomorrow's high-performance unions.* Westport, CT: Quorum Books.

Hendricks, J. & Baume, P. (1997). The pricing of nursing care. *Journal of Advanced Nursing, 25*(3), 454–462.

Kiser, J.J. (1988). The role of the financial managers: How much has it changed? *Healthcare Financial Management, 42,* 72–76.

Needles, B.E., Anderson, H.R. & Caldwell, J.C. (1984). *Principles of accounting.* Boston: Houghton Mifflin.

Porter-O'Grady, T. (1987). *Nursing finance, budgeting strategies for a new age.* Rockville, MD: Aspen Publishers.

Pyhrr, P.A. (1973). *Zero base budgeting: A practical management tool for evaluating expenses.* New York: John Wiley & Sons.

Stone, P.N. (1998). Methods for conducting and reporting cost-effectiveness analysis in nursing. *Image-Journal of Nursing Scholarship, 30*(3), 229–234.

West, D.J. (1994). Involving physicians in cost reduction strategies. *Healthcare Financial Management, 48*(4), 46–47.

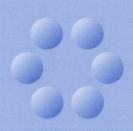

CHAPTER *15*

# Informatics and Nursing Management

## LEARNING OBJECTIVES

*After completing this chapter, the reader will be able to:*

- List the components of successful nursing information systems.
- Describe existing nursing nomenclatures and taxonomies.
- Discuss the advantages and disadvantages of implementing computer-based patient record systems.

- Outline the use of technology in nursing management.
- Discuss the function and future of telehealth.

## TEST YOURSELF

**Are you ready to answer questions about informatics?**

*Try responding to the following scenarios before you read this chapter. Review your answers after reading the chapter.*

### Scenario I

You have just assumed your first nurse manager position. In your previous position (in another healthcare facility), the chief nursing officer was extremely innovative and the organization's computerized patient record system was outstanding. This new agency has only limited use of the computer and no standard patient record system or nomenclature. When you approached the chief nursing officer and asked permission to present some of your ideas at the next nurse managers' meeting, she refused, saying, "Computerized charting is just a fad—I don't want to spend money on that. Besides, nurses need to be creative in their charting to best represent the patient." How will you respond?

### Scenario II

You are applying for your first position as a nurse manager. You consider yourself an outstanding clinician and a real "people person." The chief nursing officer is deciding between you and another well-qualified candidate. She asks you, "How do you view the use of technology in health care today?" What will you respond in order to demonstrate your knowledge of technology in health care?

---

As we enter the twenty-first century, computerized information systems, electronic monitoring devices, microprocessor implants, automated imaging systems, telehealth, and robotics have already permeated the health care system. Nurse leaders-managers are now expected to utilize information systems technology in planning and implementing nursing care (Travis & Brennan, 1998). Even though the healthcare information superhighway is still under development, nurse leaders and managers are expected to be familiar with:

- accessing patient records in real-time online.
- using a bedside or portable computer to document patient data and nursing care and access information from other team members.
- holding conferences with other healthcare providers via the Internet.
- accessing global databases, listserves, and library holdings.
- delivering healthcare services and information via the Internet to clients in remote areas (Bachman & Panzarine, 1998).
- using computerized databases to monitor budgets, schedule staff, evaluate the quality of care given and assess the effectiveness and efficiency of the care systems under their leadership and management.

Information has become one of the most critical sources of power in health care. The ability to access and disseminate information quickly and accurately can empower staff in many ways, including making timely, informed, cost-effective decisions for their clients (see Figure 15–1).

> *An individual without information cannot take responsibility; an individual who is given information cannot help but take responsibility.*
> —J. Carlzon, quoted in Wall Street Journal, 1999

In this chapter we will discuss the concept and components of nursing informatics including databases and data sets and the use of nursing nomenclature and taxonomies. We will identify the characteristics of successful computer systems and the issues surrounding the computer-based patient record. Nurse manager department planning activities using computer software will be identified as well as security and audit issues. The chapter

| | | | | | |
|---|---|---|---|---|---|
| **Problem** | **Prescription drug costs** are rising 16% to 18% annually | **Doctor bills vary wildly** across the nation for identical services | **Administrators are flooded** with non-urgent phone queries about drugs, appointments, and health care | **Health-insurance costs** to businesses are on the rise, by an average 18% to 20% nationwide | **Between 10% to 15% of patient tests** must be repeated because of lost or misread records |
| **Solution** | **Kaiser's in-house network** suggests cheaper drug alternatives or less dangerous medications | **Kaiser's in-house network** taps into a database that suggests standard treatments aimed at containing excessive charges | **Kaiser's web site** lets patients check their appointments and e-mail pharmacists with routine queries | **Kaiser's in-house network** cuts client paperwork and customizes premiums by offering real-time quotes | **In-house network** creates digital records that can easily be accessed by authorized personnel |
| **Payoff** | **Drug costs** dropped 20% at some clinics; legal costs are down; and incorrect prescriptions have been reduced | **Health-care costs** are reduced by 5% to 10% across Kaiser's operations | **Kaiser's Northern California division** expects a $4 million decrease in phone bills this year, and to cut support staff by one-fourth | **Kaiser's 4,000-plus insurance brokers** can calculate quotes and notify clients in minutes | **Duplicate tests** are virtually eliminated in some clinics, for a cost savings of an estimated $1 million in Kaiser's Northwest unit last year |

**Figure 15–1**   How informatics can be used to cut costs without reducing quality: Examples from Kaiser Permanente. *Source:* Gantenbein, D. & Stepanek, M. (2000/February 7) Kaiser takes the cyber cure. *Business Week,* EB80–85. Reprinted with permission.

ends with a discussion of telehealth and the implications for nursing.

## ● INFORMATICS

The term **informatics** was defined in 1983 as "computer science plus information science." Adding the name of the discipline, informatics denotes the application of computer and information sciences to the data management, knowledge, development, and classification of information within that discipline (Graves & Corcoran, 1989, p. 227).

The idea of "medical informatics" began in the 1970s as technology advances made it possible to enter data concerning patient care into computers. The term **health informatics** was later applied to information encompassing medicine, nursing, dental, pharmacy, and other healthcare disciplines. As members of each discipline identified the distinct information needed for professional practice, multiple informatics systems were developed (Graves & Corcoran, 1989). In the late 1960s nurses began to use electronic tools to assist in the collection and management of nursing information. Although slow to develop at first, the field is now advancing rapidly (NINR, 1999).

### Nursing Informatics

Nursing informatics is defined as the "combination of computer science, information science, and nursing science designed to assist in management and processing of nursing data, information, and knowledge to support the practice of nursing and the delivery of nursing care" (Graves & Corcoran, 1989, p. 227). As defined by the American Nurses Association (1994), nursing informatics includes: identifying, acquiring, preserving, managing, retrieving, aggregating, analyzing, and transmitting data, information, and knowledge to make it meaningful and useful to nurses (p. 6). Effective application requires (1) use of computers and understanding of computer technology, (2) identification of conceptual issues and key concepts related to nursing knowledge, and (3) development of computerized information management systems to enhance nursing practice through the entering, organizing, and retrieval of information. The interaction of these three requirements constitutes the core of nursing informatics (Turley, 1996).

Economics and the knowledge explosion continue to drive the need to advance nursing informatics. The major economic concerns are the need to maximize nursing productivity, achieve efficiency, and ensure satisfactory patient outcomes. In addition, informatics supports nursing research, which continues to expand nursing's knowledge base while the increasing complexity of patient care forces nurses to utilize increasing amounts of information when making decisions (Zielstorff, Hudgings & Grobe, 1993).

Using an integrated information system, patient-specific data, collected only once, could be used in many different situations (see Table 15–1). For example, once the patient is admitted to the hospital, a computerized patient record can be ini-

tiated. Using an integrated information system, the insurance company is billed electronically, eliminating the need for printing and mailing statements, thus saving money. Staff of the Quality Improvement department can collect data on patients and look for trends in cost and patient outcomes. Also, the need to copy and mail client records or referral forms to other agencies or to individually code and enter data from each paper chart is unnecessary. The software used to access the computerized patient record can automatically search for needed information.

## Databases and Data Sets

The development of computer systems to handle nursing data may well be the easy part. Historically, nurses have had difficulty articulating what nurses actually do and what impact nurses have on outcomes. The problem becomes more acute when the information is computerized. As early as 1986, the American Nurses Association (ANA) supported the development of a national nursing database for clinical practice. In response, the Steering Committee on Databases to Support

---

**Table 15–1** Multiple Uses of Patient Data

| User | Data | Scope |
|------|------|-------|
| Caregiver, insurer, individual agency | Patient-specific data: assessments, diagnoses, interventions, test results, procedures, treatments, patient care hours, outcome | Individual client data |
| Administrators, researchers, accrediting bodies, QI departments | Cost by patient categories, number of patients with specific diagnoses, tests, procedures, interventions by volumes, diagnostic group patient outcomes | Organization wide data |
| Analysts, public health departments, researchers | Comparisons of treatment, outcomes, costs, incidences, and prevalences | Community and regional data |
| Policy makers, researchers, lawmakers, insurers | Trends related to incidence, prevalence, outcomes, costs, diagnosis | Nationwide data |
| World health officials, national policy makers and lawmakers, national research organizations | General health-related information of individual nations | Worldwide data |

*Source:* Adapted from Zielstorff, R., Hudgings, C. & Grobe, S. (1993). *Next generation nursing information systems.* Washington, DC: American Nurses Publishing.

Clinical Nursing Practice was formed in 1989. This committee recommended adoption of the Nursing Minimum Data Set (NMDS), originally developed by 64 nursing experts during a three-day invitational conference in 1985. The NMDS is a minimum set of essential informational items concerned with nursing care supported by standardized definitions and categories. This information is entered into a computerized patient record. The NMDS provides a common language of nursing that can be used in healthcare information systems, in nursing research and outcomes assessment, and in support of the move toward third-party reimbursement (ANA, 1995). Using a common language facilitates sharing information across disciplines. Elements of the NMDS can be found in Box 15–1.

## Nursing Nomenclature and Taxonomies

In addition to the NMDS, the ANA supports the development of scientifically based naming systems that define the scope of nursing and address the uniqueness of nursing practice (ANA, 1994). The holistic nature of nursing phenomena and the use of multiple conceptual frameworks have contributed to difficulty in standardizing nursing data. The question arises not only as to what data to include, but also as to how one defines commonly held concepts. Descriptions such as "copious," "frail," or "weak," for example, are difficult to specify in a data set that will be produced by a "point and click" computer application. This fuzziness of clinical terms and the use of clinical judgments in nursing are critical nursing information issues (NINR, 1999). The development of a system to collate, integrate, compare, and monitor computerized patient data is essential. In 1994 the ANA Steering Committee published a set of policy statements related to developing a single comprehensive system for classifying nursing practice (see Box 15–2).

The predominant nursing classification systems in use today are:

- North American Nursing Diagnosis Association (NANDA)
- The Omaha System
- The Home Health Care Classification
- The Nursing Interventions Classification

### North American Nursing Diagnosis Association (NANDA)

Work on the NANDA taxonomy began in the early 1970s as part of a demonstration project that required patient data to be computerized and discipline-specific. The nurses involved in the project soon realized that they were unable to do either. They recognized what a difficult task they had undertaken and sought assistance and advice from other nurses. Their efforts at problem solving soon led to the initial 1973 meeting of the National Conference Group for the Classification of Nursing Diagnoses. The initial group decided to hold more formalized meetings. After five yearly conferences, members of the group were still unable to agree on a classification scheme so a decision was made to list the nursing diagnoses alphabetically. During the fifth annual meeting, the North American Nursing Diagnosis Association (NANDA) was formed. NANDA is recognized by the ANA as the group responsible

---

**Box 15–1    National Minimum Data Set for Collecting Uniform, Standard, Compatible Nursing Data**

Nursing diagnosis/problem
Nursing intervention/treatment
Nursing-sensitive patient outcome
Intensity of nursing care
Patient personal identification
Patient date of birth
Patient sex
Patient race and ethnicity
Patient residence
Unique facility service number
Unique health record number of patient
Unique number of principal registered nurse provider
Episode admission or encounter date
Discharge date
Disposition of client
Expected payor for most of the bill

*Source:* American Nurses Association. (1995). *Nursing data systems: The emerging framework.* Washington, DC: American Nurses Publishing.

for the maintenance and development of a standardized nursing taxonomy (ANA, 1995).

## Omaha System

The Omaha System was developed by the Visiting Nurse Association of Omaha through a series of research projects. The system is a method of describing and measuring client problems, interventions, and outcomes. It has been found to be useful in home care, public and school health, correctional facilities, and outpatient facilities.

## Home Health Care Classification

Development of the Home Health Care Classification System began as a project at Georgetown University in the early 1990s. The purpose of the original study was to determine the resources required to provide home care services to Medicare clients and to identify the expected outcomes of those services. Today this system is used as the basis for measuring outcomes and effectiveness in many home health and community health agencies.

## Nursing Interventions Classification (Iowa Intervention Project NIC and NOC)

Nurse researchers at the University of Iowa have been working since 1987 on developing the Nursing Interventions Classification (NIC) and the Nursing Outcomes Classification (NOC) (University of Iowa, 1999). In 1995, the Center for Nursing Classification was established at the University of Iowa to facilitate the research and development of NIC and NOC. The Center supports a web page, an active listserve, a newsletter, and several other publications. NIC includes 433 interventions organized into 27 classes and 6 domains; it is linked to the NOC.

A computer program that would link these different systems so that common meanings across terms can be identified is also being developed. This common language or Unified Nursing Language System (UNLS) is an important step in organizing and classifying nursing-related information. By using accepted terms nurses can move towards a system for evaluating the quality and effectiveness of nursing care and services

(ANA, 1995). Guidelines and outcomes established by such agencies as the Health Care Financing Administration (HCFA), Agency for Healthcare Research and Quality (AHRQ), and Centers for Disease Control (CDC), as well as private insurance companies, can also be linked to the UNLS to further support the evaluation of nursing outcomes.

## CHARACTERISTICS OF SUCCESSFUL SYSTEMS

Useful nursing information systems do not come about easily or automatically. Implementation of a successful nursing information system requires the following conditions:

- *An explicit nursing knowledge base:* A nursing information system provides a means to accurately and succinctly describe nurses' actions and client outcomes. Data should be available for nurses to use during clinical decision making. The system should also support a variety of nursing conceptual frameworks.
- *Administrative support:* No matter how comprehensive the database of information is, if administration does not provide financial support to purchase upgrades or training for staff, it will quickly become useless. An administration that rewards users for creatively using the system, remaining open to new ideas, and making changes as needed will keep the system current and useful.
- *Standard vocabularies and data communication protocols*
- *Integrated system using common terminology:* If systems cannot "talk" to each other they become useless. To communicate they have to use the same language (software). If they do not, data cannot be transferred from one system to another or from one agency to another. In order to have a successful nursing information system, agreement must be reached on how computer systems can represent common types of clinical nursing information. Nursing definitions must mean the same to each computer that is "reaching out" to another. Unless both patient-specific (nursing assessment, diagnoses, and interventions) and agency-specific data

(standard medical diagnosis) mean the same to all the computers in the network, data will not be transferrable from one to another.
- *The use of nursing informatics specialists:* These knowledgeable nurses have the skills needed to manage and analyze the data, supporting full utilization of the system.
- *Collaboration between nursing personnel and computer systems personnel:* Nursing personnel and information systems personnel can work together, looking at what is needed "through different eyes" to create the most useful nursing information systems (Zielstorff, Hudgings & Grobe, 1993, pp. 35–42).

## NURSING INFORMATICS AND NURSING MANAGEMENT

### Computer-Based Patient Records (CPR)

One example of using technology to access and disseminate information quickly and accurately is the electronic patient record. Several benefits of using an electronic medical record include:

- Accessing the medical record from several different locations at the same time as well as by different levels of providers
- Allowing for access to data for use in research
- Decreasing error potential while improving communication
- Decreasing documentation time thereby increasing time for client care (Hebda, Czar & Mascara, 1998, p. 7)

Decision support software can be integrated into the computerized patient record. These decision support tools notify the clinician of possible concerns or omissions using a variety of alerts and reminders. For example, when a drug is ordered an alert will notify the primary care provider of any known allergies or even potential interactions with other drug orders.

*Patients used to wait up to eight days for lab test results. Now, they can see them in as little as several hours.*
—Gantenbein & Stepanek, 2000, p. EB85

The computer-based patient record (CPR) is an electronic patient record that stores the information entered by a variety of healthcare providers. The data specified in the NMDS should be included. The Institute of Medicine has identified 12 major characteristics they consider to be a "gold standard" for an effective CPR system (Andrew & Dick, 1996):

- A problem list that indicates the client's current clinical problems for each episode; provision for evaluation of patient health status and functional level using standardized definitions of these outcomes
- Documentation of the clinical reasoning/rationale for diagnoses and conclusions
- Link to other client data and records
- Confidentiality, privacy, and audit trails
- Continuous and simultaneous access for authorized users
- Links to local and remote information resources
- Access to decision analysis tools to facilitate clinical problem solving
- Direct entry of client data by providers
- Mechanisms for monitoring the cost and quality of care
- Flexibility and expandability of the system

The "gold standard" is still a goal to be accomplished. Many healthcare systems have automated part or all of the patient record but automation alone does not constitute a fully functional CPR as described. A truly longitudinal CPR, which can be accessed by all providers, provides links to other client data and records, allows for the documentation of outcomes, and allows for assistance with decision making, is probably within five to ten years of becoming a reality (Hebda, Czar & Mascara, 1997, p. 178).

### Benefits

A well-developed CPR used by a staff that is adequately trained in the system can be of benefit to the entire healthcare team. On CPRs, information is more readable, better organized, and should be more complete. Access to client information is available at multiple locations at any time of the day or night. Decision trees and other systems for decision analysis allow caregivers to logically plan care and identify appropriate interventions and outcomes. Use of CPRs can facilitate the automation of critical pathways and allow easy access to current and historical data.

Less space is needed for record storage and the chance of losing the record is decreased (Hebda, Czar & Mascara, 1998).

> *Technology has brought about changes in the delivery of health care and in the amount and kind of information available for decision making in nursing.*
> —King, 1998, p. 1

### Caregiver Resistance

Resistance to implementation of a CPR is not uncommon. The end user, whether a registered nurse, physician, or other staff member, may feel totally overwhelmed by the need to learn an entirely new system. Some healthcare providers still do not use a computer in their personal life. Their unwillingness to use the CPR may be due to lack of familiarity with computers, the complexity of the software, availability of the computer terminals, disruptive effect on their preferred workflow pattern or even an inability to type (Simpson, 1997).

> *Cyberphobia—"fear of computers." Characterized by panic, terror, heart palpitations, breathing difficulties, dizziness, trembling, going crazy, or losing control.*
> —Siegel, 1998, p. 69

Managers responsible for facilitating the introduction of CPRs should be sure they recognize and understand the needs of each team member as they begin using the CPR. Team members include not only the professional nursing staff but also physicians and others who will be accessing the record (Hebda, Czar & Mascara, 1998). A description of one way to recommend the introduction of a new system can be found in Chapter 10 on change. See Perspectives . . . Informatics and the Human Side of Nursing.

## Management Applications
### Department Planning Activities

Planning and monitoring the unit's budget are usually the nurse manager's responsibility. Ability to access budget information from the organization's

## PERSPECTIVES . . .

### Informatics and the Human Side of Nursing

Many individuals who enter nursing are "people persons" who enjoy and need the daily face-to-face interactions with their coworkers and patients. Through interpersonal interactions we discover the patient and one another. It is also through these interpersonal interactions that we deliver much of our nursing care to our patients and clients. Brennan (1996) says that this core function is not replaced in the electronic environment, only revised. What do you think? How could it be revised?

*Source:* Brennan, P. (1996, October 11). The future of clinical communication in an electronic environment. *Holistic Nursing Practice, 1,* 97–104.

database provides you with valuable data that you can aggregate and compare over time. You can also create reports from the database. By tracking such data as unit census, patient acuity, staffing levels, and patient outcomes you will be able to develop a useful, realistic budget. Having "real" information to share with staff will assist them in understanding the process behind your decisions. Sharing historical data with staff is a useful method of helping them to look at a situation differently. For example:

*You are the nurse manager for a 60-bed oncology unit. The vice president of nursing informs you that your predecessor had run over his projected budget for the past two years. Because you have only been in the position for three months, you were not part of past budget planning. The vice president of nursing has a reputation for being a real "stickler" when it comes to the budget process. You want to impress her but at the same time do what is best for your staff and your clients.*

*Once you learned how to decipher the budget data from the previous two years, you could see where your predecessor went over allowable expenses. Knowing where your predecessor ran into trouble helped you create a plan to avoid doing the same thing. With this plan in place, you can monitor how well you are doing*

*staying within budget by periodically calling up the budget data for your unit from the database maintained by the finance department.*

A number of commercial software packages can be useful adjuncts in management (Microsoft, 1999). These packages allow you to develop your own databases and spreadsheets. They also help you monitor projects and manage your personal information. You can develop a database of names and addresses of staff and vendors to print mailing labels on your department printer.

Using project management software, you can map out an entire project including personnel needed, tasks, hours worked versus hours assigned, and staffing issues related to time away from actually providing patient care. Project management software can help you

- carefully delineate a plan.
- identify and monitor schedules and tasks associated with a project.
- detect inconsistencies and problems in the plan.
- communicate the plan to others.
- track progress and detect potential difficulties.

*The trick is to view technology as more than "just" an information system with which one must stay involved . . . the savvy nurse executive will look at technology as a way to "plug in" to more and more information—both personally and professionally—to advance his or her own knowledge base, connections and personal or professional network . . . to do more in less time and with a whole lot less cumbersome paper.*

—*Simpson, 1995, p. 89*

### Security Issues

As a rule, upper-level managers and information systems department personnel work together to develop policies and procedures related to security functions. As a first-line manager, you can set a positive example related to protection of client privacy and confidentiality. Your staff also needs the following information on this subject (Hebda, Czar & Mascara, 1998):

- Policies and procedures related to levels of access to patient and administrative databases
- User authentication
- Guidelines for secure data entry
- Training and service support available to staff
- Handling incorrect data entries, data tampering, and system failures
- Procedure for reporting security concerns or breaks in security

Security of confidential information should be a high priority in the design and implementation of any information system.

### Audit Trails

An audit trail is a record of all who have accessed the computer system. Audit software records access to any part of the system by user name or password to identify unauthorized entry into client records or other organizational information. The software searches for unusual activity of any kind. In many organizations employees are asked to sign a document stating they understand they will be terminated for inappropriate system use (Hebda, Czar & Mascara, 1998). Users must also be made aware of the danger of giving their password and/or user ID to another person.

## Telehealth

Telehealth is "the use of telecommunications equipment and communications networks for transferring health care information between participants at different locations" (Chaffee, 1999, p. 27). A well-known telehealth service is the poison control center. Telehealth has expanded to include such applications as client monitoring, diagnostic evaluations, client education, and file transfer and storage (Perednia, 1995; Ensminger, 1996). The largest users of telehealth in the United States are NASA and the military (Telemedicine Research Center, 1996). For some examples in primary care, see Perspectives . . . Using the Internet to Facilitate Primary Care.

As issues concerning cost containment and access to healthcare services continue to increase, telehealth has become an attractive means for saving healthcare dollars. Savings are achieved by (1) allowing earlier access to care, (2) decreasing travel expenses, (3) providing easier access to spe-

cialists and experts, and (4) providing easier access to continuing education for both consumers and professionals (Chaffee, 1999; Perednia, 1995).

> *. . . getting the right in to [sic] the right place can be a matter of life and death.*
> —Gantenbein & Stepanek, 2000, p. EB80

Management-related issues continue to arise as the practice of telehealth grows. Some of these include the following:

- Under what circumstances are health professionals subject to the licensing requirements of a distant state when providing services electronically to a client in another state?
- What obligations accompany licensure in another state (e.g., public health reporting require-

1. The basic standards of professional conduct governing each healthcare profession are not altered by the use of telehealth technologies to deliver health care, conduct research, or provide education. Developed by each professional, these standards focus in part on the practitioner's responsibility to provide ethical and high-quality care.
2. A healthcare system or healthcare practitioner cannot use telehealth as a vehicle for providing services that are not otherwise legally or professionally authorized.
3. Services provided via telehealth must adhere to basic assurance of quality and professional health care in accordance with each health care discipline's clinical standards. Each healthcare discipline must examine how telehealth affects or changes its patterns of care delivery and what modifications to existing clinical standards may be required.
4. The use of telehealth technologies does not require additional licensure.
5. Each healthcare profession is responsible for developing its own processes for ensuring competencies in the delivery of health care through the use of telehealth technologies.
6. Practice guidelines and clinical guidelines in the area of telehealth should be developed based on empirical evidence, when available, and on professional consensus among all involved health care disciplines. The development of these guidelines may include collaboration with government agencies.
7. The integrity and therapeutic value of the client-healthcare practitioner relationship should be maintained and not diminished by the use of telehealth technology.
8. Confidentiality of client visits, client health records, and the integrity of information in a healthcare information system are essential.
9. Documentation requirements for telehealth services must be developed that ensure documentation of each client encounter with recommendations and treatments, communication with other healthcare providers as appropriate, and adequate protections for client confidentiality.
10. All clients directly involved in a telehealth encounter must be informed about the process, the attendant risks and benefits, and their rights and responsibilities. Clients must provide adequate informed consent.
11. The safety of clients and practitioners must be ensured. Safe hardware and software, combined with demonstrated user competency, are essential components of safe telehealth practice.
12. A systematic and comprehensive research agenda must be developed and supported by government agencies and healthcare professions for the ongoing assessment of telehealth services.

*Source:* American Nurses Association. (1999). *Core principles on telehealth.* Washington, DC: American Nurses Publishing.

ments, state investigative authority, jurisdiction for lawsuits)?
- What standards govern the confidentiality of telehealth transmissions?
- Which state's legal requirements govern the disclosure and retention of the medical records of a patient in another state seen via telehealth when they conflict?

- Should unique CPT codes for services be provided through telehealth?
- How can reimbursement for telehealth care be secured from private payors and state programs?
- What telehealth equipment should be considered a "medical device" subject to FDA regulation? (Pacemaker monitoring devices that hook to the telephone are a common example of this telehealth equipment.)
- What standards have been adopted by the medical and nursing profession on the appropriate uses of telehealth and maintenance of the quality of care? (The American Nurses Association has established Core Principles on Telehealth; see Box 15–3.)

Current activities related to telehealth include the 1995 creation of the Joint Working Group on Telemedicine (JWGT) and the 1998 establishment of the federal government Office for the Advancement of Telehealth (OAT) to provide administrative support of telehealth to improve access to health care for low-income, medically underserved, or geographically isolated persons (Chaffee, 1999, p. 12).

---

## C A S E   S T U D Y

### The Electronic Record

An elderly man who lived alone began to have severe chest pain and shortness of breath. He quickly pressed a button on his phone which signaled 911 to send a rescue team to his prerecorded address. Information on his current medications and family members to contact was also available on his computerized patient record. His daughter was immediately notified so she could meet her father at the hospital. His EKG was sent via computer to the emergency department (ED) physician and treatment was begun en route to the hospital. Because his health record was immediately available, emergency personnel were aware of vital information.

Upon his entry into the ED, the nurse verbally entered her assessment of the patient into the health record through a voice recognition system. The attending ED physician communicated online to the patient's cardiologist via a small microphone attached to his lapel. The cardiologist was able to see and hear the ED physician as he discussed his patient with the ED team from his home. The patient was attached to a cardiac monitor that continually entered information into his electronic patient record. Lab results were also entered electronically so they were available immediately on the computerized record. A pacemaker was inserted and the man was prepared to return home. During the man's hospitalization, his physician could access his record from home, office, or hospital computer.

After the man was discharged, the home health nurse used a hand-held recording device to input information on the same patient's record. She instructed the patient how to use his telephone to hook a device to the pacemaker and the telephone to check the battery on the pacemaker. Once a week, the clinical nurse specialist calls the patient to discuss his diet, activity, and concerns and works with the visiting nurse on updating the care plan.

### Questions for Critical Reflection and Analysis

1. Discuss the privacy and confidentiality issues that could arise in this case.
2. Discuss the advantages and disadvantages of having a single electronic patient record that can be accessed by any healthcare provider.
3. Given the advantages and disadvantages that you listed in the previous question, do you think that all patient information should be recorded on a single electronic record? Do the advantages outweigh the disadvantages?
4. If you were a chief nurse executive, would you support the cost of implementing such a system? Why or why not?

*People can now reach 100 times more people in the course of a day. But the skills of social bonding—the skills needed to have a high-quality conversation in a team producing results—have hardly increased at all. The result is disproportionate increases in scale, with more and more people contacting each other, but less and less chance to think and reflect.*

—*Engelbart, 1999, p. 454*

Nursing opportunities in telehealth include providing nursing care for clients at distant sites, designing telehealth education programs for clients and professionals, and participating in research.

## SUMMARY

The ability to access and disseminate information quickly and accurately electronically can empower both staff and managers. The term **nursing informatics** refers to the combination of computer science, information science, and nursing science. Much progress has been made in the development of a standard language for use in computerized patient records, outcomes assessment, and research. Examples are the Nursing Minimum Data Set, NANDA, the Omaha System, Home Health Care Classification, and Nursing Intervention Classification (NIC and NOC). Computerized patient records should be easily accessible yet secure, linked to other sources of patient data, and provide decision-making support. For successful implementation a system requires administrative as well as technical support.

Access to databases and appropriate software can also support the nurse manager's planning and budgeting activities. Finally, telecommunication and the Internet can be used for patient monitoring, patient and staff education, and research.

## REFERENCES

American Nurses Association. (1994). *The scope of practice for nursing informatics.* Washington, DC: American Nurses Publishing.

American Nurses Association. (1995). *Nursing data systems: The emerging framework.* Washington, DC: American Nurses Publishing.

American Nurses Association. (1997). Position statements: Classification for nursing practice. *http://www.nursing world.org/readroom/position/uap/uapclass.htm*

American Nurses Association. (1999). *Core principles on telehealth.* Washington, DC: American Nurses Publishing.

Andrew, W. & Dick, R. (1996). On the road to the CPR: Where are we now? *Healthcare Informatics, 13*(5), 48–52.

Bachman, J.A. & Panzarine, S. (1998). Enabling student nurses to use the information superhighway. *Journal of Nursing Education, 37*(4) 155–160.

Brennan, P. (1996, October 11). The future of clinical communication in an electronic environment. *Holistic Nursing Practice,* (1), 97–104.

Carlzon, J. (1999, June 21). Former Scandinavian airlines system. *The Wall Street Journal,* R14.

Chaffee, M. (1999). A telehealth odyssey. *American Journal of Nursing, 99*(7), 27–33.

Engelbart, D. & Engelbart, C. (1999). Bootstrap principles. In P. Senge et al. (1999). *The dance of change.* New York: Currency/Doubleday, 453–456.

Ensminger, P. (1996). Telemedicine. Northwest Parallel Architectural Center, Syracuse University. *http:// www.npac.syr.edu/users/ensminger/TIMED/html1# issue1*

Gantenbein, D. & Stepanek, M. (2000, February 7). Kaiser takes the cyber cure. *Business Week,* EB80–85.

Graves, J. & Corcoran, S. (1989). The study of nursing informatics. *Image: Journal of Nursing Scholarship, 21*(4), 227–231.

Hebda, T., Czar, P. & Mascara, C. (1998). *Handbook of informatics for nurses and health care professionals.* Menlo Park, CA: Addison-Wesley.

King, I. (1998). Nursing informatics: A universal nursing language. *The Florida Nurse, 46*(1), 1–2.

Microsoft (1999). Microsoft Office 2000, CD-ROM. Microsoft Corporation.

National Institute of Nursing Research. (1999). Report of priority expert panel: Nursing informatics: Introduction. *http://www.nih.gov/ninr/vo14/Intro.html*

National Institute of Nursing Research. (1999). Report of priority expert panel: Nursing informatics: Overview. *http://www.nih.gov/ninr/vo14/overview/html*

Perednia, D. (1995). Telemedicine technology and clinical applications. *Journal of the American Medical Association, 273*(6), 483–488.

Siegel, J.P. (1998). Inner guide to office automation. In L.D. Eigen & J.P. Siegel (Eds.). *The manager's book of quotations.* New York: Amazon.

Simpson, R. (1995, Summer). Getting wired for success. *Nursing Administration Quarterly, 19*(4), 89–91.

Simpson, R. (1997, Winter). Are staff nurses prepared for the new information-based hospital enterprise? *Nursing Administration Quarterly, 21*(2), 85–88.

Telemedicine Research Center. (1996). Telemedicine Research Center, Portland: OR. *http://www.tie.telemed.org/scripts/getpage.pl?client=text&page=history*

Travis, L. & Brennan, P. (1998). Information science for the future: An innovative nursing informatics curriculum. *Journal of Nursing Education, 37*(4), 162–167.

Turley, J. (1996). Toward a model for nursing informatics. *Image: Journal of Nursing Scholarship, 28*(4), 309–313.

University of Iowa. (1999). Center for Nursing Classification, University of Iowa. *http://www.nursing.uiowa.edu/cnc*

Zielstorff, R., Hudgings, C. & Grobe, S. (1993). *Next generation nursing information systems.* Washington, DC: American Nurses Publishing.

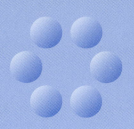

# CHAPTER 16

# Project Planning
# and Evaluation

## LEARNING OBJECTIVES

*After completing this chapter the reader will be able to:*

- List and explain the three stages of planning.
- Outline a plan for a health-related project.
- Identify situational variables that would affect a project plan.
- Suggest ways to generate creative alternative approaches.

- Use a simple rating system to evaluate alternative solutions.
- Present a project plan in a persuasive manner.
- Use a Gantt or similar chart to monitor implementation of a project.

**Project planning methodologies use a lot of terms that are unfamiliar to those encountering the field for the first time.** *Are any of the following terms familiar to you? Can you explain them in your own words? Or use them in a sentence?*

1. Breakpoint

2. Brainstorming

3. Synectics

4. Nominal Group Technique

5. Work Breakdown Structure (WBS)

6. Gantt

7. PERT

8. Critical Path

9. Formative Evaluation

10. Summative Evaluation

*Explanations of these terms can be found in the chapter on the following pages:*

*1. Breakpoint, p. 329, 2. Brainstorming, p. 335, 3. Synectics, p. 335, 4. Nominal Group Techniques, p. 335, 5. Work Breakdown Structure, p. 338, 6. Gantt, p. 341, 7. PERT, p. 341, 8. Critical Path, p. 342, 9. Formative Evaluation, p. 343, 10. Summative Evaluation, p. 344.*

Planning is a dynamic, future-oriented process. Although the sequence of events has its foundations in the problem-solving process, planning involves far more managerial activities, most of which are usually not necessary for solving an individual problem. Whether it is done on a small scale to get a project underway or on a broad, organizationwide basis, planning is one of the distinguishing characteristics of the effective manager.

As you read this chapter, you may want to refer to the planning model in Box 16–1 from time to time to keep the phases of planning and their specific steps clear in your mind. You will also find that many of the individual activities described in this chapter, such as brainstorming or synectics, are useful in other situations as well.

## ● PLANNING

### Types of Planning

**Project planning,** the focus of this chapter, involves a nonroutine set of activities designed to accomplish a specific goal. It is a time-limited responsibility rather than ongoing, usually with a specific start and end date (Lowery & Ferrara, 1998).

**Strategic planning** focuses on the future direction of an organization or its component parts. It is often marketing oriented and may include consideration of political, social, and economic changes affecting the healthcare system (Reeves, 1993; Christensen, 1997). **Healthcare planning** is a broad, survey approach to determining the health needs of a specified population, a community, or even an entire nation. The healthcare issues discussed in Chapter 20 illustrate healthcare planning at the national level.

All of these are important to nurse leaders and managers because failure to engage in formal planning can leave any unit or institution unprepared to respond to change. However, first-line managers are most likely to be responsible for project planning.

### Involvement in Planning

The needs and interests of everyone who will be affected by a plan should be represented. When they are not, some interesting problems may arise:

*University Health Science Center's planning was customarily done by a three-member committee appointed by the chancellor. Imagine the reaction of the students and faculty of the School of Nursing when they discovered that their school had been left off the design for the new classroom building. As the plan stood, they would have no space when it was implemented: no offices, no classrooms, no laboratories. The school's director had not even known that a new building plan was being developed.*

**Box 16–1 Project Planning and Evaluation**

**Stage I. Preparation**

*Phase 1. Conceptual Development*
Clarify the Purpose
Verify the Problem
Identify Stakeholders
Define Outcomes

*Phase 2. Detailed Plan*
Analyze Alternative Approaches
Specify Objectives
Identify Needed Resources
Prepare a Design for Action

*Phase 3. Approval*
Present Proposal
Obtain Resources

**Stage II. Action**

*Phase 4. Implementation*
Allocate Resources
Sequence and Schedule Activities
Direct Implementation

*Phase 5. Monitoring Implementation*
Conduct Formative Evaluation
Track Progress
Review Costs
Check Quality
Update-Revise-Adjust Plan

**Stage III. Completion**

*Phase 6. Evaluation of Outcomes*
Prepare a Summative Evaluation
Compare with Projected Outcomes
Share Results with Stakeholders

*Phase 7. Institutionalization or Termination*
Revise, Apply to New Situation, or Terminate and Redeploy
Resources

*Overbedding (more hospital beds than are needed in a community) has occurred in many places. This problem has been the impetus for a great deal of organizationwide strategic planning. Imagine the reaction of the psychiatric-mental health nurses when they found out that their highly acclaimed inpatient alcohol and substance abuse unit had been deemed "redundant." It would close in two weeks, and they would be laid off permanently.*

*An urban medical center received a large donation to build a spinal cord treatment center. The design team for this project consisted primarily of administrative personnel with a token physician, but no nurses or therapists. Imagine the caregivers' reaction when they found that standard wheelchairs could not go through the narrow bathroom doors in the new center because no one on the design team had anticipated this need.*

The patient's viewpoint has also been neglected in healthcare planning. Greater recognition of patients' preferences has come from the need to attract the patient as consumer in an increasingly competitive market.

## Impetus for Planning

**Reactive planning** is done in response to an existing problem, such as an increase in medication errors, competition from another agency, a drop in the number of patients seeking a particular service, an increase in the cost of staff or equipment, or failure to achieve approval by a regulatory agency. Any of these situations would provide sufficient impetus to initiate planning.

> *Just because few managers do much planning does not mean that project managers should abandon planning. If you have no plan, you have no control!*
>
> —Lewis, 1998, p. 19

In some cases, the problem that stimulates planning is of crisis proportions. It may even be a breakpoint in the existence of the organization. A **breakpoint** is a sudden, radical change that is so rapid and so fundamental that past experience is irrelevant, even useless in formulating a response (Strebel, 1992). An abrupt reduction in Medicaid reimbursement, for example, could create a crisis for a family clinic serving indigent patients. Likewise, a drastic cut in support for medical residents could leave a teaching hospital severely understaffed. Although motivation may be high in such circumstances, the disadvantage of crisis planning is that urgency can lead to carelessness. The "do something, anything, fast!" mentality can easily take over in a crisis (Nutt, 1984).

**Proactive planning,** on the other hand, is done before the problem occurs. It may be done in anticipation of changing needs or to promote growth and excellence within the organization. Its major advantage is that it can be done in an atmosphere of calm instead of chaos. The disadvantage is that it is more difficult to keep interest high enough to move ahead when the pressure of an immediate need or impending crisis is absent.

Bateman and Crant (1993) describe proactive planners as people who "take it upon themselves to have an impact on the world around them," and contrast them with the passive reactors who "fail to identify, let alone seize, opportunities to change things . . . [who] passively adapt to, and even endure, their circumstances" (p. 105).

Planning may also be **opportunistic.** Instead of waiting for a breakpoint to occur, an organization's administration may create one:

> *The CEO of Hospital A noted an increase in the number of young single adults in the community and accompanying drop in the number of families with children. Based on these figures, the CEO projected that a 25 percent decrease in deliveries could occur in the next five years. The CEO made an opportunistic move, closing the entire maternity service and opening a sports medicine clinic in that space. The CEO created a breakpoint in the life of this organization.*
>
> *The CEO of Hospital B looked at the same demographics but arrived at a different solution. Yes, the number of families with young children was decreasing but their average income level was rising. This CEO proposed the creation of luxury suites. Each suite would have a different theme: Tropical Paradise, Super Bowl, Country Comfort, Royal Splendor. Anxious relatives would wait in comfort, helping themselves to light refreshments rather than sitting on cracked plastic couches and fighting cranky vending machines. This CEO engaged in proactive planning.*

In actual practice, many projects are implemented with little planning. Too often, much of the process is skipped over or done in great haste. A common shortcut is to adopt a plan that has worked well somewhere else. This format ignores the uniqueness of each organization, the community within which it operates, and the population it serves. Another common shortcut is to ask a few key people for their opinions and then move immediately into implementation. Some people admire this "bold" approach, mistaking precipitate action for decisiveness, which can lead to expensive or even fatal mistakes.

## ● STAGES OF PROJECT PLANNING

The entire planning process can be divided into 3 stages: **preparation, action,** and **completion** (see Box 16–1). Sometimes the preparation stage takes as long as implementation and completion combined. Other times, the preparation is simple but the implementation phase is complex and lengthy. It all depends on the type of project involved.

Each of these three stages has a number of phases. In the **preparation stage,** the idea for a project is first studied carefully, then a detailed plan is created and approval to proceed with implementation is obtained. Once these steps are done, you move into the **action stage** in which the work is carried out. Implementation is closely monitored to be sure that it is done in a timely, cost efficient (keeping costs within the projected budget) and effective manner. Finally, the project is brought to **completion.** An evaluation of the outcome is essential at this stage. Some projects are complete at this point and termination is appropriate. Others are integrated into the routine functions of the organization, becoming institutionalized rather than terminated. The three stages and multiple phases within them are illustrated in Box 16–1. You may want to refer back to this list as you read the chapter.

Who leads this process? First-line managers are often given this assignment along with their usual responsibilities. For larger projects or projects that require a certain type of expertise, a project manager may be designated by administration. When a project is of sufficient magnitude, the project manager may be relieved of other responsibilities in order to concentrate on the newly assigned project. For example, if a new institutionwide quality improvement program has to be put into effect before the next accreditation visit, a full-time project manager may be assigned to be sure it is done on time.

## Stage I. Preparation

Impatient people have trouble with this stage. So do project managers who are under pressure from administrators to show results quickly. But rushing through this stage can result in long delays and massive cost overruns later if the project was not well thought out before it is implemented. You might even create a solution to the wrong problem! The following is an example:

> *"Attendance at our weight loss clinic is down,"* the outpatient division coordinator was told. *"Would you get a team together to redesign the program?"* The coordinator did just that, bringing in diet and exercise consultants to design an up-to-date weight loss program that was the envy of other hospitals and health centers in the community.
>
> Six months later, the coordinator was called in again to review attendance figures for the Weight Loss Clinic. To his dismay, attendance had not improved.

What happened? The coordinator had not thoroughly investigated the problem before designing the solution. The real problems, he found out later, were the hours the clinic was open, which precluded attendance by anyone who worked during the day, and the cost, which was far higher than the cost of other clinics in the community. The coordinator had solved the wrong problem.

### Phase 1. Conceptual Development

This thinking (as opposed to doing) phase of project planning begins with making sure that everyone understands the purpose of the project and the need for it.

***Clarify the Purpose.*** The first step in project planning is to clearly establish the purpose of this whole process (Box 16–2). It is *not* necessary to be specific about the objectives of planning at this point. In fact, it would be premature. Being somewhat general allows the planner more flexibility and is especially necessary if the perceived problem differs from the actual problem found when an assessment is done.

Most planning is initiated when a **break-point** occurs or a **performance gap** of some type is recognized. The problem may be an existing one or one that is probable in the near future. It becomes the *raison d'etre* of the planning process; it is the spark that sets fire to the latent interest in doing some planning and initiating a project.

Although the original idea for a project may come from anyone in an organization, the okay to proceed with planning, including inviting people to work with you, usually comes from someone in authority. A few examples:

- The vice-president for nursing was asked to call together all department heads to begin discussion of a project to increase the effectiveness of their total quality management (TQM) initiative. "I know we're doing a lot of work but I'm not seeing any results," the CEO told her. "We need to take an institutionwide approach to making TQM more than an academic exercise."
- Several nurse managers and pharmacists were invited to a meeting with the chief nurse executive (CNO) and quality improvement (QI) coordinator. "Our medication error rate has been trending upwards over the last three months. We want to see it go down, not up. I would like you to review the data, decide whether we really have a problem. If yes, identify the reasons for it and come up with a plan to reverse the trend," the CNO told them.
- "We are expanding our department," the outpatient director told the nursing coordinator. "One of the projects under consideration is a new chronic pain center. Would you put together a group to evaluate the feasibility of this idea? If your plan looks good, I think we can get support to implement it."

- "Our area agency on aging has asked us to lead an initiative to reach all live-alone older people in the city who should have an emergency call system installed in their home. They estimate that less than 10 percent have one now. They are also concerned about how much time it takes to have a system installed after a referral is received. If our plan is a good one, I think they will support it financially" (based on Powers, Pegelow & Williams, 1998).
- "A donor has given us enough money to completely renovate the pediatric unit playroom. It has always been an interest of yours. Would you like to lead this project?" the nurse manager asked the pediatric unit clinical specialist.

In each example, a general idea of the purpose of the project is evident in what was said. But a greater understanding about the reasons for initiating the project in question is required. Let's return to the pediatric playroom project to illustrate what else the project leader needs to know:

- Do you want me to put together a team to redesign the playroom or to do it myself? May I choose the team members? How much of my time will be set aside to do this? Who will pick up my other responsibilities? How soon do you want this done?
- How much money is available to spend on the renovation? Will all of it be spent on furnishings and redecoration or will some be set aside for materials (toys, books) or staffing the playroom? Could some of the funds be spent on a part-time recreational therapist who can visit patient rooms as well? Should the emphasis be on functional design or on an eye-pleasing design?

We will return to some of these examples to illustrate other phases of project planning later in this chapter.

*Verify the Problem.*   It is often a mistake to assume that the problem as originally described is an accurate representation of the situation. In the medication error example, an examination of the error rates over a longer period of time may show that the rates are all within the normal range for that institution. Or you might find that the upward trend in errors began six

| Table 16–1 | Verify the Problem: Emergency Response System |
|---|---|

**SYSTEMS-BASED FRAMEWORK**
(based on Nadler in Nutt, 1984)
***Function of the System*** is to alert others when the older person needs help.
***Outputs*** are the signals or messages transmitted electronically.
***Inputs*** are the equipment installed in the older person's home and the central receiver that directs the message to appropriate emergency response services.
***Sequence*** of events begins with identification of need for the system, followed by referral to installer, installation and testing of the system, instruction of the older person, activation of the system, and use of the system.
***Environments*** involved are the older persons' homes and the response center.
***Physical Catalysts*** are the relatively inexpensive, easy-to-use, reliable pieces of equipment used.
***Human Catalysts*** are the skilled installers and those who make the referrals.

**SERVICE-ORIENTED FRAMEWORK**
(based on Kola & Kosberg, 1981)
***Demand:*** How many people need/want this system compared with the number who have it?
***Current Resources***: What is available at present? A private contractor is presently installing the systems. Fees are charged on a sliding scale based on income and ability to pay.
***Adequacy of Resources:*** Are the current resources sufficient? The average time from referral to installation is three weeks. The contractor is doing the installations in his spare time. In addition, the number of referrals received falls far short of estimated need for the system.
***Priorities.*** How important is this system? For many older people, the system gives them sufficient security to remain in their own homes. It also reduces the need for 24-hour assistance, further reducing cost to the healthcare system.

months before when an automated dispensing system was implemented. These two different findings would lead to distinctly different projects, wouldn't they?

The choice of assessment methods depends on the data available and the type of project under consideration. To illustrate how two different frameworks for assessment (system-based and service-oriented, as shown in Table 16–1) could be used, the emergency response system project is used.

Alternatively, a fishbone diagram can be used to do a cause-and-effect analysis of the problem (see Figure 16–1). When a problem is a

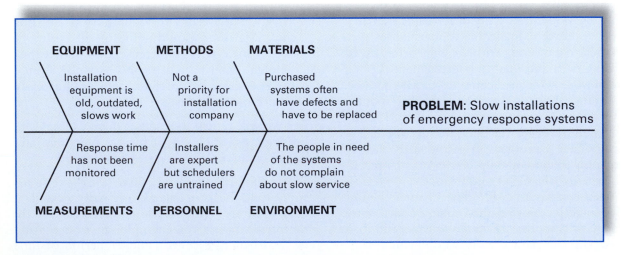

**Figure 16–1** Sample fishbone diagram for cause-and-effect analysis of emergency response system installation. *Source:* Kerzner, H. (1998). *Project management.* New York: Van Nostrand Reinhold. Reprinted with permission.

**Table 16–2** A Simple Affinity Map Illustrating the Emergency Response System Problem

| Response Time | Priorities | Equipment | Coordination |
|---|---|---|---|
| Not being closely monitored | Installer is working on system in his spare time | Installation equipment old, outdated | No one is designated to handle problems or questions |
| Very slow completion time (three weeks) | Installers are untrained | Defects in systems require second visits to homes | No one oversees entire process |

*Source:* Lepley, C.J. (1998). Problem-solving tools for analyzing system problems: The affinity map and the relationship diagram. *Journal of Nursing Administration, 28*(12), 44–50.

particularly difficult and complex one, Lepley (1998) suggests drawing an **affinity map** on which all of the various pieces of data are grouped under headings that indicate their relationships (see Table 16–2). From the affinity map, a relationship diagram can then be created that illustrates the various factors that either cause or are a result of the problem (see Figure 16–2). The factors that contribute to the slow installation of emergency response systems have been synthesized and summarized to illustrate the primary reasons for slow installation of the systems. These diagrams can be far more complex than the ones illustrated. Once the problem has been clearly defined, it can be analyzed in terms of six basic categories or aspects of the situation: equipment, methods, materials, measurements, personnel, and the environment in which the problem occurs (Kerzner, 1998). Each of these categories will have differ-

ent degrees of relevance and importance in different situations.

Whichever framework is used, it is important to take a holistic approach, considering as many factors as possible, and to avoid doing a superficial assessment. Often the context or environment in which the project is to be implemented is as important as the other factors.

*Identify the Stakeholders.* Stakeholders are *all* the people who have an interest in and/or will be affected by the project under consideration. Most health-related projects have a number of stakeholders of different kinds. Consider the following list of stakeholders for the playroom project, that is, people who would have an interest in the pediatric playroom renovation project:

- Nursing staff of the pediatric unit
- Housekeeping and maintenance staff who work on the unit

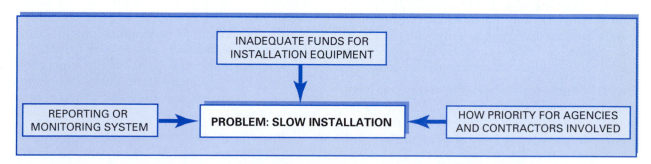

**Figure 16–2** Simple relationship diagram illustrating the emergency response system problem. *Source:* Adapted from Lepley, C.J. (1998). Problem-solving tools for analyzing system problems: The affinity map and the relationship diagram. *Journal of Nursing Administration, 28*(12), 44–50.

- Physicians, therapists, and other formal caregivers of the units' patients
- Families of the patients
- Patients
- Contractors who would be hired to do the work
- The donor
- Administrators of the hospital
- Public relations staff
- Staff on other units who also want to refurbish their dayrooms and waiting rooms

Included in the list of stakeholders should be the **sponsor** or **process owner,** the individual or individuals who have the authority to tell people to go ahead with the project and to give them access to the resources needed to do the work. Sometimes the sponsor is also the **champion** of the project. The champion is the person or persons who are enthusiastic about the project, who will make sure that the project has support (including enough resources to carry out the plan) (Emmett, 1999). If the sponsor is not a champion of the project, you need to identify, sometimes even create, champions for the project whose enthusiastic support can carry it over the unevitable rough spots you will encounter on the road to implementation and eventual completion of the project.

Why is it important to identify the stakeholders? To be successful, the needs and interests of all these people have to be considered in designing the project. Their needs and interests constitute the **motivating forces** behind the project. Without them, the project lacks crucial support. Reconciling their interests can be quite a challenge when the needs and interests conflict. For example, the donor might want a schoolroom atmosphere for the playroom but your patients might prefer cartoon characters and the administration might want a modern decor in harmony with the rest of the institution. Can you please all of them at once? You would have to be creative to do so.

*Define Outcomes.* Now that you and your team better understand the motivating forces behind the initiation of the project, who the stakeholders are, and what the real purposes are, you can identify the desired outcomes. These outcomes will be more general than the objectives specified in the next phase. The statement of outcomes should make clear why the project is being undertaken and what is to be gained from it. Some examples:

*In the playroom example, an appropriate outcome would be that pediatric patients have a safe and comfortable place to play.*

*In the emergency response system example, an appropriate outcome would be that older adults who live alone are able to call for help if they fall or have a medical emergency.*

### Phase 2. Detailed Plan

Although the steps in this second phase are described as if they occur sequentially, a more dynamic, holistic process involves considering all aspects of the design at once. Approaching the project in this way ensures that every aspect, from objectives to budget, is congruent with every other aspect.

> **Our linear-causal view of the world just does not fit the reality in which we live.**
> —Lewis, 1998, p. 7

*Analyze Alternative Approaches.* It is finally time to focus on solutions. Creativity, open-mindedness, expertise, and adequate information are all vital to this step. Consultation with internal and outside experts, a search of the literature, and surveys of clients and other stakeholders are often useful at this stage.

**Generating Solutions.** Too often the alternatives suggested are only variations of the current situation rather than real solutions. The sponsor, project team, and other stakeholders may be pessimistic about a positive outcome when monetary resources are scarce, the performance gap is long-standing, or no amount of tinkering in the past has had any effect. The planner's leadership skills become particularly important at this point for creating a climate of discovery and positive thinking.

It is also important to avoid the temptation to adopt a ready-made solution, which is analogous to borrowing someone else's shoes: they rarely fit well.

> **Insanity is defined as continuing to do what you've always done and expecting to get a different result.**
> —Lewis, 1998, p. 108

Brainstorming, nominal group technique, idealized redesign, and synectics are all useful techniques to generate ideas. These methods are discussed next.

**Brainstorming.** Brainstorming sessions are designed to encourage people to break out of their old patterns of thinking. The rules are simple. Every idea put forth by a group member is acknowledged by recording it on a chalkboard, flip chart, or the equivalent. The group is told that all relevant suggestions are to be received without criticism or challenge of any type. Any misgivings about the ideas offered are to be ignored for the time being, but other members of the group may expand on an offered idea. Wild, crazy, unrealistic ideas are encouraged because they may contain the core of a realistic solution or be a stimulus to another idea that can actually be implemented.

Idea generation ends after a specified amount of time or when the group has exhausted its ideas. The leader should encourage the group to generate as many ideas as possible and ensure that all have participated. The fact that some people may have difficulty "letting loose" in a work situation should be taken into consideration in leading the group.

The composition of the brainstorming group is another point to consider. Each member must have sufficient background information and expertise to participate intelligently. On the other hand, a fresh perspective is quite valuable and may be gained from people with little prior contact with the problem. Too large a group will limit individual participation and may inhibit creativity. More than 15 people is probably too many, but the dynamics of the group are more important than the actual number.

It is important that the group see this process as a serious undertaking, not a silly exercise, and that you do it only if it offers a possibility that a creative new approach could be accepted.

After ideas have been generated, they are evaluated in terms of what would work most effectively. This evaluation is done without reference to the originator of the idea (not easy to do in some groups). Any critique should be constructive and without criticism of the idea's originator. The final product should be a small list of the best approaches to achieving the outcomes from which the best one can eventually be selected (Beal, Bohlen & Raudabaugh, 1962; Leebov & Ersoz, 1991).

**Nominal Group Technique.** The nominal group technique is a more formal way to encourage free thinking. It is particularly useful in an organization that is formal or where status and power differences are likely to lead to the dominance of a few people (Delbecq & Van de Ven, 1971).

It is a quieter process than brainstorming. Group members are asked to think carefully about the problem and then make a list of possible solutions without discussing them with anyone else. When participants are finished writing, the leader asks each group member to read one item from his or her list, and records it on a chalkboard or flip chart. Alternatively, the leader may collect and read the suggestions in order to keep the sources anonymous. This process continues until all of the ideas have been recorded.

The ideas are then discussed in terms of how they might provide a solution to the problem and how they may or may not work. Then the group is asked to create a list of preferred options, as was done after brainstorming.

**Idealized Redesign.** In idealized redesign, the stage is set for creative thinking by asking participants to imagine that their organization, department, or unit was destroyed overnight. None of it exists any longer, so it must be entirely rebuilt. Anything can be done differently this time. The group is free to replace the former organization with whatever they wish.

Once the group has redesigned their organization, department, or unit, they are asked to work backwards from this ideal endpoint to the present situation in order to discover how these changes can be made. Working backwards transforms one's concept of what is possible, according to Ackoff (Flower, 1992).

**Synectics.** The fundamental idea behind synectics is that new ideas need to be nurtured, protected, and given a chance to develop before they are subjected to evaluation (Prince, 1970). The opposite usually happens in a group. People almost automatically criticize embryonic ideas, responding to them as if they should be born fully developed instead of being in need of development.

Each of us is, to differing degrees, sensitive to criticism, especially in front of a group of colleagues or supervisors. This sensitivity inhibits many to the point where they will offer no suggestions in groups. Others become aggressive and attack tender new ideas to avoid being attacked themselves. These attacks can be quite subtle. They can, for example, be disguised as "helpful suggestions" or "concerned questions," but their effect is to kill the new idea. Obviously, none of these responses enhance creativity.

In contrast, the synectic response encourages creativity by nurturing the new idea and protecting its source. The group is asked to build on each other's ideas rather than tear them down. Instead of challenging a new idea, group members try to contribute to its development. Questions and comments that would nurture rather than discourage an idea include the following:

- "May I add to your suggestion? I think we could also . . ."
- "Let's talk about how this could work."
- "Can you elaborate on your idea? Tell us how you see . . ."
- "Your suggestion has possibilities. Let's talk about how it could be done."

Such an approach not only gives the new idea a chance but encourages other people to share in its development. Without this encouragement, many potentially worthy ideas die in their formative stage.

Brainstorming focuses on bringing out the greatest variety of ideas possible, while synectics focuses on protecting and developing the ideas that are brought up within the group.

Refraining from criticism until each idea has been given full consideration is quite difficult. The sponsor, in particular, may become quite impatient at this point and wish to get on with the implementation of his or her favorite option.

**Weighing Pros and Cons.** Once ideas have been generated, some methods are available for making the selection of one to implement. These methods include paper-and-pencil or computer simulation, scenarios, and pilot projects (Nutt, 1984).

**Simulation.** Paper-and-pencil simulation is the most common way to analyze the pros and cons of each option. Each option is analyzed in terms of its requirements (resources needed) and anticipated outcomes. The requirements differ somewhat depending on the project, but most projects will require some space, staff, equipment, supplies, specialized expertise, legal or regula-

tory approvals, and time in which to accomplish the implementation. All these elements are calculated as accurately as possible for each option. Then the options are rated on the basis of the least difficulty in implementation for the greatest gain. This method is somewhat oversimplified and far from flawless, but it does help to reduce the subjectivity of the decision-making process.

Computer simulation programs are available for some common decision-making processes. Forecasting costs of most projects can be done by entering the data onto an electronic spreadsheet and then changing the numbers (such as the cost of staff or equipment) to reflect the budgetary needs of each option. The spreadsheet then shows how much each option would cost. One way to visualize it is to think of the spreadsheet as answering financial "What if . . ." questions such as "What if I add five more employees—how much will that increase the budget?" and "Will it cost more than if I purchase new equipment?"

**Scenarios.** Scenarios are especially useful when the human and organizational factors in project implementation are likely to be more important considerations than cost. (Will people accept this new routine? Are they willing to try it? Can they figure it out? How much resistance will there be?)

The implementation of each option may be actually acted out or just walked through mentally by the people who are analyzing the options. Imagination and creativity should be encouraged because the purpose of creating the scenario is to uncover the unanticipated advantages and disadvantages of each option. The scenario is a means by which we can ask, "What would happen if we actually implemented this option?" before the choice is made.

Returning to the pediatric playroom example, suppose your project team has come up with three options:

1. An ultra modern decor that makes liberal use of strobe lights and neon signs. Pipe in popular music and contract with a fast food outlet to sell snacks around the clock.
2. Use cartoon characters and bright primary colors on the walls. Have juice, milk, and cookies available around the clock. Stock the room with videos of favorite children's stories.

3. Use an outdoor theme for the decor with a fountain in the center, birds in cages, and lots of plants. Have spring water and fresh fruit available around the clock.

In working through scenarios for each of the suggested renovation options, the following are examples of the questions that need to be asked:

*What is the age of the children who will use the playroom? How will they be feeling? What will they want to do? What will they be able to do? How much time will they spend in the playroom? How many will use it more than once?*

*Who will accompany the children to the playroom? Will the children need supervision? What adaptations need to be made to assure the children's safety and well-being? Who will stock and maintain the playroom?*

Once participants become actively involved in the process, working out scenarios is not only stimulating but often raises a lot of questions that would otherwise go unasked.

**Pilot Projects.** Pilot projects are small-scale representations of the suggested options. They have the advantage of most closely reflecting the reality of implementing the option, but they can be expensive in both time and money. Because it is expensive to pilot more than one or two options, a decision as to which option is most favorable may be made before all of the information is available. Despite its drawbacks, the pilot project is a powerful means of analyzing an option.

The existence of criteria for analyzing the value of each option has been implied in the examples given. How you select criteria to evaluate each option should go back to the purpose and objectives of the planning process. The criteria may include cost reduction without a loss of quality, more efficient use of staff time, or an improvement in the quality of care given. Whatever criteria are chosen, it is important that they be clearly spelled out and agreed on before the analysis of the options is done.

*Specify Objectives.* Now that the situation has been thoroughly assessed, it is possible to develop specific objectives for the project. The ob-jectives should be written as **measurable outcomes** so that they can later serve as guidelines for evaluation.

The acronym SMART may help you remember how to write objectives:

**S** pecific

**M** easurable

**A** chievable

**R** ealistic

**T** ime specific (Emmett, 1999; Kerzner, 1998)

Two additional points need to be kept in mind while writing objectives. The first is to avoid writing solutions into the objectives. People often do not realize that they are making this error unless it is pointed out to them. An example:

*An objective such as "to increase playtime by making the playroom more attractive" includes a solution as well as an outcome. "To redecorate the playroom" describes a solution, but not a desired outcome. A more appropriate objective for the pediatric playroom project would be "to increase patient participation in pleasurable activities" or "to increase positive parent-child interaction during hospitalization."*

Second, it is important to achieve an appropriate level of specificity when writing objectives. If they are too specific, it could become necessary to write hundreds of objectives; if they are too broad, they will offer little guidance to the rest of the planning process. The following illustrates this difference:

| | |
|---|---|
| **Too Broad:** | To improve emergency response time. |
| **Too Specific:** | To hire Mergi-Stat, Inc., to install 500 clear-brite alarm systems in the next six months. |
| **About Right:** | To reduce the wait time from referral to completion of emergency response system installation to five workdays. |

You may have noticed that the overly specific objective also includes a solution.

***Identify Needed Resources.***   What kind of resources will you need to execute the selected option? If you have been involved with similar projects in the past, you will probably have a good idea of what will be needed. If not, you will want to talk with people who have some experience if possible. If none are available, you will have to estimate on the basis of your best judgment. Consider the following categories in deciding what resources will be needed:

| | |
|---|---|
| People: | expertise, availability, interest in the project; include the amount of time they will have to spend on the project |
| Equipment: | any mechanical supports from computers to CAT scanners |
| Materials: | expendable items from paper and postage to disposable catheters |
| Information: | given the expertise of the people on the project team, what additional skills and knowledge will be needed? |
| Money: | given all of the preceding needs, how much money will |

be needed to complete the project (Powers, Pegelow & Williams, 1998)?

***Prepare a Design for Action.***   Now that the preparatory work has been done, it is time to prepare a **work breakdown structure** (WBS). The WBS "defines all effort to be expended, assigns responsibility . . . and establishes schedules and budgets for the accomplishment of the work (Kerzner, 1998, p. 543). It is not any easy task. The WBS does not need to include every little detail but should outline the project in sufficient detail that schedules, checklists, and budgets can be developed from it. Tree diagrams, flow charts, or lists can be used to describe most projects. Table 16–3 illustrates a work breakdown for the playroom example after a modification of the cartoon decor option was selected. This WBS uses a simple listing of the major steps with space for completion dates and estimated costs.

## Phase 3. Approval

***Present Proposal.***   Most often you will have to present the plan for approval before you can proceed. Some of the people to whom you present the plan may have acted as sponsor, supporting your work up to this point. Even with this support, however, the sponsor usually re-

---

**Table 16–3**   Simple Work Breakdown Structure (WBS) Project: Playroom Renovation

| | Completion Date | Cost |
|---|---|---|
| **Step 1. Design Renovation** | 01-00-00 | $00.00 |
| a. Hire interior decoration consultant | 01-00-00 | $00.00 |
| b. Complete design | 01-00-00 | $00.00 |
| c. Obtain approval for design | 01-00-00 | $00.00 |
| **Step 2. Select Contractor** | 02-00-00 | $00.00 |
| a. Obtain bids | 02-00-00 | $00.00 |
| b. Negotiate contract | 02-00-00 | $00.00 |
| **Step 3. Renovate Playroom** | 03-00-00 | $00.00 |
| a. Complete construction | 03-00-00 | $00.00 |
| b. Order new furniture and equipment | 03-00-00 | $00.00 |
| c. Hire part-time recreation therapist | 03-00-00 | $00.00 |
| **Step 4. Reopen Playroom** | 07-00-00 | $00.00 |
| a. Begin recreation therapy (6 hours/day) | 07-00-00 | $00.00 |
| b. Invite stakeholders to opening party | 07-00-00 | $00.00 |
| c. Evaluate children's and families' responses | 07-00-00 | $00.00 |
| d. Alter as indicated by evaluation | 07-00-00 | $00.00 |

tains his or her right to approve, modify, or reject the completed plan.

In order to achieve approval, you will have to be persuasive. Sometimes, you will have to be *especially* persuasive. At other times, seeking approval for the plan is pro forma, that is, a matter of following established procedures and lines of authority with approval virtually assured ahead of time. When approval is not assured, however, you will want to make the proposal as attractive and acceptable to the sponsor as possible.

It may be helpful to think of this part of the process as "selling" your proposal. It is your job to get the sponsor to "buy" your plan. The quality of the work you have done up to now (the content) will, of course, have a great influence on the decision, but the way in which you sell your plan (delivery) may be the deciding factor.

The sponsor and other stakeholders will support the project if they believe that it is of some benefit to them. Keep this motivation in mind when seeking support for the project. It is called the "What's in it for me?" or WIIFM principle (Lewis, 1998). To answer this question successfully, of course, you need to remember what motivates the sponsor and stakeholders.

> ### People don't do anything unless there is something in it for themselves.
>
> —Lewis, 1998, p. 24

**Content.** In order to be credible, your proposal must be well supported, not only by your carefully thought-out arguments but by facts. Accurate statistics, however simple, are very persuasive (See Perspectives Box 16–1, Maps Bring Data to Life). You could, for example, survey postcoronary patients, asking them four or five simple questions about the causes of myocardial infarction and how to prevent further damage. It is safe to predict that many will not have these answers and that your survey would strongly support the need for patient education. Your own survey should be further supported by statistics from the literature on patient education.

> *In the emergency response system example, reporting an average 3-week delay between referral and installation strongly supports the need for a new approach.*

## PERSPECTIVES . . .

### Maps Bring Data to Life

A community group in Vallejo, California, called "Fighting Back" had tried unsuccessfully to convince the city council to increase its alcohol and drug-related crime prevention efforts.

To convince the city council of the need for crime prevention, they charted rates of alcohol and other drug-related (AOD) arrests and the location of liquor stores on a map of the city. Using the map, they demonstrated that you might ordinarily see 6 AOD arrests in a year in a given neighborhood. With two liquor outlets in the same neighborhood, however, the rate rises to 18 AOD arrests a year. When the number of outlets goes to three, the rate climbs "exponentially."

The city council responded to the maps. They "make crime real for people," said the project director Michael Sparks. Maps bring data to life in a way that pie charts and graphs cannot.

---

*Source:* Larkin, H. (1997). Geography gaining power as a tool for shaping health and social policy. *Advances* (newsletter of The Robert Wood Johnson Foundation) Issue 3.

When presenting information, Boettinger (1979) suggests that you never underestimate the intelligence of your audience nor overestimate their knowledge of the subject. In other words, do not talk down to your audience. On the other hand, do not assume that your audience already knows as much as you have learned in the process of developing the plan.

Boettinger suggests a framework that you may find helpful for organizing your presentation. This framework follows the way your audience needs to think about the proposal: first, describe the situation as it currently exists in general terms, then add detail, and finally, present your plan for the resolution of the problem (or prevention of the problem in proactive planning).

**Delivery.** The audience to whom you present the plan may be as small as one or as large as several hundred. Usually the plan is prepared in written form, which includes the purpose, objectives, proposed action, and means for evaluation. The following are some characteristics of a well-presented proposal:

1. *Persuasive.* Emphasize the ways in which the plan meets the needs, concerns, and goals of the sponsor and other stakeholders (remember WIIFM).
2. *Concise.* People become impatient with unnecessary detail and overly long explanations so get to your point directly. A descriptive slogan, symbol, or title, especially for a large-scale project, can increase appeal.
3. *Professional.* Sloppy work may be rejected before the quality of your ideas has been given a chance. Your proposal should be clear, well organized, and appropriately formal but not humorless, unenthusiastic, or pedantic. You can admit to the inevitable gaps in information without being apologetic or defensive. You can also list the shortcomings of previous attempts to solve the problem without putting other people on the defensive.
4. *Personalized.* Personalizing the proposal is a way to engage your audience. You can talk about how the plan will affect the stakeholders, especially the sponsor. For example, you can say that when a new computer system is installed, Ms. X will be the project director and Mr. Y and Ms. Z will spend one half of their time working on the installation for the next six months. The nurses on Units 1, 2, and 3 will then be able to do a, b, and c in half the time.

   Specific examples also help a great deal. For example, you can say, "Let's follow Patient X through the new Primary Care Clinic. When he first telephones the clinic for an appointment . . ." It is much easier for your audience to identify with Patient X or Mr. Y than with 200 clients or a whole project staff.

   Don't forget to give credit where it is due to the people who have contributed to the plan.
5. *Imaginative.* A descriptive analogy, attractive audiovisuals, charts, graphs, memorable title, and personalized examples are just a few of the ways in which you can exercise some imagination and creativity. Your efforts lend uniqueness to your presentation and capture your audience's interest and attention.

***Obtain Resources.*** Remember that list of needed resources you created in Phase 2? To implement a project, these resources have to be made available: people released from other responsibilities, funds made available to purchase equipment, and so forth. Do not try to begin a project without confirmation that the resources needed to complete it are available to you.

## Stage II. Action

### *Phase 4. Implementation*

Implementation must be planned in terms of the sequence of activities, target dates for completion of various tasks, and assignment of responsibility for continuing these activities. Once these aspects are taken care of, the leader of the project will direct the actual implementation, monitor implementation, and revise the plan as needed (Box 16–3). These last steps involve a broad range of general leadership and managerial knowledge and skills dealt with in other sections of this book, so they will only be outlined briefly here.

As a project is implemented, adjustments often have to be made when roadblocks are encountered. You could, for example, find that a vital piece of equipment is temporarily unavailable or that a family emergency has made a key team member temporarily unavailable. In some cases, a substitute can be found; in others it cannot and a delay becomes inevitable. For this reason, experienced planners often allow extra time in a schedule for such contingencies.

---

**Box 16–3 Action Stage**

**Phase 4. Implementation**
    Allocate Resources
    Sequence and Schedule Activities
    Direct Implementation

**Phase 5. Monitoring Implementation**
    Conduct Formative Evaluation
    Track Progress
    Review Costs
    Check Quality
    Update-Revise-Adjust Plan

***Allocate Resources.*** Allocation of resources focuses primarily on selecting staff, securing space and equipment, and working within a given budget. Although the details of budgeting are considered in a separate chapter, it must be kept in mind during implementation of the plan because it can be a serious constraint.

***Sequence and Schedule Activities.*** This step can become complex if the project is an elaborate one involving many people and many different activities over a long time.

A number of useful techniques have been developed to organize and monitor all these details. Among these are simple schedules; Gantt charts; the program, evaluation, and review technique (PERT); and the critical path method (CPM) (Rosenau, 1998). Each of these methods can also be used to organize and monitor routine work. The planner's major concerns at this point are:

1. The activities and sequence in which they must be done.
2. The target dates for completing each activity.
3. Matching tasks to particular individuals.

**Schedules.** Schedules are probably the simplest and most familiar of the methods described here. Schedules organize work on the basis of time and assigned staff members, leaving out any details of the tasks that must be done. Their simplicity makes them easy to construct and use. Additionally, they form the basis for the more complex methods.

A **routine schedule** would be staff assignments to a pediatric unit for the next month, indicating days off and vacation or holiday time. **Project schedules** differ somewhat in that they usually list the tasks instead of the staff, with dates for starting and completing them.

**Gantt Charts.** Gantt charts are highly developed schedules in which the tasks are detailed, with some indication of their relationship in time (Table 16–4). These charts usually do not indicate which tasks depend on the completion of earlier ones. They derive their name from their developer, Henry L. Gantt, an early management theorist.

Table 16–4 illustrates a Gantt chart that could be used for a simple project, the implementation of a new courier system in a healthcare institution. Note that two activities, developing the new reporting slip and hiring couriers, will be done at the same time, but the hiring is scheduled to be completed sooner. Note also that a column has been added to indicate the people responsible for completing each task. Although not always included, this information is vital for the entire project team. A chart such as the one illustrated can serve as a useful reminder of the multiple tasks that need to be done and can be helpful in monitoring whether project activities are completed on time.

**PERT Charts.** The PERT chart includes more detail on the relationships between the various activities of a particular project than do Gantt charts. A PERT chart graphically illustrates the sequence of events and their interrelationships, using circles for events and arrows for the activities leading up to those events. This format can

**Table 16–4  Gantt Chart, Example Illustrating Implementation of a New Courier System**

| Task | Assigned Responsibility | Jan | Feb | Mar | Apr | May | June |
|---|---|---|---|---|---|---|---|
| A. Develop new report forms | PQ KL | ----------------→ | | | | | |
| B. Hire couriers | AM | --------→ | | | | | |
| C. Train couriers | CB | | --------→ | | | | |
| D. Pilot new system on two units | PB KL | | | --------→ | | | |
| E. Implement on all units | PB KL | | | | --------------------→ | | |
| F. Evaluate | AM | | | | | | -----→ |

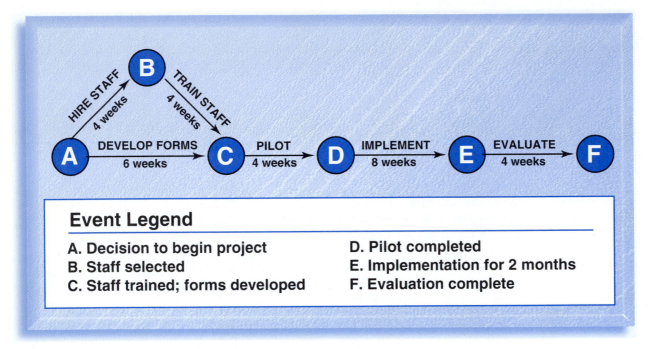

**Event Legend**

A. Decision to begin project
B. Staff selected
C. Staff trained; forms developed

D. Pilot completed
E. Implementation for 2 months
F. Evaluation complete

**Figure 16–3**   PERT chart: Example illustrating implementation of the courier system shown in Table 16–4.

be confusing when you first try to create a PERT chart. Figure 16–3 illustrates a simplified PERT chart for the same courier system shown in Table 16–4. Under each arrow is the time expected to complete this activity.

The PERT chart is more systems oriented than the Gantt chart. From the PERT chart, you can see how the work must flow from one event to the next and how one activity depends on another. It helps the project leader and staff see the project as a whole with interrelated activities and goals, each contributing to the final outcome. On the other hand, the Gantt chart is easier to construct and simpler to follow. Because many variations of these network diagrams are possible, the choice should be dictated by its usefulness for your particular project. These charts can become far more complex than the ones illustrated. Commercially designed software packages for creating these charts are readily available.

**Critical Path Method.** This method is similar to PERT except that it also identifies the critical path, that is, the path that takes the longest time

to complete. Returning to Figure 16–3 for a moment, you can see that path A-B-C is estimated to require 8 weeks, whereas path A-C requires only 6 weeks to complete. Path A-B-C is the **critical path** because it is the one most likely to delay completion of the project.

**Allowing for Contingencies.** Another helpful device in planning for implementation is to calculate not only the *most likely* but also the *most optimistic* and *least optimistic* estimates of time needed to complete the project (usually 20 percent more and 20 percent less than the most likely amount of time). These outside estimates can make the charts a more realistic representation of what will occur and prevent unrealistic expectations about completion of the project. Many activities are dependent on one another for completion, with a great number of variables affecting completion time. A number of these variables are outside the control of the project leader. For example, a low unemployment rate could make it difficult to find couriers, or the printing of the forms might be delayed due to a printers' strike.

**Research Example 16–1** *Program Evaluation of a Redesign Project in an Acute-Care Setting*

The purpose of the Patient-Centered Redesign (PCR) Project at Hartford Hospital was to "create an innovative, patient-centered, hospital-wide delivery system that continuously improves quality and utilizes resources cost-effectively" (p. 232). This broad project focused on improvements in quality, cost, caregiver/manager relationships, and decision making, continuity, and communication.

Measuring progress in such a broadly defined project is a challenge the authors described as a "moving and, at times, ambiguous target" (p. 233). Each aspect had to be operationally defined before they could decide what data should be collected. For example, achieving quality was operationally defined as higher patient satisfaction survey results and decreases in unplanned readmissions, complications, and deviations from critical paths.

Results of these surveys were reported back to stakeholders and were used to identify areas in need of improvement. For example, the patient satisfaction surveys were used to identify aspects of care rated unsatisfactory by the patients who responded to the survey. Graphic displays were often used to report the data in a concise, user-friendly manner. The authors noted that this approach is quite different from the experimental research design but more appropriate for their "moving target": a dynamic project encompassing a large number of complex, interrelated activities.

*Source:* Stetler, C.B., Creer, E. & Effkin, J.A. (1996). Evaluating a redesign program: Challenges and opportunities. In K. Kelley (Ed.). *Outcomes of affective management practice.* Series in *Nursing Administration, 8,* Thousand Oaks, CA: Sage.

---

Whichever method you use, by the end of this step you should have a clear plan of action that informs you and the project staff about what needs to be done and by when. Along with this plan you will need a congruent budget. The budget and your plan of action become the guidelines for directing and monitoring implementation.

**Direct Implementation.** Once the previous steps have been completed, the actual implementation of the project can begin. The project still needs the support of the sponsor and the direction of the project team leader because it is new and represents a change, whether welcome or not, for all involved. At this point, the skills needed are primarily those of the leader involved in bringing about change. The plan now becomes a reality.

*Phase 5. Monitoring Implementation*

- *Conduct Formative Evaluation.* This type of evaluation is concerned with improving the implementation of a project, not its final outcomes. It should continue throughout the action stage

of project planning and evaluation (see Research Example 16–1. Formative evaluation is usually the responsibility of the project leader.

- *Track Progress.* The WBS, GANTT, PERT and critical path diagrams can be used as guides to determining whether the project work is proceeding on schedule.
- *Review Costs.* The budget can be used to determine whether costs are in line with the original projections or if you are going over budget and need to make some adjustments.
- *Check Quality.* The quality of the work being done must also be evaluated. Supervision of team members is always part of the leader's role.

*Not to be accountable for results is to be seriously out of touch with reality.*
—DePree, 1992, p. 30

- *Update-Revise-Adjust Plan.* As the project work progresses, it is natural to discover ways to improve upon the original plan. Overly strict adherence to the original plan is unnecessary and often counterproductive. In other words, you cannot anticipate everything ahead of time

> **Box 16–4 Completion Stage**
>
> **Phase 6. Evaluation of Outcomes**
>     Prepare a Summative Evaluation
>     Compare with Projected Outcomes
>     Share Results with Stakeholders
>
> **Phase 7. Institutionalization or Termination**
>     Revise, Apply to New Situation, or
>     Terminate and Redeploy Resources

and have to be prepared to make adjustments when indicated.

## Stage III. Completion

This final step demonstrates once more the circularity of the planning process. Continuous revision, improvement, enhancement, and updating of any project are signs of a healthy, growth-oriented organization. The process may lead back to revision of the objectives, the action plan, even the purpose of the original plan (see Box 16–4).

### Phase 6. Evaluation of Outcomes

- *Prepare a Summative Evaluation.* When the project has been completed, a summative evaluation determines the success of the project in terms of time, cost, and outcomes. All these factors need to be considered in evaluating the success of a project. Although the outcomes are the most important, cost and time are critical elements as well. Imagine, for example, if it took three years to renovate the pediatric unit playroom or to develop a more timely system for getting the emergency response systems installed. It's obvious that such a lengthy process should have been unnecessary and would probably be too costly as well (Table 16–3).
- *Compare with Projected Outcomes.* Evaluation at this stage is usually more formal and more exhaustive than the ongoing (formative) evaluation was. The original outcomes and specific objectives of the project should serve as your guide in evaluating the success of a

project. Evaluation procedures are discussed further in Chapter 19.

- *Share Results with Stakeholders.* The results of the evaluation should be shared with all involved, not only to keep communication lines open but also to provide lessons for future projects.

### Phase 7. Institutionalization or Termination

- *Revise and Apply to a New Situation or Terminate and Redeploy Resources.* Once the evaluation is complete, the work of the project team is usually done. Some project teams continue on to a new project. Most are disbanded or regroup in different configurations for new projects. A sense of sadness almost always accompanies this disbanding but the group should also feel a sense of satisfaction in having completed a project successfully.

## ● SUMMARY

Planning is a dynamic, future-oriented managerial responsibility. It may be reactive, proactive, or opportunistic in nature. Comprehensive planning consists of three major stages: (1) preparation, (2) action, and (3) completion. During the preparation stage, the idea behind the project is carefully studied: the purpose is clarified and the problem, which could be a crisis point or an anticipated problem, is verified through assessment of the situation. Then the stakeholders are identified and the desired outcomes of the project are clearly defined. Once this conceptual work is done, the details of the plan are worked out: alternative approaches are generated and sorted to select the best one. Brainstorming, nominal group technique, idealized redesign, and synectics can be used to generate alternatives. Simulations, scenarios, and pilot projects can be used to guide selection of the optimal approach. Specific outcome-oriented objectives and the resources needed to complete the work are then listed. Approval to proceed with the plan is obtained before proceeding to the action stage.

In the action stage, resources (people, money, equipment, and so forth) are obtained and the

# C A S E   S T U D Y

## Project: Research Center

This time would be different. Oscar Rivera had seen the unfortunate results of haphazard planning many times in his five years as nurse manager. He had to admit that some of those results were his doing.

"Too little time." "This is an emergency." "We have a deadline." "The boss wants it ASAP." "We already know what we want." "It worked last time, why shouldn't it work this time?" These were the excuses he'd heard for not planning or hurrying through the process. Oscar was determined to go through every step of the process carefully and thoroughly on this new project to which he'd been assigned.

The project was an interesting one. The new CEO of the 450-bed acute-care facility where Oscar was employed wanted to increase the status and prestige of the institution. When the hospital became part of a regional for-profit system, the money that had been donated to the hospitals by community groups and individuals in the past was transferred into a charitable foundation. Some of this money would be used to support the establishment of a research center at the hospital. Oscar was selected to head the project because of his ability to work with people across disciplines and his success in implementing smaller projects in the past.

At present, no research at all was being done at the hospital. In the past, a few employees, primarily nurses and social workers, had done small studies while they were in school but that was about it. Oscar literally had to start from scratch.

## Questions for Critical Reflection and Analysis

1. Create three different scenarios for a research center at the hospital. Use your imagination.
2. Evaluate the pros and cons of each scenario. Select the one that you predict would be the most likely to succeed and meet the CEO's expectations.
3. Write specific objectives and develop a budget and time frame for establishing the research center. Include external resources that would be needed as well as the internal resources Oscar will need to accomplish this goal.
4. Go back to the objectives and describe the desired outcomes of this project and how you would obtain the needed data to determine whether they were achieved.

Note: If you have time, instead of answering the specific questions above, go back to Box 16–1 and work through each phase of project planning and evaluation for development of a research center at a 450-bed acute-care facility.

---

work is broken down into details, scheduled and assigned to various people. The progress of the work is monitored carefully in terms of the quality of the work the cost and adherence to the projected timetable for completion. Formative evaluation is done during the implementation of the plan. Revisions and updates of the plan are made as indicated by this evaluation.

In the last stage, the project is completed and end-of-project (summative) evaluation is done. At this point, the project work is either terminated or integrated into the routine of the institution.

## REFERENCES

Bateman, T.S. & Crant, J.M. (1993). The proactive component of organizational behavior: A measure and correlates. *Journal of Organizational Behavior, 14*(2), 103–118.

Beal, G.M., Bohlen, J.M. & Raudabaugh, J.N. (1962). *Leadership and dynamic group action.* Ames, IA: Iowa State University Press.

Boettinger, H.M. (1979). *Moving mountains: The art of letting others see things your way.* New York: Collier Books.

Christensen, C.M. (1997, November/December). Making strategy: Learning by doing. *Harvard Business Review,* 141–156.

Delbecq, A. & Van de Ven, A. (1971). A group process model for problem identification and program planning. *Journal of Applied Behavioral Science, 7,* 466–492.

DePree, M. (1992). *Leadership jazz.* New York: Dell Publishing.

Emmett, M. (1999, March 6). *Outcomes-based quality improvement:* A method for creating and managing changes. Paper presented at the American Society on Aging, 45th annual meeting, Orlando, Florida.

Flower, J. (1992). New tools, new thinking: A conversation with Russell L. Ackoff. *Healthcare Forum Journal, 35*(2), 62–67.

Kerzner, H. (1998). *Project management.* New York: Van Nostrand Reinhold.

Kola, L.A. & Kosberg, J.I. (1981). Model to assess community services for the elderly alcoholic. *Public Health Reports, 96,* 458–463.

Larkin, H. (1997). Geography gaining power as a tool for shaping health and social policy. *Advances* (newsletter of The Robert Wood Johnson Foundation) Issue 3.

Leebov, W. & Ersoz, C.J. (1991). *The health care manager's guide to continuous quality improvement.* Chicago: American Hospital Association.

Lepley, C.J. (1998). Problem-solving tools for analyzing system problems: The affinity map and the relationship diagram. *Journal of Nursing Administration, 28*(12), 44–50.

Lewis, J.P. (1998). *Mastering project management,* 3rd ed. New York: John Wiley and Sons.

Lowery, G. & Ferrara, R. (1998). *Managing projects with Microsoft® Project 98.* New York: Van Nostrand Reinhold.

Nutt, P.C. (1984). *Planning methods for health and related organizations.* New York: John Wiley & Sons.

Powers, J., Pegelow, B. & Williams, J.K. (1998, March 6). *Quality improvement: Making it work in your organization.* Paper presented at the American Society on Aging, 45th annual meeting, Orlando, Florida.

Prince, G.M. (1970). *The practice of creativity: A manual for group problem solving.* New York: Collier Books.

Reeves, P.N. (1993). Issues management: The other side of strategic planning. *Hospitals and Health Services Administration, 38*(2).

Rosenau, M.D. (1998). *Successful project management,* 3rd ed. New York: John Wiley & Sons.

Stetler, C.B., Creer, E. & Effkin, J.A. (1996). Evaluating a redesign program: Challenges and opportunities. In K. Kelley (Ed.). *Outcomes of affective management practice.* Series in *Nursing Administration, 8,* Thousand Oaks, CA: Sage.

Strebel, P. (1992). *Breakpoints.* Boston: Harvard Business School Press.

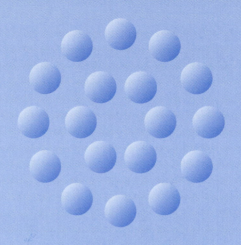

UNIT **IV**

# The Workplace

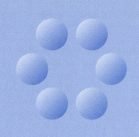

*CHAPTER* **17**

# Organizational Dynamics

## LEARNING OBJECTIVES

*After completing this chapter, the reader will be able to:*

- Differentiate the various types of healthcare organizations.
- Describe the characteristics of healthcare organizations as complex, open systems.
- Compare the structure and function of a bureaucratic structure and an organic one.

- Address both the formal and informal levels of operation.
- Differentiate authority, accountability, and responsibility.
- Identify the patterns of relationships found in organizations.

## TEST YOURSELF

1. **What does the word *bureaucracy* mean to you?** Write down all the words and phrases that come to your mind when you hear this word. Do not stop until you have written down at least 10.

2. What does the word democracy mean to you? Again, write down all the words and phrases that come to your mind when you hear this word. Do not stop until you have written down at least 10 words and phrases.

3. Now, think about which list of descriptive words and phrases attracts you and which list repels you. What does that tell you about the type of organization in which you would be most comfortable working?

Up to this point, the organization as a whole has often been mentioned but has not been the focus of our attention. Most organizations are so large and complex that it is not possible to directly observe everything that is happening in these systems. It is possible, however, to identify and evaluate the system's structure and operations once you know what to look for. It is also possible to learn how to function more effectively within these larger systems.

A healthcare organization is a human-made system of interrelated subsystems arranged to achieve a common goal. The flow of human (employees, patients, clients) and nonhuman (money, equipment, supplies, information) resources in, out, and within the organization constitute the dynamics of these complex systems (Kerzner, 1998). They are important because the way in which they are structured and how they operate have a great effect on the people who work within them and the quality of the service they provide. In fact, they are so important that organizational well-being is said to be directly related to employee well-being (DHHS, NOISH, 1999).

In this chapter we consider the different types of organizations in which healthcare professionals work, the characteristics of organizations as open systems, the ways in which organizations can be structured, how they actually operate compared with their formal structure, and some patterns of relationships that are found within them, with emphasis on the distribution of authority, accountability, and responsibility.

## ● HEALTHCARE ORGANIZATIONS

Nurses practice in many different types of organizations. Most of these are healthcare organizations: hospitals, clinics, health maintenance organizations, home healthcare agencies, public health departments, rehabilitation centers, mental health centers, and neighborhood health centers. Others are organizations in which health care is just one of many functions, a service offered to their clients or to the people employed by the organization. Schools, camps, day-care centers, prisons, and businesses of all kinds are some examples of this second category.

Healthcare organizations vary widely in the type of services they offer, the people they serve, and the way in which they are financed. Some are highly specialized, offering only renal dialysis, services for AIDS patients, or family planning, for example. Others offer a wide range of services, from prenatal classes to day surgery and intensive care. Despite this wide range of services, the organization that offers truly holistic health care is still rare.

Many healthcare and social services are designed for a limited population. They may be available only to employees of a particular company or to children in a particular school district. Some are designed only for the aged, for women, or for people with a particular problem, such as alcoholism or drug abuse. Some are available only to the poor, whereas others are available only to those who can afford them or to those who are enrolled in a particular kind of health plan. These limitations frequently result in people being excluded and, therefore, unable to obtain needed service.

Healthcare organizations can also be classified as for-profit or not-for-profit. The money needed to form and operate for-profit organizations comes from the same sources as any other business. Payment for the services that they provide comes from private insurance, government reimbursement, or out of the pocket of the person receiving the care. Because they are operated for a profit, proprietary organizations usually cannot survive for long if they are losing money. They also provide little or no service for those who cannot pay unless these services are reimbursed by the government.

The not-for-profit, or nonprofit, category includes **voluntary** organizations and **public** agencies and institutions. Public agencies are directly supported by funds from the local, state, or federal government. Their services are often free or offered at a reduced rate to those who cannot afford to pay the full cost (the medically indigent). Although they are not operated for a profit, their administrators are directly answerable to the sponsoring government agency and indirectly answerable to elected officials and the taxpayers who provide the money for their support. The amount of support they receive is strongly influenced by public opinion and the prevailing political climate. Shifts in the political climate have a direct impact on these organizations, their staffs, and the people for whom they provide care.

The term **not-for-profit** does not mean that these organizations do not have to be concerned with their financial well-being. They still must be concerned with having adequate money to expand, to be prepared for inflation or for hard times, and to be able to pay back the money they borrowed for new buildings, equipment, and so forth. Maintaining financial health has become more difficult as both private insurers and government sources of reimbursement increasingly limit coverage and scrutinize every charge for service. As a result, not-for-profit hospitals and other healthcare organizations have begun to operate more like businesses in order to keep costs under control. An unforeseen result of the emphasis on the bottom line is increasing public skepticism of their claim to serve the community (Reeves, 1993).

## ● ORGANIZATIONS AS COMPLEX OPEN SYSTEMS

Like the smaller systems we have already studied, organizations exhibit wholeness, individuality, hierarchy, complexity, openness, identifiable patterns, and growth.

## Wholeness

As large and complex as they are, organizations also have characteristics as a whole that are different from and greater than the sum of their parts. For example, even when many people join or leave, the organization as a whole can continue to function and retain its identity. It also means that a change in one part of the organization has an effect on the whole. For example, a change in the operating hours of the radiology department could affect the work of inpatient units, the operating room, ambulatory surgery, and the clinics.

## Individuality

Organizations also exhibit individuality; no two organizations are exactly alike. It is both interesting and informative to ask people who work in an organization to describe its culture or "personality." People may describe their organization as "open and informal," "schizophrenic," "suffering from growing pains," "old and traditional," or "hungry" (looking for more clients or money). You may get different answers if you ask several people, but a definite pattern will eventually emerge from the answers to this question.

Morgan (1997) suggests using an image such as an animal or familiar object to characterize the organization. For example, an organization could be described as a huge tortoise moving slowly and ponderously or a rudderless boat, drifting in no particular direction. Each of these images captures the essence of the organization as a whole.

You can also observe people's behavior in an organization and your own response to the organization. Some have a climate that is warm and friendly, open to new people and new ideas. Others present themselves as cold, hostile, and suspicious of new people. Imagine what your first impression of these two mental health centers would be:

*First Organization:* When you approach the door, a guard blocks your way until you explain that you are a community health nurse here to consult with the psychologist treating one of your clients. When the guard finally says, "Go ahead," you enter a bare lobby and head for the glass window at the far end. The switchboard operator slides back the glass and says, "Yes?" You repeat your explanation, and the operator slides the glass closed without another word. A minute later, the glass is reopened and the operator says, "Room 203 on your left," and slides the window shut again.

*Second Organization:* As you approach the door, the guard steps forward and says, "Good morning, may I help you?" On hearing your response, the guard opens the door for you and directs you to the receptionist seated at a desk in the center of a lobby that contains comfortable-looking chairs and small pots of flowers. The re-

## Research Example 17–1  *Being Sane in Insane Places*

In this provocative and frequently quoted study, Rosenhan (1973) asked whether the characteristics that lead to a diagnosis of mental illness are found in the patients themselves or in the organizational context (i.e., in the environment). Eight "sane" people, five men and three women (three psychologists, a graduate student, a pediatrician, a psychiatrist, a painter, and a housewife), presented themselves at the admissions offices of hospitals in five different states. Each person complained of hearing strange voices that were often unclear or sounded "empty" or "hollow." All eight were admitted immediately and placed in a psychiatric ward. Seven were diagnosed as schizophrenic.

Once on the psychiatric wards, these "pseudopatients," as the researcher called them, no longer claimed to hear voices and behaved as they usually did. Except for giving false symptoms and false names, they related their own ordinary life events when asked for their life history. But once they had been labeled as sick, the label stuck—all were discharged with the diagnosis of schizophrenia in remission after an average stay of 19 days (the range was 7–52 days).

Many of the real patients detected the pseudopatients and accused them of being journalists or evaluators checking up on the hospital. But staff members, including the psychiatrists, nurses, and attendants, reportedly never questioned the assumption that they were genuinely ill, despite patient records describing them as friendly, cooperative, and exhibiting no abnormal behavior.

The researcher found that the staff's perceptions of the pseudopatients' behavior, no matter how normal it was, was so strongly shaped by the diagnosis that it was considered disturbed. An example of this effect is the staff's response, or more accurately nonresponse, to the fact that the pseudopatients took notes. The staff never questioned this behavior although the real patients did. One physician told a pseudopatient that he did not have to write down the name of his medicine but could ask if he forgot it. Another pseudopatient had the comment, "Patient engages in writing behavior" written in his chart. Apparently, the writing was presumed to be part of the disturbance.

The researcher also found that the source of any disturbance was always assumed to be the patient and not the staff's behavior or the effect of the environment. For example, when a pseudopatient was found walking the halls, a nurse asked him if he was nervous. Actually, he was bored. The researcher concluded that the staff's perceptions of behavior were affected by the organizational environment. It doesn't appear that much critical reflection was being done by these staff members.

*Source:* Rosenhan, D.L. (1973). On being sane in insane places. *Science, 179,* 250.

---

ceptionist smiles at you, pages the psychologist, and tells you to make yourself comfortable; the psychologist will be out in a just a moment.*

Can you imagine how differently clients would feel about walking into these two places? The powerful and pervasive effect of the organizational climate on the perceptions and behavior of people within that organization is described in Research Example. . . . Being Sane in Insane Places.

The work climate of healthcare organizations can differ in other important ways as well.

For example, research studies have shown that the level of anxiety among staff members varies from department to department and from one organization to another. The degree of alienation in the staff has also been found to differ substantially from one organization to another. Effective leadership interventions can influence the prevailing climate. Respect for the dignity and worth of the individual employee, open communication, administrative support, and taking action on problems as needed have been found to affect the climate of the organization in a positive way (McClure, 1972; Revans, 1972). These differences have important implications not only for leadership and management action but also for selecting an organization in which you want to work.

## Hierarchy

Complex organizations are made up of many levels of systems and subsystems that are given names such as divisions, areas, units, departments, groups, and teams. In most organizations, people are ranked according to their job classification, their status, and the amount of authority that they have. This hierarchy is traditionally depicted as a pyramid having the smallest number of people with the greatest amount of authority at the top, and the largest number of people with little or no authority at the bottom (see Figure 17–1). The traditional pyramid actually oversimplifies the structure and the patterns of interaction that occur within an organization. Although it would not be as clear, a hierarchy of intersecting circles would be a more accurate model of most organizations. Some variations in the structure of organizations are discussed later in this chapter.

Some organizations have a structure and climate that encourage the free movement of information up and down the hierarchy. Others have limited communication networks in which few people know what is happening or feel as if they have anything to say about what is happening.

## Complexity

As the number of people in a system increases, the number of different relationships possible between people increases geometrically. For example, there are four different relationship combinations possible in a group of three people, 11 in a group of four people, and 9,801 in a group of 100 people (the first two sets of combinations are illustrated in Figure 17–2).

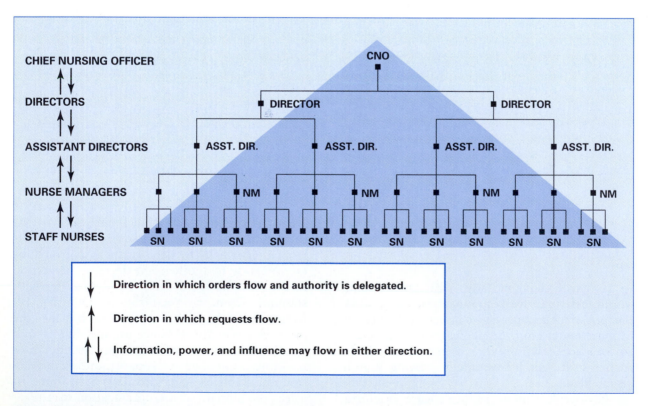

**Figure 17–1**   Traditional nursing hierarchy in hospitals and long-term care facilities.

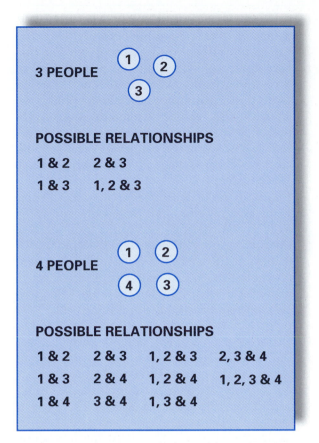

**3 PEOPLE**

**POSSIBLE RELATIONSHIPS**

1 & 2      2 & 3
1 & 3      1, 2 & 3

**4 PEOPLE**

**POSSIBLE RELATIONSHIPS**

1 & 2      2 & 3      1, 2 & 3      2, 3 & 4
1 & 3      2 & 4      1, 2 & 4      1, 2, 3 & 4
1 & 4      3 & 4      1, 3 & 4

**Figure 17–2**   Illustration of relationship combinations.

Complexity is evident in almost every aspect of the structure and operation of organizations. Most organizations have multiple goals rather than a single goal, goals that may be in conflict with one another (Huse & Bowditch, 1977). For example, cost cutting done to increase profits may conflict with the goal of delivering high-quality care.

## Openness

Every open system, including organizations, affects its environment and is likewise affected by its environment. For example, hospitals located in high crime areas may experience higher demands for their emergency services, especially for treatment of traumatic injuries. This demand in turn affects the emergency department's need for staff.

An organization exchanges information and energy with its environment. The organization's contributions are specialized skills and information needed to promote or restore health. These skills are exchanged for money and recognition.

These exchanges between the organization and its clients are influenced by many factors in the environment, such as the number of other organizations offering the same services, the actual and perceived need for the service, and government regulation. Some healthcare organizations cannot find sufficient skilled staff to offer needed services. Others find that their service is not valued and that people are not willing to pay for it. In still other cases, insufficient knowledge is available about a problem to be able to offer satisfactory care. All of these factors and many more interact to produce a complex healthcare system.

## Patterns and Growth

Like other systems, organizations have identifiable rhythms and cycles. For example, hospitals operate 24 hours a day, every day of the year. Within those 24 hours, the day shift is usually the busiest and the night shift usually has the least number of people working.

The most typical growth pattern for successful organizations is early, rapid growth followed by a slower rate of growth in the later stages of its life cycle. The alternative is failure, which happens to an incredible 80 percent of new businesses (Woerner, 1994). Eventually all of them experience some kind of decline and cease to exit.

Four specific stages in the organizational life cycle have been identified (Kolb et al., 1995):

Inception:          The start-up phase, usually characterized by a very free, open structure and operation in which everyone pitches in to get done whatever needs to be done.

High Growth:        A time of great energy and enthusiasm for the prospects of the organization. Stresses and strains are likely to appear

|            |                                                                                                                                                      |
| ---------- | ---------------------------------------------------------------------------------------------------------------------------------------------------- |
|            | and the structure and operation usually become more formal.                                                                                          |
| Maturity:  | Growth slows but operations usually run smoothly at this stage of the life cycle. By this time, numerous rules and regulations govern its operation.  |
| Decline or Renewal: | Many organizations become rigid, complex, and top heavy (too many people at the top of the hierarchy). Some fail to respond to changes in their environment and become dinosaurs, both literally and figuratively. |

Do these stages sound familiar? In many ways, they are like the forming-storming-norming-performing-adjourning stages of group development discussed in Chapter 5.

## ● ORGANIZATIONAL STRUCTURE

### The Bureaucracy

Before comparing the classic or traditional organizational structure with the organic or matrix design or structure, it would be helpful to review the basic characteristics of a bureaucracy. Max Weber (in Etzioni, 1969) defined a bureaucracy as having the four following characteristics:

1. *Division of Labor.*   Specific parts of the job to be done are assigned to different individuals or groups. For example, nurses, physicians, therapists, dietitians, and social workers all provide portions of the health care needed by an individual patient.
2. *Hierarchy.*   All employees are organized and ranked according to their degree of authority within the organization. For example, administrators and directors are at the top of most hospital hierarchies, whereas aides and maintenance workers are at the bottom.
3. *Rules and regulations.*   Acceptable and unacceptable behavior and the proper way to carry out various tasks are defined, often in writing. For example, procedure books, policy manuals, bylaws, statements, and memos prescribe many types of behavior, from acceptable isolation techniques to vacation policies (see Perspectives . . . Would You Like to Work Here?).
4. *Emphasis on technical competence.*   People with certain skills and knowledge are hired to carry out specific parts of the total work of the organization. For example, a community mental health center will have psychiatrists, psychologists, social workers, and nurses to provide different kinds of therapies and clerical staff to do the typing and filing.

Some degree of bureaucracy is characteristic of the formal operation of virtually every organization, even the most deliberately informal, because it promotes smooth operations within a large and complex group of people.

In the traditional bureaucracy, the emphasis is on the vertical rather than the horizontal relationships. This is called the **chain of command.** Within the chain of command, the CEO at the top of the pyramid delegates authority to people in middle management and so on down the line. Support staff have relatively limited power compared with those who have this **line authority,** which extends all the way down to the first-line manager.

An organization is subject to varying degrees of bureaucracy. A highly bureaucratized approach is based on the belief that employees must be told what to do and closely supervised in order to ensure that they will do it. It also assumes that some employees are more skilled and responsible than others and should, therefore, have authority over the other people. An organization that is managed according to these beliefs (which hearken back to the mechanistic perspectives of Fayol and Taylor) would have many detailed rules and regulations, close supervision of employees, and allow little autonomy to individual employees, even to professionals capable of functioning independently.

## Would You Like to Work Here?

The SAS Institute outside Raleigh, North Carolina, is a software company run by what some may call a "benevolent dictator." Family-friendly policies that build employee loyalty are emphasized. Some examples:

- A free health clinic staffed by two physicians and six nurse practitioners.
- Two day-care centers for employees' children.
- Coffee break rooms stocked with free sodas, fresh fruit, M&Ms, and pastries.
- An ergonomics specialist who helps employees choose correct office furniture.
- An artist-in-residence who advises employees on the selection of paintings for their offices.
- A pianist in the cafeteria.
- A 35-hour work week in an industry known for 60 to 80-hour work weeks.

On the other hand, salaries are modest and many of the policies are deliberately designed to keep employees at the SAS Institute. For example, the company does not provide tuition assistance because employees often seek new positions after finishing an advanced degree.

Do these policies have their intended effect? The turnover rate at SAS is 4 percent per year compared to 20 percent across the software industry. But not everyone is happy with the paternalistic atmosphere. One former employee remarked that "a gilded cage is still a cage" (p. B4).

*Source:* Schellhard, T.D. (1998, November 23). An idyllic workplace under a tycoon's thumb. *Wall Street Journal,* B1, B4.

One of the greatest frustrations people experience in trying to relate to a bureaucratic organization, either as employees or as clients, is trying to find someone who can give you an answer or solve your problem. For example, to get something done in some organizations, you need the approval of six different people on six different forms, and each of the six people refuses to give you approval until the other five have given theirs. This scenario is not true of every bureau-cratically structured organization, but it is one common negative outcome of bureaucratic organization, known as "bureaucratic red tape."

With their long lines of delegated authority and decision making, you often cannot identify exactly who in an organization is responsible for blocking a decision or holding up progress. Arendt (in Greene, 1977) calls this "rule by nobody" because the source of these decisions and rules is faceless. No one takes responsibility for outcomes and nobody seems to know where rules and decisions have originated. In extremely bureaucratic organizations, employees come to believe that they are controlled by impersonal rules and have no influence on decisions. This environment is a perfect breeding ground for powerlessness and alienation.

Another negative effect of bureaucratization is particularly relevant to health care. An extreme division of labor extends the rule by nobody to responsibility for the end product. When 12, 15, or even 20 people in one healthcare organization have given care to a patient, how can you say who is responsible for the outcome? Another problem arises from an extreme division of labor: how can people derive any satisfaction or pride from their work when it is difficult to identify their contribution? The following is one example of this fragmentation:

> *In a school clinic, a nurse observed that a youngster was flushed, restless, and had some abdominal pain. The child was immediately referred to a physician, who diagnosed the problem as appendicitis.*
>
> *The child was admitted to the hospital and prepared for surgery. The operating room nurse and recovery room nurse both offered support and reassurance when the child seemed frightened by this new experience and strange environment.*
>
> *Several nurses cared for the child on the pediatric unit until the child was sent home. The child recovered quickly at home and returned to school in two weeks.*
>
> *However, the clinic nurse's original assessment was not confirmed to the nurse until the child returned to the clinic a year later. The operating room and recovery room nurses never found out whether their intervention*

*had left the child less fearful, and the nurses on the pediatric unit never found out whether the child did well at home and upon returning to school.*

Each of these nurses had an important but limited part in the child's care. The lack of involvement in the whole process and lack of feedback about the child's progress to recovery meant that not one of them received confirmation of the ultimate effectiveness of their intervention.

## Traditional Structural Design

The traditional organizational design, which has survived for more than 200 years, is based on bureaucratic principles (Kerzner, 1998; Purser & Cabana, 1999). New, small organizations of traditional design usually have simple structures consisting of a chief executive officer (CEO) and a few additional executives forming the strategic apex at the top of the hierarchy; few or no people in the middle ranks; and the rest of its employees at the bottom forming the **operating core** (Mintzberg, 1983), (shown in Figure 17–3). Supervision and coordination are done directly from the top by the CEO, who acts as the leader and manager of the whole organization. Much of the communication within the organization is quite informal.

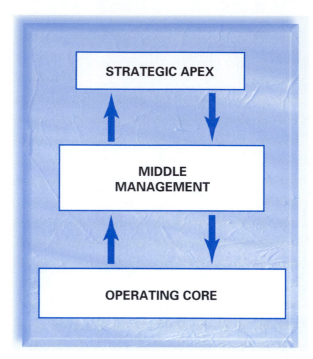

**Figure 17–4**    Structure of a growing organization. *Source:* Adapted from Mintzberg, H. (1983). *Structure in fives: Designing effective organizations.* Englewood Cliffs, NJ: Prentice-Hall.

As the organization grows larger, this simple structure no longer works well. The operating core of employees becomes too large for one or two people to direct. As a result, the work is divided up into smaller components, and many leadership and management functions are delegated to people lower in the hierarchy. These people form a new level of middle management (Figure 17–4).

As this bureaucratic organization grows, it may become even more complex. Two other components are often added: support staff and technical staff. **Support staff** provide services to the employees of the organization. In a large hospital, support staff would include the people who run the cafeteria, payroll, media department, and the employee health service department. They provide services to the staff rather than to the patients or clients themselves. The second component is the **technical staff**. These people are expert in a particular area and act as internal consultants to the operating core. Examples of technical staff in a

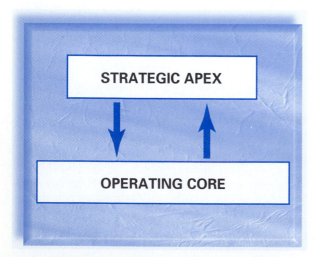

**Figure 17–3**    Structure of a small new organization. *Source:* Mintzberg, H. (1983). *Structure in fives: Designing effective organizations.* Englewood Cliffs, NJ: Prentice-Hall.

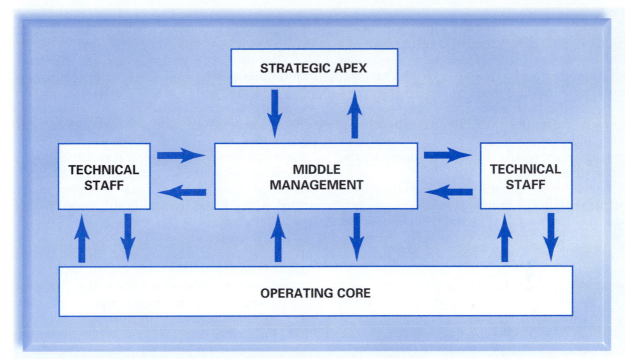

**Figure 17–5** Four components of a fully developed organization. *Source:* Adapted from Mintzberg, H. (1983). *Structure in fives: Designing effective organizations.* Englewood Cliffs, NJ: Prentice-Hall.

hospital would include hospital information system employees, risk management, and staff development. This complex organization now has all five components of Mintzberg's model (Figure 17–5).

## Matrix or Organic Designs

If linear relationships epitomize the bureaucratic organization, then circular relationships epitomize the matrix or organic organizational designs. These designs were created to allow people to break free of the limits of the bureaucratic design, particularly of its rigidity, linearity, and top-down control. Instead of a pyramid, the organic network might be compared to a system of interconnected clusters like a spider plant with its offshoots (Morgan, 1997). Increased flexibility of the organizational structure, decentralized decision making, and autonomy for working groups or teams are the hallmarks of an organic design.

*Once there were pyramids, departments, leaders, troops; now there are webs, nodes, communities, networks. Once there was continuous improvement and incremental change; now we see continuous discontinuous change.*

—S. Wimby in Purser & Cabana, 1999, p. ix

More and more people recognize that organizations need to be not only efficient but also adaptable and innovative. Organizations need to be prepared for uncertainty; for rapid changes in their environment; and for rapid, creative responses to these challenges. In addition, they need to provide an internal climate that not only allows but also motivates employees to work to the best of their ability.

Ideally, organic organizations are loose, flexible, and decentralized. Decisions are made by the people who will implement them, not by their bosses or by their bosses' boss. Rigid department or unit structures are reorganized into autonomous teams. Each team is assigned a specific task or function to carry out (common examples would be an infection control team or a child protection team). These teams are given much more authority than in a bureaucratic organization. They are responsible for their own self-correction and self-control. Together, team members make decisions about work assignments and how to deal with any problems that arise. In other words, the teams supervise and manage themselves.

Supervisors, administrators, and support staff have different functions in an organic network. Instead of spending their time observing and controlling other people's work, managers and supervisors become planners and resource people. They are responsible for providing the conditions required for the optimal functioning of the teams and are expected to ensure that the support, information, materials, and budgeted funds needed to do the job well are available to the teams. They also provide more coordination between the teams.

Because of its dynamic nature, an organic organization is harder to understand than a pyramid (bureaucratic organization). It is also harder to control. Staff may move from one cluster to another, or the entire configuration of interconnected clusters may be reorganized as the organization shapes and is being shaped by its environment. People with a great need for control, predictably, are often uncomfortable with the organic design.

## Variations in Design

In reality, the structural design of most organizations falls somewhere in between these two extremes. Figure 17–6 illustrates the continuum of designs from the highly controlled bureaucracy to the loosely connected, ever-changing organic organization.

The **bureaucracy with a top management team** (Design 2 in Figure 17–6) is a favorite design for organizations faced with an increasing need to respond to changes in the environment. In this design, a top management **team** is formed to better use the talents of upper-level management and to devise more creative strategies to deal with change. As the synergies of this pooled

expertise at the top become fully appreciated, consideration is often given to using teams at lower levels as well, leading to Design 3.

The **project team design** (Design 4) is even more fluid and has much less of the traditional hierarchical structure, which can weigh down the bureaucratic team design. This design promotes a fluid deployment of staff and extraordinary opportunities for cross-fertilization of ideas. People may work on several different teams at a time. A physician, for example, may be part of both the orthopedic-rehabilitation team and the surgical team. A psychiatric-mental health nurse may be part of both the drug treatment team and the crisis intervention team.

In the **organic matrix** (Design 5), the various teams become virtually independent satellites of the central team. The team at the center directs the overall organizational strategy and channels the needed resources to its many satellite teams. In effect, the central team subcontracts all other responsibilities to the satellites, which become more autonomous. Although the satellite teams are usually dynamic and highly responsive to change, they do lose many of the opportunities for cross-fertilization of ideas provided by the project team design (Design 4) unless the central team or roving team members assume this responsibility.

*There is no such thing as a good or bad organizational structure; there are only appropriate or inappropriate ones.*
*—Kerzner, 1998, p. 95*

Selection of the best design would depend on an analysis of the organization's goals, its environment, the work to be done, and the type of staff available to do the work. The ideal contemporary healthcare organization would have egalitarian leadership, a creative climate, flexible structure, technologically current expertise and equipment, a philosophy of continuous improvement, and a client-focused mentality (Hodgetts, Luthans & Lee, 1994). Some of the qualitative differences between traditional bureaucratic and organic structures are outlined in Table 17–1.

While many innovative organizational designs have been proposed—a "plethora of novel ideas" is one description of the recent explosion

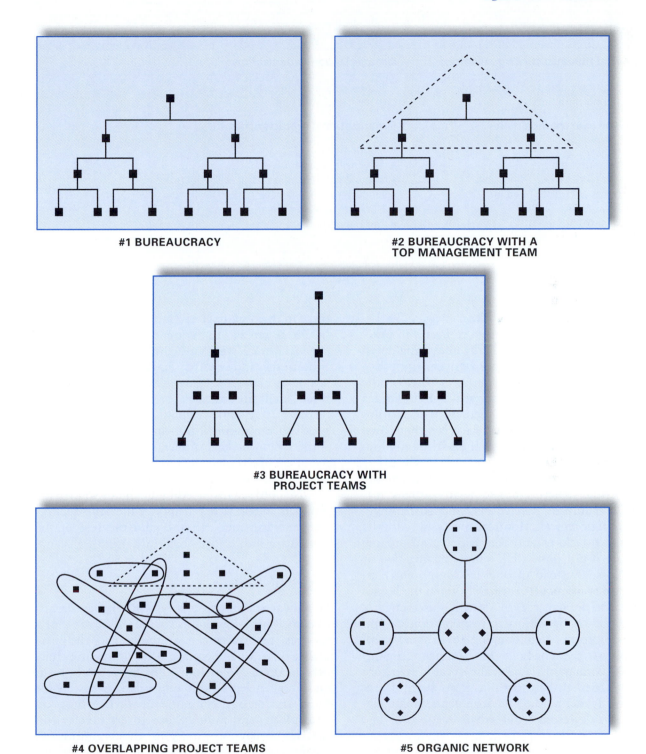

**Figure 17–6**   Organizational designs from the bureaucratic to the organic. *Source:* Adapted from Morgan, A. (1997). *Imaginization: The art of creative management.* Newbury Park, CA: Sage.

**Table 17–1**    Qualitative Differences between Traditional Bureaucratic and Organic Structures

| Traditional Bureaucratic Organization | Organic Design Organization |
|---|---|
| Simple jobs are created within a complex organizational structure. | Complex jobs are created within a simple organizational structure. |
| **Organizational characteristics** | **Organizational characteristics** |
| • Competitive<br>• One person-one task<br>• Specify tasks as much as possible<br>• Employees as cogs to be fit into the machine<br>• Stable, unchanging<br>• Rigid, controlled | • Cooperative<br>• Self-managed team<br>• Allow employees to use their skills, discretion<br>• Employees as learners with multiple skills<br>• Constant, dynamic change<br>• Flexible, responsive |

*Source:*  Adapted from Purser, R.E. & Cabana, S. (1999). *The self-managing organization.* New York: The Free Press (Simon & Schuster, Inc.).

of new designs (Senge et al., 1999, p. 364)—fewer successful examples can be found in practice than one might expect. Why? Breaking down centralized controls and lines of authority is notoriously difficult to do. It requires **trust** on the part of management, that is, trust that employees can make good decisions and will work to improve the organization, not just for their own gain. It also requires trust on the part of employees, trust that managers really mean it when they say "do what you think is best." Second, the bureaucratic structure has some advantages: it is stable, organized, predictable, and surprisingly efficient if done well. Contrast this result with the potential for chaos and confusion of an organic structure if not done well. Simply having two or three bosses instead of one has the potential to confuse any employee, especially when the bosses are inconsistent in regard to demands (Senge et al., 1999). Yet the ability to respond quickly and effectively to an ever-changing environment will continue to be a challenge for healthcare organizations (Gilmartin, 1998). The organic structure was designed to help organizations be more responsive to demanding environments. Some elements of this design are clearly needed.

## Medical Staff

The way in which members of a medical staff relate to the organization as a whole is peculiar to healthcare organizations. Although a major force in the organization, most are not employed by the organization. They also have a separate organizational structure, different credentialing procedures, and separate leadership, but this situation is changing. Many larger hospitals have hired medical directors or vice-presidents for medical affairs and a small number of medical staff office personnel, but the chief of staff, who is the senior medical officer, is usually elected by members of the medical staff (Williams & Ewell, 1996). The introduction of intensivists and hospitalists, physicians hired by hospitals to provide inpatient medical care, may reduce the separation between medical staff and the rest of the acute-care staff (Noyes & Healy, 1999).

## Board of Trustees

Healthcare organizations typically have a board of some kind—known as the board of directors, trustees, or governors—at the top of the hierarchy. Board members are often influential business people, professionals, or community leaders. They are legally and ethically responsible for the operation of the organization. Their function is to set general policies, not to get involved in the day-to-day operation of the organization. Health care is a highly complex and technologically advanced field, and the professional administrator usually has the time and training needed to thoroughly assess the situation and make these decisions.

Traditionally, the board, administration, and medical staff formed a triad of power and authority at the top of the organizational hierarchy. A number of trends have challenged this triad. More physicians are employed directly by organizations. Governmental regulation has become an increasingly powerful influence on healthcare organizations, and managed care has altered many of the traditional relationships within healthcare organizations.

## Nurses

Nurses have also challenged the traditional organizational triad. Nursing service administrators are leaders of the largest group of healthcare professionals in most healthcare organizations (approximately 50 percent of the staff of most hospitals). Many have moved up into influential positions and are no longer satisfied with the limited amount of power and authority that they had in the past.

It is important to also point out that nurses are neither powerless nor at the bottom of the hierarchy. Depending on the particular organization, nurses have positional authority over other nurses, practical nurses, nursing assistants, other unlicensed assistive personnel, and people from other professions and departments. It is also worth noting that many other healthcare professionals (physical therapists, dietitians, social workers, and so forth) are located in similar positions in the organizational hierarchy and face many of the same conflicts as nurses do in promoting the practice of their professions.

Research on organizations has shown that people at all levels in organizations tend to attribute more power to others than to themselves (Lindquist & Blackburn, 1974). In a survey at one university, for example, the faculty felt that the students and administration had most of the power, the administrators felt that the faculty and students had most of the power, and the students felt that the faculty and administrators had all of the power. It may help you to remember these survey results when you are dealing with persons above or below you in the hierarchy of your organization: these people probably feel much less powerful than they seem to you.

No single person's power or authority in an organization is absolute. Each person, no matter how high up in the hierarchy, is susceptible to the power of others either within or outside the organization. Nor is anyone, no matter how low on the hierarchy, completely without power. Although people at lower levels of the hierarchy have little or no authority, they have other sources of power that can counterbalance the authority of people above them in the hierarchy. People in high-level positions depend on their staffs to carry out their decisions: a nurse manager could not carry out all of the work that must be done if the staff left.

## ● ORGANIZATIONAL OPERATIONS

The original idea of a **formal** or public set of rules, relationships, and goals as well as an **informal** or "shadow" set of norms, relationships, and goals (Kolb et al., 1995; Purser & Cabana, 1999) came from research studies such as the famous Hawthorne series described in chapter 2. These studies clearly indicated that more was going on in an organization than was spelled out in its formal rules and regulations. In fact, an entire system of interpersonal relationships, unwritten work rules (norms), values, and shared meanings had developed and were quite different from those prescribed by management (Fleeger, 1993; Schwartzman, 1993). The classic approach to organizations focused only on the formal aspects, but it eventually became apparent that such an approach ignored too many important factors.

### Formal and Informal Goals

The two kinds of goals in an organization are the **officially stated goals** and the **actual operative goals** (Perrow, 1969; Kolb et al., 1995). The formal, official goals of an organization are those that appear in public statements about the organization. Official goals tend to be general, public-spirited, and idealistic. They are designed to sound benevolent and impressive. The following are examples:

• Promote the health and well-being of the clients we serve.

- Protect the people of this city.
- Foster a spirit of cooperative concern for those in need of our services.

Most organizations want the public to know about their official goals, making an effort to publicize them because they promote the desired image. However, the official goals do not explain the behavior of an organization, much of which is directed toward achieving another set of goals—the operative goals.

The informal, operative goals of an organization are those the organization and its people are actually pursuing in day-to-day operations. They are usually not verbalized and may be less rational or public-spirited than the official goals. They are also more difficult to determine than official goals because they are implicit. In fact, stating them directly can provoke denial and an insistence on the exclusivity of the official goals. Careful observation of behavior in the organization is needed to identify the operative goals. In particular, you need to look at the decisions that are made; what kind of behavior is rewarded; and the actual, unstated priorities that are implied by these actions.

Operative goals not only differ from official goals but often are in conflict with them. They focus primarily on the survival and growth of the organization rather than public benefit. Healthcare organizations depend on their environments for a continuous supply of clients, money, and personnel. Without these elements, they cannot continue to exist. These needs are reflected in their operative goals, which are commonly aimed at achieving financial gain, efficiency rather than effectiveness, quantity rather than quality, maintenance of a positive public image, avoiding public criticism and legal problems, especially expensive and embarrassing lawsuits. The personal needs and ambitions of people who have power and authority in the organization also affect the operative goals. Some examples:

- *Financial Gain.* A system's basic drive to continue to exist often leads to the placing of financial gain above other, more humanitarian goals even in not-for-profit organizations. The pursuit of profits can subvert caregiving goals, which becomes more evident to the public when, for example, managed care corporations limit ac-

cess to specialists or substitute generic for brand name drugs to save money.
- *Efficiency.* Efficient operation means greater output per dollar spent. Staffing patterns may reflect this operative goal. The functional mode of organizing nursing care (in which one person gives all of the medications, another does all of the treatments, and so forth) is one example. Another example is hiring the person with the least amount of skill, such as a nursing assistant, rather than the person who is better prepared to do the job best but commands a higher salary.
- *Quantity Versus Quality.* The priority of quantity over quality leads to the "numbers game" in organizations. Departments are asked to report the numbers of things done rather than how well they are done and then are rewarded for producing quantity rather than quality. The tendency to emphasize quantity over quality translates into valuing how many people a nurse practitioner can see in a day rather than the effectiveness of the care given, or counting the number of home visits made in a day rather than evaluating the effectiveness of these visits. Getting food trays delivered to patients and picked up quickly often seems to be more important than providing assistance or making a diet palatable.
- *Public Image.* A positive public image attracts attention, clients, investors, and benefactors. This aspect can influence a wide range of decisions. For example, what happens to an individual patient is much less apparent to a hospital's potential clients and contributors than is an attractive, modern building, so money needed for additional staff may be spent on renovation and landscaping instead.

On the other hand, it is sometimes possible to take advantage of this operative goal. For example, to gain support for a birthing room, you can point out that it would be the first in the community, and that it would create favorable publicity for the organization.
- *Survival.* Most healthcare organizations go to great lengths to avoid anything that would threaten their existence. For example:

*A county health department hired a pediatric nurse practitioner to conduct child health clin-*

*ics. The clinics were well attended and the parents were satisfied with the family-centered care they received. In fact, they were so satisfied that many reduced their pediatrician visits, which provoked a strong protest from influential area pediatricians. In response to the protest, the pediatric nurse practitioner's clinics were limited to families who could not pay for a private physician.*

Concern about legal repercussions is also related to the survival goal. Some examples:

*Ambulatory day surgery patients are usually not permitted to walk into surgery because of concern about legal responsibilities (Petzinger, 1999).*

*Older patients are often restrained for fear they may fall and the institution be sued.*

This operative goal can also be turned into an advantage, however. For example, if discharge planning is inadequate, you can point out that the organization could be held legally responsible if patients are given insufficient information about self-care before discharge and injure themselves as a result.

• *Needs and Ambition of Influentials.* The personal needs, desires, and ambitions of people with power and authority in organizations often influence the decisions. For example:

*Surgeons may perform unnecessary operations to keep their skills sharp or their practices busy.*

*Administrators may propose purchasing expensive equipment because they want to be associated with a technologically advanced organization.*

These individual needs can set in motion activities that are in conflict not only with the official goals but also with some of the other operative goals of the organization.

## Formal and Informal Operations

### Formal Operation

Like the formal goals, the **formal level of operation** is the official written, publicly announced manner in which one organization is suppose to function. It includes all of the written rules, regulations, and policies that are eventually created in most organizations. If you asked an administrator to describe the organization to you, the administrator would probably describe only the formal level of operation. Here is an example from an ambulatory care center:

*In the main clinic, we have our administrative offices as well as our comprehensive ambulatory care clinic. Clients can see the physicians, nurses, social worker, dietitian, or community worker as needed here. We have three satellite clinics staffed by nurse practitioners and a social worker. We also have an outreach team that is based here at the main clinic but travels to different locations each day of the week and responds to emergency calls. Clients who need to see a physician or dietitian must come to the main clinic. Also, the bookkeeping and billing are done from the main office, but people can call the satellite clinics to make appointments.*

The description would go on to say who is in charge of each clinic, who manages the entire organization, the specific services offered, the fees charged, the hours each clinic is open, and so on.

If you expressed interest in further information, the administrator might give you a **table of organization.** The table of organization is a diagram showing the formal relationships between employees of the organization, the way in which they are grouped together, and who reports to whom (Figure 17–7).

On the formal level, communication is supposed to flow along the established lines shown in the diagram; for example, from the administrator to the assistant administrator to the director of the main clinic to the supervisors, the rest of the staff, and back again. This flow is often referred to as the **proper channels of communication** and to some extent, it is the way much information travels in an organization. It is often said that the orders come down and the requests go up in a traditionally structured organization. The board of trustees delegates authority to the administrator, who in turn delegates some authority to the assistant administrators and so on down the line. Staff members who are at the bottom of the pyramid have authority over no one except perhaps the clients served by the organization,

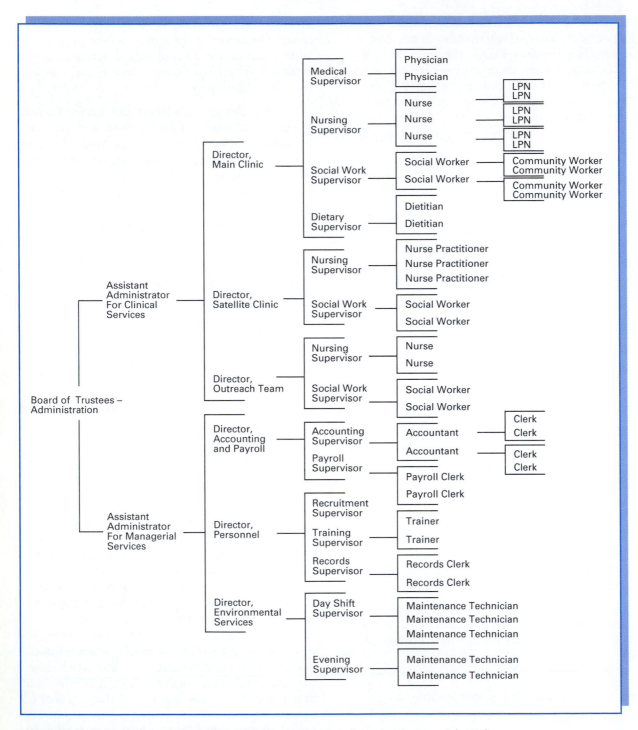

**Figure 17–7**   Formal table of organization for an ambulatory care center. *Source:* Adapted from DelBueno, D.J. (1987). An organizational checklist. *Journal of Nursing Administration, 17*(5), 30–33.

who do not even appear on most tables of organization. Work assignments and directions are passed down the line in the same way.

## Informal Operation

The **informal level of operation** or **shadow organization** includes all those unwritten, unofficial relationships that develop in an organization but are not reflected in the official structure of the organization. The most difficult to detect are the underlying assumptions, those unconscious or taken-for-granted beliefs, perceptions, and feelings about the purpose of the organization and how it should function. It is the **culture** of the organization (Schein, 1999). It includes norms and traditions about the way people work together and has a strong influence on what actually happens in an organization, existing alongside and intertwined with the formal level of operation.

The informal level of operations exists even in the most highly controlled organization. The following is an extreme example:

> A prison is a highly controlled organization: its clients (the prisoners) are not even allowed to leave without permission. Many restrictions are placed on the behavior of both the guards and the prisoners about who can visit, what possessions the prisoners are allowed, and so forth. Yet some prisoners are able to buy and sell drugs, liquor, and sex, all absolutely forbidden by the formal organization. They are able to do these things through the shadow organization or informal level of operation.

The formal and informal levels of operation can be complementary and facilitative, or conflict and obstruct each other. Rules and regulations may be circumvented, the hierarchy may be ignored, someone high up in the hierarchy may have little power or influence, or lines between specific jobs may be blurred in actual operation. Alternative paths are created by which requests are made and filled without multiple approvals; tasks are completed quickly and messages are communicated across and around the so-called proper channels of communication.

*A strong corporate culture is the invisible hand that guides how things are done in an organization. The*

*phrase, "You just can't do that here," is extremely powerful, more so than any written rules or policy manuals.*
—A. Grove, 1987, in Eigen & Siegel, 1989

Many efforts to bring about improvement or change have failed because the person planning them thought it could be done by just setting up a formal procedure. The following example illustrates the difference between using only the formal level and using both formal and informal levels:

> Two different nurses working in a large city hospital had what they thought were good ideas for improving patient care in that hospital. The first nurse had some ideas for improving the patient assessment form and asked the nurse manager how a suggestion is supposed to be sent to the vice-president for nursing services. The nurse manager told the nurse to put the idea in writing, including reasons why the nurse thought it would improve nursing care, and to give two copies to the supervisor, who would keep one and send the other to the vice-president.
>
> The nurse typed a three-page report explaining the idea and how it would increase efficiency and promote better patient care. The nurse gave the report to the supervisor as requested.
>
> Three months later the nurse received a note from the vice-president expressing appreciation for the suggestion and saying that it would be shared with the nurse managers and supervisors to find out if they thought it would work. By the time the nurse received this note, the idea was almost forgotten; and it was apparently received without enthusiasm because it was never implemented.
>
> The second nurse followed the procedure that other people had used successfully in that hospital. The second nurse talked with the nurse manager and one of the supervisors at lunch one day about an idea for improving admission procedures and why the nurse thought it would work. Both seemed interested, so the nurse asked them, "How can we try this out?" They suggested that the nurse ask to be included on the agenda for their next meeting and come to explain the idea to the group.

*The nurse asked the nurse manager and supervisor to help plan the presentation. They worked out the details of the plan with the assistance of one of the hospital's staff educators. At the meeting, the idea received sufficient support to try it out on several units to see whether it would work.*

The first nurse used only the formal channels of communication, and the idea moved along without attracting any support or having any impact. The nurse failed to observe how the informal level operated in the implementation of an idea or to attempt to interest people in the idea in order to gain some support.

In contrast, the second nurse had observed that many ideas came from the nurse managers and supervisors and that the particular ones the nurse had spoken to were often interested in new ideas. This is only the first phase in bringing about a change, but it is an important one. Without the use of the informal level of operation, it is likely that the second nurse's idea would also have been ignored.

The informal level of operations provides a lively and often efficient informal communication network commonly known as the **grapevine**. Although the grapevine is best known for spreading rumors, it is not always a negative force. The grapevine can provide employees with necessary information that the formal system is slow or neglectful about sharing with them. It is also useful as a way to test a new idea or change without having to go through the frequently cumbersome channels of the formal level.

Informal role expectations can be blended with formal ones so that people are not overly restricted by their job descriptions. This combination provides needed flexibility, but it can cause some confusion, especially for the new employee who does not yet understand the informal system. The informal level can provide support for people in an organization that fails to provide support on the formal level. However, when this support is extended to protecting or covering up for inept employees, it reduces the organization's effectiveness. Another way in which the informal level can reduce effectiveness is when employees informally agree to limit the amount of work they do and put pressure on their co-workers to do the same.

Incongruency between the informal and formal levels can lead to difficulties for those who do not understand the difference between the two levels. The following is an example:

*A community health agency officially prohibited payment for overtime, but staff members often had to stay late to finish their work. Informally, their supervisors allowed them to leave early when things were quiet or when they had an appointment in order to compensate for the extra time they had worked.*

*The director of the agency was aware of this informal procedure and tacitly allowed it to continue because it resulted in staff members feeling that they were being treated fairly. However, when a naive staff member went to the director to demand compensation time in the middle of a busy week, the staff member was told that the agency had no such policy as compensation time.*

This staff member made the mistake of trying to make use of informal procedure as if it were a formal agreement. As a result, no staff member was granted any compensation time until the formal and informal levels had been clearly differentiated again.

A conflict with the formal level in a critical area can sometimes lead to serious problems. The following is an example:

*Officially, nursing assistants are not allowed to give medications to patients, but occasionally, a busy nurse will informally ask a nursing assistant to take an oral medication to a waiting patient or to stay with the patient who takes a long time to swallow several pills.*

*One day, a nursing assistant gave a medication to the wrong patient, who experienced some serious side effects from the drug. As required, the incident was reported and both the nurse and the nursing assistant were fired for failing to obey the official rules.*

A sampling of the kinds of information you would seek in trying to understand the informal goals and level of operations in an organization (the "shadow organization") can be found in Box 17–1. As was illustrated in the examples, knowledge of the informal level of function can contribute considerably to your effectiveness within that organization.

**Box 17–1  Understanding the Shadow Organization: Some Questions You Can Ask to Reveal How It Operates**

- How much money is spent on decor, landscaping, public relations, and other amenities?
- Are employees expected to become involved in community activities? Is this involvement rewarded?
- Is socializing with coworkers encouraged or discouraged?
- Are ethnic or sexist jokes encouraged, tolerated, or frowned upon?
- What types of status symbols are evident? Do badges, uniforms, office furniture, titles, or special privileges indicate people's status in the organization?
- Who is most likely to receive a promotion or raise in pay? Is it people who have seniority, advanced preparation, excellent evaluations, or "connections" with people in powerful positions?
- Where do the most important discussions and decisions take place? Do they take place in formal meetings, informal situations, or in private meetings with administrators?
- Are any subjects "touchy" or taboo, such as unions, the work of a particular physician, or certain inadequacies in the operation of the organization?

*Source:* Adapted from Del Bueno, D.J. (1987). An organizational checklist. *Journal of Nursing Administration,* *17*(5), 30–33.

## Breaks in Communication

It is not unusual to find that communication does not flow as freely as it should from top to bottom or back again (Morgan, 1997). A break in communication between upper-level management and the rest of the organization on issues of importance can be a serious problem. Typically, miscommunication occurs when upper-level management shows some hesitation in trusting the rest of the staff with sensitive information. Lower-level employees are quick to sense this reluctance and, therefore, avoid discussing these issues with man-

agement. This failure to communicate is particularly unfortunate when they could help solve the problem. The following is an example:

*In a strategic planning session, the senior management team of a large suburban hospital struggled with a puzzling problem: the patient satisfaction index had dipped perceptibly for the third month in a row. As far as anyone on the senior team knew, nothing had changed. They reviewed some of their other quality indicators: infection rates were under control, staff vacancy rates were low, and mortality rates were quite low. Services were at the same level: maintenance was excellent, staff morale was good, and the dietary department was proud of the compliments received from patients about the meals. What was wrong? The team ended the meeting without a solution.*

*On the way back to her office, the chief nursing officer (CNO) met one of her best managers. "Ted, how are things going on your unit?"*

*"Oh just fine, Ms. Bailey."*

*"No new problems?"*

*"No, why do you ask?"*

*"Well, the patient satisfaction index is down across the whole hospital, and we're not sure why."*

*"Maybe it's because B.J. left," Ted answered.*

*"B.J.?"*

*"Yes, our ombudsman. He was so good. Patients loved him and the staff listened to him. He was a true diplomat."*

*"I think you may have solved the mystery, Ted. Thank you." Further investigation by the CNO confirmed Ted's hunch that the new ombudsman was not effective. If the senior management team had shared their concerns with first-level management, the problem would have been solved a lot earlier.*

## Relationship Games

Games are repetitive, unproductive patterns of relating to others. Like individual people, organizations also play games.

### *Paternalism*

Many organizations treat their employees as if they were children instead of mature adults. Unfortunately, this is likely to provoke childish behavior in return. An example is the use of an authoritarian style of decision making based on the assumption that managers know what is best for their employees and that employees are not capable of making wise decisions.

Paternalism can appear to be benevolent. For example, many organizations show interest and concern for what happens to their employees outside of working hours. When this commendable concern is extended in paternalistic fashion into telling or even requiring employees to conduct their lives in a certain way, it is no longer benevolent.

Paternalistic organizations are likely to give their employees turkeys on Thanksgiving or to hold expensive celebrations on such occasions as the anniversary of the organization. The paternalistic aspect of this behavior becomes more apparent when you realize that many employees would prefer to make their own decisions about how to spend the money that was used to hold these celebrations.

Organizational paternalism can become much more restrictive and suffocating. Ashley's (1976) history of hospitals' paternalistic treatment of nurses provides a good background for this more serious kind of paternalism:

> Until the 1950s, many hospitals employed only a limited number of graduate nurses and used student nurses for most of the hospital nursing staff positions. Nurses were poorly paid, poorly educated women who accepted society's definition of them as servants and physicians' helpers. For example, it was considered more important for nurses to get meals served while the gravy was still hot than for nurses to know anything about their patients' needs. Physicians continually exerted control over nurses and nursing education, denying their value at the same time that they depended on nurses to care for their patients 24 hours a day. Many of the nurses who held positions of authority in hospitals supported this status quo instead of fighting it, which reinforced the pattern of poor self-image and passivity that others have capitalized on since the 1900s.

Although much has changed since then, the approach of many healthcare organizations toward nurses is still paternalistic.

## Karpman Triangle

Another counterproductive game that service organizations play with both clients and employees is called the Karpman Triangle. It offers three different roles to choose from: victim, persecutor, or rescuer. Participants move from one role to another around the triangle to play this game. The following example shows how an organization can play these different roles in relation to clients:

> A health department decided to offer free immunizations to people who were going to travel in foreign countries, most of whom could afford to pay for this service (rescuer). When they were overwhelmed by the crowd of people appearing at their door for the first travelers' clinic, the health department announced that further clinics would be canceled, claiming that people who could really afford to pay for the service were taking advantage of the health department (persecutor).

Organizations also play these games with their employees, as in the following examples:

> An agency had harsh personnel policies, including the immediate dismissal of any employee caught taking home even a pencil (persecutor). When questioned about these extreme policies, a spokesperson for the agency said it was necessary because so many of its employees were not interested in the welfare of the organization (victim).
>
> Because of inadequate planning for summer vacations, a hospital suffered a serious shortage of maintenance workers and asked its maintenance workers to work two double shifts per week all summer to cover the shortage (victim). These employees had a union contract, so they were paid time and a half for the extra shifts. When this group was due for a salary increase in the fall, the hospital said it would not grant an increase because the maintenance workers had taken so much overtime all summer (persecutor).

As with paternalism, refusing to play any of these roles is one way to counteract this game. It is often necessary, however, to use change or power-based strategies to improve an organization's pattern of relationships with its employees.

## ● PATTERNS OF RELATIONSHIPS IN ORGANIZATIONS

### Distribution of Power and Authority

**Authority** is a specific type of power granted to certain individuals within an organization. In bureaucratic organizations it is specifically related to the person's position within the hierarchy. This power exists only because other people are willing to accept and obey the decisions made by the person who holds it (Merton, 1969).

**Responsibility** is an obligation that employees have to do their jobs well (i.e., to perform effectively). **Accountability** can be defined as answerability for completing one's assignment. Authority and responsibility can be delegated to people further down in the hierarchy but accountability rests with every employee. Kerzner (1998) suggests this formula to explain the relationship of authority, responsibility, and accountability in organizations:

Accountability = Authority + Responsibility

Why is this important? Healthcare professionals are expected to be accountable for their actions, yet in many organizations, particularly bureaucratic ones, managers are reluctant to grant them the authority they need to do their jobs well.

### Challenging the Traditional Distribution of Authority

Several approaches to redistributing power and authority within healthcare organizations have been developed.

One model is to **create a nursing staff similar to the medical staff** so that a hospital would have a board of trustees at the top and, immediately below the board, a board of medical examiners, a board of nursing governors, boards of other professions, and the hospital administration (Johnson et al., 1983). The board of nursing would handle such matters as credentials, standards, and cooperation between staff and private practitioners. This model promotes a proliferation of administrative-level personnel, which is inefficient and counter to the drive for cost containment. If not carefully designed, it may lead to problems similar to those caused by the separate medical staff.

Another model is **contracting for nursing services.** In this model, nurses take responsibility for scheduling and self-management, including peer review (Dear, Weisman & O'Keefe, 1985). This model supports primary care and the expansion of the nurse's role to include increased responsibility for discharge planning and follow-up after discharge.

**Shared governance** is a third model that is designed to transfer power and authority to the nursing staff rather than to nursing administration (Porter-O'Grady, 1992). A clinical rather than administrative base of organization is used. The congressional approach is the most sweeping change. Composed of the entire professional nursing staff, the congress develops bylaws, elects representatives, and forms committees for the purpose of governing the nursing staff. The committees are charged with responsibility for overseeing practice, quality improvement, education, staffing, research, and other professional issues (Anderson, 1992). Nursing staff need to be prepared for these new responsibilities (Jenkins & Ladewig, 1996) and implementation requires commitment of an enormous amount of time, energy, and support from administration. The outcomes, however, could be worth the effort in terms of staff improvement and organizational change.

> *Managers love empowerment in theory, but the command-and-control model is what they trust and know best.*
> —C. Argyris, 1998, p. 98

It is important to note that without a real transfer of power, any form of shared governance would be an empty exercise (Porter-O'Grady, 1992). Research Example 17–2, Innovative Models for Nursing Care, looks at the effects of these different models on job satisfaction, staff retention, and patient satisfaction.

## ● SUMMARY

Healthcare organizations vary in the type and comprehensiveness of services offered and populations served. They can be categorized as either

## Research Example 17–2    *Innovative Models for Nursing Care*

Are job satisfaction, staff retention, and patient satisfaction affected by the model of nursing care used? Weisman and associates (1993) reported the results of a study designed to test the effect of an innovative model of nursing practice at the Johns Hopkins Hospital in Baltimore, Maryland.

Eight patient care units that chose to adopt the professional practice model (PPM) were compared to eight units that retained their more traditional model of organization. The nursing staff of the units that chose the PPM contracted with the hospital to assume full responsibility for providing nursing care to the patients of that unit for the next year. Their responsibilities included the conduct of peer review, self-scheduling and staffing, maintenance of standards of care, salary agreements, and gainsharing. The comparison units used primary nursing without these additional elements of self-management (Gordon, 1993).

Questionnaires were distributed to 259 nurses on the eight experimental and eight comparison units. About 80 percent of the questionnaires were returned to the researchers for analysis.

No differences in patient satisfaction were found except that patients on the experimental units could name their nurse. Both pay and work satisfaction were found to increase retention, whereas longer hours reduced retention. Teamwork and the degree to which patient care was well coordinated within the nursing team and with the interdisciplinary team had a positive effect on staff nurses' work satisfaction. Surprisingly, neither increased autonomy nor increased decision-making authority contributed to work satisfaction. The researchers noted that staff nurses on the comparison "traditional" units had also been given some control over their schedules, so the differences may have been too small to have any effect on work satisfaction.

In their conclusion, the researchers pointed out that the emphasis on improving patient care through better coordination of all caregivers' efforts was consistent with the goals of total quality management.

---

*Sources:* Gordon, D.L. (1993). *Unit model for reorganizing hospital nursing resources.* Paper presented at the ANA Council of Nurse Researchers 1993 Scientific Session, Washington, D.C.; Weisman, C.S. et al. (1993). The effects of unit self-management on hospital nurses' work process, work satisfaction and retention. *Medical Care, 31*(5), 381–393.

---

not-for-profit (voluntary or publicly financed) or for-profit (proprietary).

Organizations are complex suprasystems made up of large numbers of people grouped in smaller systems and subsystems. Because of their size and complexity, they frequently have multiple purposes, goals, and functions. They also have identifiable characteristics and exhibit patterns of behavior such as growth, activity cycles, and interaction.

The characteristics of a traditional bureaucratically structured organization are hierarchy, division of labor, rules and regulations, and emphasis on technical competence. Alternate models utilize a more organic structure, which incorporates more flexibility, innovation, and team and project orientation.

The official goals of an organization are the stated goals. The operative goals are the unstated

ones that the organization is actually pursuing in its day-to-day operation. These goals are usually harder to identify and generally less idealistic. Financial gain, efficiency, quantity over quality, maintenance of a positive public image, and survival are common operative goals in healthcare organizations.

The informal level of operation is the unwritten, unofficial set of relationships, norms, and traditions that develop within an organization. They may complement and support the formal level, or they may be in conflict with it. It is important to know and use both levels of goals and operations in order to work effectively within an organization. Paternalism and the Karpman Triangle are unproductive relationship patterns often found in healthcare organizations. In paternalism, the organization acts as parent to the employee "children"; in the Karpman Triangle, the organization

# C A S E   S T U D Y

## A MISFIT?

Kelly Langford could not understand what had happened. For the second time, she had been passed over for promotion to nurse manager. Kelly had five years of experience on medical and surgical units, which was well over the three-year minimum for promotion in her hospital. She had excellent clinical skills, good evaluations, was rarely late or absent, and got along well with other staff members. She liked to joke around and would sometimes play harmless practical jokes on other staff members. She wore bright green on St. Patrick's Day and bunny ears during Easter week. "I'm really a frustrated clown," she would explain to people who remarked on her costumes.

Kelly worked in a small (150-bed) hospital located in a well-to-do suburb of a midwestern city. All patient rooms were private; the menu was a gourmet's delight, and room service was available around the clock. Soft music was piped into the rooms. Carpeted halls added to the hushed elegance of the facility.

Kelly took a few minutes in the staff lounge to compose herself after hearing that she had been denied a promotion again. "What's the matter, kid?" an older private duty nurse asked her on seeing Kelly's face.

Kelly explained the situation to her older colleague, ending with "I just don't understand! What did I do wrong?"

"You didn't do anything wrong. It's just who you are."

"What do you mean?"

"I've been here a long time. Seen it happen before to good people. You just don't fit the image of this snooty organization, kid," she explained. "You're a beer-and-pretzels gal in a champagne-and-caviar setting. Downtown, you'd be running the place now."

### Questions for Critical Reflection and Analysis

1. Do you agree with the private duty nurse's explanation of Kelly's situation? Why or why not?
2. Explain the "misfit" the private duty nurse saw between Kelly and the organization. What is operating here?
3. What actions could Kelly take to improve her chance of promotion to nurse manager at this hospital?
4. If you were Kelly, would you stay at this hospital or would you seek a position at the downtown hospital the private duty nurse mentioned? Explain your choice.

plays the roles of victim, rescuer, or persecutor. Upper-level management may also fail to share concerns with the rest of the organization.

Authority, which is derived from holding certain positions within the organizational structure, is generally greatest at the top of the hierarchy and lowest at the bottom. Confrontation and change strategies can be used to repattern these organizational behaviors.

Responsibility is the obligation to do one's job well; accountability is answerability for one's actions and/or inaction. Bureaucratic organizations typically withhold the authority employees need to fulfill their responsibilities. The tradi-

tional board, administration, and medical staff triad at the pinnacle of power and authority in healthcare organizations is under attack from several different directions. Different approaches to redistributing power and authority within organizations include creating a nursing staff similar to the medical staff, contracting nursing services, and implementation of a shared governance model.

## REFERENCES

Anderson, B. (1992). Voyage to shared governance. *Nursing Management, 23*(11), 65–67.

Argyris, C. (1998, May/June). Empowerment: The emperor's new clothes. *Harvard Business Review, 98,* 107.

Ashley, J. (1976). *Hospitals, paternalism and the role of the nurse.* New York: Teachers College Press.

Dear, M.R., Weisman, C.S. & O'Keefe, S. (1985). Evaluation of a contract model for professional nursing practice. *Health Care Management Review, 10,* 65–77.

DelBueno, D.J. (1987). An organizational checklist. *Journal of Nursing Administration, 17*(5), 30–33.

DHHS, NOISH. (1999). *Stress at work.* (DHHS Publication #99–101). Cincinnati, OH: Publication Dissemination, EID, National Institute for Occupational Safety & Health.

Eigen, L.D. & Siegel, J.P. (1989). *The manager's book of quotations.* New York: AMACOM.

Fleeger, M.E. (1993). Assessing organizational culture: A planning strategy. *Nursing Management, 24*(2), 39–41.

Gilmartin, M.J. (1998). The nursing organization and the transformation of health care delivery for the 21st century. *Nursing Administration Quarterly, 22*(2), 7–86.

Gordon, D.L. (1993). *Unit model for reorganizing hospital nursing resources.* Paper presented at the ANA Council of Nurse Researchers 1993 Scientific Session, Washington, D.C.

Greene, M. (1977). Self-consciousness in a technological world. In M.L. Fitzpatrick (Ed.). *Present realities/future imperatives in nursing education.* New York: Teachers College Press.

Hodgetts, R.M., Luthans, F. & Lee, S.M. (1994). New paradigm organizations: From total quality to learning to world class. *Organizational Dynamics, 22*(3), 5–13.

Huse, E.F. & Bowditch, J.L. (1977). *Behavior in organizations: A systems approach to managing.* Reading, MA: Addison-Wesley.

Jenkins, L.S. & Ladewig, N.E. (1996). A self-efficacy approach to nursing leadership for self-governance. *Nursing Leadership Forum, 2*(1), 26–30.

Johnson, L.M., Happel, J.R., Edelman, J. & Brown, S.J. (1983). Nursing Administration Quarterly forum. *Nursing Administration Quarterly, 8,* 30–46.

Kerzner, H. (1998). *Project management: A systems approach to planning, scheduling and controlling.* New York: Van Nostrand Reinhold.

Kolb, D.A., Osland, J.S. & Rubin, I.M. (1995). *Organizational behavior.* Englewood Cliffs, NJ: Prentice-Hall.

Lindquist, J.D. & Blackburn, R.T. (1974). Middlegrove: The locus of campus power. *American Association of University Professors, 60,* 367.

McClure, M. (1972). *The reasons for hospital staff nurse resignations.* Unpublished doctoral dissertation. New York: Teachers College, Columbia University.

Merton, R. (1969). The social nature of leadership. *American Journal of Nursing, 69,* 12.

Mintzberg, H. (1983). *Structure in fives: Designing effective organizations.* Englewood Cliffs, NJ: Prentice-Hall.

Morgan, A. (1997). *Imaginization: The art of creative management.* Newbury Park, CA: Sage.

Noyes, B.J. & Healy, S.A. (1999). The hospitalist: The new addition to the inpatient management team. *Journal of Nursing Administration, 29*(2), 21–24.

Perrow, C. (1969). The analysis of goals in complex organizations. In A. Etzioni (Ed.). *Readings on modern organizations.* Englewood Cliffs, NJ: Prentice-Hall.

Petzinger, T. (1999). *The new pioneers: The men and women who are transforming the workplace and marketplace.* New York: Simon & Schuster.

Porter-O'Grady, T. (1992). *Implementing shared governance: Creating a professional organization.* St. Louis: Mosby Year Book.

Purser, R.E. & Cabana, S. (1999). *The self-managing organization.* New York: The Free Press (Simon & Schuster, Inc.).

Reeves, P.N. (1993). Issues management: The other side of strategic planning. *Health and Health Services Administration, 38*(2).

Revans, R.W. (1972). Psychological factors in hospitals and nurse staffing. In E. Levine (Ed.). *Research on nurse staffing in hospitals.* Washington, DC: U.S. Department of Health, Education, and Welfare.

Rosenhan, D.L. (1973). On being sane in insane places. *Science, 179,* 250.

Schein, E. (1999). How to set the stage for a change in organizational culture. In P. Senge (Ed.). *The dance of change.* New York: Currency/Doubleday, 334–342.

Schellhard, T.D. (1998, November 23). An idyllic workplace under a tycoon's thumb. *Wall Street Journal,* B1, B4.

Schwartzman, H.B. (1993). *Ethnography in organizations.* Newbury Park, CA: Sage.

Senge, P., Kleiner, A., Roberts, C., Ross, R., Roth, G. & Smith, B. (1999). *The dance of change.* New York: Currency/Doubleday.

Weber, M. (1969). Bureaucratic organization. In A. Etzioni (Ed.). *Readings on modern organizations.* Englewood Cliffs, NJ: Prentice-Hall.

Weisman, C.S. et al. (1993). The effects of unit self-management on hospital nurses' work process, work satisfaction and retention. *Medical Care, 31*(5), 381–393.

Williams, S.J. & Ewell, C.M. (1996). Medical staff leadership: A national panel survey. *Health Care Management Review, 21*(2), 29–37.

Woerner, L. (1994). Business risk and the health entrepreneur. *Holistic Nursing Practice, 8*(2), 22–27.

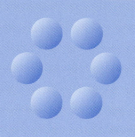

CHAPTER *18*

# Workplace Health and Safety

## LEARNING OBJECTIVES

*After completing this chapter, the reader will be able to:*

• Identify the most common risks to employee health and safety in healthcare settings.
• Suggest strategies for reducing health and safety risks in healthcare settings.
• Distinguish employee and employer responsibilities for workplace health and safety.

• Outline the process for designing risk reduction programs.
• Discuss redesign of the social and technical environment in healthcare organizations.

## TEST YOURSELF

*WHAT IS YOUR SAFETY IQ?*

**Mark each statement True or False. Then check the answers at the end of the quiz.**

_____ 1. In comparison to other workplaces, hospitals are safe places to work.

_____ 2. Pregnant employees are especially at risk from radiation exposure.

_____ 3. Healthcare and social service workers have a high rate of nonfatal injury from on-the-job assaults.

_____ 4. Too much noise, light, and caffeine can disrupt sleep patterns.

_____ 5. Sensitivity (allergy) to latex is a recognized risk for healthcare workers.

_____ 6. OSHA regulations are designed primarily to protect patients, not employees.

_____ 7. Impaired nurse programs help nurses with disabilities to find employment.

_____ 8. The harmful effects of work stress are highly overrated.

_____ 9. Sudden, unexplained increases in absence before and after days off or holidays may be a sign of a substance misuse problem.

_____ 10. Taking shortcuts and being too rushed often lead to injury on the job.

*Answers*

1. F  2. T  3. T  4. T  5. T  6. F  7. F  8. F  9. T  10. T

A considerable portion of our waking hours is spent in the workplace. For this reason alone, the quality of the workplace environment should be of interest to us all but it is still a low priority in many healthcare organizations. Administrators who would never allow peeling paint or poorly maintained equipment often are willing to leave their most costly and valuable resource, their employees, at risk. The "do more with less" thinking increases risks as nurses are pressed to work harder and faster than ever (ANA, 1997; Chisholm, 1992). Improvement of the workplace environment is difficult to accomplish under these circumstances but more important than ever.

Much of the responsibility for enhancing the workplace environment rests with upper-level management (administrators) who have the authority and resources to bring about organizationwide change. However, staff nurses and first-line managers can do a number of things to protect themselves and coworkers and foster a safer, healthier work environment.

## ● THREATS TO HEALTH AND SAFETY

A wide range of potential threats to the safety and well-being of healthcare workers exists, from exposure to potentially lethal chemical, infectious, and radioactive agents to the stress of job uncertainty (Hurrell, 1998). The following are examples:

- A survey of 1,450 Milwaukee nurses found that many of them had experienced physical or verbal abuse. Fifty-three percent of the nurses responding to the survey said that they had been hit, pushed, or had something thrown at them by patients. Another 6 percent said that they had had the same experience with physicians. Verbal abuse was even more common: 58 percent said that they had been verbally abused by patients, 51 percent by physicians, and 22 percent by their supervisors (AJN, 1993).
- Every year, somewhere between 150 and 200 healthcare workers in the United States die

from Hepatitis B infections acquired at work in spite of the fact that it is a preventable illness for which immunization is available (Henderson, 1997).

• Of the 51 documented cases of occupationally acquired HIV infection in the United States, 39 percent were traced back to one of the most common procedures done in healthcare, phlebotomy (Mendelson et al., 1997).

The degree of exposure to these and other risks varies considerably from one setting to another. Individual staff members may also differ considerably in their vulnerability: the pregnant staff member, for example, is more vulnerable to the risks from radiation. In general, however, all staff members need to be made aware of these risks and how to avoid them. First-line managers need to be proactive in taking steps to protect staff health and safety.

> **The costs of work-related illness, both in terms of human and economic loss, justify devoting substantial resources to understanding, preventing and controlling workplace exposures.**
> —Fay, 1997

Some of the most common threats to the health and safety of healthcare workers, particularly nurses, are described in the next section.

## Workplace Violence

Any verbal threat or physical attack that occurs in the course of one's employment falls under the category of workplace violence (Elliott, 1997). Intimidation, harassment, and other inappropriate behavior that threatens or frightens other people at work are included in this definition (Schneid, 1999). The Bureau of Labor statistics indicate that healthcare workers experience a surprisingly high rate of nonfatal assaults when compared to private industry: 38 cases per 10,000 employees in nursing and personal care facilities compared with three cases per 10,000 in industry. Particularly high risk areas in healthcare institutions are the emergency department, lobby, radiology, outpatient pharmacy, cafeteria,

substance abuse and psychiatric treatment areas, and the executive suite (Elliott, 1997).

What is it about healthcare settings that increases the risk of violence? Troubled people, distressed family members, public access, confined quarters, and frequent crises all contribute to the increased risk as does the increase in violence within the broader society. Specific factors include:

• 24-hour access to the building
• Availability of drugs
• More weapons in patients' possession
• Distraught family members
• Long waits
• Low staffing levels
• Restrictions on movement within the facility (Elliott, 1997)

In areas of high risk, staff should receive specific training in crisis intervention, verbal deescalation, limit setting, and handling people in possession of a weapon (see Box 18–1). They may also be taught secure holds, take downs, and carries. Additional preventive measures may include panic buttons and alarms and coding the records of patients who have a history of violent behavior to alert staff.

Employees also need to know how and when to report any violence-related incident (including threats), including how to call for assistance from security "code orange," for example, or the police (911), getting emergency treatment, and follow-up documentation. The aftereffects of an episode of violence go well beyond any physical injury that has occurred. Debriefing and counseling of everyone involved should be part of any plan to respond to workplace violence.

## Safety in Community Settings

Community-based nurses are also finding themselves confronted with drugs, weapons, and violence-prone individuals in the clinics, neighborhoods, and homes of their clients (Nadwairski, 1992). The following are some general suggestions for increasing personal safety in community and home care:

• Know where you are going before you start out; carry a detailed map.

## Box 18–1   Coping with Threats and Violence

**For an angry or hostile customer or coworker**

- Stay calm. Listen attentively.
- Maintain eye contact.
- Be courteous. Be patient.
- Keep the situation in your control.

**For a person shouting, swearing, and threatening**

- Signal a coworker or supervisor that you need help. (Use a duress alarm system or prearranged code words.)
- Do not make any calls yourself.
- Have someone call security or the local police.

**For someone threatening you with a gun, knife, or other weapon**

- Stay calm. Quietly signal for help. (Use a duress alarm or code words.)
- Maintain eye contact.
- Stall for time.
- Keep talking, but follow instructions from the person who has the weapon.
- Don't risk harm to yourself or others.
- Never try to grab a weapon.

**Telephoned threats**

- Keep calm. Keep talking.
- Don't hang up.
- Signal a coworker to get on an extension.
- Ask the caller to repeat the message and write it down.
- Repeat questions, if necessary.
- For a bomb threat, ask where the bomb is and when it is set to go off.
- Listen for background noises and write down a description.
- Write down whether it's a man or a woman, pitch of voice, accent, anything else you hear.
- Try to get the person's name, exact location, telephone number.
- Signal a coworker to immediately call security or the local police.
- Notify your immediate supervisor.

*Source:* Schneid, T.D. (1999). *Occupational health guide to violence in the workplace.* Boca Raton, FL. Lewis Publishers.

- Inform your client that you are coming and when to expect you.
- If you drive, keep your car in good mechanical condition and park as close as possible to your destination. Lock the car and do not leave any personal possessions within view.
- If you use public transportation, select a route that brings you as close as possible to your destination.
- When walking, keep to well-lit, busy streets, and avoid dark quiet side streets or alley ways.
- Carry a cellular phone to report emergencies or call for help.
- Do not carry a purse or medical bag.
- Arrange for a security escort in unsafe neighborhoods, especially at night.
- Do not raise your voice or turn your back on a threatening dog; instead back away slowly.

**Research Example 18–1**  *Substance Use and Nursing Specialty*

Do nurses in some specialties engage in more substance use than nurses in other specialties? It was the question researchers Trinkoff and Storr (1998) asked in their study of several thousand nurses in 10 states. Their sample of 4,438 nurses (a 78 percent response rate) was primarily female (96 percent) and white (94 percent). Most were married, and half had at least a bachelor's degree. Their average age was 44.

The substances under study included marijuana, cocaine, alcohol, cigarettes (at least half a pack daily), and psychoactive prescription drugs taken "on your own" (amphetamines, opiates, sedatives, or tranquilizers). Altogether, 32 percent of the sample had used one of the substances in the defined manner over the last year.

Although the rate of substance use was similar to the rate in the general population, the rates varied substantially by clinical specialty. Overall use of these substances was highest in oncology nurses (42 percent), psychiatric nurses (40 percent), and emergency and critical care nurses (both 38 percent).

Psychiatric nurses were most likely to smoke. Binge drinking was highest among oncology, emergency, and adult critical care nurses. Lower substance use was found in nurses in pediatrics and women's health. Some of this behavior was thought to be a coping mechanism related to the stresses of particular specialties. The subculture of the specialty and availability of drugs may also have played a part. It is interesting to note that these patterns of substance use are similar to the patterns found in physicians in parallel specialties.

*Source:* Trinkoff, A.M. & Storr, C.L. (1998). Substance use among nurses: Differences between specialties. *American Journal of Public Health, 88*(4), 581–585.

- Always knock, call out, or ring the doorbell before entering a home or apartment.
- If threatened, scream, kick, use a chemical spray or whistle.
- Look for slip, trip, spill, electrical, fire, and other physical hazards.
- Follow agency-recommended procedures for infection control and waste disposal in the home.
- Provide instructions to the patient, family, and other caregivers in infection control, safe lifting, fire prevention, and other safety concerns (Tweedy, 1997).

These sensible precautions are worth the time, effort, and expense in terms of increasing personal safety. They should not be ignored. When the risk of violence is high, community-based healthcare workers should receive the same training described in the previous section for institution-based employees and may, in some cases, need an escort for additional protection.

## Substance Misuse

While no evidence indicates that substance misuse is higher among nurses than it is in the general population, it nevertheless represents a potential danger in healthcare settings. When substance misuse affects the employee's ability to function, it becomes a threat to patients and a serious concern for employers. Estimates from the American Nurses Association are that 6–8 percent of nurses have a drug or alcohol problem (Trinkoff & Storr, 1998) (see Research Example 18–1, Substance Use and Nursing Speciality). Signs of substance misuse include the following:

- An increase in sick days, especially before and after weekends and days off
- Signs of increased tension, "nervousness," anxiety, or depression
- Frequent complaints of headaches, gastritis, or other malaise
- High injury, accident, and error rates
- High rate of reportable incidents
- Overreactions to criticism
- Withdrawn or overly talkative demeanor
- Missing drugs, unexplained shortfalls in drug inventories

It is most important that the problem of chemical impairment be confronted rather than ignored until it is so bad that a serious incident occurs, one that could harm staff or client. Often, the impaired individual is relieved that he or she no longer has to hide the problem and that support and understanding are offered. The staff member's colleagues may be relieved that they no longer have to cover for the impaired person. Many states have developed impaired nurse programs that offer guidelines for employers and treatment to the impaired person. International Nurses Anonymous is an organization that provides an opportunity to network with other recovering nurses (Loyd, 1997).

## Job-Related Stress

Job-related stress is broadly defined by the National Institute for Occupational Safety and Health (NIOSH) as the "harmful physical and emotional responses that occur when the requirements of the job do not match the capabilities, resources, or needs of the worker" (1999, p. 6). Being **challenged** by our work is energizing. It motivates us to work harder and to learn new skills. When we accomplish something new or complete a difficult task successfully, we usually feel satisfied. Being **stressed,** as defined by NIOSH, can lead to illness and injury. Common adverse outcomes of job-related stress are cardiovascular disease (hypertension, for example), musculoskeletal disorders (carpal tunnel syndrome, low back pain, for example), depression, burnout, cancer, ulcers, impaired immune function, and suicide (Wells, 1998). Some of the circumstances that contribute to job-related stress and ultimately to these adverse outcomes are listed in Box 18–2.

A stress-free work environment is probably impossible to achieve. Intermittent stress at tolerable levels is usually not harmful to a healthy individual. But when high levels of stress become continuous, it places the individual in a constant state of arousal (preparation for fight or flight). Eventually, the body's ability to respond to and defend itself in the face of stress is exhausted and the risk of illness or injury escalates rapidly (DHHS, NIOSH, 1999).

In health care, life-or-death situations are faced constantly. Shift work, overtime, distraught families, staff shortages, and pressure to do more with less contribute to the stresses placed on nurses. Exposure to biological and chemical hazards, po-

tentially violent patients or families, and overburdened coworkers add to the risk for stress-related illness or injury (Gold et al., 1992; Tweedy, 1997; ANA, 1999).

Warning signs that job-related stress may be reaching critical levels for an individual include the following:

- Chronic headache
- Insomnia
- Difficulty concentrating
- Short temper
- Gastrointestinal upsets
- Mood changes
- Relationship difficulties

Increased absence, tardiness and resignations are additional signs that stress is escalating in a team, unit staff or even throughout the organization.

Of the two fundamental approaches to reducing the harmful effects of job-related stress, the first places most of the **responsibility on the employee.** It is probably the most common approach. It includes teaching employees about stress management techniques using sessions about sources of stress and stress reduction; time management strategies; relaxation/meditation; improved diet; exercise; reducing caffeine, alcohol, and other substance use; relationship-building and leadership skills; and job-related skills. Many organizations also have employee assistance programs (EAPs) that offer confidential counseling.

Stress reduction and stress management strategies have some limitations. One is that the benefits may be short-lived. Symptoms often return, sometimes with a vengeance. More important, however, is the fact that stress management often does not deal with the primary cause of the stress, particularly when it lies outside the individual. For this reason, the second approach, **organizational change,** is often indicated. The changes are targeted at improving working conditions, thereby relieving the stress on individual employees. The following are a few examples of the kind of organizational changes that can reduce work-related emotional stress:

- Reduce employee career uncertainty (job security) (Ferrie et al., 1998).
- Clearly define employees' responsibilities.

**Box 18–2    Job Conditions That May Lead to Stress**

**The Design of Tasks.** Heavy workload, infrequent rest breaks, long work hours and shift work; hectic and routine tasks that have little inherent meaning, do not utilize workers' skills, and provide little sense of control.

*Example:* David in physical plant works to the point of exhaustion. Theresa is a unit secretary tied to the computer, allowing little room for flexibility, self-initiative, or rest.

**Management Style.** Lack of participation by workers in decision making, poor communication in the organization, lack of family-friendly policies.

*Example:* Theresa needs to get the boss's approval for everything, and her boss is insensitive to her family needs.

**Interpersonal Relationships.** Poor social environment and lack of support or help from coworkers and supervisors.

*Example:* Theresa's physical location reduces her opportunities to interact with other unit secretaries or receive help from them.

**Work Roles.** Conflicting or uncertain job expectations, too much responsibility, too many "hats to wear."

*Example:* Theresa is often caught in a difficult situation trying to satisfy both the patients' needs and the organization's expectations.

**Career Concerns.** Job insecurity and lack of opportunity for growth, advancement, or promotion; rapid changes for which workers are unprepared.

*Example:* Since the reorganization at David's hospital, everyone is worried about their future and what will happen next.

**Environmental Conditions.** Unpleasant or dangerous physical conditions such as crowding, noise, air pollution, or ergonomic problems.

*Example:* David is exposed to constant noise at work in the physical plant department.

*Source:* DHHS, NIOSH. (1999). Stress at work. (DHHS Publication #99-101). Cincinnati, OH: Publications Dissemination, EID.

- Keep communication channels open and do not punish "whistle blowers."
- Keep individual workloads reasonable.
- Establish people-friendly, family-friendly work schedules and leaves of absence.
- Design jobs to provide opportunities for individual development and promotion.
- Encourage collegiality.
- Recognize and reward good work performance.
- Develop and nurture an organizational culture that values individual employees.

The value of these actions is obvious from a humanistic viewpoint. In fact, they really encompass many of the principles of effective leadership and management.

Are these changes also cost effective? You might not think so, but NIOSH points out that several research studies indicate they are cost effective. For example, one 700-bed hospital reduced medication errors 50 percent after introducing stress prevention activities. In a larger study, 22 hospitals that implemented stress prevention programs reduced the number of malpractice claims (lawsuits) filed against them by 70 percent, while 22 comparison institutions saw no reduction in the number of malpractice claims filed against them (DHHS, NIOSH, 1999). Reductions in absenteeism substantial enough to produce positive financial returns have also been achieved (Maes, Verhoeven, Kittel & Scholten, 1998). It would appear that organizational change focused on reducing job-related stress can benefit both employer and employees.

## Infectious Hazards

Bacteria, viruses, fungi, and other organisms can cause acute and chronic infections, some of them debilitating, even life threatening. Any job that exposes healthcare workers to bodily fluids, wastes, or secretions poses a risk for infection. Laboratory, clerical, and maintenance workers as well as direct care staff are at risk. Bloodborne and airborne infections are of particular concern.

Accidental needlesticks expose healthcare workers to more than 20 different bloodborne infections including HIV and hepatitis B and C. An estimated one million accidental needlesticks occur every year in health care. Of these, 18,000 will sero convert and more than 100 will die from the consequences of them every year (Algie, 1997).

> *I've been stuck. I re-live it each time I counsel. You grieve and feel anger and denial. You feel like life has ended.*
> —E. Murray in Algie, 1997, p. 10

Many of these accidental needlesticks are preventable. Safety devices such as needleless and automatically retractable systems can prevent many of these accidents (Mendelson et al., 1997). Yet many healthcare organizations have been slow to adapt them, primarily due to their concerns about cost (*Wall Street Journal*, 1999).

> *The American Hospital Association encourages use of safer needles, but "you can't just throw a switch," says Dr. Jack Lord, chief operating officer.*
> —quoted in the Wall Street Journal, *1999*

A number of other preventive measures should also be taken:

- Hepatitis B vaccination of employees (employers are required to offer this free of charge)
- Personal protective equipment including protective clothing, gloves, masks, and so forth must be supplied to employees
- Proper handling of contaminated wastes and cleaning of work surfaces and reusable items

- Labeling of biohazardous materials
- Implementation of engineering controls (procedures for reducing exposure) and work practice controls (safe work methods)
- Adherence to universal precautions under which blood and certain other body fluids are treated as if known to be infectious (OSHA, 1998a)

All employees need to be well trained and have access to the most current information regarding infection control. Most important, of course, is that this information be put into practice.

If an accidental needlestick or other exposure does occur, the employee should be offered postexposure diagnostic evaluation, prophylaxis/therapy, and follow-up care (Henderson, 1997). The incident should be thoroughly documented. The patient's blood should be tested if possible, and counseling should be made available to the employee. If illness results, the employee would be eligible for treatment, follow-up care, and compensation. Workers' compensation provides workers with a percentage of their usual salary and payment for healthcare costs if they are injured on the job. Benefits are not dependent on employer fault and are not endangered by employee negligence (Schneid, 1999).

## Allergy and Hypersensitivity

Frequent prolonged contact with latex has increased among healthcare workers since the introduction of universal precautions. With it has come an increased incidence of sensitivity to natural rubber latex, which is found in as many as 40,000 products, many used in healthcare. It is estimated that 8 percent to 12 percent of all healthcare workers are sensitive to latex (Gritter, 1998).

Sensitization to latex is progressive. For some, it can lead to asthma and life-threatening anaphylactic reactions. Early recognition of the problem and avoidance of the substance is essential for those who are sensitive. To avoid latex products, however, the employer must supply alternative products not only for the sensitive person but also for the individual's coworkers. Use of low-allergen, powder-free gloves, in particular, is necessary because latex-laden powder is released into the air when gloves are put on or removed; subsequent inhalation of the powder is virtually unavoidable.

> *Given the poor understanding many nurses have of latex allergy, many may not even realize they are becoming sensitized.*
> —ANA, 1999, p. 12

In some instances, opposition to this remedy from manufacturers of powdered latex gloves has been fierce (Toland, 1997). Nursing organizations have been fighting for supportive legislation, and NIOSH has released alerts on the subject, but some nurses have been hesitant to admit to their allergies for fear of losing their jobs (McAndrew, 1999).

> *These are your peers who bring their own non-latex gloves to work, who cough, sneeze, and have red eyes while doing patient care. . . . frequently taking antihistamines and using inhalers to work. . . . The vow of silence compromises one's health, and perhaps ultimately, a life or career.*
> —McAndrew, 1999, p. 7

Prolonged exposure to chemical-filled surgical smoke (Sloane & Holcomb, 1997), anesthetic gases, disinfectants, cleaning agents, detergents, solvents, and other substances commonly found in healthcare environments can also sensitize employees (Fay, 1997). Many are toxic; some are potentially carcinogenic as well. More effective surveillance (collecting, analyzing, and disseminating information about the risks present in the workplace) and identification of those who have already become sensitized is still needed. In the meantime, sensitized individuals need diagnostic evaluation and follow-up treatment. Efforts should also be made to reduce or eliminate future exposure for them (Fay, 1997).

Smoking by employees is another potential health hazard. Tobacco smoke poses a risk to people sharing space with a smoker. For additional discussion of this hazard, see Perspectives . . . Smoking at Work: Whose Rights Should Prevail?

## PERSPECTIVES . . .

### Smoking at Work: Whose Rights Should Prevail?

In an editorial in the *American Journal of Public Health,* Lester Breslow and Robert Elashoff (1998) discuss some of the issues related to smoking in the workplace.

Is there any risk in working alongside people who smoke? "Side-stream" or environmental tobacco smoke amounts to passive smoking and is a risk to one's health. Yet the editors note five reviews of studies on the risks of environmental tobacco smoke that concluded no relationship existed between workplace exposure and lung cancer (Wells, 1998). How could this be? Those five reviews were done by consultants to or employees of the tobacco industry. Breslow and Elashoff suggest that they may have been done "as part of the lawyer-directed research sponsored by tobacco companies in order to counter the accelerating moves toward tobacco use control" (pp. 1011–1012).

Do people have a right to smoke at work? Individual rights, especially the right to individual liberty, is a cherished tradition in the United States. The opposing value is to protect the common good, in this case the health of those sharing the space of the would-be smoker. Whose rights should prevail? These authors believe the risk from passive smoking justifies a ban on smoking in the work environment, declaring that "those of us [who are] concerned with health must insist on preserving the common good and oppose any danger to the health of others created by individual actions" (p. 1012).

Do you agree with their strong statement on the right to protection from risk to one's health? Can you think of situations where this right is not protected?

*Sources:* Breslow, L. & Elashoff, R. (1998). Editorial: Significance of workplace smoking. *American Journal of Public Health, 88*(7), 1011–1012; Wells, A.J. (1998). Lung cancer from passive smoking. *American Journal of Public Health, 88*(7), 1025–1029.

## Injury

Back injuries are the most common physical injury incurred by nursing staff. Most occur during patient transfers, a frequent event when providing nursing care (Rogers, 1997). Nursing aides and LPNs have more than twice the back injury rate of other female workers (Denton, 1997). Risk factors for back injury include:

- Incorrect technique
- Poorly designed or broken equipment
- Inadequate and/or insufficient equipment (lifts and assistive devices especially)
- Lack of help from coworkers, often related to poor staffing (Rogers, 1997)

Similar factors contribute to the occurrence of other injuries in healthcare environments. The following is a list of common risk factors for injury on the job (Tweedy, 1997):

- **Inadequate Supervision:**
  *Poor training/instructions*
  *Rushing or overloading employees*
  *Failure to provide needed equipment, supplies*
- **Employee Error:**
  *Taking shortcuts*
  *Disregarding instructions*
  *Inexperience*
  *Inattention*
- **Unsafe Equipment:**
  *Broken, poorly repaired*
  *Inappropriate for the job*
  *Poor design*
- **Unsafe Working Conditions:**
  *Poor lighting, ventilation*
  *Crowded, cluttered work areas*
  *Poor housekeeping*
  *Slippery floors*

Clearly, both employee and employer have some responsibility in preventing accidents and the injuries that result. In the next section, efforts to make the workplace environment a safer and healthier place to work will be discussed.

## ● ENHANCING THE QUALITY OF WORK LIFE

### Programs to Reduce Risk

The primary objectives of any workplace health and safety program are to keep employees well and protect them from harm and to protect the organization from liability related to that harm.

Essential elements of an effective program include the following:

- Management commitment to employee health and safety
- Comprehensive worksite risk analyses
- Employee participation in the program
- Effective hazard prevention and control
- Safety and health training (OSHA, 1998b)

The first step in the development of a workplace health and safety program is for management of the organization to **recognize** potential hazards. A considerable amount of information about such hazards is available from state and federal agencies. Many of these agencies also enforce regulations concerning employee health and safety. The Occupational Safety and Health Act of 1970 covers any workplace in the United States that has at least one employee and is in some way involved in interstate commerce. Government employees and domestic workers are not covered by this law. The purpose of the act was to provide employees with a workplace environment free of hazards likely to cause serious harm or death. In effect, employers "were placed on notice that unsafe and unhealthful conditions/acts would no longer be permitted to endanger the health . . . of American workers" (Schneid, 1999, p. 39). Federal agencies involved in some way in employee health or safety protection include:

OSHA:  Occupational Safety and Health Administration

EPA:  Environmental Protection Agency

FDA:  Food and Drug Administration

CDC:  Centers for Disease Control and Prevention

Failure to comply with their standards can be costly to employers (Schneid, 1999).

The Joint Commission on Accreditation of Healthcare Organizations (JCAHO) incorporates the standards of these agencies and others, such as fire codes, into the accreditation process (Tweedy, 1997). Professional organizations such as the American Nurses Association are also concerned about employee health and safety, as are unions that represent the employees. In many cases, initial warnings about hazards come from these organizations.

The second step in the development of a workplace safety program is a **thorough assessment** of the degree of risk entailed. Staff members have a right to be informed of any potential health hazards in their place of employment and to be provided with as much protection from these hazards as possible. This assessment may require considerable data gathering to document the incidence of the problem and consultation with experts before a plan of action is drawn up. Healthcare organizations often create formal committees composed of experts from within the institution and representatives from departments affected to identify potential risks, assess these risks, draw up a plan, and put the plan into action.

The third step is the **development of a plan** to provide optimal protection for staff. Staff may become fearful in situations that do not warrant such fear or they may be complacent about such risks as tuberculosis or radiation, which cannot be seen or felt as one works with patients. It is not always a simple matter to protect staff without interfering with the provision of patient care. For example, some devices that can be worn to prevent transmission of tuberculosis interfere with communication with the patient (TNH, 1993). Also, some attempts to limit visits or withdraw visiting nurses from high-crime areas have left homebound patients without care (Nadwairski, 1992). Some actions taken to reduce staff injuries from violent behavior may affect the therapeutic nature of staff-patient relationships.

The following are some actions to be considered in the development of a workplace health and safety plan:

- Develop a written policy to protect personnel and maintain patient care standards.
- Refer to federal, state, and local regulations in development of the plan.
- Inform staff of the potential risks.
- Educate staff about safe procedures.
- Provide the necessary supplies and devices to protect staff and patients.
- Modify the environment to protect staff and patients.
- Provide administrative support and enforcement of the developed policies.

- Monitor adherence to control and safety procedures.
- Protect patient and staff confidentiality.
- Calculate the costs of the program.
- Evaluate the effectiveness of the program and modify as needed (CDC, 1992; Jankowski, 1992; TNH, 1993).

Unfortunately, hospitals and other healthcare organizations have not been in the forefront in protecting staff from health and safety hazards in the work environment. In order to promote these changes, reference to regulations, to liability for sick or injured employees, union support, and concerted effort on the part of nursing leaders and managers may be needed. Some of these tactics are described in Chapter 21 on power, empowerment, and political influence.

It is not just the physical environment that affects employee health. The social environment is considered next.

## The Social Environment

### Working Relationships

The social environment within which people work can also be either deleterious or beneficial to their health. We consider working relationships and professional growth in this section. Team building, effective communication, and development of leadership skills, all discussed earlier, are also essential to the development of effective working relationships.

### A Supportive Environment

The difference between a supportive environment and nonsupportive environment is keenly felt by most employees:

*Ms. B. came to work already tired. Her baby was sick and had been awake most of the night. Her team expressed concern about the baby when she told them she had had a difficult night. Each team member voluntarily took an extra patient so that Ms. B. could have a lighter assignment that day. When Ms. B. expressed her appreciation, her team leader said, "We know you would do the same for us." Ms. B. worked in a supportive environment.*

*Ms. G. came to work after a sleepless night. Her young son had been diagnosed with leukemia and she was very worried about him. When she mentioned her concerns, her team leader interrupted her saying, "Please leave your personal problems at home. We have a lot of work to do and expect you to do your share." Ms. G. worked in a nonsupportive environment.*

Support from peers and supervisors involves professional concerns as well as personal ones. In a supportive environment, people are willing to make decisions, take risks, and "go the extra mile" for team members and the organization. In contrast, in a nonsupportive environment, they are afraid to take risks, will avoid making decisions, and usually limit their commitment.

## Involvement in Decision Making

The importance of having a voice in decisions made about one's work and one's patients cannot be overstated. **Empowerment** is the antithesis of apathy and powerlessness. A number of actions can be taken to empower nurses: remove barriers to their autonomy and participation in decision making, publicly express confidence in their capability and value, reward initiative and assertiveness, and provide role models who demonstrate confidence in their efficacy and capability. The following illustrate the difference between empowerment and powerlessness:

*Soon after completing orientation, Nurse A heard a new nurse aide scolding a patient for soiling the bed. Nurse A did not know how incidents of potential verbal abuse were handled in this institution, so Nurse A reported it to the nurse manager. The nurse manager asked Nurse A a few questions and thanked her for the information. The new aide was counseled immediately after their meeting. Nurse A noticed a positive change in the aide's manner with patients after this incident. Nurse A felt good about having contributed to a more effective patient care team. Nurse A felt empowered and will be willing to take action again when another occasion arises.*

*A colleague of Nurse B was an instructor at a nearby community college. This colleague asked Nurse B if students would be welcome*

*on her unit. "Of course," replied Nurse B. "I'll speak with my nurse manager about it." When Nurse B spoke with her nurse manager, the response was that the unit was too busy to accommodate students. In addition, Nurse B received a verbal reprimand from the supervisor for overstepping her authority by discussing the placement of students. "All requests for student placement must be directed to the education department," she said. The supervisor directed Nurse B to write a letter of apology for having made an unauthorized commitment to the community college. Nurse B was afraid to make any decisions or public statements after this incident. Nurse B felt alienated and powerless.*

## Professional Growth and Innovation

The difference between a climate that encourages staff development and one that does not can be quite subtle. Many people are only vaguely aware of whether they work in an environment that fosters professional growth and learning. Yet the effect on the quality of the work done is pervasive and it is an important factor in distinguishing the merely good healthcare organization from the excellent healthcare organization.

Much of the responsibility for staff development and promotion of innovation lies with upper-level management people who can sponsor seminars, conduct organizationwide workshops, establish educational policies, promote career mobility, develop clinical ladders, initiate innovative projects, and reward innovative suggestions.

Some of the ways in which the first-line manager can develop and support a climate of professional growth are to encourage critical thinking, provide opportunities to take advantage of educational programs, encourage new ideas and projects, and reward professional growth.

## Encouragement of Critical Thinking

If you ever find yourself or other staff members saying, "Don't ask why, just go ahead and do it," you need to evaluate the type of climate in which your staff is functioning. An inquisitive frame of mind is relatively easy to suppress in a work environment. Staff members quickly perceive a team leader's or manager's impatience or defensiveness when too many questions are raised. Their response will be to simply stop asking these questions.

On the other hand, if you encourage the critical thinker and act as a role model who adopts a questioning attitude, you can encourage others to do the same. Interest and curiosity are intrinsic. The manager's responsibility is to stimulate and reward their occurrence.

### Supporting Education

Team leaders and first-line managers can make it either easier or more difficult for staff members to further their education. They can make it easier by being flexible in scheduling and allowing an occasional day off to finish a paper or study for an examination. They can be supportive, and they can include the pursuit of further education in performance appraisal reports. Or they can make things difficult for the staff member who is trying to balance work, home, and school responsibilities. Unsupportive supervisors have been known to attack staff members who pursue further education, criticizing every minor error and blocking their advancement. Obviously, such behavior should be dealt with quickly by upper-level management because it is a serious inhibitor of staff development.

### Creativity and New Ideas

Intellectual curiosity is a hallmark of the professional. In addition, the increasingly rapid accumulation of knowledge in the healthcare field mandates continuous learning for safe practice.

The first-line manager can do much to create an environment in which every staff member is both intellectually challenged and rewarded for meeting these challenges. Informal or formal brainstorming, nominal group technique, synectics, problem-solving conferences, and problem discussions all encourage the generation of new ideas.

The first-line manager can also encourage staff to develop and implement new projects to improve patient care services or the management of the unit. New ideas need to be nurtured. The team leader or manager can ensure that they at least get a fair amount of consideration even if some cannot be implemented. The success of one new idea can have a synergistic effect, encouraging the generation and testing of many more ideas.

### Reward for Professional Growth

Specific mention of innovative suggestions and active involvement in continuing education should be a part of every professional employee's performance appraisal. Some organizations have special incentive programs in which they reward innovative or cost-saving suggestions.

The intangible rewards of positive feedback and widespread recognition of a staff member's contribution are effective in encouraging pursuit of professional growth and change.

## Technical Environment

This aspect of workplace improvement is not as well developed as the social aspect, especially in nursing. However, with the pressure to increase efficiency, we are seeing more attention directed to this facet of work.

### Job Redesign

Job redesign or reengineering is an exciting concept that has been receiving increased attention. The traditional nursing unit was really designed to provide a convenient workshop for the physician. Even today, patients are assigned to units primarily on the basis of their medical diagnoses and only secondarily on the basis of their nursing care needs. Also, despite much tinkering, virtually the same structure is used for all units within an organization, regardless of patient characteristics or staffing needs.

The pressure for redesign comes from the need to provide more effective care for more people with reduced resources. It also comes from increasing recognition that we have not been flexible or creative enough in our thinking about these designs. Two examples of some more flexible and creative designs are the following:

*Example 1:* *A quality improvement survey noted that efforts to encourage early discharge of stroke patients were being thwarted by the traditional ways in which physical therapy, occupational therapy, and assistive devices were ordered. The orders had to be written in the chart before anything could be done and only physicians were allowed to write these orders. However, the physicians frequently forgot to do it and often were not the first caregivers to recognize a patient's readiness for these services.*

*The unit's interdisciplinary team suggested a different approach. At the discretion of the patient's primary nurse or the interdisciplinary team, physical therapy and occupational therapy could be requested by a telephone call to the respective department. Customized wheelchairs and assistive devices could be obtained in the same manner well in advance of discharge so that patients could practice with their own equipment. Despite administrative concerns that this option would lead to enormous cost increases, cost was actually decreased because patients left an average of two to three days earlier and were more independent at discharge. At the time that they made this change, the team thought it was revolutionary. Now, when they hear of other institutions not using this format, they are amazed that anyone would want to make it so difficult to accomplish a simple goal.*

***Example 2:*** *A survey at another hospital revealed that a simple chest X ray required 45 steps and involved 10 staff members, taking a total of 87 minutes, only 13 of which were spent with the patient. They also found that they had 558 job classifications with an average of only 6.2 people in each category. Clearly, care was fragmented, in part because it was organized around specialized services, not around the patient. The workflow was redesigned by a multidisciplinary committee to put the patient in the center and bring services to the patient rather than the other way around. Services such as X ray, pharmacy, electrocardiography, and laboratory work were brought to the unit. Radiology and respiratory technicians were assigned to nursing units (Pillar & Jarjoura, 1999). Caregivers were cross-trained (taught each other's jobs) to increase flexibility and the unit was renovated. Three nurses' substations replaced the central one, a movable supply cart was purchased, and nurse servers (containing dressings and other supplies) were installed in patient rooms. Unit personnel were reduced to five clas-*

*sifications: unit representative (information processing), unit support assistant (transport, cleaning, supply ordering), team care specialist (bedside caregiver), pharmacist, and clinical manager (a nurse with managerial experience). The new unit was designed to reduce complexity and inefficiency and increase continuity and time spent on direct care (Farris, 1993).*

An additional example of extensive reengineering can be found in Perspectives . . . A Case Study in Reengineering the OR.

The blurring of the lines between different professions in the second example may be reason for some concern. However, the innovative nature of the work redesign should stimulate even more creative ways to provide patient care. These innovations would not have occurred in organizations lacking a climate conducive to change. In fact, Flarey and Smith (1999) have said that radical change is inherent in reengineering. As with any change initiative, open communication and trustworthy leadership are essential to support the risk taking and creativity needed to successfully reengineer the way in which care is provided in most organizations.

## Physical Environment

Reduced steps, easier visual and auditory scanning of patients from the nurses station, better light and ventilation, unified information systems, automated drug dispensing, and reduced need for patient transport are all possible with changes in the physical environment. Several changes were mentioned in the previous example: relocation of supplies closer to patient rooms to reduce time to obtain them and substations closer to patient rooms to reduce steps.

Comfort, safety, and efficiency can be improved with changes in the physical environment. Pediatric units can have specially designed play areas for children with different types of problems, places for parents to sleep and shower when they stay overnight with their children, and provision for families to have a meal together. Nurses are increasingly being consulted about physical design *before* construction begins. Patient units can be made easier to clean, safer for patients with a high fall risk, easier to navigate for those with cognitive or physi-

## A Case Study in Reengineering the OR

Can reengineering save money and increase staff satisfaction? In this case, it did. The reeingineering project described by Moss (1999) occurred across the 30 surgical suites of a 950-bed healthcare facility in the United States.

When the project began, the organization functioned in the manner of a traditional bureaucracy, one that had ossified over time. A question from staff about policies or procedures "would take a long and slow trip up the administrative ladder" (p. 232) and back down again to the staff person. Nurses were mopping floors and answering telephones instead of engaging in clinical practice. The inventory of supplies was unnecessarily large and difficult to monitor. Staff turnover was an astonishing 38 percent. In all, operation of the 30 surgical suites was inefficient, unwieldy, and dissatisfying to staff.

In the process of reengineering, the number of levels of management in the OR was reduced from five to two (just vice-president and nurse manager). Teams were charged with solving their own problems. Managers were expected to function as "servant leaders" who really listen to the people they lead in order to learn about the stumbling blocks in the way of their performance. Sweeping changes in operation were made. The following are some examples:

- Just-in-time (JIT) inventory maintenance was implemented so supplies were delivered daily instead of weekly.
- "Mother's Hours" from 9:00 A.M. to 2:00 P.M. were instituted for nurses with school-aged children.
- Charting and patient charges were done by exception.
- A colleague of the month award was instituted, and included the physicians.
- The CEO of the facility was persuaded to spend $500,000 for additional surgical instruments to reduce waiting time between cases.

The results are impressive. Staff turnover dropped to 2 percent. The time between cases dropped from a range of 110–300 minutes to an average of 34 minutes. The overall profitability of the OR was increased by trimming expenses and improving its reputation. In this case, reengineering did save money and increase staff satisfaction.

*Source:* Moss, M.T. (1999). Creating a process-oriented organization. In S.P. Smith & D.L. Flarey (Eds.). Process-centered health care organization. Gaithersburg, MD: Aspen, 223–241.

cal disabilities, and more pleasant to stay in or to visit.

## ● SUMMARY

Workplace safety in healthcare organizations is a subject of increasing concern. Staff have a right to be informed of any potential risks in the workplace and a responsibility to follow guidelines designed to reduce risk and prevent harm. Employers have a responsibility to provide adequate programs and policies to minimize risk to the extent possible.

Among a number of concerns for employee health and safety in healthcare organizations, the most important are workplace violence, safety in community settings, substance misuse, job-related stress, infectious disease, allergy and hypersensitivity, and physical injury. The relative risk varies by setting and vulnerability of the individual employee. Factors that increase risk and specific suggestions for reducing the risk for each of these concerns were discussed.

Risk reduction programs not only protect employees but also reduce employer liability. Essential to their development are the recognition of potential hazards, an assessment of the type and degree of risk involved, development of a workplace health and safety plan, and implementation of the plan. As with other plans, its effectiveness should be monitored and modifications made as necessary.

Two additional aspects of the workplace to consider in improving the quality of work life are the social environment, especially working relationships and a climate for professional growth and for innovation, and the technical environment, especially work redesign and modification of the physical environment.

# CASE STUDY

## Do We Need Infection Control?

After graduation, JoEllen Diaz worked in a big city hospital on several different services, finally finding her niche on an infectious disease unit. The challenge of fighting a range of virulent, highly contagious infections in an age of increased resistance was one she relished. She often thought of returning to school for an advanced degree in infection control.

A change in family circumstances led to a move to a rural county. Somewhat reluctantly, JoEllen accepted the only open position she could find near home, as director of a small residential facility. Most of the residents were old and frail but some were younger adults with a history of psychiatric or substance abuse problems.

After settling in, JoEllen asked to see the infection control plan. She was appalled by the limited information available at the facility. "We need to have someone responsible for infection control here," she told the owner of the facility.

"Why?" he asked.

"It's for everyone's protection," she began to explain.

"You're just going to make more work for everyone," he groused.

"Not at all. We don't even know if one our residents has an infectious disease."

"What kind of infectious diseases?"

"Well, tuberculosis, hepatitis, HIV infection . . ."

"Old people don't get AIDS!" he exclaimed.

"Yes, they can and we need an infection control program to protect both staff and patients. In fact, I think we need to look at all of the health and safety risks and develop a comprehensive program."

## Questions for Critical Reflection and Analysis

1. How would you suggest JoEllen go about establishing a comprehensive health and safety program in this small facility?
2. What kinds of health and safety concerns do you think would be most common in a small, rural residential facility with a mixed population such as the one in the case study?
3. What types of resistance do you think JoEllen might encounter? Where do you think she would find support for her proposed program? Suggest strategies for overcoming the sources of resistance. What should she do first?
4. Once the plan is complete, can JoEllen be certain that the health and safety of the residents and employees are protected? Why or why not?

# REFERENCES

Algie, B.A. (1997, August 19). Accidental needle sticks. *Vital Signs,* 10.

American Journal of Nursing (AJN). (1993). RNs cite physical and verbal abuse. *American Journal of Nursing, 93*(1), 81–84.

ANA. (1997). Health and safety on the job: Nurse protect thyself. *The American Nurse, 29*(5), 1, 12, 22.

Breslow, L. & Elashoff, R. (1998). Editorial: Significance of workplace smoking. *American Journal of Public Health, 88*(7), 1011–1012.

Centers for Disease Control and Prevention (CDC). (1992). Surveillance for occupationally acquired HIV infection—United States, 1981–1992. *Morbidity and Mortality Report, 41*(43), 823–825.

Chisholm, R.F. (1992). Quality of working life: A crucial management perspective for the year 2000. *Journal of Health and Human Resources Administration, 15*(1), 6–34.

Denton, W.G. (1997). Occupational hazards. In D.K. Henderson (Ed.). *Sharing the challenge: Risks in health care practice.* Oxford G-1 Britain: Blackwell Science.

DHHS, NIOSH. (1999). Stress at work. (DHHS Publication #99-101). Cincinnati, OH: Publications Dissemination, EID, National Institute for Occupational Safety & Health.

Elliott, P.P. (1997). Violence in health care: What nurse managers need to know. *Nursing Management, 28*(12), 38–41.

Farris, B.J. (1993). Converting a unit to patient-focused care. *Health Progress, 74*(3), 22–25.

Fay, M. (1997). The era of allergens. In D.K. Henderson (Ed.). *Sharing the challenge: Risks in health care practice.* Oxford G-1 Britain: Blackwell Science.

Ferrie, J.E., Shipley, M.J., Marmot, M.G., Stansfeld, S.A. & Smith, G.D. (1998). An uncertain future: The health effects of threats to employment security in white-collar men and women. *American Journal of Public Health, 88*(7), 1030–1036.

Flarey, D.L. & Smith, S.P. (1999). Management and organizational restructuring: Reforming the corporate system. In S.P. Smith & D.L. Flarey (Eds.). *Process-centered health care organizations.* Gaithersburg, MD: Aspen, 141–159.

Gold, D.R., Rogacz, S., Bock, N., Tostegon, T.D., Baum, T.M., Speizer, F.E. & Czeisler, C.A. (1992). Rotating shift work, sleep and accidents related to sleepiness in hospital nurses. *American Journal of Public Health, 82*(7), 1011–1013.

Gritter, M. (1998). The latex threat. *American Journal of Nursing, 98*(1), 26–32.

Health-care workers seek state actions to curb needle sticks. (1999, March 9) *Wall Street Journal,* 1.

Henderson, D.K. (1997). Viral Challenges. In D.K. Henderson (Ed.). *Sharing the challenge: Risks in health care practice.* Oxford G-1 Britain: Blackwell Science.

Hurrell, J.J. (1998). Editorial: Are you uncertain? Uncertainty, health and safety in contemporary work. *American Journal of Public Health, 88*(7), 1012–1013.

Jankowski, C.B. (1992). Radiation protection for nurses: Regulations and guidelines. *Journal of Nursing Administration, 22*(22), 30–34.

Loyd, B.M. (1997, November 17). Nurses in recovery. *The Nursing Spectrum,* 18.

Maes, S., Verhoeven, C., Kittel, F. & Scholten, H. (1998). Effects of a Dutch work-site wellness-health program: The Brabantia Program. *American Journal of Public Health, 88,* 1037–1041.

McAndrew, M. (1999). The vow of silence (letter to the editor). *Journal of Nursing Administration, 29*(2), 7.

Mendelson, M., Solomon, R. et al. (1997). Evaluation of safety devices for preventing percutaneous injuries among health-care workers during phlebotomy procedures. Minneapolis-St. Paul, New York City, and San Francisco, 1993–1995. *Morbidity and Mortality Weekly Report, 46*(2), 21–25.

Moss, M.T. (1999). Creating a process-oriented organization. In S.P. Smith & D.L. Flarey (Eds.). *Process-centered health care organizations.* Gaithersburg, MD: Aspen, 223–241.

Nadwairski, J.A. (1992). Inner-city safety for home care providers. *Journal of Nursing Administration, 22*(9), 42–47.

The Nation's Health (TNH). (1993). Federal agencies clash as TB workplace safety debate rages. *The Nation's Health, 23*(1), 1, 24.

Occupational Safety and Health Administration (OSHA). (1998a). Occupational exposure to bloodborne pathogens—precautions for emergency responders, OSHA 3130, Washington, D.C.

Occupational Safety and Health Administration (OSHA). (1998b). Industrial hygiene, OSHA 3143, Washington, D.C.

Pillar, B. & Jarjoura, D. (1999). Assessing the impact of reengineering on nursing. *Journal of Nursing Administration, 29*(5), 57–64.

Rogers, B. (1997). Is health care a risky business? *The American Nurse, 29*(5), 5.

Schneid, T.D. (1999). *Occupational health guide to violence in the workplace.* Boca Raton, FL: Lewis Publishers.

Sloane, M.M. & Holcomb, C.B. (1997, August 25). Where there's smoke. *The Nursing Spectrum,* 6–7.

Toland, P.A. (1997). ONA intensifies campaign against hazardous powdered latex gloves. *The American Nurse, 29*(5), 13.

Trinkoff, A.M. & Storr, C.L. (1998). Substance use among nurses: Differences between specialties. *American Journal of Public Health, 88*(4), 581–585.

Tweedy, J.T. (1997). *Healthcare hazard control and safety management.* Delray Beach, FL: St. Lucie Press.

Wells, A.J. (1998). Lung cancer from passive smoking. *American Journal of Public Health, 88*(7), 1025–1029.

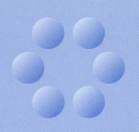

CHAPTER *19*

# Quality Improvement

## LEARNING OBJECTIVES

*After completing this chapter, the reader will be able to:*

- Discuss the similarities and differences between quality assurance, quality improvement, continuous quality improvement, and total quality improvement.
- Distinguish structure, process, and outcome variables in formal evaluation procedures.

- Participate in the development and implementation of a continuous quality improvement program at the unit level.
- Participate in the implementation of total quality management within a healthcare organization.

## TEST YOURSELF

**Nursing impact on the quality of care.**

1. Which of the following adverse patient outcomes do you think are *significantly affected* by the amount or the quality of the nursing care provided?

       a. Pressure ulcer (decubitus)
       b. Wound sepsis
       c. Anaphylactic shock
       d. Graft rejection
       e. Dehydration

       f. Fall with injury
       g. Pneumonia on admission
       h. Bowel impaction
       i. Radiation burns
       j. Urinary tract infection

2. The following is a list of diagnosis-related group (DRG) categories. Expert nurses have ranked these from high to low in terms of nursing intensity (the amount of nursing care needed). Rank them from 1 (low) to 10 (high), then compare your answers with the experts' opinions.

       a. Seizure and headache
       b. Multiple sclerosis and cerebellar ataxia
       c. Acute leukemia under age <18
       d. Unexplained cardiac arrest
       e. Uncomplicated peptic ulcer

       f. Vaginal delivery
       g. Chemotherapy
       h. Circumcision under age <18
       i. Psychosis
       j. Bronchitis and asthma

*Answers*

Question 1. a. Yes b. Yes c. No d. No e. Yes f. Yes g. No h. Yes i. No j. Yes
Question 2. a. 4 b. 6 c. 9 d. 10 e. 1 f. 2 g. 7 h. 3 i. 5 j. 8

Concern about maintaining the quality of health care while keeping costs under control has intensified efforts to improve the methods of evaluating health care. As a result, these methods are becoming increasingly sophisticated and their use is widespread (Clancy & Eisenberg, 1997).

Involvement in quality improvement (QI) begins at the staff nurse level and extends to top management. It is a process that demands clarification and articulation of what nurses do and what impact their actions should have on the outcomes of care. What was once a relatively neglected aspect of nursing leadership and management has emerged as a force for change.

The formal evaluation procedures discussed in this chapter are used for evaluating and improving the quality of care given by particular units or departments and by the organization as a whole. We will be concerned here primarily with evaluation of the quality of **nursing** care, but most of the discussion is applicable to other healthcare professions as well.

Quality improvement (QI), continuous quality improvement (CQI), and total quality management (TQM) are acronyms you will hear in almost any healthcare setting in the United States. Each refers to a particular approach to evaluating and improving the quality and efficiency of the care given within the organization. In this chapter, we sort out the various terms, consider the different players in each of these processes, and discuss some of the basic activities that are involved. Then we will work through an example illustrating continuous quality improvement.

**Quality assurance,** or **QA,** is an older term for a system of procedures used to evaluate nursing care and to give feedback to the providers of this service. **Quality improvement,** or **QI,** is a newer term used for a more comprehensive, broader-based approach to evaluating care. One important difference between the two is that quality improvement focuses on whole systems, not just the performance of individual practitioners, which is the primary focus of quality assurance. Quality improvement procedures may be used to find out what the patient care outcomes are on a particular unit, whether the incidence of nosocomial infection has declined, whether nursing intervention includes patient and family teaching, and whether these activities have an impact on the length of stay of patients on the unit. The performance of the unit may also be compared with an institutional standard of cost effectiveness. Or the entire organization's function may be compared with a healthcare systemwide standard or with a **benchmark,** the results at another organization of similar size and scope known for its high quality of care (Simpson, 1994).

The time frame used in a quality improvement program can be **retrospective** (evaluating past performance), **concurrent** (evaluating current performance), or **prospective** (future oriented, collecting data as they come in). Whichever is used, the approach will incorporate many of the familiar elements of the problem-solving process.

Quality improvement procedures are used to address not only whether the appropriate interventions took place and the desired outcomes occurred, but also how long it took and how much it cost:

*Medicare's diagnostic-related group (DRG) system of reimbursing for hospital care is based on the development of standards for what is* *"reasonable and necessary" in order to achieve the desired result for a comprehensive list of diagnoses from craniotomy to appendectomy. The hospital will not be reimbursed for care that exceeds the DRG limits. For example, it may be possible for a patient to recover full use of the lower extremities after an auto accident, but if it takes a year of intensive physical therapy at home, it is unlikely to be considered a reasonable and necessary investment of resources to be reimbursed by Medicare. (The patient and family may have a different opinion on whether this investment is reasonable and necessary.)*

Quality improvement programs are becoming integral parts of healthcare institutions' functions, because they can be used to identify areas in which cost savings can be found without adversely affecting the processes and outcomes of care. Another reason is that regulators and accreditors, including the Joint Commission on Accreditation of Healthcare Organizations (JCAHO), are calling for increasingly sophisticated and effective systems to evaluate the quality of care, particularly the outcomes of care.

## ● QUALITY DEFINED

On the subjective level, most nurses would agree that they recognize high-quality care when they see it. More objectively, however, quality in nursing care has been difficult to define. Quality improvement challenges us to articulate what constitutes an acceptable level of care and acceptable outcomes for a given set of patients or for a particular patient problem. In fact, involvement in quality improvement projects has led many nurses to pursue research studies to better define effective nursing interventions and acceptable outcomes.

> *Quality is never an accident; it is always the result of intelligent effort.*
> —John Ruskin (1819–1900) in Eigen & Siegel, 1989, p. 384

Deming defined quality as the achievement at low cost of the level of uniformity and dependability demanded by the market (1982). For Deming, quality improvement is a continuous cycle of review and improvement, a journey rather than a destination (Zabada, 1998). Quality also can be defined as conformance to the needs of the client when the outcome meets or exceeds the client's expectations (Carman et al, 1996; Crosby, 1979).

In health care, quality encompasses effectiveness, efficiency, optimality (a balance between cost and effectiveness), acceptability, legitimacy (conformance to social norms and ethical principles), and equity (Donabedian in Mark, Salyer & Geddis, 1997).

> *In health care, we have a special obligation to strive for perfection because instead of making products, we serve people . . . anything less than pushing for perfection is unjustifiable.*
>
> —*Leebov, 1991, p. 17*

> *We have to grant quality its moral dimension. . . . It should be recognized as a virtue—something to be sought for its own sake—not just a profitable strategy.*
>
> —*Edward Tenner, quoted in Eigen & Siegel, 1989, p. 384*

## ● GOALS OF QUALITY IMPROVEMENT

The long-term goals of quality improvement are both complex and lofty: they are to achieve optimal patient outcomes in terms of both improved well-being (to the extent possible given the patient's condition) and patient satisfaction with care within a well-functioning system while keeping costs to a minimum. Given the complexities of both our patients' needs and of our healthcare system, these goals are not easy to achieve. In fact, their achievement requires the full commitment and involvement of everyone in a healthcare organization.

The more immediate purposes of any quality improvement activity are to improve the efficiency and the effectiveness of the services rendered. Even these shorter-term goals present a challenge to nursing staff. (See Perspectives . . . When Is Care Good Enough?)

---

## PERSPECTIVES . . .

### When Is Care Good Enough?

Should we strive for perfection in health care? Is it good enough to provide just adequate care? Leebov (1991) asks us to consider the following before answering these questions.

- How many babies is it okay to drop?
- How many medication errors are allowable in a week or a month?
- How many rude comments to patients is too many?
- How long can a call light be ignored?

Is it good enough to drop just one baby, make just one med error, be rude to just one patient, and ignore just one call light? Or should we aim for perfection: no dropped babies, no med errors, no rude comments, no call lights ignored? These questions are difficult to answer. What do you think?

---

Source: Leebov, W. (1991). *The quality quest: A briefing for health care professionals.* Chicago: American Hospital Publishing, Inc.

---

## ● CONTINUOUS QUALITY IMPROVEMENT

**Continuous quality improvement,** or **CQI,** is an "ongoing effort to provide services that meet or exceed customer expectations through a structured systematic process" (Carman et al, 1996, p. 48). It can be contrasted to small, unconnected QI projects that have no relationship with each other and little continuing impact after they are completed.

Continuous quality improvement consists of four basic elements (Kinlaw, 1992). The first is **teamwork,** a subject that was discussed in detail in Chapter 5. A team approach, especially the ability to function as part of an interdisciplinary team, is essential to effective continuous quality improvement. Training in teamwork, problem solving, and data analysis may be necessary before undertaking any continuous quality improvement projects.

The inclusion of the **patient perspective** is the second element. In the past, the patient's point of view was often omitted from evaluation of healthcare service (Elrod, 1991), an omission that would surprise an expert in marketing and should have dismayed any nurse who claimed to provide patient-centered care. Both patient outcomes and patient satisfaction should be considered in evaluating healthcare services.

The third, and perhaps most essential, element of continuous quality improvement is **measurement of work structures, processes and outcomes.** It includes both baseline measures and measures after changes have been instituted. **Structure** includes the preparation and experience of staff. **Process** measures actions, such as how many times a patient receives colostomy care instruction; **outcome** measures the results, such as the patient's satisfaction with his or her ability to care for the colostomy at home. The data collection and evaluation are meant to be as objective as possible and may involve the use of statistical analysis. Some of these procedures may become quite complex, but the majority are relatively straightforward.

The final element is the adequacy of the **resources** available for implementation of any improvements. For example, administrative support for any needed improvements indicated by the results is essential to the success of a continuous quality improvement program. Other needed resources may include adequate staff time to participate in CQI, adequate equipment, sufficient data to perform the evaluation, consultation about resolving a problem, and so forth.

## ● TOTAL QUALITY MANAGEMENT

When the idea of continuous quality improvement becomes a management philosophy that permeates every aspect of a healthcare organization, continuous quality improvement becomes **total quality management, or TQM.** TQM is a holistic, organizationwide approach to maintaining and improving quality. All of the organization's activities and resources are directed toward the achievement of the goals stated earlier: (1) optimum patient outcomes in terms of both patient well-being and satisfaction with the care given, and (2) a well-functioning system that provides high-quality care while keeping costs to a minimum (Dienemann, 1992).

Total quality management requires a highly proactive, highly participative style of management. Earlier quality assurance models tended to focus the evaluative portion on the performance of individual staff members and, therefore, could easily create a punitive impression despite assurances that a negative focus was not the purpose (Cound, 1992). Quality improvement's focus on the patient perspective and emphasis on improvement of all aspects of patient care tend to create a more positive climate and greater staff satisfaction with their work. In theory at least, the older quality assurance methodology primarily evaluated staff while the newer quality improvement empowers staff to bring about positive changes.

> *Unless a total quality culture develops in the micro and macro environments of an organization, TQM will appear to be another passing "management fad."*
> —Wong, 1998

The primary advantage of total quality management lies in its organizationwide approach. Although each department within an organization can do a great deal to improve its patient care processes and outcomes, the interdependent nature of most departments within a healthcare organization may limit the effectiveness of many single-department quality improvement projects. For example, the nursing department can improve the speed with which new medication orders are noted, but it cannot improve the speed with which a new medication is obtained without the cooperation of the pharmacy department. Likewise, optimal reduction of postsurgical infections requires involvement of operating room, recovery room, and surgical unit staff.

In order to be most effective, total quality management crosses both departmental and disciplinary lines. Cooperation between nurses and physicians in adherence to strict infection control procedures, for example, will reduce a unit's postsurgical infection rate far more than would an effort by nurses or by physicians alone.

Often the solution to a problem lies in changing organizationwide policies or procedures. For example, linking data from the laboratory, radiology, pharmacy, nursing, and other departments in a single patient record can only be done on an organizationwide basis. W. Edwards Deming, a guru of quality management, believed that 85 percent of all quality problems were the result of harmful management practices (Hunt, 1992). Only 15 percent of the problems are said to be under a worker's control (Bernard, Bestor, Karsner & LeMay, 1994). Although this statistic may be an exaggeration, total quality management recognizes that administrative policies and procedures can be as much of a barrier to quality as the attitude or performance of the individual staff member.

Implementation of total quality management clearly requires the support of administration and participation of every employee including members of the medical staff. Successful implementation of total quality management requires considerable time and energy, and the commitment of everyone involved.

## ● ASPECTS OF HEALTH CARE TO EVALUATE

The classic approach to evaluation of health care is based upon Donabedian's structure-process-outcome model (1969, 1977, 1987). When fo-cused on nursing care, the independent, depen-dent, and interdependent functions of nurses may be added to the model (Irvine, 1998). Each of these dimensions is described here and their interrelationship is illustrated in Table 19–1.

## Structure

Structure refers to the **setting** in which the care is given and the **resources** (human, financial, and material) that are available. It is the easiest of the three aspects to measure although sometimes over-looked in evaluation procedures. The following structural aspects of a healthcare organization can be included in a formal evaluation.

- *Facilities:* comfort, safety, convenience of lay-out, accessibility of support services, adequate light, air quality
- *Equipment:* state-of-art equipment, staff abil-ity to use it
- *Staff:* credentials, experience, staff mix, assign-ment patterns, staff-patient ratios
- *Finances:* salaries, adequacy of resources, supplies

While none of these structural factors alone can guarantee that good care will be given, they do make good care more likely to occur. A higher

**Table 19–1**   Dimensions of Quality Improvement in Nursing: Examples

|  | Independent Function | Dependent Function | Interdependent Function |
|---|---|---|---|
| Structure | Pressure ulcer risk assessment form available | High-speed automatic dial-up system puts nurses in touch with physicians rapidly | Nursing case management model of care adopted on rehabilitation unit |
| Process | Assesses risk for development of pressure ulcer and implements preventive measure | Order to increase dosage of pain medication obtained and processed within one hour | Communicates with therapists about need for customized wheelchair |
| Outcome | Skin intact at discharge | Relief from pain | Able to enter narrow doorway to bathroom unassisted |

*Source:* Adapted from on Irvine, D. (1998). Finding value in nursing care: A framework for quality improvement and clinical evaluation. *Nursing Economics, 16*(3), 110–118.

level of nurse staffing (i.e., more nurses on staff) and a higher proportion of registered nurses in the skill mix are structural factors that are associated with shorter lengths of stay; higher proportions of registered nurses are also related to fewer adverse patient outcomes (Lichtig, Knauf & Milholland, 1999).

A common pitfall in evaluating structural factors, however, has been to neglect the other two aspects (process and outcome). The following example illustrates the problems that occur when evaluating only structure.

*One hospital measured the quality of nursing care given in its eight-bed critical care unit by comparing its staffing ratio with a standard (expected level) set by the hospital of one nurse to two patients. The inadequacy of using this structural measure alone became apparent during a period when the unit had six (out of a total of eight) patients who each required the care of one nurse. Operating under the standard that was set by the hospital, only four nurses were on duty, which created a severe staff shortage because seven nurses were actually needed to provide adequate care.*

## Process

Process refers to the **actual activities** carried out by healthcare providers. More specifically, it includes all activities carried out and decisions made from the time an individual approaches the healthcare system through assessment, diagnosis, treatment, and follow-up care (Irvine, 1998). Examples include the following:

- Setting an appointment
- Conducting a physical assessment
- Ordering an X ray and MRI
- Administering a blood transfusion
- Completing a home environment assessment
- Preparing the patient for discharge
- Telephoning the patient postdischarge

Each of these processes can be evaluated in terms of timeliness, appropriateness, accuracy, and completeness (Irvine, 1998). Process variables include psychosocial interventions, such as teaching and counseling, as well as physical care measures. It can include leadership activi-

ties such as interdisciplinary team conferences. Curtin (1997) suggests adding access to care and affordability of care to questions of quality of the care actually provided. Whether cost should be an outcome measure is a subject of some debate (Curtin, 1997; Kleinpell, 1997) as it may distract from the concern about the quality of the care provided. (See Perspectives . . . Defining Lousy Care.)

> *A lot of decisions have not been made in the best interest of patients, but on financial imperatives—and that's a shame.*
> —Speck, quoted in Curtin, 1997, p. 8

# PERSPECTIVES . . .

## Defining "Lousy Care"

Leah Curtin, editor of *Nursing Management*, writes that while we may find it difficult to define "improved patient outcomes," we all know what "lousy care" is. For example, lousy care is having to make 16 phone calls and wait for hundreds of minutes to get "authorization" when you're so sick you can barely hold your head up. Lousy care is having some clerk force you to go across town to get "emergency" care because your neighborhood hospital isn't part of the network. Lousy care is having to wait 6 weeks to see your primary physician when what you really need is to see a urologist. Lousy care is being told to watch your I.V. when you can't even see it. Lousy care is being sent home to fend for yourself when you have multiple wounds, drains, and dressings. Lousy care is having someone who doesn't know what he/she is doing "caring" for you.

*Source:* Curtin, L.L. (1997). Looking for outcomes in all the wrong places. *Nursing Management, 28*(4), 7–8.

When process data are collected, a set of objectives, procedures, or guidelines is needed to serve as a standard or gauge against which to compare the activities. This set of objectives can be highly specific, such as listing all the steps in a catheterization procedure, or it can be a general list of objectives, such as "offer information on breast-feeding to all expectant parents" or "conduct weekly staff meetings."

## Outcome

Outcome refers to the **results** of the activities in which the healthcare providers have been involved. Outcome measures evaluate the effectiveness of these nursing activities by answering such questions as: Did the patient recover? Is the family more independent now? Has team functioning improved?

These questions are general and reflect overall goals of healthcare providers and the organizations in which they work. The outcome questions asked during an actual evaluation should be far more specific and should measure observable behavior such as the following:

Patient:　Wound healed

　　　　　Blood pressure within normal limits

　　　　　Absence of infection

Family:　Increased time between visits to the emergency department

　　　　　Food stamps application completed

Team:　Decisions reached by consensus

　　　　　Attendance at meetings by all team members

You can see that some of these outcomes, such as blood pressure, attendance, or time between visits, are easier to measure than are other equally important outcomes, such as increased satisfaction or changes in attitude. Although these less tangible outcomes cannot be measured as precisely, it is still important to include them so that the full spectrum of biologic, psychologic, and social aspects are represented (Strickland, 1997). For this reason, considerable effort has been put into identifying the patient outcomes that are affected by the quality of nursing care. Examples include communication ability, hydration, bowel continence, grief resolution, infection control knowledge, wound healing, thermoregulation, and spiritual well-being (Johnson & Maas, 1997). The American Nurses Association (1996) has developed a

much shorter list of outcomes thought to be sensitive to the proportion of registered nurses on a nursing staff and the total staff-patient ratio in acute care:

- Nosocomial infection rates
- Patient injuries from falls
- Patient opinion of care received
- Maintenance of skin integrity
- Pain management
- Self-care knowledge

Consumers, employers, and legislators have called for objective measures of the quality of health care from various providers. The measures in the preceding list can be used to develop a nursing-specific report card for acute-care facilities.

Another problem in using and interpreting outcome measures in evaluation is that outcomes are influenced by many factors. For example:

*The outcome of patient teaching done by a nurse during a home visit is affected by the patient's interest and ability to learn, the quality of the teaching materials, the presence or absence of family support, the information given by other caregivers (which may conflict with the information given by the nurse), and the environment in which the teaching is done. If the teaching is successful, can the nurse be given full credit for the success? If it is not successful, who has failed?*

You can see that it is necessary to evaluate the process as well as the outcome in order to determine *why* an intervention such as patient teaching succeeds or fails. A comprehensive evaluation would include all three aspects: structure, process, and outcome and, when focused on nursing care, the independent, dependent, and interdependent functions of nurses (illustrated in Table 19–1).

Eventually we will have access to large data sets from which we can draw information on the typical or average length of stay and outcomes for every subset of patients, neonate to post-traumatic brain injury victim (Simpson, 1997a). Standard terminology for diagnoses, interventions, and outcomes will be needed to compare them across institutions and regions (see Research Example 19–1).

**Research Example Box 19–1**   *Linking Data Sets to Learn More about Healthcare Quality*

Even with the abundance of data out there, it is surprisingly difficult to translate it into useful information about the quality of health care. The results of a program to help states improve their health-related data systems have demonstrated the benefits of this effort.

- A small town in South Carolina used the results of its data analysis to convince the city council to reroute its buses. The analysis revealed that the neighborhoods where most of the people who used Medicaid-related services lived were not on the original bus routes.
- Wisconsin found that while some HMOs reported that up to 90 percent of their Medicaid

enrollers had received appropriate prenatal, primary, and dental care, less than 50 percent actually had received appropriate levels of service. By linking birth, hospitalization, Medicaid claims, and other databases, they were able to check the accuracy of the HMO reports.

Program participants found that the work of linking their databases had been more difficult and time consuming than anticipated but in the end they concluded that it was a worthwhile endeavor.

*Source:* Gillespie, K. (1998). States strive to turn data into health policy information. *Advances, 1,* 3, 9.

## Nursing Management Minimum Data Set

Work is also being done on standard definitions and data collection methods related to nursing management (Simpson, 1997b). The Nursing Management Minimum Data Set focuses on nursing-related structural factors, or the context within which nursing care is given, including financial resources, human resources, and the environment (see Figure 19–1).

## ● DATA COLLECTION PROCEDURES

The procedures used to collect data in a quality improvement program will depend on the purposes of the program. Usually a variety of methods are employed in order to obtain the information needed, including record audits, observation, interviews, questionnaires, and focus groups (Emmett, 1999).

## Record Audits

Record audits of various types are one of the most commonly used procedures for collecting data in healthcare organizations. Using standards developed by the CQI team, records are

evaluated to determine whether care plans are being developed for patients, whether they are being implemented as directed, and whether the expected outcomes have resulted. Audits may be done **concurrently,** while the patient is receiving care, or **retrospectively,** some time after the patient has been discharged (Phaneuf, 1976).

Record audits are limited by the amount of information that has been documented, which does not necessarily include everything that has occurred. Other methods should be used to supplement the record audit. Ideally, record audits occur while the care is being rendered rather than retrospectively. Concurrent audits provide immediate feedback on the adequacy of care while the opportunity to make corrections benefit the patient is still present.

## Observation

Observation—actually watching the care that is being given—is one of the more reliable but labor intensive ways to collect data. Observation can tell us whether complete assessments are being done, whether care is actually being given as planned, whether interventions are being done appropriately, and whether desired outcomes actually have occurred. This method of gathering information about the quality of care rendered

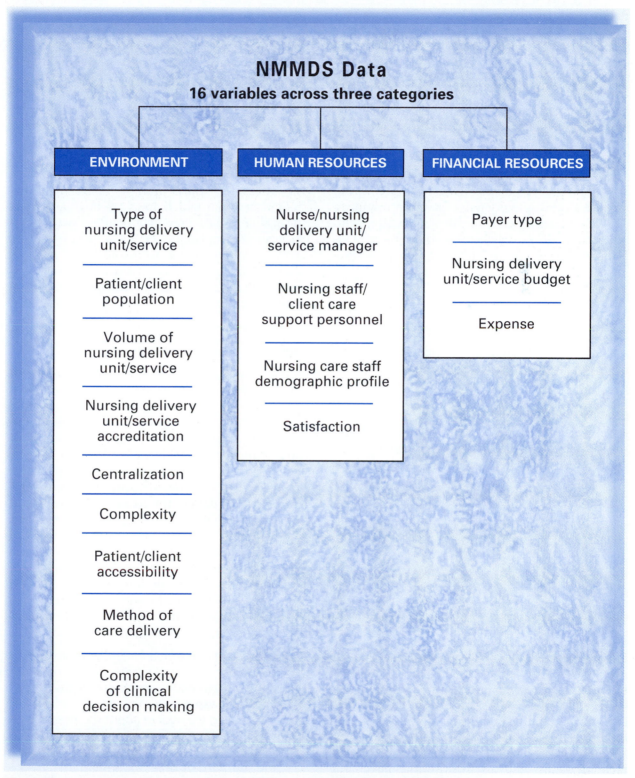

**Figure 19–1** Nursing management minimum data set. *Source:* Simpson, R.L. (1997). The nurse management minimum data set initiative needs you! *Nursing Management, 28*(6), 20–21. Reprinted with permission.

requires clear categories for recording data that should be tested for their reliability, or consistency among observers.

## Interviews and Questionnaires

Personal interviews or written questionnaires distributed to patients, families, and other caregivers can provide otherwise unavailable information about the care provided and the outcomes that resulted. Data on patient opinion, knowledge level, and emotional responses are best captured in interview or by questionnaire in most instances. This method may be used in conjunction with other methods, especially when the subjective effects of memory, anxiety, and individual interpretation are expected to be a concern.

## Focus Groups

In contrast to the methods already described, the focus group methodology provides a great deal of information from a small number of people, usually 10–15 in a single group. In some instances, experts are invited to come together to discuss an important issue or to combine their experience and knowledge. In other cases, consumers (patients or clients) are invited to the group to discuss their experience and opinions regarding that experience. An effective leader is needed to guide this process and to avoid it becoming either a gripe session or a social gathering. Focus groups are used widely in marketing to tap into consumer preferences.

## ● QUALITY IMPROVEMENT AT THE UNIT LEVEL

In this section, we consider the process of quality improvement at the unit level. For the sake of simplicity, we focus almost exclusively on nursing's effect on patient care but it is generally recommended that quality improvement be interdisciplinary at the unit level as well as at the organizational level.

After the policies and procedures for implementing quality improvement projects have been defined at the organizational level, much of the responsibility for carrying them out may be delegated to the staff of each unit. At the unit level,

the first step is to assign responsibility to various staff members. All staff members may be brought together to act as a quality circle, or a representative group may be appointed to a committee to implement quality improvement activities in consultation with the rest of the nursing staff. It is preferable to have as high a level of staff participation as possible, including representation from all three shifts in an inpatient setting.

Once staff members understand the purpose of quality improvement, they can begin to identify areas for study. Staff may use their own judgment about which areas are in greatest need of evaluation, or they may conduct preliminary surveys to determine the most problem-prone areas. Some guidance from the nurse manager may be needed to select a priority area and to prevent avoidance of a difficult problem or one that is hard to define.

## Scope

Some examples of broad areas of study might include the highest-risk patients, the most common patient problems, or the source of a high number of incident reports (Elrod, 1991). Other more selectively focused areas might be physical restraint usage, management of dysphagia, ventilator-assisted breathing, respiratory treatments, preoperative teaching, or urinary incontinence. Each of these defines the **scope** of the problem to be evaluated (Duquette, 1991). Once the scope is defined, the problem itself is further analyzed in terms of its important aspects, the generally accepted **standards of care** for these aspects, **indicators** (evidence) that these standards have been met, and the **criteria** (threshold) for determining whether they were met (Box 19–1). These terms are further explained in the following example:

*Let's say that one area for study chosen by an outpatient clinic staff is patient teaching with newly diagnosed hypertensive patients. Three important* **aspects** *of this area of care would be teaching the patient about the disease process, lifestyle modifications, and pharmacologic treatment. In regard to lifestyle modifications, the* **standard of care** *would state that the "Patient will receive information about exercise, dietary modifications, smoking, alcohol use, and stress reduction."* **Indicators** *for the*

---

**Box 19–1　Unit-Level Quality Improvement Process**

Assign Responsibilities
Identify area for study
Define scope of care
Analyze area in terms of:
　Aspects
　Standards
　Indicators
　Criteria
Measure actual performance and patient outcomes
Evaluate performance and outcomes
Recommend and implement actions
Evaluate degree of improvement

*Source:* Adapted from Hunt, V.D. (1992). *Quality in America: How to implement a competitive quality program.* Homewood, IL: Business One Irwin.

---

*dietary modification portion would be that the patient is able to describe the recommended modifications, modifies the diet as recommended, and maintains weight within*

*10 percent of ideal weight. A **criterion** or threshold for this last indicator would be that at least 50 percent of patients would achieve this level within six months of the original recommendation (Figure 19–2).*

## Standards

A **standard of nursing practice** describes what nurses do for or with patients and their families. It is in contrast to a **nursing standard of care** that describes the kind of care patients can expect and receive from nurses (JCAHO, 1993).

The major reason for setting standards is to increase objectivity by defining as clearly as possible what is acceptable and what is not acceptable. Without these standards, judgments made in the evaluation process may be variable, subjective, and susceptible to the whims and biases of the evaluators. Consistent application of these standards of care is essential for continuous quality improvement.

A second function of these standards is to communicate clearly to everyone involved (including staff, administrators, consumers, accreditors, and regulators) what level of service is expected in

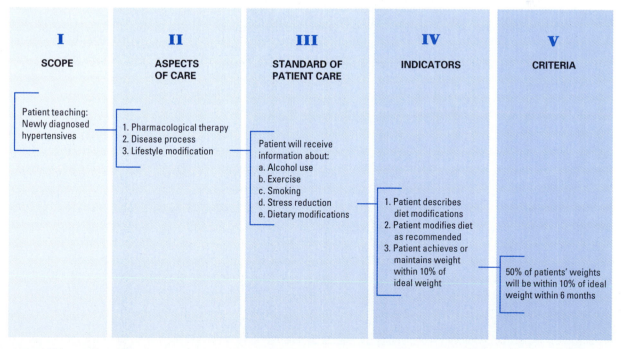

**Figure 19–2**　Example of quality improvement guidelines.

**Table 19–2** Sample Quality Improvement Work Sheet for Collecting Data in a Prospective Study

| Patient Identification Number | Weight at 1st Visit | Ideal Weight | Ideal vs. Acutal Weight Difference (percent) | Weight at 2nd Visit | Weight at 3rd Visit | Weight at 4th Visit | Weight at 5th Visit | Weight at Six Months | % Difference from Ideal Weight |
|---|---|---|---|---|---|---|---|---|---|
| #01723 | 135 | 130 | 5 (4%) | 136 | 137 | 135 | 133 | 130 | (0%) |
| #01799 | 210 | 145 | 65 (45%) | 205 | 204 | 201 | 199 | 197 | (36%) |
| #23045 | 175 | 165 | 10 (6%) | 173 | 175 | 176 | 178 | 185 | (12%) |

that organization. This function can only be carried out if the standards are made available to all of these people. In the past, these standards have not been made available to the consumer, but some evidence indicates that this gap in communication may change in the future.

The standards and measurements used for evaluating them may vary with the institution, the purpose of the evaluation, and the evaluators. They should be reviewed regularly so that they continue to reflect current nursing knowledge, practice, and research (Short & Bair, 1990). Outdated standards can perpetuate the use of ineffective practices and make the evaluation results useless at best.

## Indicators and Criteria

An **indicator** is an objective, measurable variable of care. The listed indicators are those variables on which data will be collected in a quality improvement project. If data are to be collected on a continuing basis, the process is usually referred to as **monitoring.** The **criterion,** or threshold, sets a predetermined level of the indicator that will be considered an acceptable level of care (Betta, 1992). For some indicators, such as documenting patient response to a blood infusion, a 100 percent level of achievement is expected. In other cases, such as weight reduction or smoking cessation, a 75 percent level of achievement would be considered excellent.

Once these variables are well defined, a plan for data collection is devised. Usually, some type of worksheet is designed to facilitate data collection.

*For example, a chart could be devised listing each newly diagnosed hypertensive patient, the weight at diagnosis, ideal weight, and weight at subsequent clinic visits (see Table 19–2). A final column for noting whether the patient was within 10 percent of ideal weight can be added to indicate how many met the criterion after six months.*

*After data are collected, the staff review the findings and evaluate the degree to which the criterion was met. If only 25 percent of the newly diagnosed hypertensive patients were within 10 percent of their ideal weight in six*

*months, the clinic staff might decide to offer weight reduction classes or a support group. They might also decide to invite the clinic psychologist and nutritionist to participate in the group.*

*A reevaluation of patient weights after a second six-month period that indicated 50 percent of the patients now were within 10 percent of their ideal weights would be evidence that the group was effective in improving the quality of the patient outcomes. As a result, the clinic staff might decide to continue the group but to work on making it even more effective and perhaps seeking other avenues to help the other 50 percent of the patients who had not met their weight reduction goals.*

## QUALITY IMPROVEMENT AT THE ORGANIZATIONAL LEVEL

Institution of a quality improvement program at the organizational level should actually precede the unit-level work just described. However, work at this macro (organizational) level is easier to understand after reading about what happens at the micro (unit) level.

Establishing an organizationwide quality improvement program is primarily an administrative responsibility. The first step is a statement of the organization's philosophy regarding quality improvement (Hunt, 1992) (see Figure 19–3). For example, a spirit of cooperation between management and staff and use of interdisciplinary teams may be important parts of the organization's philosophy of quality improvement.

Next, the mechanisms to implement quality improvement need to be set up. For example, an organizationwide quality council might be created with representation across departments and disciplines. Subcouncils and unit teams are also set up. Grassroots involvement, that is, participation of everyone who comes into contact with the patient, including unlicensed assistive personnel and housekeeping staff, is a hallmark of total quality management.

Once the mechanisms are in place, continuous quality improvement work begins. The quality council or other administrative body evaluates

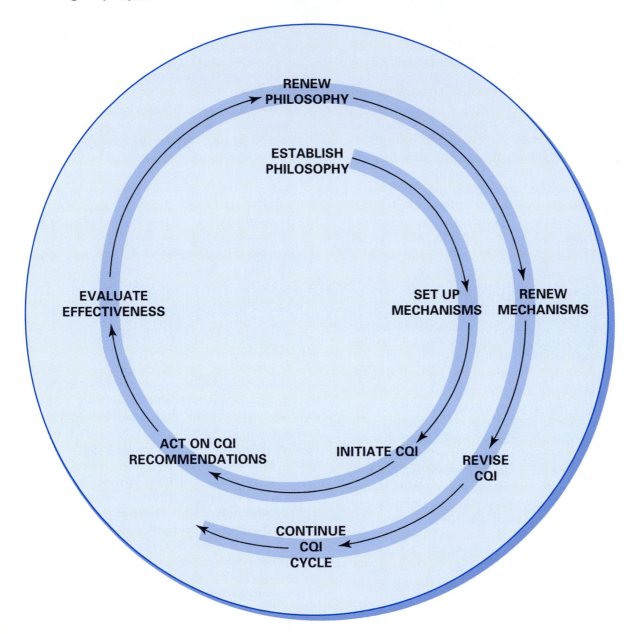

**Figure 19–3**   Continuous Quality Improvement (CQI) cycle.

the effectiveness of the organization's continuous quality improvement efforts and results, revises the process as needed, and proceeds through the cycle as illustrated in Figure 19–3.

## Quality Circles

The origin of quality circles is uncertain, but they began to receive some attention when Theory Z was introduced (see Chapter 2). Quality circles are usually composed of employees who perform the same tasks or who are responsible for achieving the same patient outcomes so that they can work on solving mutual problems. The circles meet regularly to identify problems (or potential problems) and brainstorm about their origins, their solutions, and how the solutions can contribute to the improvement of the product or service. They have been introduced in human service settings with some degree of success.

*In an institution for the care of the developmentally disabled, the staff in one of the group homes identified the use of toothpaste tubes as presenting a problem. They saw that a lot of toothpaste was wasted because of residents' carelessness or lack of dexterity, and it caused problems in keeping bathrooms clean. Furthermore, the tube posed a danger at times because the cap of the toothpaste tube got lost, sometimes down the drain where it might clog the plumbing, sometimes on the floor where it might cause someone to fall, as well as the possibility that a resident might swallow the cap.*

*The quality circle decided to do a study to determine whether toothpaste pumps might be more economical and reduce some of the inconveniences and dangers of the tubes. They methodically tested the two containers and documented the number of "brushes" that could be obtained from each, then brainstormed all the advantages and disadvantages of the toothpaste pump and compared them to those of the tube. The cost saving, when projected for the entire state, was quite impressive. (Quality Circles in Human Services, Wassaic Developmental Disabilities Office, 1986).*

The cost of quality improvement efforts in terms of both time and commitment to the process is considerable. If not carefully administered, quality circles may become still another task imposed with no more time in the day to get the additional work done. The manager who watches a group casting about for a suitable problem for brainstorming may have qualms about the cost effectiveness of the process even though it is enhancing the group process and the effectiveness of the work group. Over the long term, however, quality improvement efforts should improve patient outcomes.

*Make no mistake: realizing significant improvement in the quality of a product or service . . . is hard, hard work.*

—*Guaspari in Eigen & Siegel, 1989, p. 379*

## Continuous Quality Improvement Example

The following example describes a continuous quality improvement project undertaken by a quality council operating in a hospital that has just begun to develop a total quality management system. It illustrates a number of the principles and activities that have been described so far.

**Background.** *Central Medical Healthcare Center was recently purchased by a large corporation. Soon after its purchase, sweeping cost-cutting measures were instituted. One that received little attention at first was the elimination of the respiratory therapy department. Those respiratory therapists who were also registered nurses were reassigned to various patient care units; the remainder were dismissed. Full responsibility for provision of respiratory treatment was returned to nursing.*

*Central Medical Healthcare Center had also adopted a total quality management philosophy. The old quality assurance approach, located within the medical records department, was gradually replaced with an organization-wide total quality improvement approach. Central Medical's quality council included representatives from the staff and administration of every department in the hospital. Each month, the quality council reviewed suggestions submitted by employees and made decisions about quality improvement initiatives.*

*Identifying an Area for Study. The first mention of a potential problem with respiratory treatments came in the form of a brief note from an anonymous night shift staff nurse who asked, "Are nurses prepared to provide respiratory treatments?" "Of course they are," sniffed the CNO and the council moved on to consideration of another employee's suggestion.*

*Three months later, however, a more assertive staff nurse wrote to the council on the same subject. This nurse did not ask a question. Instead, this nurse requested that the council review the quality of the respiratory treatments being given. The nurse suggested that treatments were being given incorrectly and that documentation was inadequate. Although the CNO again said that, as far as she knew, no problem with the adequacy of this area of care had developed, the council asked her to look into it and report back at the next meeting. They suggested that she begin by contacting the nurse who wrote the second letter.*

At this point, the reader will note that the action so far has occurred at the organizational level. The stimulus for this action, however, came from the grassroots level, from two concerned staff nurses.

*At the next meeting, the CNO reported that some subjective evidence from staff nurses and nurse managers indicated that reassumption of full responsibility for providing respiratory treatments had caused some problems: increased workload, lack of familiarity with hospital policies and procedures for respiratory treatment, and some confusion over where the treatments should be documented in the chart. "There may be more of a problem here than I thought," concluded the CNO.*

*The consensus from the council was that sufficient evidence warranted further study of the problem. A task force composed of a nursing quality improvement coordinator, a pulmonary physician, a staff nurse who had been a respiratory therapist, and one who had not was convened. The council asked the task force to plan and conduct a hospitalwide survey of respiratory treatment and report back to council members with its findings and recommendations. The task force was encouraged to involve anyone who had an interest in the subject and as many disciplines as possible. Task force members were also encouraged to interview both staff and patients as well as collect data from patient records.*

*Define Scope of Care. The nursing quality improvement coordinator assumed leadership of the task force. The coordinator was familiar with traditional survey techniques and wanted the task force to conduct a chart review. Other members of the task force, however, wanted to explore some of the issues surrounding the problem before designing their survey. At the first meeting, they spent some time becoming better acquainted with each other and discussing the issues raised at the quality council meeting. They also agreed to review the existing policies and procedures for respiratory treatment in order to discuss them at their next meeting.*

As with other working groups, quality improvement task forces and quality circles need to work through the stages of group development and other issues involved in putting together a new team.

*Define Aspects of Care, Standards, Indicators, Criteria. Having done their homework, the task force felt ready to discuss the survey at their second meeting. They created a work sheet that listed the major points of information that should be documented on the patient record, which included such items as patient teaching, amount of medication, sputum production, breath sounds, pulse, respirations, and so forth. They agreed to meet once more before conducting the survey to discuss their data collection techniques.*

*At the presurvey meeting, task force members discussed what they would look for in the records, what constituted an acceptable level of care, and what criterion they should use for each item. Did it have to be 100 percent? Would 90 percent be acceptable? Did the desired percentage vary for each item? The quality improvement coordinator assured the group that all of this information could be retrieved from the respiratory treatment flow sheet that had been devised when the transfer of responsibility to nursing had occurred. The flow sheet would either be found at the bedside or in the patient's chart, she said. "Just ask the nurse manager where they keep them," she told the group. The pulmonary physician volunteered to review the medical portion of the chart: appropriate prescriptions, accuracy of order transcriptions, timely renewal of medication orders, adequate documentation of patient response in the progress notes. The task force accepted the offer and created another survey form for the physician. The group divided up the units to be surveyed and left with a packet of forms to fill out.*

The reader will note that the task force's initial approach was similar to the traditional chart audit.

*Review Results. The postsurvey meeting was long and lively. The nurses found only three units out of a total of 15 were actually using the flow sheets at all. Of these, about half of the flow sheets were complete. Technically, the compliance rate was 10 percent, but even this disturbing figure did not really reflect the na-*

ture or scope of the problem, they said. Of even greater concern to them than the inadequate documentation were problems with administration of the treatment. Nurses in the intensive care units were documenting on their own forms but felt well prepared to provide respiratory treatments. Several nurse managers and staff nurses on the other units, however, pointed out that they were not familiar with the new medications and equipment because they had not been using them until recently. Those who were well prepared (including two other nurses who had been respiratory therapists) observed colleagues making some errors in the way medications were dispensed, in their patient teaching, and in cleaning the equipment. In addition, they had concerns about the apparently poor communication between nurses and physicians regarding patient response to treatment. Often, patients remained on ineffective treatment regimens because no review or even informal discussion of the effectiveness of these treatments was occurring. Finally, they had also found that some alternative medications, including some that were particularly appropriate for patients with cardiac problems, were not available in the hospital pharmacy.

Revise Approach. *"We learned more from the interviews and our observations than we did from the chart reviews,"* concluded one nurse. *"So did I,"* added the pulmonary physician. *"Medication orders were accurately transcribed but no one questioned those that were out of the usual range. I also saw patients maintained on the same regimen despite their failure to improve and am not certain where the breakdown in communication really is."*

*"We need to rethink this survey,"* said one of the nurses. *"This is a far bigger, far more serious problem than I had imagined it to be."* *"We need to involve the pharmacy and biomedical engineering department the next time,"* said the coordinator. *"Yes, and interview and observe staff and patients more systematically as well as audit charts."* *"We may need to involve administration at some point because there may also be a problem with work overload for the staff nurses."*

*"That may be reflective of a larger problem,"* added the coordinator. *"Perhaps more than*

one,"* agreed the physician. *"Both staff burden and communication breakdowns may be systemwide problems as well."*

*"I will report our preliminary findings and concerns to the quality council,"* said the coordinator. *"All of you are welcome to come with me to the meeting. I expect that the council will encourage us to expand the task force membership and our data-gathering approaches in order to more fully understand the dynamics of the problem."* Group members agreed. Two said they would also attend the next quality council meeting.

*"This issue is much bigger than I had thought it was,"* reported the coordinator when she shared the task force's findings with the CNO. *"More serious and, actually, more interesting."* *"This is what CQI is all about,"* responded the CNO. *"When I think about the potential organizationwide problems as well, I realize we're just beginning to understand what TQM can do to improve patient care. None of us could do this alone. Divided into pieces by department or by discipline, we wouldn't be able to see the whole picture."*

The quality council supported the task force's proposal and encouraged the group to maintain the organizationwide perspective they had adopted. With renewed energy and a larger membership, the task force designed a more comprehensive survey that involved both quantitative and qualitative data from records and interviews and observation of both patients and staff including physicians.

Often the impediments to quality care and optimal patient outcomes lie outside the nursing unit. Building into the data collection process some means of identifying the nature of the problem can be helpful in beginning to determine where the solutions may lie. A need to improve the orientation of new employees, for example, or for an inservice program on a new procedure may be indicated. Some problem with the environment (overcrowding or a poorly planned transport system, for example) or policies or procedures that interfere with the desired performance may surface. The quality improvement process may provide the documentation needed to demonstrate the need for new equipment or a new procedure.

Results of the quality improvement studies can also stimulate research efforts within the institution, particularly research on the relationship between interventions and expected outcomes.

# ● ISSUES RELATED TO CQI AND TQM

Some of the structural and functional characteristics of healthcare organizations present obstacles to the successful implementation of TQM (Zabada, 1998). These obstacles include the following:

- Bureaucratic organizational cultures that limit employee empowerment
- Underinvolvement of physicians, the majority of whom are not employed by the organization
- Status of the patient as both "product" and consumer of the service provided
- Limitations on consumer choice of healthcare institution
- Reports that employees who make suggestions for change or support consumer rights are subjected to harassment, even loss of their position

Certainly not all of these points apply to every healthcare institution, but they do inhibit the full implementation of TQM where they do apply.

*The healthcare organization's culture must have precedence over any other professional subgroup's culture for TQM to be successful*

—Zabada, 1998, p. 3

The cost of the quality improvement process is also an issue. Staff time required to investigate the quality of services provided by the organization must be counted as a cost in the provision of those services. The time given to developing tools, planning methods, collecting and interpreting data, identifying problems, and solving them all need to be included in this cost. The same questions asked about patient care must be asked about the quality improvement program itself: "Is it accomplishing what we want it to accomplish? What are the outcomes? Are they the ones we want?"

If increased effectiveness results—for example, reductions in lengths of stay, improvements in patients' self-care ability after discharge, and reduced wound infection rate—and these outcomes occur because problems previously identified have been addressed and improved procedures or outcomes of care have resulted, then it can be said that the quality improvement program itself is cost effective. Some methods may ultimately be too time-consuming for the results obtained. On the other hand, failure to invest adequate time in the process of accounting for the quality of care provided may result in great waste in the long run if the quality of care is poor, costly in terms of resources, or both.

# ● SUMMARY

Quality is defined as conformance to the needs of the client, as opposed to nonconformance. The process of quality improvement follows a pattern based on problem solving. It may be retrospective, concurrent, or prospective and may focus on structure, process, outcomes, or all three. When focused on nursing care, it should include the independent, dependent, and interdependent functions of nurses. Data collection procedures include record audits, observation, interviews, questionnaires, and focus groups.

The goal of quality improvement is to achieve optimal patient outcomes while keeping costs reasonable. Continuous quality improvement is a continuing, cyclical process. Total quality management is an organizationwide philosophy. Its implementation requires the commitment of administration and the participation of every employee from every department and discipline.

At the unit level, a quality improvement project begins with assignment of responsibility and identification of an area for study. Once the scope of care is defined, the problem is further analyzed in terms of its important aspects, generally accepted standards of care, indicators that the standards have been met, and criteria for deciding whether those standards were sufficiently met.

At the organizational level, implementation of TQM begins with its adoption by the admin-

# C A S E  S T U D Y

### Nursing and Outpatient Pharmacy

"Did you review the latest patient satisfaction ratings?" the CEO asked the CNO.

"Yes." Something like a sigh escaped from the CNO. "At least we're not dead last in department averages. Outpatient pharmacy's rating is even lower than ours. Seriously, I am frustrated. Nothing we do seems to improve our ratings. Social work, speech therapy, respiratory therapy, psychology, discharge planning—all have improved. Most have met or exceeded their benchmark but our ratings haven't budged."

"What do you think happened to outpatient pharmacy? Their ratings dropped like a stone."

"They had a big staff cut last fall, remember? I hear the waiting times have zoomed from 15 minutes last year to a 40-minute average wait this year."

"That makes sense. We'll have to review the advisability of that cut we made. Maybe it was too big. Now, what's the problem with nursing? Is it as obvious?"

"I don't think so but let me think about it awhile and review the ratings with the staff. Is it okay if I get back to you by next Monday?"

### Questions for Critical Reflection and Analysis

1. Why are patient satisfaction ratings important? What do they tell you about the quality of nursing care? What *don't* they tell you?
2. In the case study, the CNO planned to talk with staff. What else could the CNO do to learn the reasons for the poor patient satisfaction ratings for nursing?
3. Compare the way nursing services are delivered with the typical mode of service delivery in pharmacy and speech therapy. What aspects are similar? What aspects are different?
4. Create a possible scenario for discovering the reasons behind nursing's low rating and the actions needed to bring it up to its benchmark.

istration as a management philosophy. Mechanisms for its implementation are then put in place and the process of identifying areas for study, measuring work processes and outcomes, and evaluating the results is begun. Management as well as staff should be included both as participants and as subjects for study.

## REFERENCES

American Nurses Association. (1996). *Nursing's quality report card OUTCOMES project.* Washington, DC.

Bernard, M., Bestor, W., Karsner, G. & LeMay, C. (1994). The role of the CFO in CQI. *Healthcare Financial Management, 48*(4), 60–72.

Betta, P.A. (1992). Developing a successful ambulatory QA program. *Nursing Management, 23*(4), 31–33, 47–54.

Carman, J.M., Shortell, S.M., Foster, R.W., Hughes, E.F.X., Boerstler, H., O'Brien, J.L. & O'Connor, E.J.

(1996). Keys for successful implementation of total quality management in hospitals. *Health Care Management Review, 21*(1), 48–60.

Clancy, C.M. & Eisenberg, J.M. (1997). Outcomes research at the Agency for Health Care Policy and Research. *Disease Management and Clinical Outcomes, 1*(3), 72–80.

Cound, D.M. (1992). *A leader's journey to quality.* Milwaukee: ASQC Press.

Crosby, P.B. (1979). *Quality is free.* New York: McGraw-Hill.

Curtin, L.L. (1997). Looking for outcomes in all the wrong places. *Nursing Management, 28*(4), 7–8.

Deming, W.E. (1982). *Out of crisis.* Cambridge, MA: MIT Center for Advanced Engineering Study.

Dienemann, J. (1992). *Continuous quality improvement in nursing.* Washington, DC: American Nurses Association.

Donabedian, A. (1969). A guide to medical care administration. *Medical Care Appraisal—Quality and*

*Utilization, Vol II.* New York: American Public Health Association.

Donabedian, A. (1977). Evaluating the quality of medical care. *Milbank Memorial Fund Quarterly, 44*(Part 2), 166.

Donabedian, A. (1987). Some basic issues in evaluating the quality of health care. In L.T. Rinke (Ed.). *Outcome measures in home care.* New York: National League for Nursing.

Duquette, A.M. (1991). Approaches to monitoring practice: Getting started. In P. Schroeder (Ed.). *Monitoring and Evaluation in Nursing.* Gaithersburg, MD: Aspen.

Eigen, L.D. & Siegel, J.P. (1989). *The manager's book of quotations.* New York: AMACOM.

Elrod, M.E.B. (1991). Quality assurance: Challenges and dilemmas in acute care medical-surgical environments. In P. Schroeder (Ed.). *Monitoring and Evaluation in Nursing.* Gaithersburg, MD: Aspen.

Emmett, M. (1999). Outcomes-based quality improvement: A method for creating and managing change. Paper presented at the American Society on Aging Annual Meeting, Orlando, FL, March 6.

Gillespie, K. (1998). State strives to turn data into health policy information. *Advances, 1, 3, 9.*

Hunt, V.D. (1992). *Quality in America: How to implement a competitive quality program.* Homewood, IL: Business One Irwin.

Irvine, D. (1998). Finding value in nursing care: A framework for quality improvement and clinical evaluation. *Nursing Economics, 16*(3), 110–118.

Johnson, M. & Maas, M. (1997). *Nursing outcomes classification* (NOC). St Louis: Mosby.

Joint Commission on Accreditation of Healthcare Organizations. (1993). *Accreditation manual for hospitals, 1993.* Oakbrook Terrace, IL.

Kinlaw, D.C. (1992). *Continuous improvement and measurement for total quality.* Homewood, IL: Business One Irwin.

Kleinpell, R.M. (1997). Whose outcomes: Patients, providers or payers? *Nursing Clinics of North America, 32*(3), 513–520.

Leebov, W. (1991). *The quality quest: A briefing for health care professionals.* Chicago: American Hospital Publishing, Inc.

Lichtig, L.K., Knauf, R.A. & Milholland, D.K. (1999). Some impacts of nursing on acute care hospital outcomes. *Journal of Nursing Administration, 29*(2), 25–33.

Mark, B.A., Salyer, J. & Geddis, N. (1997). Outcomes research: Clues to quality and organizational effectiveness? *Nursing Clinics of North America, 32*(3), 589–601.

Phaneuf, M. (1976). *The nursing audit: Self-regulation in nursing practice.* New York: Appleton Century-Crofts.

Quality Circles in Human Services. (1986, August 6). Presented by Wassaic Developmental Disabilities Service Office, New York.

Short, N.M. & Bair, L. (1990). Standards of care: Practicing what we preach. *Nursing Management, 21*(6), 32–39.

Simpson, R.L. (1994). Benchmarking MIS performance. *Nursing Management, 25*(1), 20–21.

Simpson, R.L. (1997a). Finally, a central place to evaluate nursing systems. *Nursing Management, 28*(7), 17–18.

Simpson, R.L. (1997b). The nursing management minimum data set initiative needs you! *Nursing Management, 28*(6), 20–21.

Strickland, O. (1997). Challenges in measuring patient outcomes. *Nursing Clinics of North America, 32*(3), 495–512.

Wong, W.Y.L. (1998). A holistic perspective on quality quests and quality gains: The role of environment. *Total Quality Management, 9*(4–5), S241(5).

Zabada, C. (1998). Obstacles to the application of total quality management in health-care organizations. *Total Quality Management, 9*(1), 57–59.

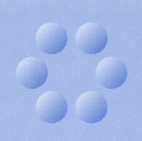

# Workplace Ethics

## LEARNING OBJECTIVES

*After completing this chapter, the reader will be able to:*

- Define personal and professional values, morals, and ethics.
- Explain the ethical principle(s) upon which decisions in the workplace are made.
- Identify the common ethical issues that arise in the workplace, particularly in healthcare settings.

- Apply personal and professional values and ethical principles in resolution of ethical dilemmas.
- Discuss the nurse manager's role in supporting ethical practice.

## TEST YOURSELF

**A personal and confidential ethics audit**

*The following "ethics audit" is designed to stimulate your thinking about the ethical side of the healthcare business and your own personal standards.*

*Personal Values*

*The most important thing in life is to decide what is most important. Look over the following list of values. Circle any values that "jump out" because of their importance to you. Then write your top three values, in order of importance. Feel free to add values if needed.*

| | | |
|---|---|---|
| truth | persistence | resources |
| efficiency | sincerity | dependability |
| initiative | fun | trust |
| environmentalism | relationships | excellence |
| power | wisdom | teamwork |
| control | flexibility | service |
| courage | perspective | profitability |
| competition | commitment | freedom |
| excitement | recognition | friendship |
| creativity | learning | influence |
| happiness | honesty | justice |
| honor | originality | quality |
| innovation | candor | hard work |
| obedience | prosperity | responsiveness |
| financial growth | respect | fulfillment |
| community support | fairness | purposefulness |
| integrity | order | strength |
| peace | spirituality | self-control |
| loyalty | adventure | cleverness |
| clarity | cooperation | success |
| security | humor | stewardship |
| love | collaboration | support |

1. _____

_____

_____

2. _____

_____

_____

3. _____

_____

_____

*Organization Values*

*Now, look at the list a second time. What do you think a healthcare organization should stand for? Again, circle the values that "jump out" because of their importance to you. Then write the top three in order of importance.*

1. _____

_____

_____

2. _____

_____

_____

3. _____

_____

_____

*Source:* Blanchard, K. & O'Connor, M. (1997). *Managing by values.* San Francisco: Berrett-Koehler.

Questions of right and wrong arise frequently in the workplace. Some of them are related to relatively minor incidents:

- Is it wrong to take home some sterile dressings and disinfectant for a scout troop project?
- An aide signed in at 7:00 A.M., but he really arrived at 7:03. Should I report him?

Others concern major issues:

- Is it wrong to go out on strike?
- Is it right to resign because staffing is so poor that it puts our patients' lives in jeopardy?
- A tech was fired for something someone else did. Should I intervene or mind my own business?
- My employer is billing for services not actually provided; should I report it? Will I be fired if I do?

These and other ethics-related questions have few if any easy answers. In this chapter we begin by defining personal and professional values, morals and ethics and considering the principles upon which ethics-related decisions are usually made in the workplace. Common issues and dilemmas that arise at work, particularly in a healthcare setting, are described next. Finally, acting in accord with one's ethical principles, resolving dilemmas, and supporting ethical practices in the workplace are discussed.

## ETHICS, MORALS, AND VALUES

### Values

Values are **judgments about the importance** of objects, ideas, attitudes, and actions. A **value system** is a set of related values. For example, one person may value (believe to be important) material things such as financial success, new cars and fashionable clothing. Another may value kindness, charity, and caring.

A person's value system affects the decisions he or she makes. For example, while one person may base a decision on cost, another person in the same situation may base the decision on kindness.

Values are learned (Wright, 1987). They can be taught directly and modeled through one's

---

**Box 20–1    American Nurses Association Code for Nurses**

1. The nurse provides services with respect for human dignity and the uniqueness of the client, unrestricted by considerations of social or economic status, personal attributes, or the nature of health problems.
2. The nurse safeguards the client's right to privacy by judiciously protecting information of a confidential nature.
3. The nurse acts to safeguard the client and the public when health care and safety are affected by the incompetent, unethical, or illegal practice of any person.
4. The nurse assumes responsibility and accountability for individual nursing judgments and actions.
5. The nurse maintains competence in nursing.
6. The nurse exercises informed judgment and uses individual competence and qualifications as criteria in seeking consultation, accepting responsibilities, and delegating nursing activities to others.
7. The nurse participates in activities that contribute to the ongoing development of the profession's body of knowledge.
8. The nurse participates in the profession's effort to implement and improve standards of nursing.
9. The nurse participates in the profession's efforts to establish and maintain conditions of employment conducive to high quality nursing care.
10. The nurse participates in the profession's effort to protect the public from misinformation and misrepresentation and to maintain the integrity of nursing.
11. The nurse collaborates with members of the health professions and other citizens in promoting community and national efforts to meet the health needs of the public.

*Source:* American Nurses Association. (1985). *Code for nurses.* Washington, DC: ANA Publishing. Reprinted with permission.

---

actions. Children learn them by observing their parents, teachers, and religious leaders and eventually adopt them as their own. Values also change with experience and maturity. As you enter the profession of nursing, for example, you will acquire a set of **professional values** in addition to your own **personal values.** Autonomy, integrity, and commitment to the profession are professional values. Strong family ties and acceptance by one's peers are personal values.

Knowing what people value is important to those who wish to lead them. At times, people take risks, give up their own comfort or security, and generate extraordinary effort because of what they value (Edge & Groves, 1994). Our values also influence our judgment of other people. For example, if you value work over leisure, you would look unfavorably on a colleague who refuses to stay late to finish a project.

## Morals

**Ethics and morals** deal with questions of the **rightness or wrongness** of human behavior and the motives behind that behavior. The term **morals** is usually used to refer to an individual's personal code of acceptable behavior. As with values, each of us has our own set of moral standards. You may find, for example, that your views on the acceptability of such behaviors as premarital sex, taking drugs, or gambling differ considerably from those of your classmates or coworkers because each of you has a different personal moral code.

## Ethics

The term **ethics** is used more frequently in the professional literature. Ethical codes are based on principles that can be used to guide decisions and judge behavior. A code of ethics is one of the hallmarks of a profession. An example is the American Nurses Association Code for Nurses, which can be found in Box 20–1.

The Code for Nurses is a dynamic, evolving document that has been revised several times to reflect changes in nursing practice and in the context in which nurses practice. In the 1968 revision, reference to personal ethics was deleted, sharpening the focus on professional ethics. The 1985 version addressed additional ethical issues such as extension of life (Fowler, 1999). Commitment to caring for people and to patient advocacy are clearly spelled out in the Code. However, the effects of economic constraints on the healthcare system and how nurses should respond to these constraints are not directly addressed.

> *Professional nurses are accountable for nursing judgments and actions regardless of the personal consequences. Providing safe nursing care to the patient is the ultimate objective of the professional nurse and the healthcare facility.*
>
> —ANA, 1985

The extent to which nurses have the power to act as moral agents or to bring about changes needed to protect their patients is a question that needs further study and discussion (Hamric, 1999). In a study, Hamric (1999) found that nurses' willingness to take action to resolve an ethical dilemma was related to their perceived degree of influence in the situation, degree of clinical expertise, ethical concern, and ethics education. As Hamric points out, many dilemmas faced by nurses arise from the power structure and political dynamics of the organization and the healthcare system overall. In many cases, resolution of these dilemmas requires a political approach.

Although they may serve as the basis for laws, ethical standards are not themselves laws. Laws are rules created by a governing body and enforced by the power of that governing body. They usually are quite specific and include punishment for disobeying them. You could say that ethical principles speak to the essence or foundation of the law rather than to the specificities of the law (Macklin, 1987).

## ● BASIS FOR MAKING ETHICAL DECISIONS

### Core Values

Certain values appear repeatedly in statements of ethics in the workplace. These include the following:

- Honesty
- Integrity
- Fairness
- Trustworthiness
- Respect
- Responsibility
- Accountability
- Good citizenship (Webley, 1997)

In healthcare settings, patient welfare and excellence in the delivery of health care are additional core values. In contrast, deception and greed are often cited as immoral and unethical values found to prevail in some organizations.

> *Business ethics . . . has to do with the authenticity and integrity of the enterprise.*
>
> —McCoy, 1997, p. 59

### Beneficence

Called a "sacred, ethical principle" in health care (Flarey, 1999, p. 3), the principle of beneficence demands that we act in the best interests of others. For nurses, it means not only doing no harm (often separated out as the principle of **nonmaleficence**) but also contributing to others' welfare, which includes advocating for patients and reporting concerns to supervisors and to others who can remedy a potentially harmful situation. (For an illustration, see Research Example 20–1,

**Research Example 20–1**   *When a Colleague Is Chemically Impaired: Ethical Decision Making by Critical Care Nurses*

Some ethical dilemmas present us with equally unsatisfactory alternatives from which to choose, which is often the case when a staff nurse is confronted with an incompetent or impaired colleague. How would most nurses respond? Hughes and Dvorak (1997) asked 82 critical care staff nurses to read a scenario about a chemically impaired colleague and then evaluate the ethical, clinical, social, legal, and professional consequences of five alternative actions:

1. Wait and see what happens.
2. Report the incident to the state board of nursing.
3. Report the incident to the state nurses association peer assistance network.
4. Report the incident to the head nurse (a friend of the impaired colleague).
5. Confront the impaired colleague privately.

Doing nothing (#1) was ranked last by 69% of the respondents. Confronting one's colleague (#5) was ranked first by 67%. This action was followed, in order, by reporting to the head nurse, calling the peer assistance network, and notifying the board of nursing.

The researchers found it disconcerting that individual confrontation ranked higher than referral to organized intervention, noting that private confrontation could encourage more secretive behavior on the part of the impaired colleague.

*Source:* Hughes, K.K. & Dvorak, E.M. (1997). The use of decision analysis to examine ethical decision making by critical care nurses. *Heart & Lung: The Journal of Acute & Critical Care, 26*(3), 238–248.

When a Colleague Is Chemically Impaired: Ethical Decision Making by Critical Care Nurses.)

The opposite of beneficence is **maleficence,** the harm that can be done if the principle of beneficence is violated. This maleficence includes physical harm, economic harm, and psychological harm. Of these, the danger of causing physical harm has been found to be of greatest concern to managers (Weber, 1996).

## General Principles

In addition to beneficence and nonmaleficence, a number of principles form the basis for making ethics-related decisions in the workplace. The following list names some common ones (Larimer, 1997; Solomon, 1997). You will probably find some of them congruent with your value system and may find others to be repellent to you:

**Egoism:** Make the decision on the basis of the greatest benefit to yourself.

*Ask yourself:* What are the consequences for me?

**Empathy:** Make the decision on the basis of compassion for others.

*Ask yourself:* If I were in [the other person's] position, what would I want? How would I feel?

**Utilitarianism:** Choose the alternative that brings the greatest good for the greatest number of people.

*Ask yourself:* Will it benefit most of the people who will be affected?

**Darwinism:** Side with the likely survivor or winner.

*Ask yourself:* Who's going to win?

**Existentialism:** Decide on the basis of what feels right, not on the basis of the consequences.

*Ask yourself:* What is my gut feeling in this situation?

**Religious Belief:** Use religious teachings and codes to guide decisions.

*Ask yourself:* What would God want me to do?

**Authority:** Look for legal precedents, professional codes, and organizational statements of values to guide the decision.

*Ask yourself:* What is the relevant rule here?

**Conformism:** Do whatever the majority would expect you to do.

*Ask yourself:* What do my colleagues think I should do?

Research indicates that managers most often base their decisions on the utilitarian principle (Weber, 1996).

## ● ETHICAL DILEMMAS

When two or more principles conflict with each other, making a decision or judgment may be difficult. Ethical dilemmas occur when a situation exists that forces a choice between ethical principles because deciding in favor of one principle will violate another. All options have good and bad aspects or consequences and no choice satisfies all principles. Ethical dilemmas occur in every aspect of our lives, personal and professional. When you are directly involved in such a situation, identification of the underlying values and principles involved is the first step in resolving the dilemma.

### Interpersonal Dilemmas

When two or more individuals or groups use different principles to guide their decision, each side may consider the other side unethical—obviously a situation full of potential for conflict (Solomon, 1997). The following is an example:

> Vicki Thomas had been employed as a home health aide for 5 months when a wealthy client invited Vicki to accompany her on a world cruise. The client needed some assistance with personal care and was impressed with Vicki's skill and calm demeanor.
> Vicki requested a 6-week leave of absence from the agency. Her supervisor thought it was

a wonderful opportunity for Vicki and recommended granting the leave (on the basis of the principle of **empathy**). The agency director vetoed the recommendation. She pointed out that leaves and vacations were not granted until the employee had worked at least 11 months. Strict adherence to the rules had always been the agency's policy and she was surprised that the manager was willing to bend the rules (the principle of **authority** is operating here). The manager thought she was being "rigid"; the director thought of herself as "principled." Each was disappointed in the other; each felt the other was wrong.

Situations such as this one call for judgment. The potential for conflict lies in the fact that the people involved used different principles to guide their decisions. The question of whether Vicki should have been granted the requested leave has no single correct answer.

### Intrapersonal Dilemmas

Another type of difficult decision arises when you find yourself in a situation where two of your own principles are relevant but in conflict. These decisions are usually between right and right rather than right and wrong. Badaracco (1998) calls these situations **defining moments** because they challenge us to further explore and weigh the relative importance of the principles that are in conflict. It is through these defining moments that we eventually shape our personal and professional identities and what we stand for. The following is an example adapted from a case suggested by Badaracco (1998).

> Imagine you are in upper-level management. A dilemma is brought to you by one of your most thoughtful, conscientious directors. KT is a highly competent, caring nurse. She is also a single parent with a child who has been having difficulty in school. RS is an ambitious, hard-driving nurse manager. She is impatient with KT's frequent requests to leave early or come in an hour late and her refusals to work overtime.
> For the director, support of KT represents support of her principles of empathy and existentialism. She can imagine herself in KT's position

**(empathy)** *and it simply does not feel right to her to be hard on KT when she is dealing with a family crisis* **(existentialism).** *On the other hand, support of RS represents support for other important principles:* **utilitarianism** *and au* **thority.** *KT's requests for time off mean that other staff nurses have to fill in for her and at times this has been difficult to do (utilitarianism). In addition, staff are expected to take turns working overtime so no one is over-burdened with it (utilitarianism and authority).*

*RS has repeatedly requested permission to fire KT. If the director grants RS's request, she is supporting a set of values that could be called her "work ethic." If she denies the request, she is supporting what is popularly called "family values." Which is more important?*

When the director makes her choice, she will be contributing to the definition of who she is and what she believes in as an administrator and as a person. It will be a defining moment for the director.

## ● ETHICAL ISSUES OF THE WORKPLACE

### Levels of Interaction

From a systems point of view, a number of different levels of interaction can generate questions of ethics in the workplace (Solomon, 1997). The first is the **intrapersonal** level. At this level, healthcare professionals can find that two or more cherished values are in conflict in a situation. At the second, **interpersonal** level, they may find that their values are not the same as those held dear by colleagues. The third level is **intraorganizational,** the interaction between individuals and the organization. At this level, individuals may find their goals and values to be in conflict with those of the organization. The next level is **interorganizational,** the interaction between various organizations such as a home health agency and referring hospital. Also of interest is the **healthcare system,** which includes many additional players: insurers, managed care organizations, private practices, government agencies, individual practitioners, individual patients, and so forth.

### Types of Issues

Across these levels, a number of ethical issues arise in the workplace. A study entitled "Sources and Consequences of Workplace Pressures: Increasing the Risk of Unethical and Illegal Business Practices" revealed that 48 percent of the employees surveyed said they had been involved in one or more unethical and/or illegal actions in the last year (Greengard, 1997). The most common of these with the percentage who mentioned them were as follows (Digh, 1998):

| | |
|---|---|
| 16% | Cutting corners (thus reducing quality) |
| 14% | Covering up incidents |
| 11% | Lying about sick days |
| 9% | Deceiving customers |
| 5% | Lying to supervisors |
| 4% | Taking credit for colleagues' ideas |

Certain ethical concerns are specific to a healthcare setting. The following is a sampling of additional issues you may confront in the workplace.

- *Gifts:* The potential effect of the gift on the receiver, particularly its effect on equality of treatment, is a concern in health care. Ask yourself whether the giver holds any expectation of a favor in return (Kaptein, 1998).
- *Theft and property damage:* These actions are not only illegal but also harmful in the sense that they raise costs when lost or damaged material and equipment needed to provide services must be replaced.
- *Cover-ups:* On occasion, employees are asked to change or destroy information that could be damaging to an individual or to the organization (Weber, 1996). Despite the legal and ethical concerns about doing so, employees are sometimes tempted to do this to protect someone or because they fear retaliation if they refuse.
- *Leaking confidential information:* Whether done through thoughtlessness or deliberate action, revealing confidential information can harm the organization as well as the individuals involved, patients or employees.
- *Inappropriate assignments:* The American Nurses Association (1997) supports nurses' obligation to reject an assignment that puts patients and/or themselves in serious, immediate jeopardy. Nurses also need to exercise judg-

ment in assigning responsibility to others. Many state nurses' associations have developed Assignment Despite Objection (ADO) forms and published guidelines for responding to inappropriate assignments (see Box 20–2).

- *Reporting fraud (whistleblowing):* Padding costs, submitting bills for services not actually given, and offering kickbacks for referring patients are some examples of the type of fraud that occurs in health care. Federal laws are in place to encourage reporting of these illegal acts and to protect whistleblowers from various kinds of retaliation, such as being fired, demoted, harassed, etc. (Kleimen, 1999).
- *Protecting patients:* Inadequate staff, incompetent practitioners, unavailable or overly expensive services, and human error can put individuals' lives in jeopardy. These situations are in violation of the principle of beneficence and the ANA Code for Nurses.

## Organizational Issues

Reiser writes that healthcare organizations "declare what really counts" by their treatment of employees, students, patients, and other stakeholders and by the way they handle controversy and conflict (1994, p. 28). Any contradictions between what they declare to be their values and their behavior produces cynicism in the staff. Reiser urges the inclusion of ethical analysis in administrative, policymaking, and interpersonal aspects of healthcare organizations' operations.

Solomon (1997) created a list of "seven deadly sins" often committed by managers. The examples following each of these "sins" are drawn from health-related situations.

1. Ignore major social problems.
   *Example:* "None of *our* patients have an alcohol or drug misuse problem."
2. Place blame on someone else.
   *Example:* "It's the insurance companies, they won't let us . . ."
3. Discredit outside critics.
   *Example:* From tobacco producers: "The research showing the relationship of cancer and smoking is flawed."
4. Fire anyone who disagrees.

*Example:* From a nursing home facing unionization: "Anyone who questions administrative decisions will be fired."
5. Suppress information.
   *Example:* From a biomedical device manufacturer that funded clinical trials on one of their devices: "We reserve the right to disseminate or suppress the results in the manner we choose."
6. Counter with a public relations campaign.
   *Example:* "Ignore the statistics: We have the BEST open heart unit in the state. We offer luxurious patient rooms with large screen TVs, round-the-clock food service . . ."
7. Deny charges.
   *Example:* From pharmaceutical manufacturers: "Those few deaths were due to preexisting conditions, not our new drug."

Many of the issues listed affect the entire organization. To a great extent, administrators of an organization set the tone for the entire organization, not only through mission statements and statements of values or principles, but also through their behavior within the organization (Blanchard & O'Connor, 1997).

## Systemwide Issues

If the seven deadly sins and the other practices listed are widespread, they can affect the entire healthcare system. One of the most critical issues at the healthcare system level is how the "bottom line," profit-oriented thinking of business (Parker, 1998) can be reconciled with the principles of beneficence and nonmaleficence that Flarey (1999) called the "sacred" principles of health care. Considerable debate on this subject has led to many statements and position papers from various scholars and interested organizations. Two of these papers, from the National Academies of Practice and the Tavistock Group, are described here.

The National Academies of Practice, an interdisciplinary association of healthcare professionals, has taken a firm position on the potential effects of cost containment on patient care: "*. . . it is unethical to compromise a patient's needs and quality care concerns to satisfy financial objectives*" (NAP, 1998).

**Box 20–2  Guidelines for the Registered Nurse in Giving, Accepting, or Rejecting a Work Assignment**

Registered nurses, as licensed professionals, share the responsibility and accountability along with their employer to ensure that safe nursing care is provided at an acceptable level of quality. This accountability is both a legal responsibility as specified in the Nurse Practice Act and an ethical one as indicated in the American Nurses Association's (ANA) *Code for Nurses*. In addition, employer requirements are outlined in the healthcare facility personnel policies and clinical guidelines/procedures.

The ANA *Code for Nurses* states, "The nurse exercises informed judgment and uses individual competence and qualifications as criteria in seeking consultation, accepting responsibilities, and delegating nursing activities to others." The nurse's decision regarding accepting or making work assignments is based on the legal, ethical, and professional obligation to assume responsibility for nursing judgment and action.

**SCENARIOS**

- Suppose you are asked to care for an unfamiliar patient population or to go to a unit for which you feel unqualified. What do you do?
- Suppose you are approached by your supervisor and asked to work an additional shift. Your immediate response is that you don't want to work another shift. What do you do?

Such situations are familiar and emphasize the rights and responsibilities of the registered nurse to make informed decisions. Yet all members of the healthcare team, from staff nurses to administrator, share a joint responsibility to ensure that quality patient care is provided. At times, though, differences in interpretation of legal or ethical principles may lead to conflict.

This document endeavors to facilitate strategies for problem solving as the staff nurse, nurse manager, chief nurse executive, and administrator operationalize practice within the complex environment of the healthcare system.

**GUIDELINES FOR DECISION MAKING**

The complexity of the delivery of nursing care is such that only professional nurses with appropriate education and experience can provide nursing care. Upon employment with a healthcare facility the nurse contracts or enters into an agreement with that facility to provide nursing services in a collaborative practice environment.

**It is the nurse's responsibility to:**

- provide competent nursing care to the patient.
- exercise informed judgment and use individual competence and qualifications as criteria in seeking consultation, accepting responsibilities, and delegating nursing activities to others.
- clarify assignments, assess personal capabilities, jointly identify options for patient care assignments when he/she does not feel personally competent

*(continued)*

**Box 20–2 Guidelines for the Registered Nurse in Giving, Accepting, or Rejecting a Work Assignment** *(continued)*

or adequately prepared to carry out a specific function. The nurse has the right to refuse an assignment that he/she does not feel prepared to assume.

**It is the nursing management's responsibility to:**

- ensure competent nursing care is provided to the patient.
- evaluate the nurse's ability to provide specialized patient care.
- organize resources to ensure that patients receive appropriate nursing care.
- collaborate with the staff nurse to clarify assignments, assess personal capabilities, jointly identify options for patient care assignments when the nurse does not feel personally competent or adequately prepared to carry out a specific function. The facility has the right to take appropriate disciplinary action according to facility policies.
- provide education to staff and supervisory personnel in the decision-making process regarding patient care assignments and reassignments, including patient placement and allocation of resources.

**It is the healthcare facility's responsibility to:**

- ensure competent nursing care is provided to the patient.
- plan and budget for staffing patterns based upon patients' requirements and priorities for care.
- provide a clearly defined written mechanism for immediate internal review of proposed assignments, which includes the participation of the staff involved, to help avoid conflict.

**Issues central to potential dilemmas are:**

- the right of the patient to receive safe professional nursing care at an acceptable level of quality.
- the responsibility for an appropriate utilization and distribution of nursing care services when nursing becomes a scarce resource.
- the responsibility for providing a practice environment that assures adequate nursing resources for the facility, while meeting the current socioeconomic and political realities of shrinking healthcare dollars.

**LEGAL ISSUES**

Behaviors and activities relevant to giving, accepting, or rejecting a work assignment that could lead to the disciplinary action include:

- practicing or offering to practice beyond the scope permitted by law, or accepting and performing professional responsibilities the licensee knows or has reason to know that he or she is not competent to perform; performing, without adequate supervision, professional services the licensee is authorized to perform only under the supervision of a licensed professional, except in an emergency situation where a person's life or health is in danger.
- abandoning or neglecting a patient or client who is in need of nursing care without making reasonable arrangements for the continuation of such care.

*(continued)*

**Box 20–2    Guidelines for the Registered Nurse in Giving, Accepting, or Rejecting a Work Assignment *(continued)***

• failure to exercise supervision over persons who are authorized to practice only under the supervision of the licensed professional.

Of the preceding issue, abandonment or neglect has thus far proven the most legally devastating. Abandonment or neglect has been legally defined to include such actions as insufficient observation (frequency of contact), failure to assure competent intervention when the patient's condition changes (qualified physician not in attendance), and withdrawal of services without provision for qualified coverage. Because nurses at all levels most frequently act as agents of the employing facility, the facility shares the risk of liability with the nurse.

**APPLICATION OF GUIDELINES FOR DECISION MAKING**

The following are some specific examples of how a nurse may apply the guidelines for decision making and the legal concepts as have been outlined in this document.

**SCENARIO—A QUESTION OF COMPETENCE**

An example of a potential dilemma is when an evening supervisor pulls a psychiatric nurse to the coronary care unit (CCU) because of a lack of nursing staff. The CCU census has risen and no additional qualified staff is available.

Suppose you are asked to care for an unfamiliar patient population or to go to a unit for which you feel unqualified. What do you do?

1. CLARIFY what it is you are being asked to do.
   • How many patients will you be expected to care for?
   • Does the care of these patients require you to have special knowledge and skills in order to deliver safe nursing care?
   • Will qualified and experienced RNs be present on the unit?
   • What procedures and/or medications will you be expected to administer?
   • What kind of orientation do you need to function safely in this unfamiliar setting?
2. ASSESS yourself. Do you have the knowledge and skill to meet the expectations that have been outlined to you? Have you had experience with similar patient populations? Have you been oriented to this unit or a similar unit? Would the perceived discrepancies between your abilities and the expectations lead to an unsafe patient care situation?
3. IDENTIFY options and implications of your decision.
   a. If you perceive that you can provide safe patient care you should accept the assignment. You would now be ethically and legally responsible for the nursing care of these patients.
   b. If you perceive a discrepancy between abilities and the expectations of the assignment, further dialogue with the nurse supervisor is needed before you reach a decision. At this point it may be appropriate to consult the next level of management, such as the house supervisor or the chief nurse executive.

*(continued)*

**Box 20–2   Guidelines for the Registered Nurse in Giving, Accepting, or Rejecting a Work Assignment** *(continued)*

In further dialogue, continue to assess whether you are qualified to accept either a portion or the whole of the requested assignment. Also point out options that might be mutually beneficial. For example, obviously it would be unsafe for you to administer chemotherapy without prior training. However, if someone else administered the chemotherapy perhaps you could provide the remainder of the required nursing care for that patient. If you feel unqualified for the assignment in its entirety, the dilemma becomes more complex.

At this point it is important for you to be aware of the legal rights of the facility. Even though you may have legitimate concern for patient safety and your own legal accountability in providing safe care, the facility has legal precedent to initiate disciplinary action, including termination, if you refuse to accept an assignment. Therefore, it is important to continue to explore options in a positive manner, recognizing that both you and the facility have a responsibility for safe patient care.

4. POINT OF DECISION/IMPLICATIONS. If none of the options are acceptable, you are at your final decision point.
   a. Accept the assignment, documenting carefully your concern for patient safety and the process you used to inform the facility (manager) of your concerns. Keep a personal copy of this documentation and send a copy to the chief nurse executive. Courtesy suggests that you also send a copy to the manager(s) involved. Once you have reached this decision it is unwise to discuss the situation or your feelings with other staff or patients. Now you are legally accountable for these patients. From this point withdrawal from the agreed-upon assignment may constitute abandonment.
   b. Refuse the assignment, being prepared for disciplinary action. Document your concern for patient safety and the process you used to inform the facility (manager) of your concerns. Keep a personal copy of this documentation and send a copy to the nurse executive. Courtesy suggests that you also send a copy to the manager(s) involved.
   c. Document the steps taken in making your decision. It may be necessary for you to use the facility's grievance procedure.

**SCENARIO—A QUESTION OF AN ADDITIONAL SHIFT**

An example of another potential dilemma is when a nurse who recognizes his/her fatigue and its potential for patient harm is required to work an additional shift.

Suppose you are approached by your supervisor and asked to work an additional shift. Your immediate response is that you don't want to work another shift. What do you do?

1. CLARIFY what it is you are expected to do.
   For example, would the additional shift be with the same patients you are currently caring for, or would it involve a new patient assignment?

*(continued)*

**Box 20–2    Guidelines for the Registered Nurse in Giving, Accepting, or Rejecting a Work Assignment** *(continued)*

- Is your reluctance to work another shift because of a new patient assignment you do not feel competent to accept? (If the answer is yes, then refer to the previous example, "A Question of Competence.")
- Is your reluctance to work due to fatigue, or do you have other plans?
- Is it a chronic request due to poor scheduling, inadequate staffing, or chronic absenteeism?
- Are you being asked to work because no relief nurse is coming for your present patient assignment? Because your unit will be short of professional staff on the next shift? Because another unit will be short of professional staff on the next shift?
- How long are you being asked to work, the entire shift or a portion of the shift?

2. ASSESS yourself.

Are you really tired, or do you just not feel like working? Is your fatigue level such that your care may be unsafe? Remember, you are legally responsible for the care of your current patient assignment if relief is not available.

3. IDENTIFY OPTIONS and implications of your decision.
   a. If you perceive that you can provide safe patient care and are willing to work the additional shift, accept the assignment.
   b. If you perceive that you can provide safe patient care but are unwilling to stay due to other plans or the chronic nature of the request, inform the manager of your reasons for not wishing to accept the assignment.
   c. If you perceive that your fatigue will interfere with your ability to safely care for patients, indicate this fact to the manager.

If you do not accept the assignment and the manager continues to attempt to persuade you it may be appropriate to consult the next level of management, such as the house supervisor or the nurse executive.

In further dialogue continue to weigh your reasons for refusal versus the facility's need for an RN. If you have a strong alternate commitment, such as no child care, or if you seriously feel your fatigue will interfere with safe patient care, restate your reasons for refusal.

At this point, it is important for you to be aware of the legal rights of the facility. Even though you may have legitimate concern for patient safety and your own legal accountability in providing safe care, or legitimate concern for the safety of your children or other commitments, the facility has legal precedent to initiate disciplinary action, including termination, if you refuse to accept an assignment. Therefore, it is important to continue to explore options in a positive manner, recognizing both you and the facility have a responsibility for safe patient care.

4. POINT OF DECISION/IMPLICATIONS.
   a. Accept the assignment, documenting your professional concern for patient safety and the process you used to inform the facility (manager) of

*(continued)*

**Box 20–2    Guidelines for the Registered Nurse in Giving, Accepting, or Rejecting a Work Assignment *(continued)***

your concerns. Keep a personal copy of this documentation and send a copy to the nurse executive. Courtesy suggests that you also send a copy to the manager(s) involved. Once you have reached this decision it is unwise to discuss the situation or your feelings with other staff and/or patients.

b. Accept the assignment, documenting your professional concerns for the chronic nature of the request and possible long-term consequences in reducing the quality of care. Documentation should follow the procedures outlined in (a).

c. Accept the assignment, documenting your personal concerns regarding working conditions in which management decides the legitimacy of employee's personal commitments. This documentation should go to your manager to discuss the incident and your concerns regarding future requests.

d. Refuse the assignment, being prepared for disciplinary action. If your reasons for refusal were patient safety or an imperative personal commitment, document this fact carefully including the process you used to inform the facility (nurse manager) of your concerns. Keep a personal copy of this documentation and send a copy to the chief nurse executive. Courtesy suggests that you also send a copy to the manager(s) involved.

e. Document the rationale for your decision. It may be necessary to use the facility's grievance procedure.

**SUMMARY**

Some specific examples of how a nurse may apply the guidelines for decision making in the actual work situation have been presented. Staffing dilemmas will always be present and mandate that active communication between staff nurses and all levels of nursing management be maintained to assure patient safety. The likelihood of a satisfactory solution will increase if prior consideration of the choices is available. This consideration of available alternatives should include recognition that professional nurses are intelligent adults who should be involved in the decision-making process. Professional nurses are accountable for nursing judgments and actions regardless of the personal consequences. Providing safe nursing care to the patient is the ultimate objective of the professional nurse and the healthcare facility.

The **Florida Nurses Association Labor and Employment Relations Commission** acknowledges:

5. the work of the **North Carolina Nurses Association ad hoc Committee on RN Work Assignments** for their initial work in developing the concepts for this publication:
**Elizabeth A. Trought, M.N., R.N., Chairman**
Betty Baster, B.S., R.N., C.N.A.
Betty Benton, R.N.
Charlotte Hoelzel, M.S., R.N.

*(continued)*

> **Box 20–2 Guidelines for the Registered Nurse in Giving, Accepting, or Rejecting a Work Assignment** *(continued)*
>
> Joyce H. Monk, B.S.N., R.N.
> Eldean Pierce, M.S.N., R.N.
> Loucille Swain, R.N.
> Gladys Warlick, R.N.
> 6. the **Florida Organization of Nurse Executives** for input and collaboration in the development of the 1989 edition of this document.
> 7. the **Florid Nurses Association ad hoc Committee on Safe Nursing Practice** for final preparation of the revised 1989 edition of this document:
> Frank Moore, R.N., Chairman
> Richard Bednar, R.N.
> Phyllis Connerley, R.N.
> Gina Giovinco, R.N.
> Sandra Janzen, R.N.
> Pamela Erb, R.N.
> Katherine Mason, R.N.
> Paula Massey, R.N.

Protecting and maintaining the welfare of the patient is a fundamental principle in Western ethics, one that has been reiterated in professional codes and contemporary, regulatory codes (National Academies of Practice, 1998). Subordinating the patient's welfare to economic considerations is a threat to this principle. Herein lies the potential for serious conflict in the healthcare system. The fundamental goal of health care is to promote health and well-being while the fundamental goal of business is to make a profit. As the delivery of health care becomes increasingly business focused, these goals may come into conflict. Silva (1998) notes that while the principles of efficiency, competition, and profit making do not necessarily violate the principle of beneficence, they can lead to such abuses as refusal to pay for needed care, penalizing consumers and providers who exceed the limits set on choice and cost, and charging for services that were never given. Nurses working in such environments can experience feelings of anger, fear, powerlessness, and guilt (Silva, 1998).

Also of interest is the work of the Tavistock Group, an international interdisciplinary group that met at Tavistock Square in London to discuss healthcare issues. This group produced a list of five principles intended to serve as a starting point for discussion and a guide to ethical decision making in our healthcare systems (Berwick et al., 1999). The five principles are:

1. Health care is a human right.
2. The care of individuals is at the center of healthcare delivery but must be viewed and practiced within the overall context of continuing work to generate the greatest possible health gains for groups and populations.
3. The responsibilities of the healthcare delivery system include the prevention of illness and the alleviation of disability.
4. Cooperation with each other and those served is imperative for those working within the healthcare delivery system.
5. All individuals and groups involved in health care, whether providing access or services, have continuing responsibility to help improve its quality (Berwick et al., 1999).

The group emphasized the preliminary nature of these principles and encouraged comment, including ideas for implementation of the principles (Henry, 1999). It is hoped that insurers, regulators, providers, employers, governments, individual healthcare professionals, and the public will use them to stimulate debate and guide work on the improvement of the delivery of health care to all in need of it (Berwick et al., 1999).

> *The pressures to contain costs and formulate policies regarding allocation of scarce resources certainly strain, if not obliterate, what many perceive to be the obligations of hospitals toward individual patients and society as a whole.*
>
> —Hilliard, Coffey & Johnson, 1999, p. 27

## ● ETHICAL DECISION MAKING

### Acting in Accord with Your Principles

Living and working in accord with one's personal and professional codes of ethics begins with **thinking** and **reflecting** on what one is asked to do. Taking action follows reflection. The following six rules for ethical thinking are based on suggestions from Solomon (1997):

1. *Consider the well-being of others.*

   This principle of beneficence may be more familiar to you as the well known golden rule: *Do unto others as you would have them do unto you.* Solomon (1997) admits that few businesses will always focus on this rule but suggests that businesses are nevertheless able to contribute to the welfare of others and to avoid doing harm.

2. *Be a member in good standing of the health-care community.*

   Honesty and integrity in dealing with other agencies as well as with individuals are central to community membership. Charging reasonable prices and offering quality care are part of being a good organizational citizen.

3. *Obey the law.*

   Ethical behavior includes but also goes beyond the law. In fact, many laws have their foundation in ethical principles.

4. *Apply rules equitably.*

   Any rule worth following should be applied at all times and on all occasions. For ex-

ample, you do not retain one employee and fire another for the same infraction. It also means you do not go to great lengths for one patient and not for another. If the consequences of applying a rule consistently appear to cause harm, then the rule should be reevaluated.

5. *Respect others' principles but not at the expense of your own.*

   Solomon (1997) suggests that when your own principles conflict with another's, the priority should be your own.

6. *Act in concert with your principles.*

   Live out your principles, do not just give them lip service.

These rules are not easy to follow. In fact, you may want to reflect on the degree to which you agree with them, follow them, and see others following them.

> *We cannot quit our jobs over every ethical dilemma, but if we continually ignore our sense of values, who do we become?*
>
> —McCoy, 1997, p. 60

### Resolving Ethical Dilemmas

A five-step values-based guide to making ethical decisions is derived from Blanchard & O'Connor (1997):

1. *Issue:* What is the issue here? What decision are you being called upon to make?
2. *Impact:* Identify the people who will be affected by your decision: coworkers, managers, patients, families, administration, stakeholders, members of the community, members of your profession, etc.
3. *Principle:* Identify the values and related ethical principles involved in this situation. If they conflict, which one has the highest priority?
4. *Reflection:* Which of the values and/or principles involved is most important to you and to the profession?
5. *Action:* What action is called for?

The following example illustrates how this guide can be used when an ethics-related question arises at work:

*Unusually heavy traffic almost made Jeri Brown late for work. She arrived on the unit just 2 minutes before seven. "The director wanted you to call him as soon as you arrive," the nurse manager told her.*

*Jeri was in the third week of a 6-week orientation for new registered nurses. She had met the director just once since she began, during the first week of orientation. What could he want?*

*Jeri was pleased to hear the director say he had heard positive comments about her work so far. "I know you are only halfway through your orientation," he added, "but we have an unusual situation this morning. Mrs. Quincy resigned yesterday, leaving 2 South without a charge nurse. I'd like you to take over there today. If it goes well .. . . who knows. We might be able to keep you in this position."*

*"Me?" Jeri responded. "Can I think about it a moment?"*

*"Sure, call me back in 5 minutes. If you don't accept, I'll have to get someone else."*

*Jeri told her teammates what the director wanted her to do. "You're not ready!" her fellow orientee told her.*

*"Oh, you're just jealous. Go ahead, give it a try. It is the way to move up in a hurry here," the licensed practical nurse on the team advised her.*

*Jeri retreated to the staff lounge to think. She pulled out the "Guide to Values-Based Decision Making" that the CNO had distributed at one of the orientation meetings. She used it to evaluate her position:*

| | |
|---|---|
| **1. Issue** | *Accept or decline the charge nurse assignment.* |
| **2. Impact** | *The director, staff in 2 South, patients on 2 South, and administration could be affected by my decision.* |
| **3. Principles Involved** | |
| *Egoism:* | *It is an opportunity to win the director's favor and earn a promotion to charge nurse faster. I don't want to appear unco-* |

*operative or afraid to accept responsibility.*

| | |
|---|---|
| *Empathy:* | *The director is in a bind. I could solve his problem.* |
| *Nonmaleficence:* | *I'm new and inexperienced. My taking this position could stress the staff and put patients in jeopardy.* |
| *Beneficence:* | *An experienced individual would be a better choice.* |
| **4. Reflection** | *Too many people could be hurt by a decision to accept the assignment. Patient welfare is more important than personal ambition here.* |
| **5. Action** | *Decline, indicating interest in such an assignment when I'm ready for it.* |

*Later, Jeri heard that 2 South had 10 admissions, 7 discharges, and a patient code that day, which she also learned was a common occurrence on this unit. She wondered why the director had considered her for the charge nurse assignment. On what basis had he made his choice?*

## Management Role

A number of actions can be taken at the administrative level to encourage and support adherence to an agreed-upon set of values and ethical principles within an organization.

- Include discussion of ethics-related issues and the organization's position on these issues in employee orientation and subsequent inservice programs.
- Review organizational policies and procedures from an ethical perspective.
- Consult with legal counsel, ethicists, and the clergy on ethics-related issues.
- Conduct ethics audits of the organization using surveys of employees and patients; re-

# C A S E   S T U D Y

## To Tell or Not to Tell?

Kamal Nasreen recently accepted a staff nurse position at the transplant center of a large university hospital. He had done an internship at the medical center during his BSN program and had been impressed with the staff of the center and the exciting advances in the transplant field. After several weeks, he began to feel comfortable at the center.

During a particularly hectic day, a fellow nurse asked Kamal to hold onto a small box of immunosuppressive medications for her. "I'll just put them in the med room for you," he said. "No. Don't do that. Keep them in your desk. I'll get them when I'm done with Mrs. Seguro."

Feeling vaguely uneasy, Kamal put the box in the desk drawer and returned to his work. His colleague came back just before quitting time and asked for the box. "Here it is," said Kamal, pulling it out of the desk drawer. "What are you planning to do with these meds? They're all prescriptions for Mr. Landon. Didn't he die last week?"

His colleague looked uncomfortable. Then she sighed and sat down at his desk. "Yes, they were Mr. Landon's meds and he did die last week. Do you know how expensive these drugs are? His wife brought them to me earlier today. She said they couldn't do him any good anymore but they might help someone else."

"You can't do that! "Kamal exclaimed. "That's illegal, unethical. . . ."

"Is it? Half of our patients can't afford the drugs they need. Some go without food to buy them. Others take them every other day to cut down the cost. One actually held up a convenience store to get money for his kid's meds he was so desperate. They'll die without them and Mr. Landon can't use them. Is that so bad?"

Kamal didn't answer. He had no idea that this underground sharing of prescription drugs had been going on in the center. Did their manager know? Did the medical center administration know? He knew that passing along a drug prescribed for another person was a violation of federal law and could jeopardize his colleague's license. Yet his colleague was right; many patients could not afford the drugs and would die without them. Could such a benevolent act be illegal or unethical?

## Questions for Critical Reflection and Analysis

1. Analyze the ethical dilemma that Kamal faced in this situation in terms of rights and wrongs. What is *right* about what his colleague is doing? What is *wrong?*
2. Should Kamal help his colleague collect and distribute the drugs, ignore what his colleague is doing, or report his colleague to their manager? On what basis (using the terms explained in the chapter) did you make your choice?
3. Is it possible to resolve the ethical dilemma that would help the patients and not violate any legal or professional code at the same time?

*Source:* Inspired by Lagnado, L. (1999, June 21). Do or die. Transplant patients ply an illicit market for vital medications. *Wall Street Journal,* A1, A8.

views of institutional statistics on theft, property damage, etc.; and observation of behavior at all levels.

- Provide a viable forum in which ethical questions and concerns can be discussed freely. The Joint Commission on Accreditation of Healthcare Organizations began requiring that a process for addressing ethical concerns be in place in 1992 (Curran, 1998; Hilliard, Coffey & Johnson, 1999; Kaptein, 1998).

Although staff nurses and nurse managers can encourage implementation and actively participate in these actions, you can see that much of the responsibility for initiating and maintaining them rests with upper-level management of the organization. Managers at all levels can ensure that the principles set forward and the expected behaviors of adherence to those ethical principles are clear, achievable, consistently enforced, and actively discussed (Kaptein, 1998).

## ● SUMMARY

Values are judgments about the importance of objects, ideas, attitudes, and actions. Morals and ethics deal with questions of right and wrong. Professional ethics are often guided by formal codes such as the ANA's Code for Nurses.

A number of core values, including honesty, integrity, fairness, trustworthiness, respect, responsibility, accountability, and good citizenship have been identified as particularly relevant to the workplace. In health care, beneficence and nonmaleficence represent the most fundamental core values. Additional principles upon which ethics-related decisions are made in the workplace include egoism, empathy, utilitarianism, darwinism, existentialism, religious belief, authority, and conformism.

An ethical dilemma occurs when two or more principles or values are in conflict. They may occur at any level: intrapersonal, interpersonal, intraorganizational, interorganizational, and across the healthcare system. Frequently arising dilemmas in healthcare settings include accepting gifts, reporting theft and property damage, cover-ups, leaking confidential information, inappropriate assignments, reporting fraud, and protecting patients. The potential for conflict between the principle of beneficence and the business ethic of for-profit healthcare organizations is a matter of some concern these days.

Working in accord with one's personal and professional ethical codes requires thinking and reflection prior to taking action. This ethical evaluation begins with identification of the issues and the potential impact on other people. Then the principles involved are identified and a choice is made and acted upon. Managers can support ethics-based practice through the encouragement of discussion and reflection on ethical principles, consultation with experts, review of organizational policies, and ethics audits. Most important, however, is the degree to which managers and higher-level administrators actually practice the principles they espouse.

## REFERENCES

American Nurses Association. (1997). *The right to accept or reject an assignment.* Washington, D.C.

American Nurses Association. (1985). *Code for Nurses.* Washington, DC: ANA Publishing.

Badaracco, J.L. (1998). The discipline of building characters (management decisions). *Harvard Business Review, 76*(2), 114(11).

Berwick, D.M., et al. (1999). A shared statement of ethical principles for those who shape and give health care: A working draft from the Tavistock Group. *Nursing Standard, 13*(19), 34–36.

Blanchard, K. & O'Connor, M. (1997). *Managing by values.* San Francisco: Berrett-Koehler.

Curran, C.R. (1998). Coping with "slippery slope" questions. *Nursing Economics, 16*(3), 109(2).

Digh, P. (1998). The "I" in ethics. *Association Management, 50*(8), 105–106.

Edge, R.S. & Groves, J.R. (1994). *The ethics of healthcare: A guide for clinical practice.* Albany, NY: Delmar.

Flarey, D.L. (1999). Above all, do no harm. *JONA's Healthcare Law, Ethics and Regulation, 1*(2), 3–4.

Fowler, M.D. (1999). Relic or resource? The code for nurses. *American Journal of Nursing, 99*(3), 56–58.

Greengard, S. (1997). 50% of your employees are lying, cheating and stealing. *Workplace, 76*(10), 44.

Hamric, A. (1999). The nurse as moral agent. *Nursing Outlook, 47,* 106.

Henry, B. (1999). Journal priorities, ethical principles. *Image-Journal of Nursing Scholarship, 31*(1), 2–3.

Hilliard, B.B., Coffey, B.S. & Johnson, R.B. (1999). Hospital executives and ethics committees: An effective collaboration. *JONA's Healthcare Law, Ethics and Regulation, 1*(1), 25–31.

Hughes, K.K. & Dvorak, E.M. (1997). The use of decision analysis to examine ethical decision making by critical care nurses. *Heart & Lung: The Journal of Acute & Critical Care, 26*(3), 238–248.

Kaptein, M. (1998). Ethics management: Auditing and developing the ethical content of organizations. Dordrecht, Netherlands: Kluwer Academic.

Kleimen, M.A. (1999). The False Claims Act: An interview with Mark Kleimen. *JONA's Healthcare Law, Ethics, and Regulations, 1*(2), 17–22.

Lagnado, L. (1999, June 21). Do or die. Transplant patients ply an elicit market for vital medications. *Wall Street Journal,* A1, A8.

Larimer, L.V. (1997). How employees decide which way to go (resolving ethical dilemmas). *Workforce, 76*(12), 109(3).

Macklin, R. (1988). *Mortal choices ethical dilemmas in modern medicine.* New York: Houghton Mifflin.

McCoy, B.H. (1997, May/June). The parable of the Sadhu. *Harvard Business Review,* 54–64.

National Academies of Practice (NAP). (1998). *Ethical guidelines for professional care and services in a managed health care environment.* Edgewood, MD.

Parker, M. (1998). Business ethics and social theory: Postmodernizing the ethical. *British Journal of Management,* 9SPI/1 P.S27.

Reiser, S.J. (1994). The ethical life of health care organizations. *Hastings Center Report,* 24(6), 23–35.

Silva, M.C. (1998, June 10). Financial compensation and ethical issues in healthcare. *Online Journal of Nursing Issues.* Available at *http://www.nursingworld.org/ojcn/tpc6/tpc6_4.htm*

Solomon, R.C. (1997). It's good business: Ethics and free enterprise for the new millennium. Lanham, MD: Rowman & Littlefield.

Weber, J. (1996). Influences upon managerial moral decision making: Nature of the harm and magnituding consequences. *Human Relations,* 49(1), 1.

Webley, S. (1997). The business organisation: A locus for meaning and moral guidance. In P.W.F. Davis (Ed.). *Current issues in business ethics.* London: Routledge, 65–75.

Wright, R.A. (1987). *Human values in health care.* St. Louis: McGraw-Hill.

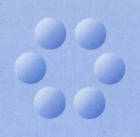

CHAPTER *21*

# Power, Empowerment, and Political Influence

Political Action: Influencing the Flow of
    Power and Decision Making
    *Entering the Decision-Making
        Channel*
    *The Agenda or Desired Change*

*Identifying the People For and Against
    Change*
*Barriers to Effective Implementation*

● SUMMARY

## LEARNING OBJECTIVES

*After completing this chapter, the reader will be able to:*

- Define power, empowerment, politics, and influence.
- Discuss the issues involved in empowering employees.
- Identify the sources of power in a given situation.
- Describe the distribution of power within an organization and in the community.
- Use power strategies to bring about change.
- Debate the advantages and disadvantages of collective bargaining from both labor's and management's points of view.

- Describe the activities of labor and management during the development of a collective bargaining agreement.
- Compare and contrast the rights and responsibilities of labor and management in a grievance procedure.
- Participate in political action to bring about change.

## TEST YOURSELF

**Self-Assessment: Personal Influence**

*What approach do you usually use to influence others? Do you do it primarily through assertiveness, through involving others, the use of persuasion or the use of logic and reason? Rate yourself on each of the following items and then score your results as shown.*

| | Strongly Disagree | Disagree | Neutral | Agree | Strongly Agree |
|---|---|---|---|---|---|
| **1.** I express my needs and opinions in a direct manner. | 1 | 2 | 3 | 4 | 5 |
| **2.** I am comfortable in a conflict situation. | 1 | 2 | 3 | 4 | 5 |
| **3.** I concentrate my energy on working toward consensus. | 1 | 2 | 3 | 4 | 5 |
| **4.** I prefer to use a team approach when working for change. | 1 | 2 | 3 | 4 | 5 |
| **5.** I use my enthusiasm to energize others. | 1 | 2 | 3 | 4 | 5 |
| **6.** I share my vision for change to inspire others. | 1 | 2 | 3 | 4 | 5 |
| **7.** I do my "homework" before presenting my position. | 1 | 2 | 3 | 4 | 5 |
| **8.** My proposals for change are thorough, well thought-out. | 1 | 2 | 3 | 4 | 5 |

Scoring:  #1 & 2   Assertiveness   _____ + _____ =
          #3 & 4   Involving Others   _____ + _____ =
          #5 & 6   Persuasion   _____ + _____ =
          #7 & 8   Reason (logic)   _____ + _____ =

*Source:* Adapted from Kolb, D.A., Osland, J.S. & Rubin, A.M. (1995). Organizational behavior: An experiential approach. Englewood Cliffs, NJ: Prentice Hall. Reprinted with permission.

Like it or not, *power* and *politics* have a significance effect on virtually every aspect of your practice, from the size of your paycheck to the amount of money made available to support research in your speciality area. **Power** and **politics** are terms that are still outside the "comfort zone" (Koerner & Bunkers, 1992) of many nurses. All organizations, including healthcare organizations, are intrinsically political (Morgan, 1997). Within them, power is unevenly divided between the various departments and disciplines and across levels of hierarchy.

In addition, much of healthcare policy development and decision making is a political process. From licensing and the legal specification of the rights, privileges, and responsibilities of nurses and other healthcare professionals to the procedures that are and are not covered by Medicare, politics enters our practice and affects our relationship with patients and clients in innumerable ways. Such diverse influences as prevailing public opinion, the lobbying efforts of special interest groups and the economic climate have important roles in shaping our healthcare system. It is naive to think that these powerful forces can be ignored. Instead, effective leaders and managers not only recognize these forces but also learn how to capitalize on them.

In this chapter, power, empowerment, and political influence are defined and the sources of power available to people in authority and to those who are not in authority are considered. Then empowerment of the individual employee and power-based strategies for change within organizations and in the political arena, including the controversial issue of collective bargaining, are discussed.

## ● POWER AND INFLUENCE

### Definitions

**Power** is the ability to change people's behavior in ways they might not otherwise change (Vecchio, 1997). An alternative definition is the ability to impose your will on others, even when they resist you (Hook, 1979). Power involves the use of some type of force, although it is not necessarily physical force. The force may be gentle or it may be harsh, but it is used to overcome resistance. If the target system is not willing to change, it may be forced to by the use of power.

**Influence** is subtler and usually weaker than power. People who are influenced by a leader or manager yield to or accept the other's attempt to change or direct them (Vecchio, 1997).

For a number of reasons, one person or group may allow others (including managers) to influence them. These reasons include internalization, identification, and compliance. An explanation of each follows:

**Internalization:** when people believe the other's ideas or suggestions are correct, appropriate, well-founded. In some instances, people are genuinely committed to the other's point of view and enthusiastically support it.

**Identification:** based primarily on desire to please the other. It usually stems from admiration, imitation, desire for approval.

**Compliance:** behavior results from seeking a reward or avoiding the other's displeasure rather than genuine belief in the suggested action (internalization) or desire to emulate the manager (identification).

An individual, group, or organization can use a number of ways to try to influence others' behavior before employing power-based strategies. Most of these methods have been discussed in earlier chapters. Consider the following possibilities:

- Use data, logic, reasoning.
- Form coalitions with others who have similar interests.
- Be direct and forceful (assertive).
- Bargain, using negotiation skills.
- Rely on goodwill, earned respect, likeability.
- Invoke wishes, preferences of those in authority.

### Sources of Power

Although power is not evenly distributed among individuals or across groups, everyone has some sources of power. The sources could be physical strength, ability to threaten harm, positional power, money, legal power, public recognition and support, expert power, the power of an idea, strength in numbers, or control of access to resources. These sources are interrelated, so the categories are not clear-cut. They do, however, provide a useful guide for assessing your actual and potential power and your opponent's actual and potential power.

> *There is an elusiveness about power that endows it with an almost ghostly quality. . . . We can "tell" whether one person or group is more powerful than another, yet we cannot measure power.*
>
> —*Kaufman, Jones, 1954, quoted in Rose, 1967*

## Physical Force

Physical force can be used to change behavior. For example, a parent will bodily remove a toddler from immediate danger rather than try to reason with the child. Police use physical force when necessary but usually try to use other powers (authority and legal power) first. Nurses occasionally use force to restrain patients in danger of doing harm to themselves or others. A manager may step bodily between two arguing staff members to break up a fight.

With these few exceptions, physical force is rarely considered appropriate for use in leadership or management situations. Its use may be illegal in some instances; it also violates a number of social norms. Another serious drawback to the use of physical force is that it can provoke return physical force and escalation into violence.

## Ability to Harm

The threat of harm does not have to be made directly to change another's behavior. For example, an employer negotiating with a union knows that the union can strike and does not have to be told this directly. In fact, the veiled, ambiguous threat of harm is often more frightening and therefore more effective than the direct threat.

The ability to inflict some kind of harm is not limited to those in authority. For example, an employer can fire an employee, but employees can also quit, leaving the employer without any-

one to do the work. Many other more subtle kinds of harm can be threatened, including public embarrassment, loss of prestige, or loss of popularity.

## Positional Power (Authority)

Positional power or authority comes from the position itself rather than from the individual who holds that position. Part of this power is delegated. For example, an elected official is given power by the voters. A supervisor or nurse manager has power that has been delegated by the administration of the agency or institution. An additional portion of this power comes from those who work under the direction of the person with positional power. They grant the person this power by respecting the position and being willing to carry out the requests made by the holder of this position. Another source of positional power is having a social position with high status. Two examples are being known as a community leader or being the spokesperson for a particular group.

Because positional power is granted by others, it is not too effective against strong resistance, especially from those who have granted this power. However, it is often effective when used in combination with other sources of power.

## Legal Power

When the behavior you want to change is contrary to an existing law, you can use the legal system to force the target system to change. For example, nurse practice acts define the legal scope of the profession and may be used to support efforts to expand nursing functions. Also, laws regulate fair employment practices, health and safety standards for employees, legal precedents in malpractice cases, and regulations defining adequate health care for reimbursement purposes. These examples are just a few ways in which laws can be used to support your efforts to bring about change. You can also challenge existing laws in the courts or work to get them changed at the local, state, or federal level of government.

Using legal power is not a simple thing to do. It requires knowledge of the law, of the way courts and legislatures operate, and money to support your effort. However, many important changes have been brought about through the legal system. Well-known examples are the civil rights laws, disabilities laws, and laws that support advanced practice nursing.

## Money

Money is thought by some to be the greatest source of power. Both the opportunity to gain monetarily and the fear of losing money affect much behavior. For example, because money is needed to purchase the basic necessities of food, clothing, and shelter, the loss of one's salary threatens these basic needs. As a result, people will usually behave in ways that keep their salary secure.

Economic motivation works at other levels too. For example, most organizations need money to survive; those that lose too much money will cease to exist. Accordingly, much behavior in organizations is aimed at bringing money into the organization or preventing the loss of money already earned.

People or groups who are able to control access to money either directly or indirectly have a tremendous source of power. Also, financial information may be used to control decisions within an organization. For example, a suggestion for change may be met with a flat refusal because "we can't afford it," without consideration of how the suggestion may earn money for the organization.

Indirect ways in which this source of power can be tapped are numerous. For example, at the organizational level information that leads the public to believe that an institution's services are inferior can result in economic losses for that institution by reducing the number of people seeking and paying for its services. On the individual level, a poor evaluation that eliminates a yearly raise for a staff member is another example of an indirect way to control economic resources.

## Public Recognition

Although public recognition may seem nebulous and unsubstantial, it can have a powerful effect on behavior. Most people and most organizations want to avoid embarrassment or disapproval and will often change their behavior to do so.

Pressure from peers can change behavior. For example, staff members who have gotten into the habit of coming in to work late will change their behavior if coworkers begin to criticize their habitual tardiness.

Most people desire recognition and approval. Letters of thanks from former patients or a favorable article in the newspaper about the high quality of care can strongly reinforce the staff's desire to function at a high level. Public recognition of this type not only raises morale but also brings in more patients and keeps the administration from interfering with success.

Hospitals and other healthcare organizations find it difficult to operate in a climate of unfavorable public opinion. Public recognition is so important that large healthcare organizations have public relations departments whose major purpose is to win public approval and recognition. Favorable public opinion about an organization brings increased numbers of clients. It also brings increased charitable contributions to nonprofit organizations.

Public sympathy can be used to bring about change. For example, you can use public sympathy for abused children to support the expansion of a family counseling and child protective services agency.

## Expert Power

Expert power is based on the education, skill, and experience of an individual or group. Patients often follow the nurse's directions simply because they believe the nurse is the expert on health matters. Well-known examples of the use of expert power by a group are the American Dental Association's endorsement of fluoride in toothpaste, the Heart Association's dietary recommendations, and the Surgeon General's warnings about smoking.

Gaining expert power first requires preparing yourself as an expert, then identifying yourself as an expert, and finally seeking recognition as an expert. By itself, expert power is not usually sufficient to overcome strong resistance, but it is useful in establishing the legitimacy of your claims to power and in combination with other sources of power.

## Power of an Idea

Ideas by themselves have considerable power. For example, a hospice staff can be depressed by the idea that they are only preparing people to die. The idea that hospice provides needed comfort and care can completely change the feelings of the staff and the climate of the agency.

> ### Knowledge is power.
> —*Sir Francis Bacon, 1597, quoted in Fitton, 1997, p. 150*

In order for an idea to have power, it must be heard. For example, the idea that hospice means comfort and care would not have any effect if it were not effectively communicated. The power of an idea is enhanced when the idea can be simply stated, easily remembered, and is accepted by a large number of people.

## Strength in Numbers

The number of people who support a change is an important source of power. The larger the number of people who support a change, the harder it becomes for others to oppose the change. When other factors are equal, the side with the most supporters appears stronger.

## Control of Access to Resources

This last source of power overlaps several of the others already mentioned. The person or group who controls access to money, communication, or information has a potentially enormous source of power available because little can be accomplished without money, communication, or information. For example, organized medicine has actively opposed increasing autonomy for advanced practice nurses (APNs):

> In one instance, the Florida Academy of Family Physicians implied that drug addiction would increase if nurse practitioners were given authority to prescribe controlled substances under protocol (Mitnick, 1998). Why would they make such a recommendation? To retain control of access. In this case, if the physicians retain control of access to these drugs, then patients must see a physician, not an APN, to obtain them.

## Power Distribution in Organizations

A number of interrelated factors determine the distribution of power within an organization. These factors are fluid, not fixed—they can and will change over time.

## Overt vs. Covert

Identifying the sources and distribution of power in an organization is not an easy task because the exercise of power is not always overt. An example of the **overt** exercise of power would be an open struggle between nursing and social work over the ownership of a new at-home counseling service for disabled children and their families.

**Covert** exercise of power has been called the "invisible face" of power and influence in organizations (Wilson, 1992, p. 54). Evidence for the covert exercise of power is usually indirect. For example, you may notice that appointments to important decision-making committees in nursing are limited to some select few people, all of whom are strong supporters of the CNO. Or you might find that every idea suggested by a particular department head is eventually approved whereas suggestions from other department heads are rarely approved.

## Upper vs. Lower Management

The primary locus of power in most organizations rests with management (Porter-O'Grady, 1992). A common countervailing (opposing) source of power are the collective bargaining units where they exist. If most of the power rests with senior management, lower-level managers and staff may have a strong sense of helplessness (Nadler et al., 1992). Additional factors contributing to perceived powerlessness are lack of resources, too much bureaucratic control, and insufficient authority to carry out one's responsibilities. Together, these factors can lead to a condition of apathy due to insufficient capacity to take action throughout the lower echelons of the organization.

The overt versus covert and upper versus lower management categories are useful but oversimplify the distribution and exercise of power in most organizations. Morgan (1997) suggested a list of indicators of the distribution of power that better reflect the complexity of power distribution in organizations:

*Formal Authority.* Who holds the top administrative positions? Is a nurse included in this group? Who reports to these people?

*Control of Resources.* Who makes decisions about spending money, granting raises and promotions, and so forth? Who can reverse these decisions if necessary? Who has the crucial skills without which the organization cannot function?

*Use of Organizational Structure.* What are the rules in this organization? Who can help you make the rules work for you? Who knows how to circumvent the rules?

*Change Arena.* Where are the most important decisions made? In the chief executive officer's (CEO's) office? In the physician's dining room? On the quality improvement council?

*Control of Decision Processes.* Who sets the agendas for important meetings? Who is capable of stopping or suppressing movement toward change? Who is capable of pushing through an unpopular idea?

*Control of Boundaries.* Who controls communication with top management? Is there a secretary who has the boss's ear?

*Management of Meaning.* What words or images evoke strong emotions in this organization? Who uses them effectively?

*Interpersonal Alliances and Networks.* Who knows what is happening in the organization? Who supports whom? Who is friendly with whom? Who knows what "strings" to pull to get something done?

*Countervailing Organizations.* Is any opposition organized? Are staff represented by unions? Do professional organizations influence the staff?

Once you have analyzed all of these factors, you will have a better picture of the distribution of power within the organization.

## Redistributing Power through Empowerment

Employees are empowered when they have not only responsibility and accountability but also authority to make the necessary decisions to get a job done. Without all three, empowerment can be an "empty business buzzword" (Bradford & Cohen, 1998, p. xviii).

What does it take to have genuinely empowered employees?

- *Capability:* the education and experience needed to make good decisions
- *Initiative:* active, as opposed to passive style of working and relating to others
- *Commitment:* see work as important, satisfying, meaningful
- *Independence:* sufficient authority to carry out the work (Kolb et al., 1995; Fullam et al., 1998)

Once guidelines regarding reasonable and ethical behavior and legal limitations have been established, the genuinely empowered professional would be free to do whatever it takes to accomplish his or her objectives (Schwertzer, 1998). For more information on factors that support staff nurse empowerment, see Research Example 21–1, Empowering Staff Nurses.

Although they support empowerment of employees in theory, many managers and upper-level administrators have a great deal of difficulty actually empowering employees. Sharing their authority makes them nervous (Bradford & Cohen, 1998). Many feel as if they are giving away their own power and do not have sufficient trust in their staff's capability and willingness to accept responsibility. They fail to recognize that most employees, particularly professionals, will rise to the occasion given the opportunity to do so. Far more can be accomplished by an empowered staff than by a staff that must wait for permission from their manager to do what they know needs to be done.

*Democracy is the empowering characteristic fundamental to all new high-performance work systems.*
—Hannigan, 1998

**Research Example 21–1    *Empowering Staff Nurses***

In this study of 537 nurses, the researchers tested the hypothesis that leader behaviors have an impact on empowerment in the work setting (Laschinger et al., 1999).

A random sample was drawn from the list of 2,200 nurses employed at two newly merged tertiary hospitals. The majority of the sample worked full time (69.47 percent). Most (83.6%) had diploma preparation in nursing. The average respondent was almost 40 years old and had 17 years experience in nursing. Questionnaires were mailed to participants. A voucher for coffee and a muffin in the hospital cafeteria was enclosed to reimburse them for their time.

On the whole, the respondent nurses found their work setting to be moderately empowering. Confidence in the employee and fostering autonomy were rated as the most empowering

leader behaviors. In addition, empowerment appeared to ameliorate their job stress and tension despite the effect of the merger. The researchers concluded that "staff members perceive themselves to be empowered when their leaders provide purpose and meaning to their work and help them understand the importance of their role in the organization, solicit their participation in decision-making processes, enhance their skills, provide the resources required for effective performance, show confidence in their ability to perform at a high level, and promote autonomous practice by removing "red tape.""

*Source:* Laschinger, H.K.S., Wong, C., McMahon, L. & Kaufman, C. (1999). Leader behavior impact on staff nurse empowerment, job tension, and work effectiveness. *Journal of Nursing Administration, 29*(5), 28–31.

## Using Power-Based Strategies for Change

Empowerment of employees is an application of the participative approach to leadership and management. In contrast, the use of power strategies is neither democratic nor participative. When using power-based strategies, people's needs, feelings, attitudes, and values may be recognized but they are not necessarily respected. Power-based strategies are used when a consensus cannot be reached through the use of the rational or participative modes of change.

The leader or manager who decides to use these strategies is entering a win-lose situation and assumes the risk of losing the contest. The target system is truly a target. Members of the target system can be resistant, sometimes actively resistant, to the change and are not necessarily included in the decisions made during the change process.

The tactics described in this section are derived primarily from the work of Alinsky (1972) and Haley (1969). Both concentrated on the use of power by people who are "have nots" as opposed to the "haves." In other words, these tactics can be used by people who do not have the

advantage of high position or great wealth to support their desire to bring about change.

> ***All power tends to corrupt; absolute power corrupts absolutely.***
> —*J.E.E. Dahlberg-Acton, 1987, in Fitton, 1997, p. 19*

> ***Powerlessness corrupts. Absolute powerlessness corrupts absolutely.***
> —*Kantor in Eigen & Siegel, 1989, p. 292*

> ***If you are unable to bite, refrain from showing your teeth.***
> —*French Proverb in Eigen & Siegel, 1989, p. 290*

The following tactics are designed to take advantage of the sources of power available to have-nots. They are presented in a logical sequence, but their actual use is usually not as orderly.

### Step 1. Define the Issue and Identify the Opponent

As with most strategies for change, you need to be clear about exactly what change is desired. In a power-based strategy you also need to reduce the change to a single issue around which you can polarize people (divide into groups for and against) and rally support.

The issue must be specific enough that people can take sides for or against it. It also needs to be expressed in a few simple words that can be easily communicated to a large number of people and can serve as a slogan or battle cry. Finally, the issue should express a realistic goal and have the possibility of being achieved (see Box 21–1).

In a power strategy, the target system becomes the opponent. This opponent is the person or group that has the ability to bring about the desired change but is resistant to doing so. The target is not necessarily the person or group who will actually implement the change but whoever controls the behavior targeted to be changed. It is important to identify the opponent as sharply as the issue in order to focus all the pressure on this point later on.

**A target is always a person. . . . Even the most powerful institutions are made up of people.**

—Bobo, Kendall & Max, 1991, p. 6

---

**Box 21–1    Checklist for Evaluating the Strength of an Issue**

As the first step in organizing people for change, the issue must be clearly defined and attractive enough to rally people to your cause. To evaluate the issue in terms of the strength of its attractiveness, ask yourself if the issue will . . .

- Be easy to understand
- Be winnable
- Have a clear target
- Be worthwhile
- Be widely felt
- Be deeply felt
- Give people a sense of their own power
- Result in real improvement if won
- Be consistent with your values and vision

*Source:* Adapted from Bobo, K., Kendall, J. & Max, S. (1991). *Organizing for social change: A manual for activists in the 1990s.* Washington, DC: Seven Locks Press.

---

The following example illustrates how healthcare providers can use a power-based change strategy to fight restrictions on their professional roles:

*Several incidents related to patient education had come to the attention of the chief of the medical staff of a private not-for-profit suburban hospital. A traditional pediatrician complained because a nurse taught several parents how to massage their sick babies. Then, an oncologist found a patient weeping and complained that the nurses had spoken to this patient about dying. Finally, one patient called the attending physician because the patient had realized during routine preoperative teaching that the scheduled surgery would be much more extensive than the patient had expected.*

*The chief of the medical staff brought these complaints to the hospital administrator and asked the administrator to do something about them. The administrator then asked the chief nursing officer (CNO) to tell the nurses that they could not do patient teaching without a physician's order. The CNO protested vigorously and pointed out that nurses were expected to teach patients as needed. The administrator was adamant and told the CNO, "If you do not take care of it, then I will." The CNO replied, "You are making a mistake."*

*The next day, a memo from the administrator was distributed to every nursing unit. The memo stated that nurses in that hospital would do no patient teaching without a physician's order.*

A nurse manager, Ms. B., who had been planning an extensive new patient teaching program with her staff, was infuriated. She decided to fight the new rule. The issue, as she saw it, was nurses' right to teach their patients. Her opponent was the administrator who signed the memo.

### Step 2. Organize a Following

As leader, you may be completely alone when you begin to implement a power-based strategy but you cannot remain alone and succeed.

Actually, two kinds of supporters are needed. The first is a small cadre of people who are strongly in favor of the change and who are willing and able to help you plan and carry out the tactics needed. This cadre is the **core group,** the key people on whom you can depend throughout the rest of the process.

The second group is a larger following of people, as many as possible, who will support you and take part in some of the tactics if necessary. These people do not have to be as dedicated or skillful as the key people, but it is important to keep up their interest and motivation. This larger number of people is needed to provide the strength of numbers. The size of the group is one demonstration of your side's power.

Some organizing tactics may be needed to develop a following. The issue and the identity of the opponent need to be clearly and simply communicated to anyone you want to recruit. The opponent is defined as the "enemy" of your following, an enemy who threatens harm to your group. Identification of a common enemy increases the cohesiveness of your following and appeals to the needs or interests of the people on your side. It is important to define your side as having the ability to bring about the desired change and as being right in demanding this change, whereas the other side is defined as wrong and as a threat to your group that can and must be overcome.

It may be difficult to attract a large following immediately. Alinsky offers a formula for dealing with this problem:

> If you have a vast number of people, "you can parade it visibly" and "openly show your power. . . ." If you have a small number of people, "conceal them in the dark but make a lot of noise so it sounds like a lot of people. . . ." If you have a tiny number, "too tiny even for noise, stink up the place." (Alinsky, 1972)

In the example so far, the nurse manager has decided to fight the new rule limiting nurses' rights to teach their patients:

> Ms. B talked with two of her friends about the memo after the nursing administration meeting. Both were angry about it but not sure what to do. Ms. B. suggested that they meet after work to talk about it some more.
>
> After work, the three nurse managers met. One had asked the evening supervisor, who was known to be in agreement, to join them. They discussed the problem for a while. They

all thought that most of the nurses in the hospital were unhappy about the memo, so they decided to collect as many signatures as possible to send with a reasonable letter stating their position to the administrator.

> The first nurse manager mentioned including the CNO, but the supervisor suggested that they wait until the signatures were collected. Each of the four nurses took a section of the hospital and began to collect the signatures immediately so that the letter could be sent within 48 hours.

### Step 3. Establish a Power Base

The following developed in the last step is the beginning of the establishment of a power base. The leader and key people need to carefully assess what types of power they have or can develop. As many as possible of the power sources listed earlier should be used to build this power base.

The power available to the opponent should also be assessed as should the opponent's weak points, which will be the targets of the power tactics in the next step. For example, an opponent's violation of a law is an obvious weak point. Or your opponent may be particularly sensitive to public opinion, which would then be a logical target. No opponent has an unshakable power base; everyone has an Achilles' heel if you search hard enough for it.

The four nurses found that most of their colleagues supported their fight for nurses' rights:

> Several other nurses offered to help them collect signatures. Within the 48 hours, they had signatures from more than half of the nurses working in the hospital. The first nurse manager also prepared a letter to the administrator that described the importance of patient teaching and pointed out that it was an independent function mentioned specifically in their state's nurse practice act.
>
> The administrator, Mr. C, was impressed with the number of signatures and began to wonder whether he had acted too hastily. However, he was concerned that if he gave in to this petition, the hospital staff would think they could always get him to change his mind by presenting a petition. So he decided to ignore the peti-

*tion. When Ms. B called his office, his secretary told her that no action would be taken.*

*The nurse manager called the key people together again to plan their next move. They reassessed their position. What could they do next? They had several sources of power available: many nurses on their side (numbers), the law supported but did not demand that they be allowed to do patient teaching (some legal power), the patients wanted teaching (potential public support), and they were good at it (expert power). Also, they could refuse to work (threat of harm) and paralyze the hospital, although they did not want to resort to this option. The administrator had the power of his position, economic power, and the support of some physicians but seemed susceptible to public opinion and pressure from others with positional power.*

## Step 4. Begin Action Phrase

In the action phase, tactics that will push the opponent into accepting the desired change are selected and implemented. These tactics are designed to create fear, confusion, and anger in the opponent. (Note that conflict and controversy are encouraged when using power-based strategies, in contrast to other approaches to change.)

Several factors should be considered when selecting tactics. First, the tactic must suit your following. For example, healthcare professionals are far more likely to be comfortable with petitions than with anything that is illegal or potentially dangerous. The tactic should also be one that your group can enjoy carrying out. One that has some drama or humor is more fun to implement and usually more effective in terms of rallying your supporters.

Alinsky (1972) was a master at creating tactics that people enjoyed. For example, he figured out a harmless way to tie up a busy airport: have people go into the restrooms and keep them occupied—for hours. Similarly, a bank can be paralyzed by large numbers of people opening up new accounts with small amounts of money.

Alinsky also used ridicule effectively. He found that it not only infuriated the opponent but is also difficult to counterattack. When obeyed to the letter, most rules become absurd;

it can be an effective way to ridicule your opponent's rule.

Threats have already been mentioned. However, if you decide to use a threat, be sure that you can fulfill it because your opponent may challenge you to carry it out. In other words, do not bluff.

Haley (1969) recommends that you set yourself up as an authority on the issue and speak to the opponent as an equal or better, never as a subordinate. It is also important to respond to any attack with either a question or another attack, never with a defensive reply that could be perceived as a sign of weakness.

At the same time, you can paradoxically define yourself as not seeking power, which makes your opponent appear to be the one who is power hungry. You can also say that you are not calling for a change and then call for a change; this tactic confuses your opponent and makes it harder to attack your side. It is a pretended meekness that makes your opponent appear to be the bad guy and builds public sympathy for your side. You cannot really be meek when implementing a power strategy says Haley. An effective strategy demands strength. Each tactic demonstrates your group's power and challenges the power of your opponent.

*Based on their assessment of the power available to them and to their opponent, the four nurses planned a tactic that they believed their following would be willing to carry out.*

*The four nurses decided to launch a campaign to publicize their fight and build more support. They distributed buttons saying "Nurses' Rights" to all nurses who would wear them. Many patients, visitors, and staff members asked what the buttons meant and expressed support for the nurses' group.*

*The administrator began to wish he had just let the nurses keep on teaching, but he was still concerned about the three physicians who had originally complained and about appearing weak by giving in to the nurses. So he decided to live with both the buttons and his memo.*

## Step 5. Keep the Pressure On

It may be necessary to continue the pressure on your opponent until your opponent agrees to the desired change, which can be done by changing tactics. The changes serve two purposes. First, they keep your opponent off balance, unable to predict your next move. Second, they keep your following interested and excited. A single tactic used for a long time becomes predictable and boring. New tactics help to keep your group's motivation high.

Although the administrator was definitely feeling the pressure, he had not agreed to change after both the petitions and buttons with the "Nurses' Rights" slogan on them had won some public support for the nurses:

> The four nurses decided that it was time to increase the pressure on the administrator by increasing public support and by using ridicule. They asked the people in their group to encourage anyone who expressed support to call the administrator. The nurses also asked every physician who supported them (and these were many) to stop by the administrator's office to tell him what they thought, as the administrator seemed to be susceptible to physicians' influence.
>
> In the meantime, the key people in the core group began telling hospital staff members that the only reason the original memo had been sent was because the administrator was afraid of one of the three complaining physicians. They quietly started referring to the administrator as "Chicken Charlie." They also decided to meet with the CNO.
>
> Because the administrator originally issued the memo in response to physicians' complaints, he assumed that he had support from most of them until they began to visit his office. The number of calls to his office increased that day to the point that his secretary threatened to resign. The administrator went home a little earlier than usual that day.

## Step 6. The Final Struggle

Neither side can continue to give or take pressure indefinitely. If the opponent has not yet agreed to the desired change despite several different tactics, it is time to increase the pressure enough to force a decision. Several new and stronger tactics are needed.

The four nurses felt that they were close to winning and wanted to force a decision:

> The four nurses met with the CNO, who had closely followed their activities and quietly supported their efforts. They asked the CNO for more direct support. With the CNO, they planned the final attack.
>
> The attack focused on two points: making the administrator look foolish by over-obeying his rules and bringing in pressure from outside the hospital for the first time. The four nurses went back to their group and asked each nurse to point out to the physicians every time a patient needed any information at all. At the same time, the CNO canceled all prenatal classes held at the hospital, declaring that they were in violation of the administrator's rule. To inform the people who attended the classes, the CNO asked the local newspaper and radio stations to announce the cancellations.
>
> After it was all over, the administrator could not remember whether it was the chief of the medical staff or the president of the board of trustees who called him first. The president of the board demanded to know why they were going to be the only hospital in the city without those popular prenatal classes. The chief of the medical staff told the administrator to stop being ridiculous and let the nurses get on with their work so that the physicians could get on with their work.
>
> The four nurses celebrated their victory with their following. Along with several members of their group, they were asked to serve on a nursing advisory committee that made recommendations about new policies affecting nurses. The CNO took advantage of the situation to strengthen the power of the CNO position in relation to the administrator so that any further policies affecting nursing would come only from the office of the CNO.

Not every power strategy will end in victory. Effective implementation of a power strategy demands time and energy from the leader and from supporters and entails the risk of losing, even of subsequent retaliation from the winners. However, because it is used when other change strategies are ineffective, deciding not to use the strategy constitutes an acceptance of defeat on an issue.

## COLLECTIVE BARGAINING

Collective bargaining is a particular type of formal, legally defined power-based strategy designed to redistribute power within an organization.

Collective bargaining is the joining together of employees for the purpose of increasing their ability to influence their employer. In labor relations parlance, the employer is usually referred to as **management** and the employees are referred to as **labor,** even if the employees are professionals. Anyone involved in hiring, firing, disciplining, or evaluating employees or in scheduling work is considered part of management and cannot be included in a collective bargaining unit. Some organizations deliberately include nurse managers in the hiring and firing process in order to keep them out of collective bargaining units.

From the manager's point of view, collective bargaining changes and regulates the employee-manager relationships. At its worst, it can be a source of constant tension between managers and their staffs. Managers often find collective bargaining an anxiety-producing subject, although it does not need to be.

The terms **labor relations** and **collective bargaining** still conjure up images of coal miners, steelworkers, and truck drivers in many people's minds. But these images reflect only half of the people who have joined organizations to represent them collectively at work. Administrators, college faculties, physical therapists, interns and residents, nurses, and other professionals are also engaged in collective bargaining for reasons that we will consider in this section.

The National Labor Relations Act and its amendments are the primary laws that protect an employee's right to engage in collective bargaining. This act established the National Labor Relations Board (NLRB), which has two major functions. The first is to ensure that employees are able to choose freely whether they want to be represented by a particular bargaining agent—for nurses, the professional association or an af-

filiate of a local or national labor union. The second function of the NLRB is to prevent or remedy any violations of the labor laws, called **unfair labor practices.**

Nonprofit healthcare organizations, including hospitals, nursing homes, visiting nurse associations, clinics, and others, have only been subject to these labor laws since 1974, making them relative newcomers to collective bargaining. Special rules designed to safeguard the welfare of patients apply to healthcare organizations. Proprietary (for-profit) organizations are also covered by these laws, but government-operated healthcare facilities are subject to an entirely different set of rules.

### Purpose

Unions exist to represent employees' interests in the workplace. As part of their representation, they engage in collective bargaining, their *raison d'etre* (Hannigan, 1998). Collective bargaining is a conflict-oriented power strategy operating on the principle of increased strength through numbers. Its fundamental purpose is to equalize the power distribution between labor and management. The majority of employees find themselves at or near the bottom of the hierarchy with little authority while people higher up (the "management") have more authority and appear to be far more powerful to people below them in the hierarchy.

*What workers really want is empowerment—real influence in the workplace. The only effective instrument for true influence in the workplace is a union.*
—Hannigan, 1998

The distribution of power is not as unequal as it appears to be. The organization depends on employees lower in the hierarchy to carry on its work; they are vital to the growth and development of the organization, even to its survival, and far outnumber the people higher up in the hierarchy. Collective bargaining takes advantage of both of these factors. A single employee who attempts to bargain with an employer is far more vulnerable to reprisals than is an entire group of employees. In health care, collective bargaining addresses economic issues, arbitrary treatment of employees, and professional/practice issues.

**Basic economic issues** such as salary are usually the first concern of people joining a collective bargaining unit. Other economic concerns covered by collective bargaining include shift differentials, overtime pay, holidays, personal days, the length of the workday, sick leave, maternity and paternity leaves, payment for uniforms, lunch and rest periods (breaks), health insurance, pension plans, and severance pay. People often assume that these elements are automatically provided by every employer, but in fact, some vital and costly ones such as health insurance are not.

Examples of **unfair or arbitrary treatment** include being the only one who has to work three weekends in a row, having been passed over for a promotion without explanation, or being fired because a physician thought your assertive protection of a patient's rights was "insubordinate." Other bargainable issues include staffing and scheduling, policies governing days off, limits on mandatory overtime, rotating shifts, being on call, promotion policies, transfers, layoffs, seniority rights, and the posting of job openings (Flanagan, 1992).

Perhaps the most important protection against arbitrary treatment is the inclusion of a grievance procedure in the collective bargaining agreement. It enables an employee to bring a complaint to management without having to fear later reprisals for his or her assertiveness. Nonprofessional support staff, including UAPs, also need this protection. For example, in a New York City hospital, support staff were sporadically paid, penalized for taking leave, and fired for union activity before a collective bargaining agreement was put in place. It took the union 10 years to gain recognition as their bargaining representative. Most telling was the union's initial goal: "Human dignity: to be addressed as a human being, to be called Mister or Miss. This was the key thing" (quoted by Ness, 1998, p. 96). For another example, see Perspectives . . . EMS Workers and Collective Bargaining).

## PERSPECTIVES . . .

### EMS Workers and Collective Bargaining

Emergency Medical System (EMS) personnel saw their salaries go from $26,000 in 1988 to $42,000 in 1992 after unionizing. With union support, they documented ambulance maintenance problems, inadequate equipment, and system faults that slowed their response time and won the right to participate in the selection of companies providing emergency services. While this change did lead to an increase in the cost of emergency services it also led to saving more lives. Can unions work with management in a cooperative manner? An organizer of EMS workers, John Dalrymple, said "In us the *good* employers have an ally they never had before—if they are willing to work with us and treat their EMS workers the way they should" (p. 96).

*Source:* Dalrymple, J. (1995). Turning privatization to advantage. In A.B. Shostok (Ed.). *For labor's sake: Gains and pains as told by 28 creative inside reformers.* New York: University Press American, Inc., 90–98.

**Maintenance and promotion of professional practice** is a third purpose, the importance of which is often underestimated by management (see Research Example 21–2, Nurses' Purposes Versus Management: Perceptions in Collective Bargaining). Proponents of collective bargaining believe that it is an effective way to maintain control over practice (Riffer, 1986). An example is putting the entire American Nurses' Association Code of Ethics into the contractual agreement with employers. Adequate staffing, acceptable standards of care, and other quality of care issues and standards can also be negotiated with employers. Research Example 21–2, Nurses' Purposes Versus Management: Perceptions in Collective Bargaining, and Research Example 21–3, Nurses' Concerns about Downsizing, Restructuring, and Deskilling, describe some sources of dissatisfaction experienced by nurses. (Also see Perspectives . . . System Problem or Individual Error? for an example of professional organization support for nurses.)

**Research Example Box 21–2** *Nurses' Purposes versus Management: Perceptions in Collective Bargaining*

Are nurses primarily concerned with economic issues when they bargain collectively? Do managers know what issues are actually important to their staff members?

Bloom, Parlette, and O'Reilly (1980) interviewed 78 public health nurses and 11 supervisory nurses from three large community healthcare agencies in California for this study. Two of the agencies had recently settled work stoppages. These nurses had worked an average of 7.5 years for the county. All county employees were represented by an international labor union.

The nurses were asked to rate the importance of 17 different issues on a four-point scale from *not a factor at all* to *a major factor* in the decision to strike. Ten top-management people, including the director of nursing, three assistant directors of nursing, the director of public health, and the county manager, were also asked to rate the same 17 issues.

Little relationship was found between the ratings of the nurses and the ratings of people in management over what issues were important (the correlation was a low .17). The nurses considered support for nurses in their unit, difficulty communicating with management, management's authoritarian behavior, a belief in collective bargaining as a way to balance the power between management and employees, and the need for more nursing positions (the only economic issue) to be most important. In contrast, the people in top-management positions thought that the most important factors in the strike decision were a pay increase, allowing two nurses to share a full-time position, a union attempt to gain power, and pressure from other nurses to go on strike. None of the four issues rated important by management were actually important to the nurses.

In their discussion, the researchers asked why people in management fail to use principles of effective communication and the basic concepts of the well-known motivational theories when dealing with collective bargaining. They concluded that management thought that the industrial type of bargaining issues such as wages and job security were the critical issues but that the nurses were actually more concerned about professional issues, especially with improving communication with management and increased participation in organizational decision making.

*Source:* Bloom, J.R., Parlett, G.N. & O'Reilly, C. (1980). Collective bargaining by nurses: A comparative analysis of management and employee perceptions. *Health Care Management Review, 5,* 25.

## Issues Related to Collective Bargaining

Most of the objections to collective bargaining stem from the conviction that it is an unprofessional activity and that some of the activities may endanger patient safety. Another concern is that it may, paradoxically, endanger job security.

### Unprofessional

For many people, collective bargaining does not fit the image of a nurse as professional. They emphasize that other means can be found to achieve the purposes of collective bargaining.

Organizers of collective bargaining units, on the other hand, argue that many other professionals are members of unions. The NLRB defines nurses as professionals because their work requires having advanced specialized training and making critical judgments. Advocates of collective bargaining add that it is unprofessional to accept low salaries and poor working conditions. Control over one's practice, they would say, is the essence of professionalism (Luttman, 1982).

### Unethical

Most healthcare professionals place patient welfare ahead of personal gain. This value system is

### Research Example 21–3   *Nurses' Concerns about Downsizing, Restructuring, and Deskilling*

What are nurses' concerns in relation to the sweeping changes in the U.S. healthcare system? A survey on patient care published in the March 1996 issue of the *American Journal of Nursing* drew responses from 7,500 nurses across the country.

Nurses from every setting and specialty reported increased responsibility and less time to care for each patient. Deskilling (substitution of UAPs for RNs) was reported by more nurses from the Pacific region. Cutbacks in RN staffing were related to the degree of penetration of managed care in various regions of the country. Increases in unplanned readmissions and complications secondary to admitting diagnosis were reported by many respondents. Only one third of nurses in subacute settings thought that care met their standard while two thirds in home care felt that way. Cuts at the management level were also reported, indicating that *speed-ups* (expecting fewer workers to do more) were not limited to the staff nurse level.

Some of the nurses who responded to the survey were clearly distressed by their working conditions and the potential effect on their patients. A few examples of what they wrote:

- The busy days don't usually allow everyone to take their break and lunch—don't even think about time to use the toilet facilities yourself. I know my staff is trying their hardest. But there are not enough hands at times to do what needs doing.

- I feel exhausted most times and what used to be a career that I loved is turning into a job that I would rather not go to.
- I'm glad I will be retiring soon. I have worked full-time in hospitals since 1959. It has always been hard, but having businesspeople run hospitals is the worst I've seen.
- We are beyond the level of "unsafe." It has become frightening. I am only concerned about patient survival in my facility. We are forced to document treatments not actually given. I fear for my license.
- There's been an increase in disciplinary actions against nurses in order to (I believe) keep the blame and responsibility from sticking to administration for poor staffing and management.
- One incident I observed occurred when an aide disconnected an IV to help a patient change gowns. The [pediatric] patient lost a large amount of blood before I got to the room to clamp the tubing.

The authors conclude that cutting the number of registered nurses while at the same time increasing their patient load and cross-training them to perform more tasks is "demoralizing at best and downright dangerous at worst."

*Source:* Shindul-Rothschild, J., Berry, D. & Long-Middleton, E. (1996). Where have all the nurses gone? *American Journal of Nursing, 96*(11), 25–39.

---

in conflict with any type of work slowdown or stoppage. Many nurses believe that they could not abandon their patients during a strike under any circumstances, that it would be unprofessional and unethical to do so.

The opposing argument is that the poor, sometimes intolerable, conditions under which many nurses work are also a threat to the patients' welfare. The threat of a strike is needed to improve these conditions. The law requires giving 10 days' notice before striking a healthcare facility to reduce the possibility of harm to the

patients. This notice allows time for management to make preparations for the patients' safety, such as reducing elective surgeries and admissions or transferring patients to other facilities.

When the American Nurses' Association had a no-strike policy (prior to 1968), nurses who tried to bargain collectively with their employers found that they had little or no success. Their employers ignored them, refused to bargain with them, or rewarded them with platitudes about how important they were while raising other people's salaries. Without the clout of a potential

## PERSPECTIVES . . .

### System Problem or Individual Error?

A well-known health columnist for the Boston Globe died after receiving a drug overdose during chemotherapy at the Dana-Farber Cancer Institute. In a related incident, a 53-year-old teacher died 3 years later after having suffered severe cardiac damage following chemotherapy at Dana-Farber. In response, the Massachusetts Board of Registration in Nursing filed charges against 16 Dana-Farber nurses in January 1999, 4 years after this incident occurred, saying that they had failed to recognize that the doses were in excess of the doses called for in the protocol. Three pharmacists had already been reprimanded in regard to this incident and the license of the physician who wrote the incorrect order was suspended for 3 years.

Both the American Nurses Association (ANA) and the Massachusetts Nurses Association (MNA) have thrown their support behind these nurses, saying the incidents were the result of system failure, not individual incompetence. ANA and MNA noted several factors that contributed to their decision to support the nurses including the high-paced environment in which the nurses worked and the fact that they had followed the Institute's policy in checking the medication order. Chemotherapy dosages vary widely, especially during Phase I testing of new drugs at which point the correct dose is still being determined through research studies. The nurses had checked the dosage against the physician order, not the research protocol. It was also noted that at the time of the incident, many clinical nurse specialists and middle level nursing management positions had been eliminated at the Institute.

This situation brings up several implications for the profession as a whole. One fundamental question is "whether the current culture of blame will drive the reporting of mistakes underground" (p. 10). In addition, responsible management should be able to distinguish between a problem with individuals who are unsafe and a problem within the system. Do all managers do this? "No," said MNA member Judith Shindul-Rothschild, "That's why you need collective bargaining" (p. 10).

*Source:* Trossman, S. (1999, March/April). Support Dana-Farber nurses facing disciplinary action. *The American Nurse,* 1, 10.

strike, nurses could not get their employers to listen to them.

### *Divisive*

Collective bargaining draws a clear line between management and labor and treats the relationship as an adversarial one. It also presents some potential conflicts for state nurses' associations (SNAs). While their membership includes both administrators and staff nurses, the SNAs may represent staff nurses at the bargaining table if they have been selected as the bargaining agent. Needless to say, it results in some negative feelings on the part of member nurse administrators. On the other hand, collective bargaining has enabled staff nurses to bring about some of the same changes that nursing administrators had been trying unsuccessfully to implement through persuasive means for years. The adversarial nature of the relationship is one that can be ameliorated given a climate of cooperation and understanding on both sides.

### *Endangering Job Security*

Paradoxically, collective bargaining may also be a potential threat to job security. People who actively engage in collective bargaining and become well known to management may find themselves targets for reprisals, particularly if the collective bargaining effort fails.

Some risk is always involved in taking action, particularly against those who have the authority to remove people from their positions. For this reason, most collective bargaining activities arise when working conditions become so adverse that people believe it is worth the risk. Initial attempts at organizing people are usually done outside the organization with representatives of the nurses' association or the union acting as spokespersons for the employees, shielding the employees from management's anger. A related concern is that a union that is too successful in gaining concessions from management can drain the organization's resources, inhibiting the organization's growth or even endangering its survival.

Although the healthcare industry offers few examples in this regard, organizations in other fields have become so restricted by union rules and so inefficient because of high union wages that they have failed to keep up with their com-

| Table 21–1    Summary of the Pros and Cons of Collective Bargaining | |
|---|---|
| **For Collective Bargaining** | **Against Collective Bargaining** |
| • Equalization of power between labor and management<br>• Prevents unfair treatment of employees<br>• Promotes professionalism<br>• Increases control of practice<br>• Economic security<br>• Improves the quality of care | • Unprofessional<br>• Leads to unethical actions<br>• Promotes conflict and interferes with effective management<br>• Inhibits organizational growth<br>• Drains organizational resources<br>• Endangers job security |

petitors. Some unions' actions have been compared to those of a parasite that lives off the organization and eventually kills it. Obviously, it is not in the union's best interest to destroy the organization that employs its members. A fair distribution of resources between the management and owners of the organization and its employees is one that can benefit both labor and management. However, in a conflict between two opposing groups (in this case, labor and management), it is often difficult to achieve this delicate balance between competing interests.

Table 21–1 summarizes the pros and cons of engaging in collective bargaining.

## Organizing

In the first phase of collective bargaining, a bargaining group is formed and recognition as the employees' bargaining agent is sought. While it is possible to form an independent group for bargaining with an employer, established professional associations (the SNAs) and unions have developed expertise on the applicable laws and multiple strategies needed to bargain effectively with management. Healthcare organizations frequently hire consultants to help them fight unionization and sometimes pool their resources with area institutions to improve their expertise and bargaining position. Their access to this expertise would put an independent group, especially an inexperienced one, at a disadvantage.

### The Organizing Council

The movement toward unionization begins when a group of interested employees forms an informal organizing council. This council becomes the core group of people who get other nurses interested and involved in joining a union. While the initiative to organize may come from a union or competing unions, the core group of committed employees is essential to the success of an organizing effort.

The organizing council usually meets outside of working hours away from the work setting to plan its organizing strategies. As they persuade other nurses that collective action is needed, core group members ask them to sign authorization cards. These cards indicate their desire to be represented by a particular labor organization (their SNA or a union). The cards are checked by a neutral third party; management does not see the signatures at any time. When a majority of the nurses employed in the organization have signed the cards, the employer is asked to voluntarily recognize the union or nurses' association as the bargaining agent. Most of the time, the employer will not recognize the union, and an election supervised by the NLRB is held.

### Elections

The preelection campaigning on both sides can become intense. Management often plays on nurses' feelings of guilt, implying that they are planning to abandon the patients who depend on them or are betraying the CNO who has worked so hard on their behalf. Other tactics may be aimed at stirring fear of reprisals, such as being fired. Actual threats or coercion, even promises of benefits for those who vote against the union, are illegal. Analysis of data from the NLRB indicates that as many as one third of the employers studied illegally fired union supporters during the preelection campaign. This figure was an increase from 8 percent in the 1960s. Half of the employers threatened to close their facility if the union won the election and 91 percent required their employees to meet with managers to discuss the issue (Bernstein, 1999, p. 43). Such actions are believed to have had a significant impact on election outcomes.

An entirely different strategy sometimes used by management is to take a positive approach. Suddenly, the pay scale for nurses is raised and supervisors become more attentive to the needs of individual employees. This attentiveness fades quickly, however, if the organizing effort fails.

The union side has its own strategies. Unions often mount educational campaigns explaining what a union is and what it can do for employees. These campaigns usually include responses to criticisms that collective bargaining is unprofessional or unethical. Unions also use fear by pointing out how vulnerable an employee is without their protection. Whatever unsatisfactory conditions exist that led to the interest in collective bargaining are emphasized. Individual incidents may be exaggerated to stir anger against management. Any threats or coercion from the union is illegal.

## Negotiating a Contract

The bargaining agent that wins the election is certified by the NLRB. The employer is required to bargain with this designated representative. Collective bargaining then enters the second phase in which an agreement on a contract is reached. Contracts can be negotiated with a single institution or a contract can be done corporatewide, thus including all hospitals or long-term care facilities or home health agencies owned by a single corporation (Hannigan, 1998). This contract is a legal document that both management and the union must abide by after it is signed. All the items listed earlier under the purposes of collective bargaining can be included in this agreement. Issues concerning union membership and payment of dues, called "union security items," are also included in the contract.

### Negotiations

Both management and labor groups form negotiating teams and designate one member of the team as their spokesperson. Before negotiations begin, each team meets separately to decide upon priorities and the items that they are willing to compromise on at the bargaining table. As with other types of negotiations, both sides typically begin by asking for a list of everything they might possibly want, but avoid making completely unreasonable demands. When an expiring contract is being renegotiated, either side may ask for something that they lost at the last contract negotiation.

As a rule, management is reluctant to give up any of its power or to spend more money; the union, on the other hand, attempts to equalize the power balance between labor and management and to gain benefits for its members. The recitations of who-wants-what can go back and forth for many meetings, but they do have some purpose. During this time, the negotiating team finds out what the other side wants and determines where they might make concessions or seek them from the other side (Walker, 1995).

Much of what happens in the early rounds of negotiation are demonstrations by each team meant to gain public support for their side. Often much posturing and showmanship characterize the early rounds of talks, and the serious bargaining is done later behind closed doors. Then common ground is established, the really difficult issues are dealt with, and necessary compromises are made to reach an agreement.

In collective bargaining each side is **obliged by law** to bargain in good faith. **Good faith** means that both parties must agree to meet at reasonable times, to send representatives with the authority to negotiate to the bargaining table, and to bargain with the other side. Presenting a take-it-or-leave-it package of demands and refusing to negotiate any changes in that package is not bargaining in good faith.

### Stalemates

Despite good-faith bargaining by both sides, negotiations may reach a stalemate, which means that the two teams are unable to reach an agreement. If this happens, both sides must notify the Federal Mediation and Conciliation Service, a government agency. One of several actions may then be taken to break the stalemate: mediation, fact-finding, binding arbitration, or work stoppages:

- *Mediation.*   A neutral party provided by the Federal Mediation and Conciliation Service may meet with each of the negotiating teams to explore the nature of the stalemate and then bring the two sides together to try to work out a settlement of the dispute. Both sides must cooperate with this federal mediator, but they do not have to accept the mediator's recommendations.

- *Fact-Finding.*   The Federal Mediation and Conciliation Service may appoint a fact-finding board of inquiry to investigate the situation and make recommendations. This board's report and recommendations are made public and can be used to pressure one or both sides to move toward an agreement.

- *Binding Arbitration.*   Like the mediator and fact-finding board, the arbitrator is a neutral party who thoroughly investigates the situation, meets with each side, and makes a decision regarding a settlement between the two. However, because both sides must accept the arbitrator's decision, both management and labor are reluctant to voluntarily limit their bargaining power by submitting the dispute to binding arbitration unless no better alternative is available. One of the risks of binding arbitration is that either side may lose something gained during previous negotiations. For example, the arbitrator could reverse a hard-won agreement to reduce the probation time of new employees from six months to two months. This change would be a victory for management because it means that benefits do not have to be paid for the first six months and it slows down pay raises for new employees.

- *Work Stoppages.*   When talks reach an impasse, employees have a fourth alternative: they can slow down or stop working. Employers can also lock out employees. The union must give 10 days' notice before striking unless management has committed an unfair labor practice. At this point, the tension builds rapidly. In fact, the prospect of a strike usually leads to more intense negotiating and often to a last-minute settlement. Generally speaking, no one really wants a strike and the decision is preceded by much discussion between the union and the membership of the bargaining unit. Unions do not want to strike unless their members are solidly in support of the action.

Nurses who strike usually do so only when they believe that all other options have been exhausted (Giovinco, 1993). While management is preparing (often frantically) for the loss of nurses' services, the union has to organize the strike, set up strike headquarters, and build support from its members, the public, and other unions for its strike. Once begun, strikes usually continue until some kind of settlement is reached. Some unions have begun to develop alternatives to strikes because strikes no longer generate the public sympathy that they once did. As an alternative to striking, for example, airline workers adopted the CHAOS (Create Havoc Around Our System) technique, consisting of random walkouts that left many flights grounded. Another technique is an organized boycott of a company's product or services (Byrnes, 1993).

- *Ratification.*   When an agreement is finally reached, the union negotiators take it back to the membership for their approval. A vote is taken and, if approved, the agreement becomes a legally binding contract under which management and labor now have to work.

## Contract Administration

Collective bargaining does not end with the signing of the agreement. The hard-won agreement now has to be enforced.

### *Grievances*

Almost every collective bargaining agreement includes provisions for a grievance procedure to deal with any dispute or complaint from the employer or any employee in the bargaining unit about implementation of the contract. The contract usually specifies certain steps to be taken and the time limits for completion of each of these steps. For example, employees may be given a limit of 5 days after an incident to file a grievance with their immediate supervisors, and the supervisors must respond within a specified number of days.

If the problem is not resolved at this first step, it proceeds through further steps. The grievance may be brought next to the director of personnel and then to the administrator of the organization. If the grievance is still not resolved at the end of these steps, it can then be taken to arbitration (Thomson & Murray, 1976).

A typical grievance begins when an employee feels mistreated and contacts the **union delegate** (a fellow employee who represents a particular work group at union meetings) or **association representative** to find out if the perceived mistreatment is a violation of the contract. The delegate then discusses the situation with the employee and decides how to handle the complaint. The following is an example:

> An employee informed the delegate about not receiving a raise that was due. The delegate spoke to the employee's manager, who said it was just an oversight, and the problem was quickly resolved.

If the problem affects other employees too, the delegate will also speak to them before deciding how to handle it. Here is an example:

> The supervisor of the intensive care units told the day shift nurses that they would have to work an extra weekend for the next 3 months. One of the nurses informed their delegate. The delegate spoke with several other nurses, who confirmed that they had been told the same thing. The delegate then went to the supervisor, told the supervisor that it was a violation of the contract, and showed the supervisor the relevant clause in the contract. The extra weekend work was removed from the schedule before it was posted and was not mentioned again.

Often the delegate needs to use his or her understanding of human behavior and some effective communication techniques to deal with a grievance, because supervisors may take a grievance personally and become defensive about having made a mistake or feel threatened by the power that the delegate represents. The following is an example of a situation that the delegate handled tactfully to avoid making the supervisor defensive:

> At the end of an unusually busy week during which the staff could not get all their work done on time and everyone was becoming tired and short tempered, an irritable supervisor decided that staff members were spending

too much time in the lavatories and tried to limit them to one trip a day. Most of the staff ignored the order, but a few became angry, and one threatened to use the supply room sink. The delegate approached the supervisor privately and told the supervisor that staff members could not obey the rule and that it could not be enforced. The supervisor realized that the head of the department would not approve of the absurd rule and dropped the whole matter after the conversation with the delegate.

As you can see, many grievances are minor and can be resolved in an informal manner by the employee, immediate supervisor, and delegate at the first step of the grievance procedure.

Any disputes of a more serious or complex nature than the previous examples are usually brought to a union staff member, often called an **organizer** or **association representative.** This individual has more experience in resolving grievances and is in a less vulnerable position than the delegate, who is an employee of the organization. The organizer is not emotionally involved in the situation, cannot be harassed by management, and can be more objective than the people directly involved. In this instance, it is an advantage to be represented by a large union or active professional association that has locally based representatives available to represent employees throughout the steps of the grievance procedure.

The organizer is likely to confront supervisors or administrators more directly than a delegate would. The following are two examples in which a problem was resolved at the first step of the grievance procedure:

> A nursing assistant, Miss M, felt that she was being treated unfairly by her nurse manager who often criticized her, never praised her, and never granted her requests for a particular assignment or day off. The assistant brought her problem to the delegate, who referred it to the organizer. The organizer was direct with the nurse manager. The organizer told the nurse manager. "You don't have any respect for this nursing assistant as a person. She's a human being." The nurse manager responded somewhat defensively but did treat the nursing assistant fairly after the confrontation.

*A nurse, Mr. P, requested a particular day off in order to take care of some important personal business that had to be done during work hours, but his supervisor denied the request. The organizer accompanied the nurse to meet with the supervisor and repeated his request. The supervisor said that he could have the day off only if he found someone to work his shift. The organizer said, "Are you asking Mr. P to do your job for you?" The supervisor backed down, rearranged the schedule, and allowed the nurse to take the day off.*

The organizer plays the same roles of mediator and defender of the employee's rights if the grievance is not resolved at the first step. The next steps involve management higher up in the hierarchy of the organization. If the grievance is a serious matter, such as the firing of an employee, it may be taken directly to the administrator of the organization.

## Binding Arbitration

When the previously mentioned steps of the grievance procedure fail to resolve the dispute, the problem can be taken to binding arbitration. This kind of arbitration is much the same as the arbitration used during contract negotiations except that it is done to resolve a disagreement over implementation of the contract.

The contract usually specifies the way an arbitrator is selected, most often from a list supplied by the American Arbitration Association, which acts like a clearinghouse. Both sides must agree with the choice. Again, both parties may be reluctant to submit to arbitration because the decision is binding and the arbitrator's fees, which are paid by both sides, can be substantial. If the employee has been offered a reasonable settlement at an earlier stage and does not have a strong case, the organizer will privately encourage the person to accept the offer. If the employee is completely in the wrong in the dispute, the organizer may refuse to proceed with the arbitration. This refusal can be appealed to the union board.

The arbitrator acts much like a judge in hearing the case except that the rules of evidence are not as strict as they are in a courtroom. The arbitrator's duty is to decide whether the contract was violated and what action is to be taken. The following are two examples in which the firing of a hospital employee was taken to arbitration:

*A shipment of perishable materials was due sometime during the day, and a pharmacy aide was assigned to unpack and store the materials. The shipment arrived just before quitting time, and the pharmacist said that the aide had to stay. The aide refused, saying, "I would have stayed if I had been asked earlier in the day." Because the aide had received disciplinary warnings in the past, the aide was fired for insubordination.*

*Because it was a serious case, the union organizer began the grievance procedure at the second step with the personnel department. Eventually, the case was brought to arbitration. The contract stipulated that management could ask employees to work overtime and this employee had been warned about insubordination in the past, so the employee lost the arbitration procedure and remained fired.*

*In another case, a new technician who was in a training program had a seizure, fell down a flight of stairs, and broke several bones. The technician was fired by the hospital for excessive absenteeism while out of work on disability. The hospital claimed that the technician was incapable of completing the training program or doing the job for which he was hired. The technician said, "I just forgot to take my Dilantin that day," but the hospital would not reinstate the employee.*

*The union brought this case to arbitration, and the arbitrator ruled in favor of the employee, noting that it was an accident, that anyone could make that kind of mistake. This employee got his job back.*

The grievance procedure provides employees with two safeguards not always available to employees who have not organized to bargain collectively. The first is a guarantee of a fair hearing and a response within a given time. The second is that employees have someone to represent and defend them and do not have to face an authority figure alone.

## Collective Bargaining from a Management's Viewpoint

### Preventing Unionization

From the management point of view, the non-unionized organization's goal in regard to collective bargaining is clear: to remain nonunionized. It would be extremely unusual to find management that did not want to avoid unionization.

We will look at two approaches to preventing unionization: a positive approach that creates a climate in which most of the workforce is generally satisfied with their working conditions and has little interest in unions and collective bargaining, and a more aggressive approach in which the organization takes deliberate steps to prevent unionization. It is generally agreed that widespread job dissatisfaction within an organization makes that organization vulnerable to unionization (Hunter et al., 1986). In fact, union organizers say that in many organizations, management has done their work for them, that "management is our best advertisement." What they mean is that poor leadership and management practices in the organization lead to a more strongly felt need for collective bargaining to equalize the power relationship between labor and management and in order to improve working conditions. Research Example 21–3, Nurses' Concerns about Downsizing, Restructuring, and Deskilling, describes some typical areas of employee dissatisfaction in hospital settings, many of which could be eliminated by effective leadership and management.

One way to avoid unionization is responsive, proactive leadership and management throughout the organization. Certainly, the first-line manager to whom this book is primarily addressed cannot do it alone. However, because upper-level management depends on first-line managers to implement this approach, we will look at the most common and generally effective approaches.

In analyzing why a strike took place at a Michigan hospital, Simms and Dalston (1984) divided the factors into those specific to collective bargaining and those of a more general nature. The more specific factors included economic issues; overtime; rotating shifts; working weekends; recruitment; retention; morale; appreciation and valuing of nurses; provision for adequate input into the quality of care, scope, and autonomy of nursing practice; relationships with other disciplines; lines of accountability; and other general working conditions. The general factors included the effect of reorganization within the institution, a restructuring of the CNO's role, and the effect of many outside parties, including politicians, other organizations, and the news media. These factors may vary from one situation to another, but they give you a good idea of how complex and far-reaching the influences can be.

Although all-round high-quality, effective leadership and management are needed to create a positive organizational climate that is resistant to unionization, focus on some specific areas can help in preventing unionization:

1. *Provide real opportunities for participation in organizational decision making.* We are going back to a basic principle in leadership and management here in saying that the participative approach is most effective. However, the participative approach also requires more effort and openness to suggestions for change, particularly when implemented at the organizationwide level. On the other hand, the professionals who work within the organization have much to contribute that can be lost in an organization with autocratic leadership. Staff members should, at the very least, have input into scheduling, quality improvement, and patient care procedures. They should also be consulted on budgetary matters and the long-range planning goals of the organization. Professionals want to have a voice in the operation of the organization. When they do not, serious discontent can develop (Flarey, Yoder & Barabas, 1992).

2. *Treat professionals as professionals.* Even though this point sounds so obvious, many nurses are not accorded the respect, value, and authority they are due. Staff members generally live up to expectations, but when little is expected of them, they often will not display as much professionalism as they could. It leads to a vicious circle in which ad-

ministration believes that their poor treatment is justified.

Just a few small examples are mentioned here. Timing coffee breaks taken by professional staff, for example, or monitoring mileage for community nurses is insulting. Professionals skip their breaks when the need arises and should be able to judge for themselves when they can extend a break. Expecting nurses to yield to physicians' demands is demeaning. In some organizations, nurses also find themselves acceding to the demands of housekeeping, dietary, pharmacy, and other departments. The relationship should be one of equals, of colleagues working together toward a common goal of good patient care. A narrow, limited view of nursing practice on the part of administration is sure to lead to a dissatisfied nursing staff that is more easily convinced to organize to bargain collectively.

3. *Pay salaries in keeping with the education required and the responsibility given.*    This is an effective way to demonstrate the degree to which nurses are valued by the organization; it will also help to reduce staff turnover.
4. *Develop a procedure for handling grievances.* One of the most attractive aspects of collective bargaining is the opportunity to appeal a decision made by one's boss if the decision is unfair. A management-initiated grievance policy should be well defined, supported by administration, and include safeguards for the employee who decides to use it. An "open door" policy that allows staff members to approach higher-level management is one component of such a policy. Another would be the organization of an appeals committee composed of both staff and management to hear any grievances that were not satisfactorily resolved through other means.
5. *Survey staff regularly.*    Another effective way to communicate administrative concern and to provide a channel of communication for all staff members is to institute a regular survey of staff opinions, asking questions such as those mentioned in Research Example Box 21–3. Such a survey is useless or worse, however, if management does not do anything about the problems that are uncovered through the survey.

Some organizations go even further in their efforts to prevent unionization. The following are some more specific actions that can be taken on an organizationwide basis to prevent unionization:

1. *Keep salaries and benefits at rates equal to or greater than those offered by unionized organizations.*    The organization regularly surveys the salaries and benefits offered at neighboring institutions and agencies and deliberately sets its salaries to keep up with the other organizations.
2. *Control communications.*    Company newsletters, bulletin boards, and other means of communication with employees are controlled by a designated department or individual. Employees are not permitted to post or distribute any kinds of advertisements or flyers, for example, without their manager's permission.
3. *Negotiate with individuals, never with groups.*    If a group of employees approaches their manager together, requesting clarification of promotion policies or some other matter, the manager is advised to agree to speak with them but only on an individual basis. This power tactic is an example of the application of "divide and conquer." It prevents employees from using one of their major sources of power, their greater number within the organization.
4. *Prohibit pro-union speakers.*    This tactic is related to the control of communication. An organization has the right to determine who is allowed to speak to its employees during work time in areas that are designated as work areas. The organization does not have the right, of course, to determine what its employees do outside of work on their own time in this regard.

All of the preceding points are allowed under the labor laws. Management is not allowed to spy on employees, to make any promises to employees to influence union elections, or to attempt to influence or threaten employees.

### Supervision and Management under a Collective Bargaining Contract

In the past, much of the management literature spoke of collective bargaining as an evil thing that interfered with their work, tied their hands, and threatened to destroy their companies. That attitude has changed a great deal as unions in general have become weaker in the United States and management has realized that they share an important goal with employees: survival of the institution that employs them. The current attitude toward collective bargaining seems to be leaning toward the feeling that it is possible to work effectively under a collective bargaining agreement and that it is not always management that ends up making concessions when a disagreement arises. Although employers' need for flexibility in staffing and employees' need for job security will continue to create some tensions between labor and management, they do share concerns about employee satisfaction and maintaining the viability of the organization (Hannigan, 1998).

> *Labor's vision of a new model workplace and management's vision are, with few exceptions, dramatically different. You can bet management dreams of union-free, intra-organization work groups.*
> —Hannigan, 1998

In order to manage effectively under a collective bargaining agreement, it is often necessary to deal first with management's feelings about the agreement. It would not be unusual for managers to feel as if the necessity for the contract implied that they were the enemy of the staff members, who had to be protected from them. Working under a legal contract also makes some managers anxious about being confronted by the delegate about a mistake or having a particular action brought up in a grievance.

It is most important to know and understand the contract well. The contract is a legal document, and violations of it are **unfair labor practices** that can be grieved, usually successfully, by the union. A thorough knowledge of the contract can prevent the majority of grievances. It is not possible to prevent all grievances because some people will grieve almost anything, even the smallest infraction. The occurrence of a grievance is not necessarily an indication of ineffective management.

When a problem does arise, it is important to react in as nondefensive a manner as you can.

Most problems can be dealt with at the manager-delegate-employee level, as in the examples given earlier. It is particularly important to avoid getting caught up in the Karpman Triangle of victim-persecuter-rescuer or other game playing.

The practice of effective leadership and management with everyone involved, including the union people, and a thorough knowledge of the contract are the most important safeguards against a high-tension, conflict-ridden management-labor relationship. When a conflict does arise that cannot be immediately resolved using these approaches, it should be brought to the attention of higher-level management or the personnel department, depending on the particular institution or agency. Labor-management councils can be formed to encourage cooperation and collaboration, as opposed to conflict, between these two groups (Hannigan, 1998).

### Handling Grievances

If informal counseling with the dissatisfied employee does not lead to resolution of the problem, the first-line manager should bring the problem to the attention of the next higher-level manager. Together they can conduct an investigation of the situation and the relevant policy in the collective bargaining agreement. At this point, it is important to evaluate the accuracy and completeness of the facts presented, whether the particular policy was appropriately interpreted and applied, and whether the policy has been applied in the same way in other situations. If all these questions are answered satisfactorily, the administrator will generally support the first-line manager's decision.

Support of the first-line manager's decision may lead the employee to decide to file a grievance. If personnel and administration support the manager, the employee may, in consultation with the union organizer or professional association representative, decide to take the grievance further, usually to arbitration.

The following list of questions has been suggested by Fay and Morrill (1985) for review of the strength of management's case before deciding to proceed to arbitration:

1. Regarding the policy or practice itself (a requirement that all staff work rotating shifts or

that promotions be based on merit ratings, for example):

- Is the policy clearly stated?
- Have the consequences of violating that policy been clearly communicated?
- Has the policy been applied uniformly in the past?

2. Regarding management's decision to pursue arbitration:
   - Does administration support continuing the action?
   - Is the cost worthwhile in terms of the money, time, effort, and potential outcome?
   - How will this action affect staff morale?
3. What is the likelihood of management winning the case at arbitration?

The organization's legal counsel and other experts in collective bargaining will probably be called in for consultation. All pertinent facts will be reviewed again and questions such as those listed will be debated. If management decides to continue to arbitration (rather than attempt to settle the grievance with the employee), a team will be assigned to handle the case.

The seriousness of the matter usually leads to some self-questioning as to whether the initial decision was correct and if all this further effort is worthwhile. However, not every grievance is justified; a failure to defend a fair decision made by a first-line manager can have a deleterious effect on the morale of all first-line managers and leave employees with the impression that management policies do not have to be taken seriously. Seen from this point of view, proceeding to arbitration can be a positive step for management under a collective bargaining agreement.

## POWER AND POLITICS IN THE COMMUNITY

### Power Distribution in the Community

We turn now to an even larger arena, the community in which healthcare professionals, their clients, and their employers operate. The question of who has the most power and who has the ability to influence decisions within a community has been a difficult one to answer. A community is far too large and complex to re-create in a laboratory, which has been done with groups. Members of a community can be observed of course, but power, authority, and influence relationships are multiple, interconnected, and at the same time subtle and, therefore, difficult to identify by an outsider.

One of the early solutions to the problem of identifying the power distribution in communities was to ask people to list the most influential leaders in their community. It was found that a small number of people were consistently named. These people, primarily from the top ranks of commerce, finance, and industry in the community, were assumed to be the ruling elite, the group that made the decisions in the community (Hunter, 1970).

However, when additional methods (such as studying actual participation in decision making; memberships in community organizations; and positions within business, government, educational, labor, and religious organizations) were used, it was found that different people were influential on different issues. Power and influence varied according to the particular issue and the particular resources controlled by the individual or group. In actuality, the power structure of a community is not a single hierarchy of the elite, but a complex network of many actors, each with varying amounts of power and influence and diverse, often conflicting, interests (Coleman, 1977; Freeman et al., 1970; Marsden & Laumann, 1977; Polsby, 1970).

One useful, although simplified, way of visualizing the distribution of power in the community is to divide those who are powerful into three major groups: the influentials, the effectors, and the activists. The institutional leaders, or **influentials,** are the people who head the largest business, government, political, educational, and other types of organizations. They are the people mentioned earlier who have a reputation for being influential based on their positions within these organizations. It is interesting to note that most of the influentials are not particularly active in community affairs. Their influence is felt primarily by their prestige and support of one side or other on an issue but also through the next group, the effectors.

**Effectors** are active in the community's decision-making processes. Although they are not heads of organizations as the influentials are, they are the professionals, government officials, and employees of corporations in a community. They often become involved in the community's decision-making processes through specific work assignments and are most influential in decisions that require technical or specialized knowledge.

The **activists** are different. They come primarily from voluntary, civic, or service organizations. Although they do not have the effectors' power base of a government agency or large corporation behind them, they influence decisions by committing their time and energy to involvement in community affairs. The activists are less likely to be involved in economic decisions than are the influentials and effectors.

The people who participate regularly in decisions that affect the community are a diverse but powerful group. Some of their power is derived from their positions and based on authority relationships, ability to control the flow of money, credit, and jobs, and expert technical knowledge unavailable to most people in the community. Additional power is derived from their reputation as people who can mediate negotiations, respect for their ability to get things done in the community, connections with other influential people, and influence in community organizations such as political parties or volunteer organizations. Outside political and economic ties are also power sources. People who are influentials, effectors, or activists usually have a cluster of these characteristics, rather than just one or two of them.

For most purposes, the leader or manager will find that the categories of influential, effector, and activist are sufficient for analysis and action. However, the power distribution in a community is actually more complex than these categories indicate, encompassing a large network of people and groups with different resources and links with the decision-making processes of the community. To complicate matters, different issues are settled in different **arenas** within the community so that certain people and groups will be close to one decision-making process but completely removed from, and not even interested in, other decisions.

Those people in the community who do not regularly participate in community decisions still have some potential for influence on decisions. When they do participate, they usually follow one of two general patterns: the high-initiative, direct-action pattern or the low-initiative pattern of participation (Litwack, Meyer & Hollister, 1977).

The **high-initiative** pattern includes group actions such as mass demonstrations, hearings, lobbying, consumer boycotts, picketing, agitation, and protest marches (Bobo, Kendall & Max, 1991). Many of these actions can also be effective as media events, especially if they are dramatic. It also includes such direct actions as hiring professional advocates (for example, lawyers) and using ombudsman organizations, consumer protection agencies, outside auditors, and investigative agencies to bring about desired change.

The **low-initiative** pattern includes group actions such as holding formal meetings and presenting formal requests for change. Individual actions include letter writing, telephoning, and meeting with those who will make the decision and presenting individual requests for change. Although these tactics are low-pressure, they can influence the outcome of community decision-making processes by providing information about community values and positions on particular issues that decision makers, especially politicians and public officeholders, know they cannot ignore without risking negative reaction.

## Political Action: Influencing the Flow of Power and Decision Making

Although often used interchangeably, politics and power are not synonymous. **Politics** includes the actions taken to acquire and use power to achieve one's goals. It can be defined as power in action (Vecchio, 1997) or the use of power (Chesney & Feinstein, 1997).

### Politics is the art of the possible.
—R.A. Butler, 1902–1984, in Eigen & Siegel, 1989

Whenever resistance is strong to a proposed change, an approach is needed that recognizes and deals with the ever-present political behavior and the relevant sources of power and influence. Bachrach and Baratz (1970) developed a model for understanding political decision making including the directions in which power and influence flow, and the major barriers encountered en route to implementing a change. This model (Figure 21–1) is applicable to a wide range of decisions at the organizational, local, state, or national level.

This model is especially useful as a guideline for analyzing a situation in which a large number of variables are involved, as it helps you to sort them out. Once the situation has been analyzed using this model, you can see more clearly where it is possible to have an impact on the decision-making process.

Once the desired change is well defined, the analysis begins with the identification of the individuals and groups who will support the change and those who will oppose it. Then it follows the proposed change through the decision-making channel past four major barriers (community values, blocking procedures, the decision-making arena itself, and administrative interpretation and enforcement) until it is finally implemented. At any barrier, the proposed change can be defeated or delayed indefinitely by the opposing group.

This model uses a combination of the elements of Lewin's analysis of force fields and the power strategies discussed earlier in this chapter in bringing about change through the political process.

### Entering the Decision-Making Channel

When entering the decision-making channel, it is important to clearly identify the most essential factors that will influence the process, which are the desired change or **agenda** and the way in which different individuals and groups involved feel about the change.

### The Agenda or Desired Change

So many different types of decisions are made that it is difficult to categorize all of them. In the healthcare field alone, myriad decisions are made about the kind of services to offer; who will be el-

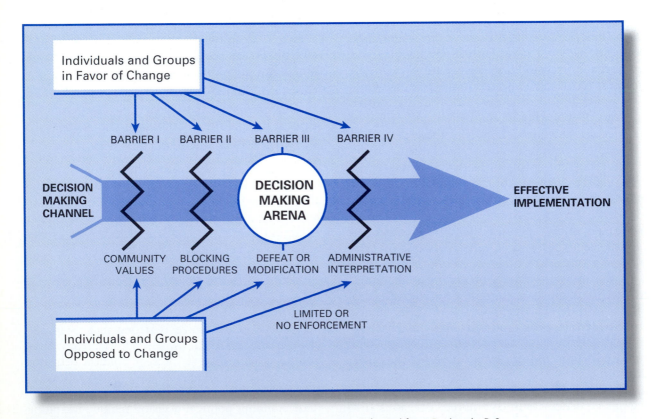

**Figure 21–1**   Flow of decision making in the community. *Source:* Adapted from Bachrach, P. & Baratz, M.S. (1970). *Power and poverty: Theory and practice.* London: Oxford University Press.

igible for them; how to support them; and how they will operate, by whom, and so forth.

The proposal for change or agenda may come from either individuals or groups, such as healthcare organizations; unions; government officials; civic, social, and religious groups; interest groups; professionals; concerned citizens; and individuals who are in need of service.

Groups with the same or different but reconcilable agendas often form coalitions, particularly when each group by itself does not have sufficient power to achieve their goal. Building a coalition requires expression of one's position, clarity on others' positions on the issue, and a search for sufficient common ground to work together (Chesney & Feinstein, 1997).

The proposal that will be followed through the decision-making channels to illustrate the use of this model is one that came from concerned professionals who lived in a particular community:

> Two community mental health nurses who were employed outside the community became concerned about reports of inadequate health care in a correctional facility located in their community. News items about problems with the county jail included stories about serious incidents arising from the neglect of the prisoners' health needs. Two prisoners had committed suicide within the past month, and one had died of a neglected perforated ulcer, although the prisoner had pleaded for medical attention.
>
> After confirming these reports and trying unsuccessfully to work with county officials to improve the situation, the two nurses decided to become involved in a political campaign to improve health services at the jail.

## Identifying the People
## For and Against the Change

Every proposal for change involves some kind of issue around which people can align themselves as being for or against it. At this early stage of the process, many people will be potential rather than actual supporters or opponents. Others will remain indifferent or uninformed about the issue.

The individuals and groups who are in favor of the proposed change will try to push it through the decision-making channel. The opposing forces will try to keep it out of the channel or, once it gets into the channel, to slow or stop its progress. Both must be identified in order to estimate their strength and the sources of their power.

In the example being used, the correctional facility was becoming a controversial issue in the community. Because of the many news stories, a number of individuals and groups had already taken sides on the issue:

> The two nurses found several groups in favor of improving conditions at the jail. A key citizens' organization in the community, the Civic Union, was considering doing a study of the situation and invited one of the nurses, who was a member of the organization, to head the study group. The Interfaith Council, which included representatives from every church and temple in the community, had been trying to introduce some counseling services at the jail and was in support of the proposed change. The major political parties were divided on the issue, but a few in the majority party of the county legislature, which provided the funds to run the jail, supported the idea of making improvements but had not yet worked out the details of any improvement plan. A number of individuals also spoke out against the present conditions in the facility and called for reforms. Among them were several inmates and the parents of a young man who had died in the jail.
>
> Opposing any changes were many individuals who believed that being in prison was supposed to be a punishment. Among them were several people who had been victims of crimes committed by people in the jail. The county sheriff, who was responsible for operating the jail, opposed any changes at the jail except improvements in the building. The sheriff was supported by most members of the sheriff's political party, which was currently the minority party in the county legislature but had only two seats less than the majority party. Two active taxpayers' groups opposed spending any more money on the jail at all.

At the time the nurses joined the movement to improve the jail, many other people in the community were beginning to be concerned about what had happened at the jail but were not sure what should be done about it.

## Barriers to Effective Implementation

### Barrier I. Community Values
Those individuals and groups who are opposed to the change will try to keep it from being considered in any decision-making arena. They will reinforce any existing community values that support the status quo (present situation). These values are the first barrier to any proposed change in the community and are already in place when the change is proposed.

You can almost always find some community values that can be called on in support of a change, but often more of the values support the status quo. The proponents of change will have to overcome the status quo.

Strong community values supported spending as little as possible on the jail, but the media focus on problems at the jail threatened to upset the status quo:

> The county jail was constructed as a place to detain people accused but not convicted of crimes and to punish those found guilty of relatively minor offenses. Those who were given long sentences for serious crimes were sent to the state prison.
>
> Most people in the community preferred to ignore the jail and to leave it to the sheriff's department to operate in such a way that it did not cost the taxpayers too much but kept the inmates securely inside. The prevailing value, then, was to provide the minimum necessary for the jail and its inmates. There was also an undercurrent of feeling that the victim of a crime was more neglected than the person who committed the crime.
>
> Values in support of improving the correctional facility were primarily based on support of humane treatment of any individual regardless of past behavior, and a belief that most people found in county jails would be more accurately described as troubled than as evil or dangerous. When people in the community heard news reports of a series of escapes from the jail, they began to wonder if even the minimal necessities were presently taken care of at

the jail. They also began to think about their own safety living in a community that had frequent escapes.

> The deaths at the facility sparked a grand jury investigation that uncovered numerous instances of inhumane treatment, including neglect of the most basic health needs and failure to provide emergency treatment. Dissemination of the grand jury findings through news stories and discussions at gathering places throughout the community upset the status quo—the community could no longer ignore the jail; too many of its values were in conflict with conditions at the jail.

The proposed change passed barrier I when it became apparent to the community that the jail was not well managed and that its inmates were treated far worse than they had imagined.

### Barrier II. Blocking Procedures
Once the first barrier has been passed, the opponents of the change will try various maneuvers to block its movement into the decision-making arena. At this stage, a working knowledge of the systems involved is needed and often includes the community and its organizations and the different levels and branches of government. This information is needed to set up blocks to the opposition or maneuver around those set up by opposing groups.

Those who oppose the change will try both **avoidance tactics and direct blocking tactics.** The specific tactics used vary according to the situation. The following is an example of those commonly found in organizations:

> If you were trying to get a change made in a particular operating room routine, but the administrator and his staff oppose your idea, the administrator would first try avoidance tactics, such as not returning your calls and not responding to your memos. When you finally succeed in speaking with him (perhaps catching him at a public meeting), he would be politely evasive. If you persist, he might claim that you do not understand the situation and therefore cannot understand why your proposal cannot be implemented. If pressed further, he would probably say he cannot make the decision alone but would not tell you who could make the de-

cision. *When you try to approach others in the institution you might find that they have been instructed to direct all inquiries back to the administrator. If you try to go around him to his superior, you would find that he has been there first and that a new policy that all requests for changes in the operating room policies and procedures must come through the administrator is about to be implemented.*

When these so-called normal channels of communication are effectively blocked, it becomes necessary to circumvent them or to open them up.

This type of avoidance and blocking is common. It succeeds in discouraging all but the most persistent agents for change. However, no person or group is completely immune to public pressure to change, so if the usual channels are blocked, you *can* break down the barrier through the use of power tactics.

In the jail situation, it became necessary to use some power tactics to finally move the issue into the decision-making arena. For this issue, that arena was the county legislature:

*At first the sheriff simply refused to comment on the news stories about the jail. When the grand jury report was released, the sheriff told reporters it was full of erroneous statements. These avoidance tactics succeeded for several months. Finally, however, the legislators felt that they had to do something about the rapidly deteriorating situation and placed the jail on the agenda of their next meeting. The sheriff came to the meeting and told the legislators that because a sheriff is a duly elected official of the county, they could not tell the sheriff how to run the county jail. This direct block succeeded, and the issue was dropped for the time being.*

*The groups supporting the proposal searched for a way around this block. The Civic Union study group, led by one of the nurses, met with several county legislators who were known to oppose the sheriff and support the proposed change. The legislators decided to bring the study group's data and the grand jury reports to the attention of the state investigation commission. At the same time, a group of former inmates decided to sue the sheriff for*

*inadequate medical care. These two actions kept the jail on the front page of the county's newspaper and kept up the pressure on the county legislature.*

*State investigators visited the jail and issued yet another critical report on conditions at the jail. Based on this new report, unidentified sources in the governor's office were quoted as saying that they were looking into ways to remove the sheriff from office. When this news story broke, county legislators were spurred into action. They found a different way to deal with the jail situation—through control of the funds needed to operate the jail.*

Supporters of the proposals to improve the jail finally had succeeded in moving the issue into the decision-making arena.

**Barrier III. The Decision-Making Arena** Once an issue reaches the decision-making arena, both the supporters and opponents are likely to become more open about their viewpoints, and the dividing lines between the groups become clearer. Movement to the decision-making arena often forces the groups or their representatives to face each other directly for the first time to debate the proposal. Evasion is more difficult at this point, but stalling and blocking tactics can still be used by opponents of the proposal for change.

The arena itself varies according to the particular issue. Legislatures at any level of government are frequent arenas, but the courts and administrative arms of government and regulatory and appeals boards are also common arenas. In the jail issue, for example, the former inmates' lawsuit could have become the decision-making channel if the county legislators had failed to respond, and the courts could have ordered improvements at the jail if the inmates won their suit. The executive branch or government can also conduct investigations and hearings that become arenas for decision making. The election process is another arena for community decision making.

Arenas also exist outside of government. Within an organization, the arena may be an appeals board, the board of trustees, or the top executive team. Schools, colleges, and a wide range of community organizations can hold meetings and forums that have the potential to be decision-making arenas. Neighborhood gatherings and formal meetings of representatives from various organizations can also become decision-making arenas. The media—especially newspapers, radio, and television stations—disseminate information, encourage debates on issues, and sometimes support one side but are not usually decision-making arenas.

The jail issue has finally been brought before the county legislature:

*At the preliminary hearing of the legislature, a number of proposals were presented. A coalition of the Civic Union group and the Interfaith Council led by the nurses presented a well-developed, comprehensive plan that called for changing the administrative structure of the jail; providing a wide range of health, social, and vocational services for the inmates; and petitioning the state legislature to remove the county prison from the sheriff's control. One of the supporting legislators presented a similar but less expensive plan.*

*Another legislator who supported the sheriff presented a proposal that simply allocated more funds for the jail, which would be used at the sheriff's discretion. The sheriff had previously requested more money to renovate the building, and this request was read to the group. A representative of one of the taxpayers' groups cautioned the legislators against getting caught up in the emotionalism of the issue and against throwing money at problems instead of trying to solve them inexpensively.*

*Now the lines were clearly drawn. Both sides supported an increase in funds for the jail, but one side wanted the money to be spent on services and to remove control of the jail from the sheriff. The other side wanted the sheriff to retain control of the jail and to spend any additional funds on construction.*

*As often happens, the positions and proposals of the two sides were reduced to two-word descriptions, and they became known as the "anti-sheriff" and "pro-sheriff" groups. The division also followed political lines, with most members of the sheriff's political party supporting the sheriff and many from the other party opposing the sheriff.*

*The sheriff was a well-known, popular figure in the community. At the legislative hearing, the sheriff spoke persuasively of a long*

*fight to maintain law and order in the community and implied that the other side wanted to coddle the prisoners and let them run loose in the community. One of the guards at the jail described the unruly behavior and abusive language guards had to deal with daily. The county engineer described the deteriorating condition of the prison building.*

*The "anti-sheriff" group, including the two nurses, described the inhumane treatment of the inmates in dramatic tones, implied that the sheriff was not capable of operating the prison properly, and warned that the sheriff's methods would turn relatively harmless people into dangerous criminals by the time they were released back into the community. The parents of the young man who died recounted their unanswered pleas for help and the way their son was treated in the hours before he died. The hearing lasted six hours and received extensive news coverage.*

*The legislature adjourned at 2:00 A.M. and reconvened the next afternoon to vote on the proposals. The coalition's proposal to expand services was approved after cuts were made in the budget section. However, the proposal to remove control of the jail from the sheriff was defeated by a small margin. Both groups claimed victory, but neither side actually felt satisfied. The sheriff retained control of the jail but was now supposed to provide more services for the inmates.*

**Barrier IV. Administrative Interpretation and Enforcements**   It would seem that once a decision is made, especially if it is in the form of a law, that the battle would be over. It is not that simple, however. As with official goals of an organization, official laws can be ignored or partially enforced if the community does not support the law and pressure a reluctant administrator to firmly and fully enforce the law. In addition, some laws are so vaguely worded that they can be interpreted in several ways.

The same is true of any decision. Any ruling, procedure, or decision can be ignored or evaded by its opponents if its enforcement is not closely followed by its supporters.

The results of the county legislator's decisions left a situation in which limited enforcement was almost a predictable outcome:

*The sheriff continued to control the jail. After the funds were appropriated, the sheriff quickly initiated renovation plans and publicized the physical improvements being made. However, the introduction of new services did not conform with the approved plan. A part-time social work student and a licensed practical nurse were hired but given little direction or support. One community group was given permission to visit inmates once a week, but the volunteers were treated so rudely that they did not want to return.*

*Although news items about the jail decreased considerably, both the coalition and supporting legislators continued to pay close attention to what was happening at the jail. When it became apparent that only token attempts to improve health, social, and vocational services were being made, they brought their data and complaints back to the state investigation commission, which renewed its pressure on the sheriff. The threat to remove the sheriff from office was a real possibility although it was a rare occurrence. The sheriff finally hired an experienced and capable administrator for the jail. The new administrator appointed several community advisory boards to develop plans for improving conditions in the jail, and within a year, most of the services described in the coalition's original proposal were implemented.*

The tremendous amount of time and energy required to implement the proposal described in the example was due not only to the strength of the opposing side but also to the community's fundamental lack of interest in what happened at the jail so long as members of the community did not feel that it affected them personally. The combination of strong opposition, initial community disinterest, and conflicting beliefs and values made it difficult to move the issue through the channels of decision making to effective implementation.

You may have noticed that the nurses in the example were only a small part of the group that finally succeeded in improving prison conditions. A number of different individuals and groups within the community and outside the community were eventually involved and brought their collective power and influence to bear on the situation. Without this convergence of power and influence from many sources, the change would not have taken place. As an individual leader, you can act as a catalyst in bringing these forces together. As an energizer in helping to keep up interest and momentum, you can greatly extend your influence in the community.

## ● SUMMARY

Power is the ability to change people's behavior despite resistance. Everybody has some sources of power available to them. These sources may include physical strength, ability to threaten harm, positional power, money, legal power, public recognition and support, expert power, the power of an idea, strength in numbers, and control of access to resources.

Power is unevenly distributed both in organizations and in the broader community within which they operate. Within an organization, the sources and distribution of power may be overt or covert. Formal authority, control of resources, use of organizational structure, the arena for change, the management of meaning, control of boundaries, interpersonal alliances and networks, and countervailing organizations are indicators of the way in which the power is distributed and exercised within an organization.

Use of a power-based strategy begins with defining the issue and identifying the opponent. Then the leader organizes a following, builds a power base, and carries out the power tactics needed to pressure the opponent into the desired change in behavior.

From the employee's point of view, collective bargaining begins with the formation of an organizing council and recognition of a bargaining agent, which is usually the professional association or a national union, by the employer, either voluntarily or after an election. Then contract negotiations begin between representatives of management and the bargaining unit. If a stalemate occurs, mediation, fact-finding, binding arbitration, or work stoppages may be used to bring about an agreement. Once a contract is signed, it must be enforced. When a problem arises concerning interpretation of the contract or fairness in treatment of an individual employee, the grievance procedure is used to work out the problem as specified in the contract.

From the management point of view, a number of actions can be taken to prevent unionization, including regular surveys of employee opinions, adequate compensation and benefits, an effective grievance procedure, opportunities for participation in decision making, and treating professionals like professionals. More specific measures include controlling communication within the organization and refusing to negotiate with employees in groups. If the organization is unionized, good leadership and management and a thorough knowledge of the contract are the most important components of an effective management strategy for dealing with unionized employees.

People who regularly influence decision making in the community can be categorized as influentials, effectors, or activists. Others in the community participate at irregular intervals and can be categorized as having high- or low-initiative patterns. The model for analyzing the flow of power and decision making in the community begins with the identification of the proposed change, its supporters, and its opponents. The four barriers in the way of effective implementation are prevailing community values, blocking procedures, the decision-making arena, and administrative interpretation and enforcement of the change.

## C A S E   S T U D Y

### The Right to Practice One's Profession

After completing a master's degree, Tawana Wright accepted an advanced nurse practitioner (APN) position in a large 75-physician medical practice. Her first week was a disappointment. She found herself functioning at the same level as the office nurses but thought it was just because she was still being oriented to the new setting. After several weeks, however, she realized that nothing had changed. She was still a glorified office nurse.

Tawana began talking with several advanced practice nurses who worked with other physicians within the practice. She soon realized that most were functioning at the same level as she was. When she asked them why, they told her that they had tried to function more independently, including seeing patients on their own, but that the resistance had been enormous and they had failed to bring about any significant change. When they met as a group with the physicians, the physicians told them that they (the physicians) were happy with the way things were and did not want to change it. Furthermore, if they (the APNs) were not happy with the situation, they could leave. "We have

to try again," Tawana declared after the meeting. "Are you with me?"

### Questions for Critical Reflection and Analysis

1. Assess the relative power of Tawana and her APN colleagues versus the physicians in this group practice. What sources of power does each group have?
2. Assume that the APNs had tried all of the other approaches to change (rational, participative, and reframing) and failed so that a power-based strategy is appropriate. Create a scenario in which the APNs use a power strategy to change their roles within the practice.
3. Assess the likelihood of success of the power strategy you designed for the APNs. What factors are essential for success? What factors would undermine (weaken) the strategy?
4. Now, assume the strategy you designed is successful. What do the APNs need to do after winning?
5. Would you be comfortable being involved in the power strategy you created? Why or why not?

# REFERENCES

Alinsky, S.D. (1972). *Rules for radicals: A practical primer for realistic radicals.* New York: Vintage Books.

Bachrach, P. & Baratz, M.S. (1970). *Power and poverty: Theory and practice.* London: Oxford University Press.

Bernstein, A. (1999, June 19). All's not fair in labor wars. *Business Week,* 43.

Bloom, J.R., Parlett, G.N. & O'Reilly, C. (1980). Collective bargaining by nurses: A comparative analysis of management and employee perceptions. *Health Care Management Review, 5,* 25.

Bobo, K., Kendall, J. & Max, S. (1991). *Organizing for social change: A manual for activists in the 1990s.* Washington: Seven Locks Press.

Bradford, D.L. & Cohen, A.R. (1998). *Power up: Transforming organizations through shared leadership.* New York: John Wiley & Sons.

Byrnes, N.C. (1993). Blue collar blues. *Financial World, 162*(23), 26–30.

Chesney, J.D. & Feinstein, O. (1997). *Building civic literary and citizen power.* Upper Saddle River, NJ: Prentice Hall.

Coleman, J.S. (1977). Notes on the study of power. In R.J. Liebert & A.W. Imershein (Eds.). *Power, paradigms, and community research.* Beverly Hills: Sage.

Dalrymple, J. (1995). Turning privatization to advantage. In A.B. Shostok (Ed.). *For labor's sake: Gains and pains as told by 28 creative inside reformers.* New York: University Press American, Inc., 90–98.

Eigen, L.D. & Siegel, J.P. (1989). *The manager's book of quotations.* New York: AMACOM.

Fay, M.S. & Morrill, A.K. (1985). The grievance-arbitration process: The experience of one nursing administration. *Journal of Nursing Administration, 15*(6), 11–16.

Fitton, R.A. (1997). *Leadership: Quotations from the world's greatest motivators.* Boulder, CO: Westview Press.

Flanagan, L. (1992, October). How collective bargaining benefits nurses. *Directions Supplement to the American Nurse.*

Flarey, D.L., Yoder, S.K. & Barabas, M.C. (1992). Collaboration in labor relations. *Journal of Nursing Administration, 22*(9), 15–22.

Freeman, L.C. et al. (1970). Locating leaders in local communities: A comparison of some alternative approaches. In M. Aiden & P.E. Mott (Eds.). *The structure of community power.* New York: Random House.

Fullam, C., Lando, A.R., Johansen, M.L., Reyes, A. & Szaloczy, D.M. (1998). The triad of empowerment: Leadership, environment, and professional traits. *Nursing Economics, 16*(5), 253–254.

Giovinco, G. (1993). When nurses strike: Ethical conflicts. *Nursing Management, 24*(5), 86–90.

Haley, J. (1969). *The power tactics of Jesus Christ and other essays.* New York: Avon Books.

Hannigan, T.A. (1998). *Managing tomorrow's high-performance unions.* Westport, CT: Greenwood Publishing.

Hook, S. (1979). The conceptual structure of power—An overview. In D.W. Harward (Ed.). *Power: Its nature, its use, and its limits.* Boston: Schenkman Publishing.

Hunter, F. (1970). Methods of study: Community power structure. In M. Aiken & P.E. Mott (Eds.). *The structure of community power.* New York: Random House.

Hunter, J.K., Bamberg, D., Catiglia, L.L., P.T. & McCausland (1986). Job satisfaction: Is collective bargaining the answer? *Nursing Management, 17*(3), 56–60.

Koerner, J.G. & Bunkers, S.S. (1992). Transformational leadership: The power of symbol. *Nursing Administration Quarterly, 17*(1), 1–9.

Kolb, D.A., Osland, J.S. & Rubin, K.M. (1995). *Organizational behavior: An experiential approach.* Englewood Cliffs, NJ: Prentice Hall.

Laschinger, H.K.S., Wong, C., McMahon, L. & Kaufman, C. (1999). Leader behavior impact on staff nurse empowerment, job tension, and work effectiveness. *Journal of Nursing Administration, 29*(9), 28–31.

Litwack, E., Meyer, J.J. & Hollister, C.D. (1977). The role of linkage mechanisms between bureaucracies and families: Education and health as empirical cases in point. In R.J. Liebert and A.W. Imershein (Eds.). *Power, paradigms and community research.* Beverly Hills: Sage.

Luttman, P.A. (1982). Collective bargaining and professionalism: Incompatible ideologies? *Nursing Administration Quarterly, 6*(2), 21.

Marsden, P.V. & Laumann, E.O. (1977). Collective action in a community elite: Exchange, influence, resources and issue resolution. In R.J. Liebert & A.W. Imershein (Eds.). *Power, paradigms and community research.* Beverly Hills: Sage.

Mitnick, S. (1998, April). Nurses as drug dealers? Organized medicine. Get real! *The Florida Nurse,* 14.

Morgan, G. (1997). *Images of organization.* Thousand Oaks, CA: Sage.

Nadler, D.A., Gersten, M.S., Shaw, R.B. et al. (1992). *Organizational architecture: Designs for changing organizations.* San Francisco: Jossey-Bass.

Ness, I. (1998). *The unions and the betrayal of the unemployed: Labor conflict during the 1990s.* New York: Garland Publishing.

Polsby, N.W. (1970). How to study community power. In M. Aiken & P.E. Mott (Eds.). *The structure of community power.* New York: Random House.

Porter-O'Grady, T. (1992). *Implementing shared governance: Creating a professional organization.* St. Louis: Mosby Year Book.

Riffer, J. (1986, January 20). Physician unions fight loss of control. *Hospitals, 82.*

Rose, A.M. (1967). *The power structure: Political process in American society.* New York: Oxford University Press.

Schwertzer, C. (1998). Empowerment by example. *Association Management, 50*(5), p.50(2).

Shindul-Rothschild, J., Berry, D. & Long-Middleton, E. (1996). Where have all the nurses gone? *American Journal of Nursing, 96*(11), 25–39.

Shostok, A.B. (1995). *For labor's sake: Gains and pains as told by 28 creative inside reformers.* New York: University Press of America.

Simms, L.M. & Dalston, J.W. (1984). A professional imperative. *Health and Health Services Administration, 29*(6), 115–123.

Thomson, A.W.J. & Murray, V.V. (1976). *Grievance procedures.* Westmead, UK: Saxon House.

Trossman, S. (1999, March/April). Support Dana-Farber nurses facing disciplinary action. *The American Nurse, 1, 10.*

Vecchio, R.P. (1997). Power, politics and influence. In R.P. Vecchio (Ed.). *Leadership: Understanding the dynamics of power and influence in organizations.* Notre Dame, IN: University of Notre Dame Press.

Walker, E. (1995). Making a bid for change: Formulations in union/management negotiations. In A. Firth (Ed.). *The Discourse of negotiation: Studies of language in the workplace.* Oxford, UK: Elseirer Science Ltd.

Wilson, D.C. (1992). *A strategy of change: Concepts and controversies.* London: Routledge.

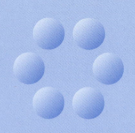

CHAPTER **22**

# Political and Economic Context of Health Care

LEARNING OBJECTIVES

*After completing this chapter, the reader will be able to:*

- Trace the evolution of the U.S. healthcare system from the mid-nineteenth century to the present.
- Assess the impact of various payment mechanisms on health care and healthcare delivery.

- Discuss the current issues and concerns related to the present healthcare system.
- Create scenarios for continued evolution of the healthcare system through the twenty-first century.

## TEST YOURSELF

**Healthcare System Quiz**

*Place either a **T** for **TRUE** or an **F** for **FALSE** in front of each of the following statements.*

_____ 1. The Social Security Act marked the beginning of federal support for social welfare programs.

_____ 2. Medicaid is a federal health insurance program for people over 65.

_____ 3. The largest percent of people without health insurance are children and the elderly.

_____ 4. The right to health care is guaranteed by the U.S. Constitution.

_____ 5. HMOs are an increasingly common form of health insurance

_____ 6. HMOs cover all healthcare costs.

_____ 7. Medicare covers all healthcare expenses for those over 65.

_____ 8. PPOs negotiate reimbursement rates directly with providers.

*Answers*

1. T  2. F  3. F  4. F  5. T  6. F  7. F  8. T

It seems that some new problem or new proposal related to our healthcare system comes up every day. While this comment may be an exaggeration, the level of interest and concern about what has been happening to our healthcare system certainly has been rising. The combination of the following factors:

1. Rapid technological advances making new treatments available across a wide range of health problems
2. Increasing costs related to these new drugs, tests, procedures, high-tech inpatient care, and specialized care
3. Changes in employers' and the various levels of government's willingness to pay the bill for health care
4. Consumers' increasing concern about what the quality and availability of health care will be when they need it and how they will pay for it

has created a tangle of issues, conflicting goals, and political pressures that no one has been able to unravel and reconstruct as a viable, cost efficient system that provides high-quality care to everyone who needs it.

Representing a substantial proportion of the healthcare workforce that supports our present system, nurses are clearly impacted by the resulting turmoil. Their role and presence within the healthcare framework have a number of implications for the kind of leadership needed to ensure professional survival and growth in an increasingly complex world.

In this chapter, we look first at the way in which our healthcare system evolved into its present form, the broad changes in society that have affected the system as a whole, and the nursing profession as a critical component of that system. Then we consider the issues facing our healthcare system today and how these factors may affect the shape of our healthcare system in the future.

## ● EVOLUTION OF TODAY'S HEALTHCARE SYSTEM

### Beginnings

Social welfare programs as we know them today did not exist in colonial America. Any help or assistance came from family, friends, neighbors, or church members. Health care was given primarily by practitioners using a variety of remedies and treatments selected by trial and error. Treatment choices were guided by folk wisdom rather than by research. Health care was not yet organized, and the hospitals and community agencies we are so familiar with today did not exist.

The modern healthcare system began in the mid-nineteenth century. In the United States, the call to attend to Civil War casualties focused attention on the need for hospitals, surgeons, and nurses. Still, most health care remained outside the walls of any organized institution and in the hands of individual practitioners.

By the 1870s, the establishment of the nation's first large hospitals, Bellevue in New York and Massachusetts General in Boston, marked the beginning of the institutionalization of health care. By the early 1900s, sanitation had substantially improved. Various voluntary organizations had been established, such as the Mental Health Society in 1909 and the American Cancer Society in 1913. Some of the organized charities, such as the Red Cross, began to be known for their contributions to the health and welfare of society (Spradley, 1990).

Most nurses worked privately, as private duty nurses do today. Hospitals used students rather than graduate nurses to staff their wards. In many cities, visiting nurses were bringing badly needed care into the homes of the ill and poor. By 1920, the larger visiting nurse associations (VNAs) had added prevention to their services, but these preventive measures were soon taken over by the nurses from the developing public health agencies (Buhler-Wilkerson, 1985).

## Scientific, Technological, and Social Expansion

Science and technology made rapid advances in the period from 1900 to 1940. Vitamins were discovered in 1912, insulin in 1922, and the 1940s saw the introduction of antibiotics. With the availability of effective antibiotic therapy, the nature of the nation's health problems changed dramatically. As improved sanitation, widespread immunization, and antibiotic therapy lessened the threat of infectious disease, chronic diseases (heart disease, cancer, stroke, diabetes, and so forth) assumed greater importance.

Until this time, hospitals were used only by people without families to care for them, by the mentally ill, and those too poor to afford private care. Those patients who could afford to pay for their care had no reason to use the hospital, because it could not offer them more care than could be provided at home by physicians who made house calls or by the readily available private duty nurses. The number of patients using hospitals changed as more technology developed and hospitals offered services of interest to paying patients and their physicians.

The financial problems of the Great Depression gave birth to many economic changes, including the beginnings of commercial health insurance. A group of Dallas schoolteachers arranged a prepaid plan to provide themselves with up to 21 days of hospitalization a year for 50 cents a month. The idea was supported by members of the American Hospital Association, who feared the loss of income they would suffer when people were having difficulty paying their bills. The idea quickly gained popularity. Before World War II, 20 percent of Americans were covered by health insurance; by the 1960s, 70 percent were covered (Torrens, 1978). By 1996, 83 percent of the population had insurance coverage (Rubin and Koch, 1999).

In 1935, Congress passed the Social Security Act. This important act provides aid to people who are totally disabled, blind, aged, poor, or families with dependent children, and is now known collectively as the Supplemental Security Income (SSI) program. Social security also provides pensions for older adults based on the contributions they made during their working years. This legislation marked the beginning of governmental involvement in social welfare programs. As we begin the new millennium, debate continues regarding what the role of government should be in the delivery of healthcare and other social welfare programs.

When World War II ended and soldiers returned home, many new families were formed. The demographic phenomenon of high birthrates now known as the "baby boom" began in 1946 and extended through 1964. The sheer size of this group has attracted attention as it moves along its life path, from entry into the public school system, then into the workplace, and now, as they grow older and need more health care. Concern about meeting their healthcare needs when they become the older generation is increasing (*Looking to the future*, 1997). It is the focus of much discussion in not only the federal and state governments, but also in the private employment sector, which faces new challenges as the workforce ages and retires, including the nursing workforce (Peterson, 1999).

The Hill-Burton Act was enacted in 1946 to increase the number of hospital beds in rural areas and to redistribute physicians so that medical care was more equally available throughout the country. This program was extended into the 1960s by the Hill-Harris amendment, which provided for the modernization and replacement of public and nonprofit facilities in both urban and rural areas. These bills were later criticized for focusing too much on construction and too little on healthcare delivery and distribution (Rydman & Rydman, 1983). They were not effective in achieving physician redistribution, a problem that persists to the present day. However, with these initiatives the federal government "became firmly and irreversibly part of the American health care system" (Hyman, 1975).

## Growth and Prosperity

The New Frontier began in 1961 with the inauguration of President Kennedy, who encouraged the development of a sense of altruism. A positive attitude toward helping the people of the world was exemplified by the founding of the Peace Corps. President Johnson, Kennedy's successor, refocused this theme on the poor in the United States and called for the creation of the Great Society. People believed that we could conquer social and health problems the way we had been able to "conquer" space; they thought that by applying our vast knowledge and resources, we would meet the goals of the Great Society.

One successful offshoot of space exploration was a tremendous expansion in research and technological development, much of which was applicable to health care. Sophisticated monitoring devices became available, making intensive care units possible. New materials and compounds were developed and found their way into replacement joints and other devices.

In this era of growth and prosperity, the concept of comprehensive medical insurance for older adults finally gained public support. Compromises were made, and in 1965, two separate programs were created, Medicare for the elderly and Medicaid for the poor. **Medicare** is a federally supported program of health insurance for those over age 65 and disabled social security recipients. It is financed by payroll deductions from employees and employer contributions. **Medicaid** is a program for the financially indigent and is administered by most states with a combination of state, federal, and local funds.

## Skepticism and Disillusionment

The controversial war in Vietnam and the resignation of President Nixon because of the Watergate scandal increased public skepticism of government. In 1975, President Ford signed the National Health Planning and Resources Development Act, designed to replace all previous planning programs, including the Hill-Burton program. This act set forth specific guidelines for health planning and the construction of new facilities. Its goals were the elimination of duplication of resources through the issuance of certificates of need (CONs) before new facilities could be built, the identification of priority goals, and the encouragement of health maintenance organizations (HMOs), a form of prepaid health coverage discussed later in this chapter. The intent was to influence supply and demand for services on a statewide level, with input from regional groups known as health systems agencies. Budgetary cuts forced the closure of these agencies by the mid 1990s.

Disillusionment with the unfulfilled promises of the Great Society and its hastily enacted programs (Schlesinger, 1988), loss of the war in Vietnam, the Arab oil embargo of the late 1970s and other brief military actions made Americans more aware of their limitations and interdependence with the world's economy. Suddenly, we were vulnerable and imperfect, facing complex social and economic problems which had no easy solutions. It seemed to be easier to send men to the moon and set up orbiting space stations than to solve the problems of poverty and ill health.

Meanwhile, taxes, especially social security taxes, continued to rise, as did the federal deficit. Healthcare costs also escalated, from $41.9 million in 1965, the year Medicare and Medicaid were enacted, to $248.1 million in 1980 (Pear, 1993). This figure accounted for 5.9 percent of the gross national product (GNP) in 1965, and 14.1 percent in 1995 (Congressional Budget Office, 1995). People began to talk about the limitations of the nation's resources and our ability to continue to finance these programs. President Reagan was elected in 1980 on a platform promising fiscal restraint and return of power to the states, a concept known as the New Federalism. This concept proposed a reduced federal obligation to serve and protect those who cannot protect themselves; it provided a safety net in times of crisis, but no new assistance to those in need. Nonetheless, the national debt grew during the Reagan years due to increased military spending, while more support for health and social welfare programs was expected to come from private, corporate, and religious philanthropy (Jones, 1985). Self-reliance had become a theme.

During the 12 years of the Reagan and Bush administrations, reducing taxes and balancing the federal budget were priorities. To accomplish these goals, spending cuts had to be made. Yet a growing cohort of older people continued to place demands on the social security system, which became a prime target for reduction measures. The aged, however, had become a large and effective lobby. So while resources shrank, social security recipients continued to receive cost-of-living adjustments to their pensions. Healthcare costs also escalated with little restraint.

In the 1980s, the public began to accept the concept of self-responsibility for health, particularly in regard to health-related behaviors, such as exercise, eating more fruits and vegetables, and lowering dietary fat intake. These habits began to be accepted as good ideas. Even the once glamorous behavior of smoking was to be banned in most public places.

The limits of self-reliance became clearer as the 1980s ended. The staggering physical, emotional, and financial burden of caring for people with Alzheimer's disease has been well publicized, as has been the care of persons infected with AIDs. Services were often fragmented or unresponsive (Nokes, 1991), and the number of people with these diseases continues to rise. Tuberculosis (TB) which has long challenged healthcare workers, had a resurgence, particularly in urban areas. Increased violence, substandard housing conditions, poverty, and chemical dependency further contributed to the demands on the healthcare system. Many questions about the healthcare system's ability to respond to these needs have remained unanswered.

## An Age of Limits

In the early 1990s, Americans began to doubt their ability to meet the numerous challenges their nation faced. After a costly skirmish in the Middle East and a multibillion dollar bailout of the federal savings and loan industry, Americans questioned their government's financial priorities. Domestic problems such as unemployment, homelessness, AIDs, drug abuse, crime, and recession worsened and healthcare costs continued to cause concern. An increasing elderly population and a rise in the number of single-parent families placed unprecedented demands on social services, particularly when extended family members were not available to help.

Even though the economy stagnated in the early 1990s, technology advanced. The human genome project was funded and genetic markers for life-threatening diseases such as cystic fibrosis and breast cancer were found. Organ transplants continued to be performed with increasing success. Many benefitted from joint replacement surgeries and cardiac procedures that not only prolonged life but offered the promise of a higher quality of life.

Employers, ever conscious of the bottom line, were redesigning the workplace. Corporate giants merged, displacing thousands of upper and middle income people, while job expansion occurred mostly at entry-level, minimum wage jobs. Other positions were redesigned to no longer be full time, resulting in the elimination of eligibility for benefits such as health insurance and paid sick leave. Health insurance is a valuable employee benefit, usually paid for by employers, and usually available only to full-time employees. Economic downturns, the expansion of lower-wage part-time positions, and in the mid-1990s the movement of many from welfare roles to lower-paying positions left many people lacking in health insurance coverage. They made too much money to qualify for governmental programs, but too little to be able to afford health insurance premiums.

Presidents Reagan and Bush made many conservative judicial appointments. These appointments left their mark when federal funds were restricted from use for abortion services. A contentious issue since the 1973 *Roe v. Wade* Supreme Court decision, the courts drifted toward a more conservative stance, eventually banning abortions in federal military facilities. In some states, parental disclosure and notification laws were passed. A "gag" rule was placed on agencies receiving federal support prohibiting the mention of abortion as an alternative to continuing a pregnancy.

At the same time, extensive lobbying by several groups brought about the passage of the Americans with Disabilities Act (ADA) in 1992. First introduced in 1989, this act was designed to prohibit discrimination against individuals with disabilities in accessing public services and employment. Persons who are qualified for a position cannot be denied that position because of a disability. Instead, employers must make "reasonable" workplace accommodations unless doing so would cause an undue hardship. The ADA also requires that all businesses and services be accessible to all people. New construction must be wheelchair accessible; older construction must be made accessible unless it would cause undue hardship. The interpretation of "reasonable" and "undue hardship" remains a point of debate (Litowich, 1999; Coit & Shapiro, 1996).

Health services research uncovered disparities between communities in the frequency of certain medical and surgical procedures. The Agency for Healthcare Research and Quality (AHRQ), formerly called the Agency for Health Care Policy and Research, was established in 1989 to study the effectiveness of various treatments and practices. This agency became the leader in the movement toward evidence-based practice and the careful examination of healthcare policies, procedures, and treatments in terms of their efficacy.

The existence of this agency was threatened in the mid-1990s when an orthopedic medical specialty group lobbied against support for chiropractic studies. Keeping such agencies free from political influence continues to be a problem. Despite these issues, AHRQ has succeeded in identifying and establishing frameworks for determining the efficacy of various treatments through outcomes-based research and evidence-based practical studies and continues to support study of healthcare delivery and financing options (Buerhaus, 1998).

The continuing increase in technology coupled with an aging population and rising expectations resulted in an increase in healthcare costs from 10 percent of the GNP in 1990 (Rheinhardt, 1990) to 14 percent in 1993, to a predicted 16–19 percent by the year 2000 (Solovy, 1994). Controlling cost while maintaining access to care raised the issue of healthcare reform, which became a major political issue in the 1992 presidential campaign.

## Reform of Health Care

President Clinton's election in 1992 marked the return to power of the Democratic party. In his first week in office, he had the "gag" rule limiting discussion of reproductive options set aside. Soon afterward, he announced the formation of a healthcare reform task force to be led by his wife, Hillary Rodham Clinton.

In the fall of 1993, the healthcare reform plan was made public, but was not well received. The healthcare reform task force's comprehensive plan was seen as cumbersome, costly, a threat to free enterprise, and too much government interference in people's personal lives. The plan failed, but the question of how to best meet people's healthcare needs remained.

As health insurance costs rose, businesses sought more economical solutions. Individuals who did not have healthcare insurance through their employers found premiums to be prohibitive. As a result, many opted to not be insured. In an effort to keep their products affordable, healthcare insurers designed new plans with more limited coverage, while Congress and the public continued to debate ways to keep both the social security system and Medicare solvent into the twenty-first century. Businesses began to offer a greater array of healthcare insurance plans for their employees, offering different coverage at varied costs. Health maintenance organizations (HMOs) became popular options.

Despite the failure of the proposed Health Care Security Act in 1993, some healthcare reforms were put in place. Pressure to reduce the number of diagnostic tests and the length of stay (LOS) in acute-care facilities increased. The average LOS in acute-care facilities has decreased steadily since 1990. In the state of Florida, for example, it dropped from 8.5 to 6.2 days for Medicare patients and from 6.7 to 5.2 for the entire patient population (FHA, 1998). Nationally, Medicare-reimbursed hospitals' stays declined in length from 8.1 to 6.6 in just three years (McGinley, 1999). The increasingly rapid discharge from these facilities left a much more acutely ill population in the hospital. Advances in technology such as laser surgeries, more potent oral antibiotics, and safer anesthesia techniques enabled 70 percent of surgeries to be done on an outpatient basis. Hospitals began to experience lower occupancy rates, and the demand for home healthcare services increased dramatically. The number of home health agencies increased from 11,097 Medicare-certified home health agencies in 1989 to 20,215 in 1996 (National Association for Home Care, 1997), but many have since closed, blaming changes in Medicare reimbursement for their financial troubles (Hicks, 1999).

Insurers began to require precertification for inpatient procedures. Larger insurers began to negotiate the amount they would reimburse to providers. The balance of power shifted in health care; physicians could no longer order unlimited tests and procedures without consideration of cost. Healthcare reform was being driven not by consumers or direct care providers but by third party payers.

Physicians increasingly resented this intrusion into their clinical decision making and into their finances, evidenced by the passing of a historic resolution at the American Medical Association's (AMA) House of Delegates 1999 meeting. This resolution gave official organizational sanction to collective bargaining efforts by physician employees. At almost the same time, the American Nurses Association (ANA) House of Delegates voted to strengthen their presence in collective bargaining on a national level by forming a new subsidiary, United American Nurses (UAN). UAN will serve in an advisory capacity to the ANA on issues such as staffing and workplace safety (ANA, 1999).

## Corporatization of Health Care

As the twentieth century ended, hospital mergers became common. Community-based hospitals increasingly merged with other facilities or agreed to be purchased by larger entities. Local boards of trustees have merged with corporate boards. Voluntary, not-for-profit hospitals that reflected the character and values of their local communities were changing, adopting the values of Wall Street rather than Main Street (Brown, 1996).

When hospitals, healthcare facilities, and insurance companies are investor owned, questions must be asked regarding who benefits: Is it the community? Staff? Individual patients? Will the drive for profits ultimately shortchange patient care? (Brown, 1996). Business models value customer satisfaction, but business also values profits. Will one win out over the other? What will the corporate mission be? How will decisions be made? Will the community remain the primary beneficiary of transactions? Who will the decision makers be? Who will monitor care and decide what is paid for? Will it be local clinicians or an actuarial company? (Anders & McGinley, 1998). Who will monitor drug practices and decide which drugs are on the formulary, a pharmacy benefit management company or local clinicians? (Ingersoll, 1998).

## Challenges in Healthcare Delivery

What are the challenges that lay ahead in healthcare delivery? The continued shift to ambulatory and outpatient services makes each patient encounter all the more important. With shorter acute stays and increasing home-based care, limited time is available to assess, diagnoses, treat, teach, and evaluate patient responses to therapies as well as the family's ability to provide care at home. Lower reimbursements may tempt providers to increase the volume of patients they see and to cut back on what they may see as the "frills," including patient education and follow-up care. How can patients be educated to care for themselves and feel "cared for" in a system that funds only a seven-minute encounter per ambulatory care patient? (Brody, 1999).

Continued technological advances are making it possible for people to live longer. The life expectancy of an infant born in America in 1996 was 76 years. Life expectancy for those already 65 was 17.5 more years (Center for Disease Control and Prevention, 1999). When Medicare was first introduced, the average life expectancy was much less. As technology advances, we can expect to see more individuals living longer lives, meaning more years in which Medicare and Social Security are needed.

The huge cohort of baby boomers will reach age 65 between 2011 and 2029. The generations that follow them are smaller, having come in years of lower birth rates. The result is that fewer workers will be paying into the social security trust fund relative to the number of new retirees as the "boomers" turn 65. The continued funding of Social Security and Medicare, as well as Medicaid and other services for senior citizens is a major concern. Numerous Congressional commissions have been formed over the years to come up with ways to "save" Social Security, but a solution acceptable to all has been elusive.

Technological advances have also enabled people to become more informed about their health care. The burgeoning use of the Internet and the ease with which people can access health-related information makes it much easier for individuals to learn about their health care. The wise provider knows that many patients are searching web sites relevant to their condition and may well be comparing what they are told against information obtained on the Internet or from printed material. The concern is that not everyone is able to evaluate the veracity of information posted on various sites. Providers can help patients evaluate the relevance of information to their particular circumstances and can provide listings of credible web sites and other sources of information to their patients.

The continued corporatization of health care may or may not be beneficial in the long run. Practitioners may also move to a corporate model. Entrepreneurial physician groups who want more control over their practice may split away profitable hospital service lines and establish their own radiology, women's health, or cardiology centers (Winslow, 1999). A danger here is that the healthiest patients will be referred to these freestanding centers, enabling them to be more profitable, while the poorer and more seriously ill patients will be left to obtain care within the traditional acute-care system.

Financing health care will remain a challenge as long as Americans disagree on whether health is a right for all citizens or a commodity available for purchase by those who can afford it. Greater agreement can be found among Americans in support of basic public health measures, such as a clean water supply, sanitary waste disposal, and communicable disease surveillance than support to either finance or to provide basic healthcare services to individuals. Wellness programs and patient education are recognized as critical to keeping the public healthy and reducing the need for costly intervention, but funding for them remains limited.

## ● FINANCING HEALTH CARE

Health care is financed in many different ways within the United States. The predominant form of payment for health care has shifted from a retrospective payment system to either a prospective payment system or a system in which reimbursements have been preset at a negotiated amount between provider and insurer. These approaches to financing health care are explained in the next section.

### Retrospective Payment

For many years, private health insurance companies and government programs reimbursed healthcare providers and hospitals on the basis of what it cost them to provide care. As costs increased, however, this format was seen to provide little incentive for either the consumers or the providers to be cautious about expenses or to seek lower-cost alternatives, because the bill was paid by a third party, usually an insurance company or government agency. Health care was given as ordered by the physician with little questioning of the physician's decisions by either the hospital, the insurer, or the consumer.

As healthcare costs escalated, private insurers, employers who paid for that insurance, and others who paid the bills began to question the costs of health care. They began to encourage more outpatient procedures, second opinions before surgery, and use of preventive services, the latter on a limited basis. Employers began to encourage employees to attend health education and fitness programs. Although this change initially appeared to mark a shift from an illness to a wellness focus, eventually the emphasis became cost savings.

## Prospective Payment

Prospective payment made its debut as part of the Social Security Amendments of 1983. In an attempt to control costs, this bill provided for prospective rather than retrospective reimbursements for hospitals. Under the **prospective** approach, payment levels were set ahead of time on the basis of the average cost for providing various types of care. To preset costs to be reimbursed, almost 500 different diagnostic-related groups (DRGs) were identified. Medicare data from prior years was used to determine a preset payment for care. If care could be provided for less than this fixed amount, hospitals could still keep the full payment, benefitting from their efficiency. However, if expenses exceeded the allowed payment, no further payment was made, and the hospital suffered the financial consequences of this discrepancy.

Medicare is financed by a payroll deduction tax on working individuals and by monthly premiums paid by enrollees. Medicare does not cover certain important healthcare expenses, such as routine vision and hearing care, dental care, and prescription medications. It also covers only limited long-term care and home healthcare coverage. Even on allowable services, enrollees must pay a certain deductible amount out of pocket. Consequently, many people on Medicare also purchase supplemental insurance policies to cover these expenses. Providers who accept Medicare or Medicaid patients agree to accept the reimbursement provided by these insurances; additional amounts cannot be charged to the patient. Medicare patients also have the option of joining a Medicare managed care plan, called a Medicare HMO.

## Health Maintenance Organizations

An HMO is a different approach to paying for health care whereby the insureds or their employers pay a set premium to cover whatever health care they need. Care is provided by a network of physicians and facilities who have agreed to the payment they will accept from the HMO. Under a **capitation** system, the HMO receives an agreed-upon annual amount "per head" and is thus motivated to provide care in a cost-effective manner (i.e., to spend as little as possible on each enrollee). Members typically have primary care physicians within the HMO. To see a specialist within or outside the network, most HMOs require that they obtain the approval of their primary care provider who acts as "gatekeeper." Even emergency care must be approved by the primary care provider within a "reasonable" time frame. Many predict a waning of the "gatekeeper" concept, with HMOs becoming more liberal in allowing tests and specialist visits. Some see gatekeepers as an additional administrative layer and expense as well as an unnecessary source of delay in receiving needed services (see Perspectives . . . Encounters with the Healthcare System).

An original goal of HMOs was that each individual would have a primary care provider who would "know" him or her and would be able to coordinate his care. Consumer choice, however, is limited to those providers who are HMO participants. Unfortunately, they may change from year to year. Some HMOs rely on staff physicians and in-house clinics to provide care (Freudenheim, 1998).

*The logic of capitation is to take a larger pool of aggregates and hope or at least develop a confidence that a low incidence of those patients will ever utilize the services, and the lower the utilization, the more profit can be claimed.*
—*Robbins, 1998, p. 222*

*. . . capitation has incentives to undertreat, delay, and undercare.*
—*Robbins, 1998, p. 189*

## PERSPECTIVES . . .

### Encounters with the Healthcare System

Families and providers unhappy with the present cost-conscious system gave vivid examples of their frustrations with the present healthcare system. Some examples:

- A child who sustained an eye injury during a Little League game received emergency treatment from an ophthalmologist who was attending the game. The child's HMO denied emergency room coverage and the recommended admission for surgery until his parents received approval from his primary care physician. Payment for care given by the ophthalmologist who provided on site emergency care was denied because he was not a member of the HMO. The child's care and subsequent surgery were delayed until necessary HMO approvals were obtained and an HMO-member ophthalmologist was found to care for the child. The child and his family, already upset and stressed by the accident, were further distressed by these delays.

- An obstetrical patient who had a cesarean section in the past suffered a ruptured uterus during vaginal delivery. The baby became a quadriplegic as a result. The family sued the hospital noting that all the nurses on duty that night had limited obstetrical experience. Their lawyer argued successfully that the hospital was responsible for the infant's injury because a conscious decision had been made to save money by staffing the unit with less experienced nurses (Robbins, 1998).

- A cancer patient had to wait four months for his HMO to approve high-dose chemotherapy recommended by his physicians. His doctors finally provided the care without the HMO's approval but it was too late. He died believing he had left his wife with a $750,000 medical bill (Court, 1999).

*Sources:* Robbins, D.A. (1998). *Managed care on trial.* New York: McGraw-Hill; Court, J. (1999, February 3). Telling verdict. *Sun-Sentinel.* West Palm Beach, FL, 217.

Some HMOs entered communities with heavy marketing and promises of low insurance premiums. However, they may have limited enrollment to younger, presumably healthier populations. As these populations age and HMO members develop more chronic health problems, premiums have risen. Some HMOs have declared bankruptcy or have left some unprofitable markets. Members who have preexisting conditions then have difficulty finding another insurer.

### Preferred Provider Organizations

In the late 1990s, Preferred Provider Organizations (PPOs) also became popular (Freudenheim, 1998). Members of PPO plans can go to any primary care provider or specialist they choose but it costs them more to see those who are not part of the network. They do not need permission to seek health care. In 1998, HMOs had 75 million members nationally while PPOs had 105 million members. From 1993–1998, PPOs added 44 million members, while HMOs added 30 million (Freudenheim, 1998).

One of the largest private insurers, Blue Cross/Blue Shield, with 69 million members, moved almost a quarter of its subscribers to PPOs in the 1990s; this figure compares with only one in 10 before that time. PPOs have become popular because they allow members more choice in terms of who provides their care.

A modified version of the PPO is the point-of-service (POS) plan. These plans are a bit less expensive than PPOs. Members can go to specialists outside the PPO network, but at an added cost. They may also need "gatekeeper" approval. However, the member has more choices than in a traditional HMO. They do not have the advantage of a single, primary care provider who coordinates their care.

Some policies regarding what is covered or not covered are inconsistent, others discriminatory. For example, for years, many forms of health insurance have denied coverage for contraceptive care. When some of these same policies chose to cover prescription medications for disorders such as male pattern baldness and erectile dysfunction, women's groups were quick to identify these inequities in coverage.

Frequently, insurers deny claims for treatments whose efficacy is not "proven," such as bone marrow transplants for cancer patients.

While policies may or may not clearly state their limitations, people may not read the fine details of their prospective coverage when choosing insurance, or they may not have a choice in coverage. Because few people anticipate that they will experience a catastrophic illness they rarely investigate the fine print of their contracts until a need arises.

> *Plans and providers say they will provide all medically necessary care and are paid up front to do so. If there is a scheme that results in denial of appropriate care, then both the government and the beneficiaries have been defrauded.*
>
> —Turner, 1999, p. 31

## Limitations in Coverage

Individuals and families become upset when their healthcare insurer denies care. Denial of care, limitations on coverage, and delays in obtaining care all contributed to what became a "consumer backlash" against the insurance industry. Nader (1999) reported that "nearly seven of 10 Americans fear that when they are sick their managed care company will be more interested in saving money than in providing the best medicine" (p. 29). Consumer demands for increased HMO accountability led to efforts to have Congress pass a "Patient's Bill of Rights," while the health insurance industry countered with claims that the demands put forth in such proposed legislation would be so costly that it would leave more Americans than ever without health insurance (Igangni, 1999). Disillusionment with HMOs helped foster the growth of other forms of health insurance.

## Consequences of the Changes

What have these changes meant to the healthcare system? First, these changes have firmly moved the delivery of health care into the context of business, where the ability to compete is essential to survival. The DRG system alone has had profound effects on all aspects of healthcare delivery. Healthcare providers have been forced to look more critically at the outcomes of their care and the efficiencies of their operations. In the course of having to become more businesslike and competitive in their operations many smaller hospitals have closed. Even larger medical centers have merged into multihospital systems to take advantage of efficiencies of scale in administrative costs, marketing, and purchasing.

All these newer forms of healthcare coverage contract with providers and facilities for agreed-upon reimbursement rates for services. By the end of the 1990s, primary healthcare providers and facilities were feeling increasingly squeezed as more and more people were covered by these forms of insurance. As specific plans became more popular in given geographic areas, insurers often reduced or stabilized reimbursement rates to control costs. When large numbers of people in a community are covered by just a few plans, the providers who refused to accept the negotiated reimbursement rates risked losing their client base. While this trend results in cost savings for the insurer and those paying insurance premiums, it can force those in private practice to close practices if revenues do not meet expenses. It can also pressure facilities to use "downward substitution" to lesser-educated, lower-cost employees, such as unlicensed assistive personnel (UAPs) to provide care formerly given by professionals. Ingersoll (1998) reports substitution of the originally prescribed drug in order to achieve cost savings, sometimes at the expense of efficacy.

The prospective payment system greatly increased the incentive to discharge patients more quickly from acute-care settings. However, if a patient is readmitted within 30 days with the same DRG diagnosis, the facility may not be reimbursed for the second hospitalization. Moving patients out of the hospital more quickly has decreased the daily occupancy rates markedly, a trend that began when DRGs were instituted in 1983. As predicted (Shaffer, 1985), decreased occupancy rates caused a decline in revenues for hospitals, while fixed costs such as utilities, salaries, and supplies continued to rise. The patients who remained were more acutely ill during their hospitalizations requiring more intensive assessments, interventions, and evaluations. More acutely ill patients consume more resources relative to their length of stay. Patient acuity has also had an effect on home health agencies and long-term care facilities, which are admitting patients who require more care than their clientele did in the past (See Perspectives . . . Healthcare Gridlock?).

---

PERSPECTIVES . . .

## Healthcare Gridlock?

Acute-care facilities have worked for years to shorten hospital stays. Their success has had an unintended effect on the long-term care sector of our healthcare system. At the same time, reductions in Medicare coverage of long-term care stays led many skilled nursing facilities to refuse to admit some patients ready to be discharged from acute care because their care could cost far more than the amount the facility will be reimbursed by Medicare. Some examples:

- A Medicare patient admitted for a six-day stay in a long-term care facility needed a prosthetic device post amputation. The device cost $3,750 but Medicare reimbursed the facility only $1,183 for both the patient's stay and the device.
- An older woman was denied admission to two long-term facilities because they had calculated that her prescription drugs alone cost more than Medicare would reimburse them for all of her care.
- In one case, a hospital agreed to buy a patient's antibiotics to persuade a long-term care facility to accept him.

Some home agencies have also closed as a result of reductions in Medicare reimbursement, further complicating hospitals' attempts to find placements for patients who no longer need acute care but are not ready to care for themselves entirely.

---

*Source:* Based on McGinley, L. (1999, May 26). As nursing homes say "No," hospitals feel pain. *The Wall Street Journal*, B1.

---

Home healthcare services were initially seen as a cost-effective way of providing care while enabling individuals to remain in their homes. The demand for home healthcare services and

nursing home care grew. Home healthcare became a "high-tech" 24-hour-a-day service. Nursing homes have a greater number of seriously ill patients than in the past, patients who require more monitoring by more professional staff. Population shifts and societal changes leading to more adults living on their own in single-person households, with few people to rely on for help, caused a demand for subacute care services. For example, an 85-year-old widow may have same-day surgery and be transferred from the recovery area to a subacute unit of a nursing home for 24–48 hours of care and monitoring prior to returning home.

At the same time, hospitals have sought ways to increase their revenue by branching out into numerous allied health services in their communities. Some offer surgicenters, pain clinics, women's health centers, rehabilitation services, subacute care centers, long-term care, and home health services. Others develop specialty area service lines in cardiology, oncology, gerontology, and the like. Satellite branches of high-volume service lines may be offered in outlying communities, providing a patient stream to the acute-care facility. Establishing a "center" is an effective marketing tool if it meets the needs of its target audience. Patients appreciate "one-stop shopping" for their healthcare needs, a place where services are delivered holistically and in an organized, comprehensive manner respectful of their time (Phillips, Himwich & Fitzgerald, 1999).

Despite the array of healthcare insurance options available, 43.4 million Americans were without health insurance in the mid 1990s (Kilborn, 1999). Who were these uninsured people? Not the elderly or disabled, because they are covered by Medicare. In fact, only 1 percent of the uninsured were over the age of 65. Relatively few are children; 15 percent were under 18. Many poor children are eligible for Medicaid; those who were ineligible were likely to be eligible for a five-year, $24 billion program for non-Medicaid-eligible children, approved by Congress in 1997 (Kilborn, 1999).

The remainder of the uninsured, 25–30 million people between the ages of 18 and 65, have the greatest chance of being unable to pay for care if they become ill. The shift of people from welfare to work in the late 1990s has been identified as one reason why so many are uninsured. Many low-paying or part-time jobs do not provide health insurance coverage, yet these individuals may no longer be eligible for Medicaid (Kilborn, 1999). In addition, one in four of those with health insurance available to them through employers declined that option (often because they could not afford it), forcing them to either pay for care out of pocket, or to forego care.

A gulf has been growing between what is medically available and what is affordable (Wielawski, 1998). The danger is that health care may be rationed by the ability of the patient to pay for care, not by need. The uninsured may avoid needed health care only to develop far more serious and costly health problems later. Medicare patients may receive treatment, but if they cannot afford the cost of their prescription medications, that treatment is ineffective.

> *Perhaps managed care should itself be treated as an experiment, in fact a potentially dangerous experiment and until such time that it can assure the same safety, honesty, safeguards, and integrity that other health care delivery options afford, it should be treated as such, rather than being prematurely and uncritically heralded as something which works and works well.*
>
> —Robbins, 1998, pp. 223–224

A prevalent myth in America portrays everyone who needs medical care as being able to get it (Wielawski, 1998). Yet in reality stories abound of children who have repeated hospitalizations for acute asthma exacerbations because their parents cannot afford to pay for their medications. Some elderly may skip medication in an attempt to make a prescription last longer. Uninsured women delay starting prenatal care. Children remain unimmunized.

It is true that many of the newest, latest treatments are costly. Yet ethical questions surround the establishment of different standards of care, based on ability to pay (Wielawski, 1998).

## ● A LOOK AHEAD
### Prospects for Future Reform

None of the plans to reform healthcare finance put forth in the early 1990s took hold. The "Jackson Hole Group" in the early 1990s had supported the concept of government assistance to finance healthcare collectives (Hubner, 1993). The American Nurses Association and 57 other nursing organizations supported a single-payer system similar to that used in Canada. But businesses and much of the public resisted anything that would increase payroll taxes. Rather than an organized, universal system of health care, Americans ended the twentieth century with a fragmented care system.

Opponents of national healthcare plans questioned the role of government in the provision of healthcare services. They pointed out that the U.S. Constitution, adopted in 1789, makes no mention of the public's health. Thus, healthcare matters, like all matters not mentioned in the Constitution, were left to the responsibility of individual states. Americans have historically favored the view that health care is not a "right" and not an obligation of the federal government. The argument that health care is not a federal responsibility ignores the federal government's critical role in disease prevention through the formation of the U.S. Public Health Service and the Centers for Disease Control and in research through the National Institutes of Health (Spradley, 1990). Such disparate views have caused conflict and lack of consensus whenever expansion of services is suggested.

Many issues are yet to be resolved when considering how to finance health care in the future. Foremost is the decision regarding who is responsible for healthcare costs: state or federal government, employers, consumers, or all of the above. Second, what level of service should be available to everyone? What services would be offered? What services would be optional? How would decisions be made regarding the addition of services as technology advances? Would supplemental insurance policies or private payment for a higher level of service be permitted? Is that fair to all? Americans accustomed to freedom of choice in their health care have already found HMOs, with their restricted panels of providers, less attractive than the PPOs (Freuden-heim, 1998). Healthcare practitioners who work within HMOs have voiced frustrations regarding lack of control over their practice (Greenhouse, 1999). Eventually we will have to answer the fundamental question behind all of these issues surrounding the financing of our healthcare system. The question remains as to how we can reconcile what is best for each individual with what is best for society (Rheinhardt, 1993).

## What Will Health Care Be Like in the Future?

The patient of the future may face many different care scenarios. The following story is one version of how health care may be delivered in the future:

> Arriving at the surgical center of the future, the client is directed to a walk-up window that resembles a present-day automatic teller. The client is instructed to place the appropriate health insurance card into the slot. A computerized voice then directs the client:
>
> "Press 1 if you are having surgery. Press 2 if you are having diagnostic tests. Press 3 if you are here to have a postoperative evaluation. Press 4 if you need further assistance. A qualified healthcare person will be with you shortly."
>
> The client is then instructed to choose the appropriate surgical procedure on the computer screen. After the selection is verified and approved, the client receives directions from the electronic voice:
>
> "You may now enter through the double doors to your right. The doors will open automatically. Please step carefully onto the moving platform. The platform is traveling at the same speed as the treatment vehicle. Kindly enter the first treatment vehicle as it approaches. Place the second finger of your left hand into the yellow circle for a blood test. A blood pressure cuff will encircle your left upper arm. Do not pull on the bar or belts. The safety bars and seat belts will lock automatically as the back of your vehicle reclines and the foot rest rises to the forward position. Your vital signs and other appropriate information will be monitored by highly sophisticated computer technology throughout your entire stay with us.

> "As you pass through Station 1, please place your right arm through the designated opening for the placement of your intravenous line. This will be inserted by an automated sensor robot. Through the use of infrared sensors and sonography, the sensor robot locates an appropriate vessel with greater skill than an actual nurse. You may feel a slight burning at this time. Do not pull your arm away. We repeat, do not pull your arm away.
>
> "You are now approaching Station 2. Please place your right hand through the designated opening to receive the appropriate medication. The computerized vehicle in which you are traveling has automatically calculated the accurate dosage of medication based on your body weight and metabolism. The medication you will receive has been determined by an analysis of your blood drawn at Station 1. This eliminates any possibility of human error. However, if at any time you feel any itching, tingling, or tightness in your throat or lungs, please press the red button on the left side of your vehicle. Our computers will automatically institute emergency measures for your health and safety. This action precludes the possible delays that can occur in the human decision-making process.
>
> "You have reached Station 3, your assigned surgical suite. Please observe the screen in front of the vehicle. Meet your surgeon, Dr. I. M. Yourfuture, from Houston, Texas. Through the use of computer technology and robotics, she will be performing seven of these procedures simultaneously in different geographic locations. Anesthesia will be administered through the mask moving toward your face. Please remain still while the robot arm securely fastens the straps around your neck. Take several slow deep breaths when the blue light on the console begins to flash. Your anesthetic dose has been predetermined through a highly sophisticated mathematical formula. Pleasant dreams. We hope you enjoy your surgery while at 21st Century Surgical Center, saving healthcare dollars for a better tomorrow."

Compare the experience of the 21st Century Surgical Center to this alternative view of the future of health care:

*Arriving at the New Age Health Center, the client walks into a central atrium, is offered a cool drink, and is encouraged to "choose a comfortable seat in the center, where you can enjoy the musical fountain or meditate in one of our quiet corners, whichever you prefer." After relaxing awhile in the atrium, the client walks down the hall to the consultation rooms. The client notices that one of the center's animal healers (a big, friendly Labrador) has joined him and is accompanying him down the hall.*

*Guides along the walkway ask the client if he knows the way or would like some assistance in choosing a healer to consult. "I'm feeling very stressed at work lately," answers the client. "Having trouble sleeping, which is unusual for me."*

*"We have several ways to approach your concerns," says the guide. "You could try our stress-reducing exercise path, our yoga path, the medicinal consultation, the sleep consultation, or all four if you'd like."*

*"I already have a good exercise program and prefer not to use medicinal therapies unless they're necessary, so I think I'll try that sleep consultation. I really need to get more sleep than I have lately."*

*The guide nods and directs the client toward the sleep center. "Ralph (the Labrador) would be happy to go with you, if you'd like." Ralph wags his tail in agreement.*

*At the end of the consultation, the client walks to the door with his sleep tapes and a video explaining how to use them as he has been shown by the sleep consultant. His sleep consultant bids him "a good night's rest tonight," and Ralph walks him back to the atrium, leaving him with a quiet "woof."*

What is your preferred view of future healthcare delivery? Do you prefer the high-tech approach of the 21st Century Surgical Center or the high-touch approach of the New Age Health Center? Which would your clients choose? Is it possible to combine the best of both approaches? Which one do you think will prevail in the future? If you or a family member were a patient, which of these scenarios would be the preferred care model?

## Nursing's Role in the Future

We don't know for sure how health care will be delivered in the future or what nurses' roles will be in the healthcare system of the future. However, we can look at the current trends in our society, their effect on today's healthcare system, and what they may tell us about the future. There we may find some clues to the future of health care and of the nursing profession.

Nursing has played a major role in the evolution of the American healthcare system. Nurses have adapted to changes in healthcare delivery in the past and will have to continue to evolve to remain an important presence in the healthcare arena. Today's nurse faces new challenges. Although these challenges can create turmoil, they also open the door to opportunity.

> *Transition management, role change and expansion, and a need for new skills such as delegation, team building and supervision of others are essential in this new marketplace.*
> —Turner, 1999, p. 42

Nurses are the largest single group of healthcare professionals; they are a major force in the delivery of health care in the United States (Cherry, 1999), spanning all practice settings in which people seek care. The skills professional nurses possess uniquely position them among the health professions to provide and manage care across the health-illness continuum. Nurses' critical thinking ability and proximity to patients make them key members of the healthcare team, both at the bedside, and in the boardroom. Nurses must accept their special societal role to not only succeed in these care arenas, but to be patient and community advocates.

To succeed, nurses need to accept the challenge of an environment that is in a state of constant change, susceptible to market and fiscal pressures. These pressures can create new opportunities for some nursing positions while eliminating the need for some others. Paying attention to the marketplace and social change, coupled with continuing education, enables individual nurses to grow and to evolve in their professional lives. The nursing profession bears the responsibility of ensuring that a nursing presence is maintained in the health care of tomorrow.

> *Nurse innovators all across the country are leading the organizational changes in their hospitals, systems, and emerging integrated delivery networks by implementing unique and creative patient care options that decrease lengths of stay, lower costs, and enhance patient outcomes.*
>
> —Turner, 1999, p. 15

## ● SUMMARY

The evolution of the healthcare system was influenced by the development and growth of hospitals, which became the favored workplace for healthcare professionals through the influence of scientific and technological advances, the effect of the introduction of antibiotics, and the introduction of health insurance, Medicare, and Medicaid. Government involvement in health care has gradually increased, but so have costs, to the point that concern is being expressed about the limitations of our resources in continuing to provide for everyone's healthcare needs. Greater longevity and a growing cohort of older adults will place even greater demands on the healthcare system in the twenty-first century. In response to this concern, prospective payment systems were introduced to attempt to control healthcare costs, which had a significant impact on many facets of the healthcare system, particularly on attitudes toward competition, productivity, and marketing.

Concerns about escalating healthcare costs and access to care became so great that by the early 1990s healthcare reform had become a promi-

---

## C A S E   S T U D Y

### Admission Denied

Mathilda Dutoit is a new staff nurse in the emergency department of a suburban hospital. Halfway through her first night shift tour, a patient told her that he intended to kill himself. Mathilda reported this incident to the supervisor, suggesting that the patient be admitted. The supervisor later advised Mathilda that the patient would not be admitted.

"But he might kill himself!" Mathilda exclaimed. "We learned in school that a threat must always be taken seriously. If he succeeded, we'd be responsible. He needs help."

"Unfortunately, his insurance company informed us that because he did not *attempt* to commit suicide, just *threatened,* they will not cover the cost of inpatient hospitalization. Instead, he is to be medicated and referred to a day center. We will give him a referral to the mental health clinic."

"That's not enough. What if he doesn't go? What if he doesn't continue to take his medication?"

"Look, we can't admit someone who can't pay for his or her care. We know his insurance company will not pay. He is not critically ill or injured and wants to leave. There is nothing we can do. I'm sorry."

### Questions for Critical Reflection and Analysis

1. Based on the information provided in the case study and in the chapter, on what principle do you think the decision was made to refuse to admit this patient?
2. What further action do you think Mathilda should take? What further action do you think the supervisor should take in this situation? Explain your answer.
3. If the patient did commit suicide the next day, who would you say was responsible? Explain your choice.
4. Create a scenario in which this patient receives the appropriate care without leaving the hospital responsible for subsidizing his care.

*Source:* Based on Robbins, D.A. (1998). *Managed care on trial.* New York: McGraw-Hill.

nent political issue. Several approaches to reform, including managed competition and single-payer systems, were considered. Important issues arose in these discussions, including the role of government in health care, access to care, rationing of care, health care as a private responsibility versus an individual's public right, the financing of health care, and individual rights and obligations in respect to maintaining one's own health.

The shift to prospective payment systems and managed care/managed competition forced economies on healthcare facilities and providers. Health care entered the realm of business, with mergers, acquisitions, and work design. Technological advances in care enabled shorter hospitalizations and more procedures done on an ambulatory basis, driving inpatient populations down while increasing the demand for home care and ambulatory facilities. Yet despite the sustained economic growth of the 1990s, the gaps between society's "haves" and "have nots" grew, while welfare reform pushed more people off Medicaid rolls and into low-paying jobs without health insurance.

# REFERENCES

American Nurses' Association (1999, July/August). ANA creates new "house" for all nurses. *The American Nurse, 31*(4), 1, 8.

Anders, G. & McGinley, L. (1998, June 15). Actuarial firm helps decide just how long you spend in the hospital. *The Wall Street Journal,* 1, a-16.

Brody, J. (1999, June 4). How to die young as old as possible. Presentation at Western Connecticut State University, Danbury.

Brown, M. (1996). Commentary: The commercialization of America's voluntary health care system. *Health Care Management Review, 21*(3), 13–18.

Buerhaus, P. (1998). Nursing's first senior nurse scholar at the U.S. Agency for Health Care Policy Research, *Image, 30*(4), 311–314.

Buhler-Wilkerson, K. (1985). Public health nursing: In sickness or in health? *American Journal of Public Health, 75*(10), 1155–1161.

Centers for Disease Control (1999). Life expectancy. *National Vital Statistics Reports, 47*(13). *http://www.cdc.gov.nchs.www/faststats/lifeexpec.htm*

Cherry, B. (1999). Nursing care delivery models. In B. Cherry & S.R. Jacob, *Contemporary nursing issues, trends and management.* St. Louis: Mosby.

Coit, J.H. & Shapiro, L.J. (1996, Spring). The ADA at three years: A state of flux. *Employee Relations Law, 21*(4), 5–38.

Congressional Budget Office (1995, February). *U.S. Congress, Health and Human Resources.*

Court, J. (1999, February 3). Telling verdict. *Sun-Sentinel.* West Palm Beach, FL, 217.

Florida Hospital Association (1998). *FHA eye on the market: Healthcare in the sunshine state 1998.* Orlando.

Freudenheim, M. (1998, September 29). (Loosely) managed care is in demand. *New York Times.* C-1, C-4.

Greenhouse, S. (1999, February 4). Angered by HMOs treatment, more doctors are joining unions. *New York Times,* A-1, B-8.

Hicks, C. (1999, February 26). The century foundation convenes group of medicare experts to chart course for reform. *The Century Foundation.*

Hubner, J. (1993, July 18). The abandoned father of healthcare reform. *New York Times Magazine,* 24–37.

Hyman, H. (1975). *Health planning: A systematic approach.* Rockville, MD: Aspen.

Igangni, K. (1999, September). "No: it's lawyers, not patients, who stand to benefit." *AARP Bulletin, 40*(8), 29, 31.

Ingersoll, B. (1998, January 6). FDA to watch drug switching, sales practices. *The Wall Street Journal,* B-1, B-6.

Jones, P.A. (1985). Reaganomics: Health policy and politics. In R.R. Wieczorek (Ed.). *Power, politics and policy in nursing.* New York: Springer, 26–33.

Kilborn, P.T. (1999, February 26). Uninsured in U.S. span many groups. *New York Times,* A-1, A-17.

Litowich, L. (1999, May/June). Overcoming hurdles. *Michigan Health and Hospitals, 35*(3), 28–29.

Looking to the future. (1997). *The Nation's Health.* Washington, DC, 1, 7.

McGinley, L. (1999, May 26). As nursing homes say "No," hospitals feel pain. *The Wall Street Journal,* B1.

Nader, R. (1999, September). Yes: HMOs currently face no liability. *AARP Bulletin, 40*(8), 29, 31.

National Association for Home Care (1997). *http://www.nahc.org*

Nokes, K.M. (1991). Applying the chronic illness trajectory model to HIV/AIDS. In P. Woog (Ed.). Illness trajectory framework: The Corbin and Strauss nursing model. *Scholarly Inquiry for Nursing Practice, 5*(3), 140–248.

Pear, R. (1993, September 3). Clinton cuts aims on mental health and dental costs. *New York Times.*

Peterson, C.A. (1999). Nursing Supply and Demand. *American Journal of Nursing, 99*(7), 57–59.

Phillips, C.R., Himwich, D.B. & Fitzgerald, C. (1999). The business of women's health: What nurses need to know now and in the 21st century. *AWHONN's Lifelines, 3*(2), 23–29.

Rheinhardt, U.E. (1993, September 10). Health care reform. "Today Show" (televised interview).

Rheinhardt, U.E. (1990). Rationing the health care surplus. An American tragedy. In P.R. Lee & C.L.

Estes. *The nations' health* (3rd ed.). Boston: Jones & Bartlett.

Robbins, D.A. (1998). *Managed care on trial.* New York: McGraw-Hill.

Rubin, R.M. & Koch, M.W. (1999). Economic issues in nursing and health care. In B. Cherry & S.R. Jacob (Eds.), *Contemporary nursing: Issues, trends, management.* St. Louis: Mosby, 145–164.

Rydman, L.D. & Rydman, R.J. (1983). The United States health care delivery system. In W. Burgess & E. Ragland (Eds.). *Community health nursing: Philosophy, process and practice.* Norwalk, CT: Appleton-Century-Crofts.

Schlesinger, M. (1988). The perfectability of public programs: Real lessons from large-scale demonstrations. *American Journal of Public Health, 78*(8), 899–902.

Shaffer, F.A. (1985). Prospective payment: A strategic plan for nursing power. In R. R. Wieczorek (Ed.), *Power, politics and policy in nursing.* New York: Springer, 33–54.

Solovy, A. (1994, March). Taming the tiger: The economics of healthcare reform. *Hospitals and Health Networks, 26–34.*

Spradley, B.W. (1990). *Community health nursing: Concepts and practice* (3rd ed.). Glenview, IL: Scott Foresman/Little Brown Higher Education.

Torrens, R. (1978). *The American health care system. Issues and problems.* St. Louis: Mosby.

Turner, S.O. (1999). *The nurse's guide to managed care.* Gaithersburg, MD: Aspen Publishers.

Wielawski, I.M. (1998). Rationing medical care: The growing gulf between what's medically available, and what's affordable. *Advances Supplement, 4,* 1–4.

Winslow, R. (1999, June 22). Fed-up cardiologists invest in own hospital just for heart care. *The Wall Street Journal,* 1, A-12.

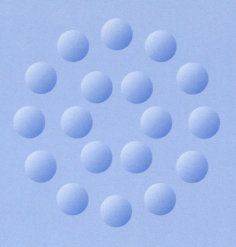

*UNIT* **V**

# Career Development

*CHAPTER* **23**

Leadership Aspects of
Career Development

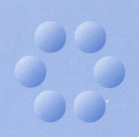

# Leadership Aspects of Career Development

## LEARNING OBJECTIVES

*After completing this chapter, the reader will be able to:*

- Conduct an effective job search.
- Design an appropriate resume.
- Participate in both traditional and competency-based job interviews.

- Describe approaches to prevention and treatment of reality shock and burnout.
- Describe a career path for a nurse who has advanced to the highest levels of the profession.

## TEST YOURSELF

**What kind of job do you really want?**

*Why are you looking for work? What is it that you really want from your job? Rate each of the following on a scale of 0 (of no importance to you) to 10 (very important to you). It does not matter how many you rate at 0 or how many you rate at 10.*

*When you have finished the ratings, look for patterns in the scores. Do you prefer a quiet, stable environment or a high pressure environment full of excitement and drama? Is patient contact most important to you? Are financial considerations important to you? Is recognition important? Think about what your ratings tell you: what* really *matters to you in regard to your work? The answer should reflect your personal preferences and values. All the following rewards are available in nursing, but not all can be gained from any one position.*

Rating Rewards

_____ A balance between work and personal life

_____ Recognition for your achievements

_____ Opportunity to work independently

_____ Colleagues with whom you make decisions jointly

_____ Slow, steady pace of work

_____ Weekends and evenings free

_____ Steady paycheck

_____ Long-term relationship with patients

_____ Opportunities to form friendships

_____ Low-stress environment

_____ Clear guidelines and established procedures

_____ Flexible schedules

_____ Highly competitive environment

_____ Financial rewards

_____ Sense of purpose, meaning from work

_____ Free time for social, recreational activities

_____ Time to be alone

_____ High pressure environment

_____ Opportunities to be part of a team

_____ Fulfillment from what you do at work

_____ Opportunities to manage others

_____ Opportunities to be creative and innovative

*Source:* Based on Double, D.L. (1998). *Assessing your career options.* Chicago: American Medical Association.

---

The term **career path** evokes many images. One is that of a journey that will take you to your eventual career destination, whatever it may be. It also reminds us that many twists and turns may be encountered along the way, even occasional detours. Along this path, you are likely to encounter a number of different people who will influence the speed and direction of your progress. Some will point out stumbling blocks you might have tripped over if you didn't know they were there. Others will suggest ways to get around barriers you find across your path. A few will give you misdirection, and you may have to retrace your steps because of them. For the most part, however, you will be making your own choices: deciding on your direction, how quickly and directly you want to reach your destination, and what you want to accomplish along the way. These personal decisions are ones you must make for yourself.

In this chapter, some guidelines for making these decisions and progressing along your career path will be offered. In keeping with the leadership/management focus of this book, the emphasis is on the intra- and interpersonal aspects of career development: the job search, employment interview, reality shock, burnout, mentoring, and career advancement. You will not find forecasts of employment opportunities in the nursing profession or descriptions of the many specialty areas from which you can choose because they are so numerous and they change so rapidly. For this type of information, it is best to obtain the most recent reports from the professional organizations and the governmental agencies that monitor the job sector. You can ask for information from these organizations, read the literature (including the news media), or do an online search. Even if you have already been employed in a healthcare position, this chapter will help you reflect on where your career path has led you so far and where you want to go in the future.

## ● OBTAINING A POSITION

### The Job Search

When you embark upon a search for a new position, reflect upon your answers to the three following questions:

1. What am I prepared to do?
2. What do I really want to do?
3. What type of positions are available?

Each of these questions is discussed in the following sections.

### Preparation

Both education and experience should be taken into consideration in evaluating the degree to which you are prepared for a particular nursing position. Some skills are relevant to almost any position: interviewing, counseling, and assessment skills, for example. Others are useful only in specific situations: preparing a patient for childbirth or administering the pneumovax vaccine, for example.

### Basic Qualifications

The basic degree in nursing and licensure in the state where you will work are the essential credentials for an entry-level position as a registered professional nurse. In addition, employers also look for the following qualities in job candidates (Shingleton, 1994).

- Oral and written communication skills
- Demonstration of responsibility
- Interpersonal skills
- Proficiency in a given field
- Technical competence
- Ability to work as part of a team
- Willingness to work hard
- Ability to assume leadership tasks
- Motivation, initiative, and flexibility
- Analytical skills
- Computer knowledge
- Problem-solving and decision-making abilities
- Self-discipline
- Organizational skills

### Levels of Competence

In her 1984 book, *From Novice to Expert,* Dr. Patricia Benner described five levels of competency in clinical nursing practice: novice, advanced beginner, competent, proficient, and expert.

1. *Novice.* The novice is the beginner; a student just learning about nursing is a novice as is the nurse entering his or her first position in nursing. Novices use rules to guide their actions. These rules are typically limited and inflexible and are related to what the person learned in school.

2. *Advanced Beginner.* The advanced beginner has handled enough challenging patient care situations to have prior experience to apply to new situations. The advanced beginner can sift through the rules more rapidly and assess situations through the eyes of past experience. Both novices and advanced beginners need support in the clinical area. They are still unable to set their own priorities and identify meaningful patterns in nonroutine situations without help from more experienced nurses.

3. *Competent.* The competent nurse usually has been in the same or similar clinical role for 2–3 years. The competent nurse is able to develop long-range plans and proceed accordingly. Although not as quick or flexible as the proficient nurse, the competent nurse is beginning to achieve efficiency, organizational skills, and ability to cope with the complex needs of multiple clients.

4. *Proficient.* The proficient nurse has learned from experience and can look at the whole picture at once. For example, the statement "he doesn't look right to me" has caused many proficient and expert nurses to take immediate action even though the objective signs of patient distress that the novices had learned from their textbooks had not yet emerged. The proficient nurse no longer has to consciously review the reasons why a client "doesn't look right."

5. *Expert.* The expert nurse has developed an extensive repertoire of skills, knowledge and clinical experience, and an intuitive grasp of each situation. This expert nurse is able to assess a situation quickly, forming an accurate picture of current and long-term implications, and devising effective solutions. Along with possessing finely tuned analytical skills, the expert nurse is a role model and mentor for novice nurses.

It is important that you recognize your own level of competence and that you allow yourself time to gain the experience needed to move to the next level. Remember, someday you will be the expert and a new novice will obtain from you the support, guidance, and nurturing needed to provide care for clients in complex situations.

## Strengths and Weaknesses

You may also want to evaluate your personal strengths and weaknesses. For example, if you are applying for a first-line nurse manager position, the following are examples of what you might consider to be your most critical strengths and weaknesses:

### Strengths
- Relevant work experience on same type of unit
- Advanced education in nursing
- Good communication/people skills
- Computer skills
- Self-directed learner
- Flexibility

On the other hand, you know you also have some weaknesses.

### Weaknesses
- History of frequent job changes
- Limited technical skills
- Poor math skills, no budget experience
- Difficulty delegating work to others

Not only should this list help you decide whether a management position is a good choice for you but also the areas you need to work on improving.

## Preferences

Now that you have a better idea of what you are prepared to do, it is time to reflect on what you really want to do. You have already chosen the nursing profession and had an opportunity to sample some of the many different positions available to nurses during your clinical experiences in school and for some, in the workplace. Your answers to the Test Yourself at the beginning of this chapter should have given you some idea of the work environment you prefer. Some more specific questions may also help you identify your career preferences:

1. What was your favorite clinical rotation? What was it that made it your favorite?
2. What age group do you particularly enjoy working with? Is it neonatal, adolescents, older people? Or do you prefer a mix of ages?

3. If you had to choose a book to read about any health-related matter, what subject would you choose?
4. What type of setting attracts you? Where are you most comfortable? In a patient's home? A clinic? The operating room?

Your answers should help direct you to the type of nursing position that you would find most rewarding.

## Opportunities

Most people go about looking for a job the wrong way according to Richard Bolles, author of the well-known guide, *What Color Is Your Parachute?* (1999). He notes that job seekers do not start their search in the same places that employers are looking for candidates for their positions. The typical would-be employer begins the search by looking at the people already known to him or to her: current employees, former consultants, temporary workers, even volunteers. If none of these look promising, the next group to be considered consists of friends, acquaintances, colleagues, and former coworkers. The typical job hunter on the other hand, often begins by reading help wanted ads in the newspaper or job listings online and sending resumes to any place that sounds promising. Both the job seeker and would-be employer will eventually turn to agencies or search firms if their initial actions prove fruitless. Eventually, they will find each other.

Instead of these traditional measures used by job seekers, Bolles (1999) suggests using more creative approaches including the following:

- Ask for job leads from anyone and everyone you know, including family members, friends, classmates, teachers, former employers, and even the people to whom you go for health care.
- Use the Yellow Pages of the telephone book to identify potential employers. If they say they have no openings when you call, ask if they know of others who are seeking nurses with your skills and interests.
- Continue to build your network. Use any contacts you have to help you get an appointment with a potential employer.

- Go after the organizations that have positions that interest you. Even if they have no opening at the time you first contact them, keep in touch, letting them know of your continued interest and availability.

## Resumes

Once you've identified potential job openings, the next step is to prepare your resume. In some cases, potential employers want to see a resume before they schedule an interview. If not, you can bring the resume with you to the interview.

### Format

Resumes usually follow one of three formats: chronological order, functional order, or a combination of the two. The chronological resume is easiest to prepare. On a chronological resume, you document your work history in reverse chronological order by dates of employment. You may also include an objective that indicates the type of work you are seeking. The chronological resume focuses on what you have done in the past, not what you can or feel you will do in the future. But it is easy to read and it can be used to show that your past work experience relates to your current job objective.

The functional resume starts with a job objective and documents your accomplishments, abilities, and transferable skills under headings such as "leadership skills" and "clinical experience." Most people prepare a combination of functional and chronological resumes by documenting their skills and abilities as well as providing a chronological education and work history (Vogel, 1993; Dadich, 1992; Collins, 1991).

### Essentials of a Resume

Whatever format you use for your resume, be sure to include the following in your resume (Parker, 1989):

- Listing of relevant education and training
- Chronological work history
- Presentation of directly relevant skills and experience
- Highlighted qualifications

If you haven't prepared a resume before, you can begin this process by writing down everything you can think of in these four categories.

## Education

Education is usually the easiest place to begin. Include the name and location of every educational institution attended, the dates you attended, and the degree, diploma, or certification attained. Start with your most recent degree. Include your license number and state(s) of licensure (if you are awaiting licensure, indicate when you will take the examination). If you are seeking additional training such as ACLS certification, include it if it is relevant to your job objective.

## Work History

Next, arrange your work history in reverse chronological order, listing your current job first. Include all your employable years. Short lapses in employment are acceptable, but longer periods should be accounted for with an explanation. Each position statement should include the employer, the dates worked (years only, i.e., 1999–2001), city, and state. Briefly describe duties and responsibilities of each position. Here you emphasize your accomplishments, any special expertise you gained, or changes you implemented. Use action verbs such as those listed in Box 23–1 to describe your accomplishments. Also, cite any special awards or committees you chaired. If the position is not health related, try to relate your

---

### Box 23–1   Action Verbs

**Management Skills**

attained
improved
increased
strengthened
developed
planned
organized
recommended
supervised

**Communication Skills**

collaborated
convinced
developed
formulated
negotiated
recruited
promoted
reconciled
enlisted

**Accomplishments**

achieved
expanded
improved
reduced (losses)
resolved (problems)
restored
coordinated
adapted
developed
facilitated
instructed
implemented

**Helping Skills**

assessed
assisted
clarified
demonstrated
diagnosed
expedited
facilitated
motivated
represented

*Source:* Adapted from Parker, Y. (1989). *The damn good resume guide.* Berkeley, CA: Ten Speed Press.

duties and accomplishments to the position you are seeking.

### Skills and Experiences

Relevant skills and experience are included not just to describe your past activities but to present a "word picture of you in your proposed new job, created out of the best of your past experience" (Parker, 1989, p. 13). Begin by jotting down the major skills required for the position you are seeking. Include five or six major skills such as:

- Management
- Problem solving
- Patient relations
- Proficiency in a specialty
- Technical skills

What if you have not been employed for many years? Explain your activities in work-related terms such as community volunteerism, personnel relations, fund raising, counseling, and teaching. College career offices, women's centers, or professional resume preparers can offer assistance with analyzing the skills and talents you shared with your family and community. If you are a student with no work experience, give examples of non-work experience that show marketable skills. Include the following (Parker, 1989; Eubanks, 1991):

- Working on school paper or yearbook
- Serving in student government
- Leadership positions in clubs, bands, church activities
- Community volunteerism
- Coaching or tutoring others

### Summary or Highlights

Now that you have noted everything relevant about yourself, it is time to develop the **highlights** of your qualifications, also called the **summary of qualifications** or just **summary**. These are your immodest one-liners designed to let your prospective employer know that you are qualified and talented and absolutely the best choice for the position. A typical group of highlights might include (Parker, 1989):

- How much relevant experience you have
- What your formal training and credentials are, if relevant

- Significant accomplishments, briefly stated
- One or two outstanding skills or abilities
- A reference to your values, commitment, or philosophy if appropriate

For example, a new graduate's qualifications could read:

- Five yeas of experience as an LPN in a large nursing facility
- Excellent client/family relationship skills
- Experience with chronic psychiatric patients
- Strong teamwork and communication skills
- Special certification in rehabilitation and reambulation strategies

Tailor the list to the job you are seeking. Include only relevant information such as internship, summer jobs, intersemester experiences, and volunteer work. Even if your previous experience is not directly related to nursing, your previous work experience can show transferable skills, motivation, and your potential to be a valuable employee.

### Additional Tips

The following are some additional tips on preparing a resume (Anderson, 1992; Rodriquez & Robertson, 1992):

- *Make sure your resume is readable.* Although most professionals recommend a resume of no more than two pages, the length does not appear to be as important as the ease with which the reader can find critical information. Is the type large enough for easy reading? Are paragraphs indented or bullets used to set off information, or does the entire page look like a gray blur? Using bold headings and appropriate spacing can offer relief from lines of gray type, but be careful not to get so carried away with graphics that your resume becomes a new art form. The paper should be an appropriate color such as cream, beige, light gray, white, or off-white. Use appropriate fonts and a laser printer. If a good computer and printer are not available to you, most printing services will prepare and print resumes at a reasonable cost.
- *Make sure the important facts are easy to spot.* Education, current employment, responsibilities, and other facts that indicate the experience you

have gained from past positions are important. Put the strongest statements at the top. Avoid excessive use of "I." If you are a new nursing graduate with little or no job experience, list your educational background first. Remember that positions you held prior to entering nursing may be relevant to your nursing career. Remember also to let your prospective employer know how you can be reached, including email address, an answering machine, or fax for leaving messages.

- *Do a grammar check.* Use simple terms, action verbs, and descriptive words. (See Box 23–1.) Check your finished resume for spelling, typing, or grammatical errors.
- *Watch for these don'ts.* Don't include pictures, personal references, or use fancy binders. Don't include hobbies (unless they have contributed to your work experience) or salary information unless required. Don't include personal information such as weight, marital status, or number of children. Don't repeat yourself just to make the resume longer.

A good resume is lean, to the point, and focused on your strengths and accomplishments. It invites a prospective employer to consider you a good candidate for the open position.

Regardless of how wonderful you sound on paper, if the paper itself is not presentable your resume may end up in the circular file (trash can). Further information about the criteria potential employers use in reviewing a resume may be found in Box 23–2.

A portion of a sample resume is shown in Figure 23–1.

> **Your resume is assumed to be an accurate mirror of who you are. You could be Einstein, but if you don't write well, you will not get an interview.**
>
> —Bolles, R.N. 1999, p. 52

## The Interview

### Preparation

Preparation for an interview is essential. If you have not already done it during your job search,

---

> **Box 23–2    Seven Key Areas Potential Employers Focus on When Reviewing a Resume**
>
> 1. *Overall Appearance:* cover letter, grammatically correct, attractive format, print, paper.
> 2. *Missing Information:* time gaps between periods of employment are "red flags."
> 3. *Work History:* relevance to current opening, evidence of advancement.
> 4. *Consistency and Accuracy:* particularly of dates and places of past employment.
> 5. *Frequency of Job Changes:* if too frequent, may be considered evidence of interpersonal difficulties or inability to meet job expectations.
> 6. *Reasons for Leaving Previous Jobs:* another "red flag" area so omit if not required and be prepared to discuss at the interview.
> 7. *Salary Requirements:* if not required, it is best to omit this point and reserve for discussion at a later time.
>
> *Source:* Based on Arthur, D. (1998). *Recruiting, interviewing, selecting, and orienting new employees.* New York: AMACOM (American Management Association).

---

it is time to learn as much as you can about your prospective employer including:

- Key people in the organization
- Size in terms of clients and employees
- Types of services provided
- Skills and experience of staff
- Organizational climate
- Reputation in the community

The importance of learning about the organization in which you might work is illustrated by the question of how to dress for the interview:

> *It would be obvious that you had not done your homework if you appeared in a well-pressed suit at a community center where the staff dress in rumpled jeans! You would not wear rumpled jeans for your interview but you would adjust your attire to the less formal environment.*

You also need to obtain information about the specific position for which you are being considered, including

**Delores Wheatley**
**5734 Foster Road**
**Middleton, Indiana 46204**
**(907) 123-4567**

**Objective: Position as staff registered nurse on pediatric unit**

**HIGHLIGHTS OF QUALIFICATIONS**

**EDUCATION:**
High School Diploma June 1996
Coral Reef High School
Dolphin Beach, Florida

Associate of Science Degree in Nursing May 1998
Howard Community College
Middleton, Indiana

Bachelor of Science in Nursing May 2001
St. Xavier College
Athensburg, Ohio
Currently enrolled in Advanced Life Support certification course at St. Xavier

**EXPERIENCE**
Special Olympics Committee 1993-1995
Nursing Assistant, Howard Community Hospital 1996-1998
Volunteer, Kids in Distress 1998-2001

**QUALIFICATIONS**
Pediatric inpatient experience
Pediatric Intensive Care Internship
Ability to work as part of an interdisciplinary team
Experience with abused children
Experience with families in crisis

**Figure 23–1** Sample resume.

- Title of the position
- Preparation and credentials required for the position
- Technical skills, certifications, and any additional qualifications necessary for the position
- To whom you would report and with whom you would work
- Description of the type and amount of work that would be expected of you (e.g., primary care nurse for 10–12 postoperative patients)

- Salary and benefits offered
- Work hours

Discussion of salary is usually delayed until both sides have decided they have some interest in the other. However, when hourly rates are standard (sometimes they are published), then you can ask about them during preliminary discussions.

## Traditional Interview

Job interviews commonly take one of two formats. We begin with the traditional format. A second type of interview, the competency-based job interview, is described following discussion of the traditional interview. The traditional job interview has four phases: (1) the initial welcome and introductions, (2) questions from the interviewer, (3) questions from the applicant, and (4) a summary before departure.

Beginning with the initial welcome and introductions is where appearance really does count. This includes arriving on time but not too early, appearing comfortable with yourself and the situation (not too nervous but also not over confident), and being dressed appropriately.

If more than two or three people are interviewing you, it may be hard to remember who they are. Don't let this throw you. Instead, pay attention to the departments they represent and try to address their various interests (such as, nursing administration, medical staff, social services, hospital administration) in your responses.

> **Be honest. Remember that, in the last analysis, you want not only to land a job, but to land the job that's right for you.**
> —*Double, 1997, p. 23*

## Interviewer Questions

The interview should be a dialogue between you and the interviewer. Neither should monopolize the discussion. Remember also that while the interviewers are trying to learn about you, you need to learn as much as you can about them, the organization, and the work you would be doing. At the same time that you are trying to demonstrate that you would be a valuable employee, they are trying to attract you to their or-

ganization. For both parties, the interview has at least two purposes: a fact-gathering mission and an opportunity for each party to persuade the other that they constitute a good match.

The typical job interview begins with general questions and proceeds to more specific ones. Usually, the interviewers ask their questions first and then in turn allow the applicant to ask his or her questions. The following are some of the most common questions asked of applicants with some tips on how to respond to them (Bolles, 1999; Double, 1997).

- *Why are you interested in this position?*
  The interviewer is looking for evidence of a good fit between the applicant and the available position. People who accept positions they really don't want usually end up unhappy and are unlikely to stay long. It is both expensive and time consuming to hire and orient new staff so this point is a serious consideration for most employers.
- *Why should I hire you?*
  A confrontive question that could take you by surprise, it requires that you first describe your preparation and skills and then relate them to the position for which you are applying. In other words, you are being asked to tell the interviewers how you would be an asset to their organization and why they should choose you over other candidates for the position.
- *Tell me about yourself.*
  This request often opens the interview. Sometimes it means that the interviewer has not studied your resume or simply didn't know how else to begin the interview. You can prepare for this question. Be ready to briefly describe your preparation and experience. Again, relate your background to the available position.
  Don't memorize your response. "Canned" responses not only sound unnatural but may make the interviewer wonder why you had to memorize an answer. Will you always have to memorize your lines?
- *What are your strengths and weaknesses?*
  Again, don't memorize a response but do think about how you would answer this question. The strengths you offer should relate to the available position. Avoid both excessive modesty and aggressive overconfidence in your response.

Be careful how you respond to the question about weaknesses. Bolles (1999) suggests mentioning a relatively harmless weakness and then pointing out its positive aspects. For example, you could say that while you do not have a highly confrontational style, you are a good listener and that colleagues seem to appreciate that.

- *Describe your* least *favorite boss.*

  This question is one of the most difficult to answer diplomatically. Keep your answer general: describe mild frustration with not being given as much responsibility as you can handle or with an organization's limited vision as to the potential of advanced practice nurses. Remember, never, ever mention people by name. The interviewer is looking for signs that you have difficulty getting along with others, especially people in authority. Don't inadvertently reinforce this concern.

- *Why do you want to leave your current position?*

  This question, too, is difficult in some cases. The interviewer is looking for indications of difficulty in your current position and for evidence that you will stay a reasonable amount of time if you are hired. Above all, avoid criticizing present or former employers (your prospective employer will be thinking, "this is what he or she will be saying about us next"). Instead of looking back, look forward in your answer. Emphasize the attractiveness of the new position: new challenges, a desire to obtain experience in a new setting or specialty area, the fine reputation of the new organization, etc. The longer you have been in your old position, the safer it is to add that you are ready for a change. Employers do not want to hire people who change jobs too often.

- *What are your long-term goals?*

  In some cases, this is another way of asking you how long you will stay if you are hired. It is also a way to find out how interested you are in developing and enhancing your skills and advancing in your profession, both of which make you a more valuable employee.

For more information on the tactics used by interviewers, see Box 23–3, and on mistakes made by interviewees, see Box 23–4.

## Competency-Based Job Interviews

You may encounter this alternative approach to job interviews in your job search. Competencies are the skills, traits, qualities, and characteristics that contribute to a person's job performance (Arthur, 1998). In relation to a beginning nursing position they would include items in three main categories: knowledge, technical skills, and leadership ability. For example:

Knowledge: Familiar with pediatric dosages of most commonly used medications.

---

**Box 23–3 Recommended Communication Tactics for Interviewers**

- Do not give away too much information about the job and desired work-related knowledge, skills, and abilities (KSAs), work requirements, and so forth early in the interview; otherwise, the applicant may try to give answers that reflect those desired factors.
- Allow the applicant to do most of the talking during the selection part of the interview; actively listen to what the applicant is saying.
- Do not show surprise or disapproval in response to any of the applicant's answers.
- Use silence, head nodding, and similar tactics to encourage the applicant to continue his or her answers.
- Use empathic statements (e.g., "That sounds like a difficult experience you had") when appropriate, such as when the applicant describes a problem situation that he or she has encountered.
- Avoid arguing with the applicant over the answers he or she provides; conversely, avoid coaxing the answers you want out of the applicant.
- Avoid using nonverbal cues (e.g., moving forward when you are starting to listen carefully) that may signal the applicant that he or she is relaying some negative information.

*Source:* Eder, R.W. & Harris, M.M. (1999). *The employment interview handbook.* Thousand Oaks, CA: Sage Publications.

|  | Able to evaluate the developmental stage of the young child. |
| Technical skill: | Able to use the audiometer in screening school children. |
|  | Able to provide routine ileostomy care. |
| Leadership ability: | Works well on interdisciplinary teams. |
|  | Is receptive to corrective feedback. |

During a competency-based interview, you are likely to be asked to give specific examples of how you have handled challenging situations and crises in the past and how often you have preformed certain tasks such as drawing blood or resuscitating a patient. In addition, the interviewer may present you with a hypothetical situation and ask you how you would handle it. A few examples:

- You are making patient rounds at the beginning of the midnight to 8:00 A.M. shift. In the second room, you find a postoperative hip repair patient is unresponsive. What would you do first?
- A new mother tells you her infant cries for a half hour every time she puts him to bed. What is an appropriate response?
- You have observed a staff member putting a patient's watch in her own pocket. What would you do?

In some instances, you may believe the information is insufficient to respond to the hypothetical situations definitively. It is better to respond that you need to know more about the situation than to make too many assumptions in crafting your response. If you are asked a question to which you really do not know the answer, tell the interviewer how you would go about getting the answer. This response accomplishes several goals: it assures the potential employer that you are honest and realistic about your capabilities and that you will not act without a sufficient basis for your actions but also that you will take the initiative to find a solution to problems that arise.

Some employers prefer this type of interview because it is more structured, job specific, and potentially a more objective way to choose the best person for the position (Arthur, 1998).

## Applicant Questions

You also need to find out as much as you can about the position for which you are applying, the people with whom you would work, and the organization in which you would work. The following are some suggested questions (Bischof, 1993):

- What would be my key responsibilities?
- What kind of person are you looking for?
- What are the challenges of the position?
- Why is this position open?
- Why did the previous person leave this position?
- To whom would I report directly?
- What is the salary for this position?
- What opportunities are available for advancement?

- Are opportunities offered for continuing education? What kind?
- What are your expectations of me as an employee?
- How, when, and by whom are evaluations done?
- What other opportunities for professional growth are available here?
- How are promotion and advancement handled within the organization?

The following are a few additional tips about asking questions during a job interview:

- *Do not* begin with questions about vacations, benefits, or sick time. To do so would leave the impression that they are the most important part of the job to you, not the work itself.
- *Do* begin with questions about the employer's expectations of you. It will leave the impression that you want to know how you can contribute to the organization.
- *Be sure* you know enough about the position to make a reasonable decision about accepting an offer when one is made.
- *Do* ask questions about the organization as a whole. The information is useful to you and demonstrates that you are able to see the big picture.
- *Do* bring a list of important points to discuss (a list can help if you are nervous).

Be alert for the following "red flags" during the interview process (Tyler, 1990):

- Lots of turnover in the position
- A newly created position without a clear purpose
- An organization in transition
- A position that is not feasible for a new graduate
- A gut feeling that things are not what they seem

### After the Interview

If the interviewer does not offer the information, ask about the next step in the process. Thank the interviewer, shake hands, and exit. If the receptionist is still there, you may quickly smile and say thank you and good-bye. Don't linger and chat, and do not forget your follow-up thank you letter.

## STAGES OF A NURSING CAREER

Each of us progresses along our career path in our own fashion, at our own pace. Some get started late in life; others take time out from their careers. Some move ahead quickly; others are content to remain in a comfortable niche. Despite these differences, some commonalities can be noted, particularly in how we experience the beginning of a career and the various stages through which we may pass.

Vance and Olson (1998) suggest that most nursing careers have as many as four stages:

Stage 1: The first 2 years during which one goes from Benner's novice to advanced beginner

Stage 2: The next 3–10 years of practice during which one becomes a skilled, confident professional

Stage 3: The next 10 years or more during which many move into advanced practice, management, education, and/or research

Stage 4: The pinnacle of one's career; those who reach this stage become the leaders of the profession

Each of these stages has its own issues. We will consider some of the most critical ones including the adequacy of orientation for every new employee and the problem of reality shock for the new graduate in Stage 1, the dangers of burnout in Stage 2, and the exciting possibilities of Stage 3. A slightly different way to think of the stages of a nursing career, including what happens before you begin your nursing education, is illustrated in Figure 23–2.

### Stage 1: Getting Started

This stage lasts about two years for most nurses. However, if you take a new position or change specialties, for a time you may feel as if you've returned to being a Stage 1 novice.

### Orientation

Everyone, even an expert, needs some orientation when beginning a new job. No matter how much experience you have, you need to become

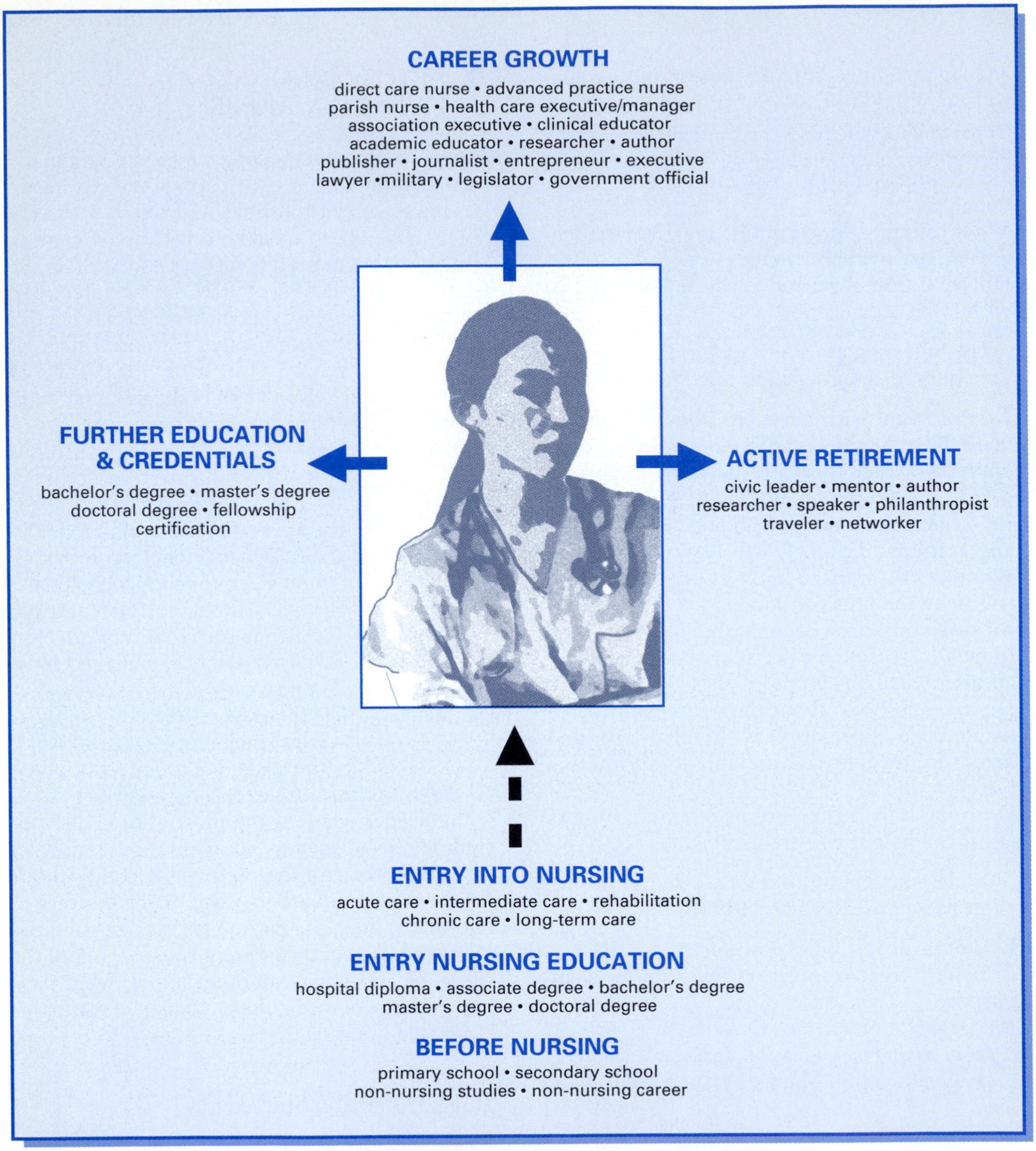

**CAREER GROWTH**

direct care nurse • advanced practice nurse
parish nurse • health care executive/manager
association executive • clinical educator
academic educator • researcher • author
publisher • journalist • entrepreneur • executive
lawyer •military • legislator • government official

**FURTHER EDUCATION
& CREDENTIALS**

bachelor's degree • master's degree
doctoral degree • fellowship
certification

**ACTIVE RETIREMENT**

civic leader • mentor • author
researcher • speaker • philanthropist
traveler • networker

**ENTRY INTO NURSING**

acute care • intermediate care • rehabilitation
chronic care • long-term care

**ENTRY NURSING EDUCATION**

hospital diploma • associate degree • bachelor's degree
master's degree • doctoral degree

**BEFORE NURSING**

primary school • secondary school
non-nursing studies • non-nursing career

**Figure 23–2** Eight skills for a health career. Adapted with permission from International Leadership Institute, Sigma Theta Tau International Honor Society for Nursing (2000). Eight skills for a healthy career. *Reflection on Nursing Leadership, 26*(1), 20–21.

acquainted with the new organization, new co-workers, new ways of doing things.

In most larger healthcare organizations, a general orientation is provided for all new employees. Over the course of a day or two of ori-entation meetings, employees are usually in-formed about the following:

- The organization's philosophy and mission
- Employee benefits

- Work hours, scheduling of breaks, holidays, and vacations
- Department structures and interrelationships
- Personnel policies, including grievance procedures (Arthur, 1998)

Orientation then continues with more specific information about the department or unit to which you are assigned and your own job duties and responsibilities. The novice nurse needs far more. It is unrealistic to expect a new graduate to be fully prepared to assume a staff position without some on-the-job preparation. Novice nurses and nurses entering a new specialty area also need an extended period of internship or apprenticeship during which they work closely with an experienced nurse who acts as teacher, guide, and mentor.

> ### . . . the new nurse should function as a protégé under the tutelage of involved, caring, supportive and experienced professionals.
> —Vance & Olson, 1998, p. 11

At this beginning stage, the novice nurse needs to develop technical skills, expand his or her knowledge base, and increase confidence in self as a professional (Vance & Olson, 1998). The new graduate should make every effort to find a position in an organization that provides the support and guidance needed for a successful beginning. Unfortunately, in some places little mentoring is available and new nurses find themselves in an unsupportive, demanding situation often described as "sink or swim."

## The Honeymoon

The first few weeks after orientation on a new job are the honeymoon phase. The new employee is excited and enthusiastic about the new position. Coworkers usually go out of their way to make the new person feel welcome and overlook any problems that arise. Everything seems rosy.

## Avoiding Reality Shock

Honeymoons do not last forever. The new graduate is soon expected to behave just like everyone else and discovers that expectations for a professional employed in an organization are quite different from expectations for a student in school. Those behaviors that brought rewards in school are not necessarily valued by the organization. In fact, some of them are criticized. The new graduate who is not prepared for this change feels confused, shocked, angry, and disillusioned.

Reality shock stems from the realization that the way the graduate was taught to do things in school is not necessarily the way things are actually done on the job.

## Conflicts

What are these differences in expectations? Kramer, who studied reality shock for many years, found a number of them. Some of the most important ones are listed in Table 23–1 and discussed in more detail in the following paragraphs.

Ideally, health care is comprehensive. Not only should it meet all of a patient's or client's needs, but it should be delivered in a way that considers the client as a whole person, a member of a particular family and community. Most healthcare professionals, however, are not employed to provide comprehensive, holistic care. Instead, they are asked to give medications, to provide counseling, to make home visits, or to prepare someone for surgery, but rarely to do all these things. These tasks are divided among

| Table 23–1 Professional Ideals and Work Realities | |
|---|---|
| **Professional Ideals** | **Work Realities** |
| Comprehensive, holistic care | Mechanistic, fragmented care |
| Emphasis on quality of care | Emphasis on efficiency |
| Explicit expectations | Implicit (unstated) expectations |
| Balanced, frequent feedback | Intermittent, often negative, feedback |

*Source:* Kramer, M. (1981, January 27–28). Coping with reality shock. Workshop presented at Jackson Memorial Hospital, Miami, FL.

different people, each a specialist, for the sake of efficiency rather than continuity of care.

When efficiency is the goal, the speed and amount of work done are rewarded rather than the quality of the work. This focus also creates a conflict for the new graduate who was allowed to take as much time as needed to provide good care in school.

Expectations are communicated in different ways. In school, an effort is made to provide explicit directions so that students know what they are expected to accomplish. In many work settings, however, instructions are brief and many expectations are left unspoken. New graduates who are not aware of these expectations (part of the informal level of operations) may find that they have unknowingly left tasks undone or are considered inept by coworkers. The following is an example:

*A new graduate nurse was assigned to give medications to all the patients cared for by the team. Because it was a fairly light assignment, the nurse spent some time looking up the medications and explaining their actions to the patients receiving them. The nurse also straightened up the medicine room and filled out the order forms, which the nurse thought would please the task-oriented team leader.*

*At the end of the day, the nurse reported these activities with some satisfaction to the team leader. The nurse expected the team leader to be pleased with the way the time had been used. Instead, the team leader looked annoyed and told the nurse that whoever passes out medications always does the blood pressures too and that the other nurse on the team who had a heavier assignment had to do them. Also, because supplies were always ordered on Fridays for the weekend, it would have to be done again tomorrow so the nurse had, in fact, wasted time.*

The example of the new graduate also illustrates some differences in the way feedback is given. The feedback given was all negative, and it was given too late. Other common problems are messages that are too vague or global such as "You're doing fine," indirect messages such as grumbling under the breath or redoing something that has just been done, or a complete lack of feedback until something goes wrong.

## Additional Pressures on the New Graduate

Many people think of their first job after graduation as a proving-ground for testing their new knowledge and skills. Some set up mental tests for themselves that they feel must be passed before they can be confident of their ability to function. Passing these self-tests also confirms achievement of identity as a practitioner rather than a student.

At the same time, new graduates are undergoing testing by their coworkers. The new graduate is entering a new group, and the group will decide whether to accept this new member. The testing is usually reasonable, but sometimes new graduates will be given tasks they are not ready to handle. Kramer (1981) recommended that you refuse to take a test you are not ready for rather than fail it. Another opportunity for proving yourself will soon come along.

The discrepancies in role expectations and the need for a feeling of competency are the top two concerns of new graduates, according to most surveys. Next in order of concern are the system that must be dealt with, self-concept, and the type of feedback that is given (or not given). Before considering ways to resolve these problems, we will look at some of the less successful ways of coping with these problems.

## Ineffective Coping Efforts

When faced with reality shock, some new graduates abandon their professional goals and adopt the organization's operative goals as their own. This behavior eliminates their conflict but leaves them less effective caregivers. It also puts the needs of the organization before their needs or the needs of the client and reinforces operative goals that might better be challenged and changed.

Others give up their professional ideals but do not adopt the organization's goals nor any others to replace them. Being devoid of goals has a deadening effect: they become automatons, believing in nothing related to their work except doing what is necessary to earn a day's pay. Some even leave the profession. Kramer and Schmalenberg (1993) believe that fewer shortages of nurses would occur if more healthcare organizations supported these professional goals.

## Preventing Reality Shock

Some of the shock experienced by the graduate can be prevented. Prevention begins with preparation in leadership and management before graduation. It should continue at the employment interview. An honest description of the organization's work environment and employee policies is the first step in preparing the new employee. After the new employee orientation has been completed, follow-up should continue but gradually decrease over the next year. Regular meetings with groups of new staff provide opportunities to share concerns and prevent the feeling that one is alone in having difficulty adjusting. Probably the worst way to handle new employees, especially new graduates, is to let them sink or swim.

Several other things can be done to ease the transition from school to work. The usual expectations of staff members may be modified somewhat to allow time for adjustment. The new employee also needs more frequent informal feedback and closer supervision until he or she is functioning well within the new environment. Assigning new staff members to work with experienced staff in a preceptor-preceptee relationship facilitates adjustment and provides extra feedback. When using this format, it is important to select staff who provide excellent role models, who function well within the organization, and who have maintained their professional ideals.

## More Effective Coping

Opportunities to challenge one's competence and develop an identity as a professional can begin in school. Success in meeting these challenges can immunize the new graduate against the loss of confidence that accompanies reality shock.

When you begin a new job, it is important to learn as much as you can about the organization's formal and informal levels of operation and goals. Such knowledge not only saves you from some nasty surprises but also gives you some ideas about how to work within the system and how to make the system work for you. The following is an example of how a new team leader figured out how to use the system.

*A new team leader realized that patient care conferences were never held in the home health agency but were needed to improve the care given. When the team leader approached team members (who were all long-term employees of the agency) about the idea, they expressed no interest in having conferences. The supervisor's response was also negative.*

*The agency was a rigid, bureaucratic organization in which team leaders had little authority, so the team leader could not begin the conferences without the supervisor's approval. (The team members would not attend them unless they were approved, anyway.) However, the agency did have a strong bias in favor of education, held many classes for its employees, and rewarded employees for accumulating large numbers of education credits or contact hours.*

*The new team leader took advantage of the value placed on education. The team leader adopted the patient care conference format to focus on the teaching and learning aspects and presented the idea to the supervisor as twice-weekly seminars for staff. The supervisor recognized the seminars' similarity to patient care conferences but felt a need to approve the plan because of the strong emphasis on education in the agency. The staff agreed to attend because it was a good way to accumulate continuing education credits on work time. The patient care conference/seminars became an accepted part of the team's operation, and the team leader was later praised for interest in meeting the educational needs of the team.*

The team leader did not abandon or even compromise the goal to improve care but adapted it to the realities of the work situation.

Keep in mind that much energy goes into learning a new job. Attempting to implement change also takes time and energy on your part, so you need to make some choices regarding any changes and improvements that you see are needed. It is also a good idea to make a list of these things so that you do not forget them later when you have become socialized into the system.

Three other actions can help to reduce the shock effects of these conflicts. The first is to **seek feedback** often and persistently. Feedback not only provides you with needed information,

## Research Example 23–1    *A Changing Workforce: What Does It Mean?*

The Families and Work Institute conducted an extensive national study of hourly and salaried workers (Schellenbarger, 1993). In-depth telephone interviews were conducted with 2,598 workers for this national study of the changing workforce supported by 15 private corporations and foundations.

### Diversity and Discrimination

One fifth (20 percent) of the minority respondents said that they had experienced discrimination on the job. This experience correlated with a tendency to feel burned out. Female managers also rated their opportunities for advancement much lower than male respondents did, although neither saw much difference in the way male and female managers functioned.

### Work Environment

Only 28 percent of the respondents expressed a strong loyalty to their employing organization,

compared with 57 percent who expressed satisfaction from doing their work well. Open communication was rated the most important factor in selecting their current jobs. The next most important factors were effect on family and personal life (60 percent), the nature of the work (59 percent), and the quality of the management (59 percent). Salary was mentioned by 35 percent.

### Work-Family Conflicts

When conflicts between work and family responsibilities occurred, the respondents reported that they were three times more likely to give up time with their family than to reduce their work time. Two thirds of those who had children said that the time they had to spend with their families was inadequate, that they wanted to spend more time with them but came home exhausted.

*Source:* Shellenbarger, S. (1993, September 3). Work-force study finds loyalty is weak, divisions of race and gender are deep. *The Wall Street Journal.*

---

but also pushes the people you work with to be more specific about their expectations of you. A second and related action is to **use confronting communication** to deal with the problems that can arise with coworkers.

The third action is to **develop a support network** for yourself. Identifying colleagues who have also held onto their professional ideals and sharing not only your problems but the work of improving the organization with them is a helpful cushion against reality shock. Their recognition of your work can keep you going while rewards from the organization are meager. A support network is a source of strength when resisting pressure to give up professional ideals and a source of power when attempting to bring about change. Working on these and other components of effective leadership can help to prevent the problems of reality shock.

Conflicts may arise in any position, even if you are not a new graduate. (See Research Example 23–1, A Changing Workforce: What Does

It Mean?) Many of these coping behaviors will help you deal with these issues as well. Additional ones are discussed in the next section on burnout in Stage 2.

## Stage 2: Gaining Experience

Stage 2 encompasses the next 3–10 years, in which time the nurse becomes a highly skilled, confident professional. During this stage, nurses often decide upon a specialty area (public health nursing, home health, pediatrics, gerontology, oncology, critical care, to name just a few). Many return to school to earn a graduate degree in their specialty area. Both peers and mentors are sought out for guidance and support. They can help Stage 2 nurses make decisions about career advancement, provide opportunities to expand their networks, and help them to find a good balance between family, personal, and professional responsibilities. Those who do not advance may ex-

**Research Example 23–2** *Predictors of Nurse Turnover*

Why do nurses leave their job? High turnover of nurses continues to be a serious problem, both in terms of its effect on patient care and the cost of replacing nurses who have left. Lucas, Atwood, and Hagaman (1993) replicated an earlier study of nurse turnover in order to retest a set of factors believed to be related to turnover. They compared the responses of 625 nurses from the original study done in the southwestern United States with a new sample of 385 nurses in the southeastern United States. Sixty-one percent of the nurses returned their questionnaires to the researchers.

The nurses in the new sample were younger, more had bachelors' degrees, and more worked on medical-surgical and intensive care units than did the nurses in the original sample. The new sample also had a higher turnover rate than did the original sample. Turnover was measured as the number of days until resignation after the nurses completed the questionnaire.

The researchers used a complex series of regression analyses to analyze the data. The results indicated that group cohesion promotes both organizational and job satisfaction. Job stress inhibits satisfaction. Group cohesion and both organizational and job satisfaction inhibit turnover. Nurses from the medical-surgical units had higher job stress than did nurses from the intensive care units.

The researchers noted that nurses' anticipation of resignation (those who expect to leave) predicts actual leaving. Awareness of this point would allow administrators time to develop strategies to retain some of these nurses. Also because the effect of job stress can be mitigated by increased job satisfaction, administrators can develop and test strategies to optimize job satisfaction, thereby reducing stress and related turnover. In addition, if stresses differ by clinical service, then strategies to reduce stress need to be targeted to specific services as well.

*Source:* Lucas, M.D, Atwood, J.R. & Hagaman, R. (1993). Replication and validation of anticipated turnover model for urban registered nurses. *Nursing Research, 42*(1), 29–35.

perience burnout, a serious impediment to work satisfaction and career advancement.

### Avoiding Burnout

The term **burnout** refers to a state of emotional exhaustion, a depletion of energies that seems to be a particular problem for people in helping professions. It begins with frustration, disillusionment, or doubts about one's work and leads to the loss of ideals, purpose, and energy.

The burned-out individual may feel apathetic, alienated, or exhausted. Stress-related physical symptoms such as headaches, backaches, indigestion, and lowered resistance to infection may be experienced. Family difficulties and social problems may also occur. Like reality shock, the cost of burnout to individuals, their families, employing organizations, and clients is enormous. The effect of job stress on nurse turnover was analyzed in the study described in Research Example 23–2, Predictors of Nurse Turnover).

People who enter helping professions usually do so with a lot of enthusiasm and idealism. They want to help people and expect that their interventions will have an impact. The system needs to be changed and they frequently intend to do something about that, too. Support and success can nourish their high hopes. But nursing environments often lack the support and nurturing of creativity that people in the helping professions need (Moch & Diemert, 1987). When they meet continuous resistance, disinterest, and failure to meet their goals, many begin to burn out.

### Factors Contributing to Burnout

Burnout is the result of the negative interaction between the expectations and behavior of the healthcare professional and the system within which the professional is working. The following is a list of the factors contributing to this negative interaction.

- *Low Pay.* In comparison with the salaries of professionals in other fields, many healthcare professionals are not well paid for their level of expertise and the degree of responsibility they are given.
- *Long Hours.* Not only is the work demanding, but many healthcare professionals find themselves working well beyond the standard 40-hour week. For example, nurses are frequently asked to work rotating shifts or 12-hour days, both of which are a considerable stress.
- *Too Much Paperwork.* People who enter helping professions derive their satisfaction from interacting with people, not with paper. When much of their time is spent on filling out forms, charts, and reports, they become frustrated by the loss of time that could be spent with their clients.
- *Client Losses.* If you commit yourself to helping people, their failure to recover can become a personal disappointment. Clients may return to destructive behavior after counseling; patients may not recover from their illnesses. These things happen to intensive care nurses, oncology unit staff, counselors, rehabilitation workers, hospice nurses, and many others. The continual loss of patients alone can result in burnout.
- *Lack of Appreciation and Understanding.* Intangible rewards (that psychological paycheck) meet the need for recognition and esteem. Although patients or clients often express their appreciation, supervisors frequently fail to comment favorably on a job well done. In addition, the public still does not fully understand what nurses do and does not appreciate how demanding the work is. Some people still think of nurses as little more than bedpan carriers and doctors' helpers until they require the services of a nurse and find out what nurses really do.
- *Lack of Support.* Many healthcare professionals find themselves working in organizations that do not support their efforts to improve the quality of the services offered. Continually fighting for the right to practice in a professional manner has left many burned out.
- *Unresponsiveness to Client Needs.* The healthcare system's lack of responsiveness to clients' needs (impersonal, fragmented care, restrictive eligibility requirements, or lack of respect for the dignity of the individual) conflicts with the professional ideals of a helping person. Finding out that the operative goals of a healthcare organization emphasize efficiency and monetary gain over the needs of the people served leads to much frustration and disillusionment.
- *Powerlessness.* The opposite of empowerment, powerlessness, can result from the failure to recognize and use the potential power available to any large group that performs a vital function. Many people in the helping professions feel that it is inappropriate to use their power and react with dismay when they find themselves the target of a power play.
- *Discrimination.* Nurses still find themselves resisting physician dominance and the myths that they are weaker, less dependable, or less intelligent. Although much progress has been made in reducing discrimination, more women and minorities still fill the lower-status, lower-paid positions in health care. This problem is quite evident in the healthcare field but not unique to it.
- *Inadequate Advancement Opportunities.* People at the lower levels in the helping professions are often discouraged by the educational prerequisites for moving up the career ladder. Those who are higher up on the ladder find that further advancement means moving into management or teaching and further away from the people they want to help. This frustration also is not unique to the helping professions.

## Counteracting Burnout

When energies are seriously depleted, it is difficult to channel them into counteracting burnout. For this reason, it is a good idea to intervene for yourself and others before burnout becomes too severe.

Several of the factors contributing to burnout are based on unrealistic expectations. A focus on one's successes rather than on one's failures helps to reduce feelings of discouragement and disappointment. People who define success in terms of having all their patients recover or all their clients rehabilitated have set themselves up for failure. In contrast, if you are able to define success as having made *some* contribution to the health and welfare of *some* of the people you care for, then you have set yourself up for success.

Partial goals are more likely to be successfully met. For example, if your staff's goals are to completely rehabilitate a stroke patient, they may fail, especially if the patient has another stroke. But if they set several partial goals or separate steps leading to the patient's full recovery, such as finding a new means of transportation or being able to prepare meals, they have a much greater probability of meeting at least some of these goals.

If you recall the victim-rescuer-persecutor roles of the Karpman Triangle (from Chapter 17), you will remember that helping professionals who take complete responsibility for what happens to a client are acting in the role of rescuer. In contrast, caregivers who recognize that their clients also have some responsibility and who allow clients to exercise that responsibility have taken some of the burden off their shoulders. At the same time, they have become more effective helping professionals. This strategy has more utility in some settings than in others, but even in intensive care units, caregivers can learn to recognize their own limits and can focus their thoughts on the people who would not have survived without their care.

Effective leadership actions are helpful in dealing with burnout as well as reality shock. It is important to learn how to use change strategies to fight back when work situations are unsatisfactory. It is also important to overcome the idea that the use of power tactics is unprofessional. Power tactics can and will be used on you by other people (including other professionals), so you will need to use them in return or at least recognize when they are occurring. Many people in the helping professions are reluctant to let go of the myth that rewards somehow come automatically to those who do their work well. Although it happens occasionally, more often the rewards go to those who know how to ask for, and even demand them.

Stress reduction, relaxation techniques, exercise, and good nutrition are all helpful in keeping energy levels high. However, while they can prepare people to cope with the stresses of a job, they are not solutions to the conflicts that lead to reality shock and burnout. It is more effective to resolve the problem than to treat the symptoms (Lee & Ashforth, 1993).

Many people in the helping professions have difficulty setting limits on their commitment. If they enjoy working extra hours and taking calls at night and on weekends limits may not be an issue, but if it exhausts them, then they need to stop doing it or risk serious burnout. For example, when you are asked to work another double shift or the third weekend in a row, you can say no. At the same time that you are setting limits at work, you can expand your outside activities so that you live in a large world in which a blow to one part can be cushioned by support from other parts. If you are the team leader or nurse manager, it is important that you recognize and accept staff members' need to do this as well.

## Stage 3: Advancement

Stage 3 nurses have between 10 and 20 years of experience in the profession. Many have become nurse managers or advanced practice nurses by this time. Others have moved into nursing administration, education, or research. It is in this stage that they become mentors themselves, sharing their extensive knowledge and experience with newer nurses who are working their way through the earlier stages. Those who have advanced to this stage and assumed the mentor role often derive a great deal of satisfaction from their accomplishments and the opportunity to share with others. Their work is "complex, requiring a high degree of interpersonal skill level, with high rewards and high satisfaction" (Vance & Olson, 1998, p. 26). Many will stay at this stage for the remainder of their careers.

## Stage 4: Influence

Those who reach stage 4 are the leaders of the profession. Called nurse-influentials, they are the chief nurse executives, deans, funded researchers, scholars, and noted practitioners within the profession. Many become mentors to other nurses. Many of the mentor-mentee relationships eventually evolve into collegial partnerships (Vance & Olson, 1998).

## Moving along the Career Path

If you reflect on how far a nurse can advance along one of the many different career paths open to nurses, you will appreciate the value of gaining clinical experience, advanced education, developing an extensive network, and having successful role models and mentors along the way. None of these aspects are helpful, however, without some thought about your eventual goals. Felton (1998) wrote that her survival and career advancement were made possible by those who were her patrons, protectors, benefactors, sponsors, advocates, and advisors. These expert nurses were her role models and career advisors. They shared with her their encouragement, recognition, honest criticism, and political savvy. The same is available to you if you know how to seek it.

*We have learned that mentoring is truly a reciprocal process. If staff and leaders are provided the time and tools to mentor one another, they will*

---

## C A S E   S T U D Y

### Go or Stay?

"I'm going to make you an offer you can't refuse," Chester Shulman, chief of neurology, said to Jenna Tompkins, nurse manager for two of the busiest trauma units in a tertiary medical center. "How does twice the pay with no nights, weekends, or holidays sound to you?"

"Sounds great," said Jenna. "What would I be doing?"

"Running my practice. I've seen the way you handle disagreements, expedite priority requests, manage an impossibly heavy workflow, and still maintain excellent patient care. You have all the skills needed to do an excellent job. The practice is growing by leaps and bounds. You can grow with it by owning a share of the practice."

"Would this position include patient contact?"

"Primarily when patients or their families have a complaint. The majority of your time would be spent on the administration side. The staff would be your "patients.""

"This is really an administrative position, isn't it?" asked Jenna.

"Yes, but you would have the opportunity to make sure that all systems support excellent patient care, from the way staff answer patients' questions to helping them deal with insurance companies. I think you'd enjoy it. I know you would do a good job. Do you need time to think about it?"

"I do. The offer is very attractive but the loss of patient contact, being in the middle of all the dramas, big and small, that occur here every day, and having an impact on the outcomes . . . I would miss that."

### Questions for Critical Reflection and Analysis

1. Why did Jenna Tompkins receive this offer? In formulating your answer, you can use your imagination to fill in details that are congruent with but not mentioned in the case study.
2. Draw an imaginary career path for Jenna Tompkins. Use solid lines to indicate how she reached her current position as nurse manager. Use dotted lines to show the choice between alternative paths she is facing right now.
3. Jenna is at a fork in the road: Which way should she go? Does she have a third choice that she might consider? What might it be?
4. What values are represented by the choices Jenna faces?
5. If you were Jenna, which scenario would be most attractive to you? If Jenna decides to consider the offer, what terms of employment should she negotiate?
6. Write three brief scenarios describing Jenna's career 10 years from now, each one representing a choice she made at the present fork in the road (include the third choice you created in question #3).
7. Now that you've analyzed the situation, if you were in Jenna's place, would you consider the offer? Why or why not?

*be successful in giving to and learning from each other and bringing our profession and our organizations into the future.*

—Fiore & Cima, in Vance & Olson, 1998, p. 102

## ● SUMMARY

When embarking on a job search your preparation, preferences, and the types of positions available should all be considered in deciding on your goal. Consider where you are in your career (novice, advanced beginner, competent, proficient, or expert), your qualifications, your primary strengths and weaknesses, and what you really want to do. Then use all possible avenues for finding the right job for you: do not depend on help wanted ads in the newspaper or online but on all your contacts and ingenuity in approaching potential employers.

A resume should include your education, work history, relevant skills, and a summary of your qualifications for the position you seek. Keep the resume simple, short, and straightforward. Avoid padding or excessive embellishments.

The job interview has the potential to present many challenges to the applicant. Be sure you know the organization, the services provided by the organization, and the specific position that is available before you go for an interview. The applicant has two goals during an interview: to impress the potential employer and to find out as much as possible about the position, the organization, and the people with whom he or she would work. In the traditional interview, the interviewer usually asks a series of questions designed to help the interviewer become acquainted with the applicant and identify his or her strengths and weaknesses. The applicant then has an opportunity to ask questions in return. Competency-based interviews, in contrast, are designed to obtain more specific information about the ability of the applicant to fulfill the responsibilities of the position available.

Once you have obtained a position, you will probably go through a general orientation and then a more specific introduction to the specifics of your position. Novice-level nurses need extensive preparation before they can assume the full responsibilities of a new position. The honeymoon phase of this first career stage usually does not last long. When the environment is unsupportive and the new nurse is unprepared, reality shock may occur.

In Stage 2, the nurse selects a specialty area, pursues advanced preparation, and may have to learn how to balance home and work responsibilities. Stage 3 nurses have 10–20 years of experience. Many are managers, advanced practice nurses, or have moved into education, administration, or research. Not everyone reaches Stage 4 in which one becomes a leader in the profession and mentor to those who are beginning their career.

## REFERENCES

Anderson, J. (1992). Tips on resume writing. *Imprint, 39*(1), 30–31.

Arthur, D. (1998). *Recruiting, interviewing, selecting and orienting new employees.* New York: AMACOM (American Management Association).

Benner, P. (1984). *From novice to expert: Excellence and power in clinical nursing practice.* Menlo Park, CA: Addison Wesley.

Bischof, J. (1993). Preparing for job interview questions. *Critical Care Nurse, 13*(4), 97–100.

Bolles, R.N. (1999). *What color is your parachute?* Berkeley, CA: Ten Speed Press.

Collins, M. (1991). Resume is key to getting a job. *American Nurse, 23*(2), 18.

Dadich, K.A. (1992). Your resume. *Health Care Trends and Transition, 3*(2), 20–21, 96.

Double, D.L. (1998). *Assessing your career options.* Chicago: American Medical Association.

Double, D.L. (1997). *The physician in transition: Managing the job interview.* Chicago: American Medical Association.

Eder, R.W. & Harris, M.M. (1999). *The employment interview handbook.* Thousand Oaks, CA: Sage Publications.

Eubanks, P. (1991). Experts: Making your resume an asset. *Hospitals, 5*(20), 74.

Felton G. (1998). Reflections on mentoring and networks. In C. Vance & R.K. Olson. *The mentor connection in nursing.* New York: Springer Publishing Co., 32–34.

Fiore, T. & Cima, L. (1998). Mentorship in a magnet nursing department. In C. Vance & R.K. Olson. *The mentor connection in nursing.* New York: Springer Publishing Co., 112–113.

International Leadership Institute, Sigma Theta Tau International Honor Society for Nursing (2000). Eight skills for a healthy career. *Reflection on Nursing Leadership, 26*(1), 20–21.

Kramer, M. (1981, January 27–28). Coping with reality shock. Workshop presented at Jackson Memorial Hospital, Miami, FL.

Kramer, M. & Schmalenberg, C. (1993). Learning from success: Autonomy and empowerment. *Nursing Management, 24*(5), 58–64.

Lee, R.T. & Ashforth, B.E. (1993). A further examination of managerial burnout: Toward an integrated model. *Journal of Organizational Behavior, 14*(1), 3–20.

Lucas, M.D, Atwood, J.R. & Hagaman, R. (1993). Replication and validation of anticipated turnover model for urban registered nurses. *Nursing Research, 42*(1), 29–35.

Moch, S.D. & Diemert, C.A. (1987). Health promotion within the nursing work environment. *Nursing Administration Quarterly, 11*(3), 9–12.

Parker, Y. (1989). *The damn good resume guide.* Berkeley, CA: Ten Speed Press.

Rodriquez, K. & Robertson, D. (1992). Selling your talents with a resume. *American Nurse, 24*(10), 27.

Shellenbarger, S. (1993, September 3). Work-force study finds loyalty is weak, divisions of race and gender are deep. *The Wall Street Journal.*

Shingleton, J. (1994). The job market for '94 grads. In College Placement Council, Inc. (Ed.). *Planning job choices.* Philadelphia: College Placement Council, 19–24.

Tyler, L. (1990). Watch out for "red flags" on a job interview. *Hospitals, 64*(14), 46.

Vance, C. & Olson, R.K. (1998). *The mentor connection in nursing.* New York: Springer Publishing Co.

Vogel, D. (1993). Writing a resume. *Imprint, 40*(1), 35–36.

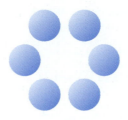

# Index